Ursel Broesskamp-Stone

Assessing Networks for Health Promotion

Politik und Partizipation

Band 2

LIT

Ursel Broesskamp-Stone

Assessing Networks for Health Promotion

Framework and Examples

LIT

Printed with the kind support of Health Promotion Switzerland

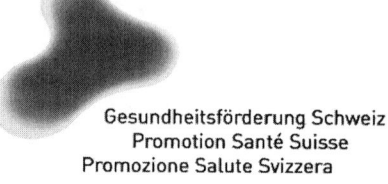

Gesundheitsförderung Schweiz
Promotion Santé Suisse
Promozione Salute Svizzera

Bibliographic information published by Die Deutsche Bibliothek
Die Deutsche Bibliothek lists this publication in the Deutsche
Nationalbibliografie; detailed bibliographic data are available in the
Internet at http://dnb.ddb.de.

ISBN 3-8258-7674-8
Zugl.: Bielefeld, Univ., Diss., 2003

© LIT VERLAG Münster   2004
Grevener Str./Fresnostr. 2   48159 Münster
Tel. 0251-23 50 91   Fax 0251-23 19 72
e-Mail: lit@lit-verlag.de   http://www.lit-verlag.de

Distributed in North America by:

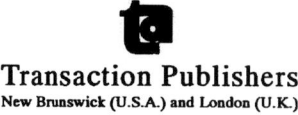

Transaction Publishers
New Brunswick (U.S.A.) and London (U.K.)

Transaction Publishers
Rutgers University
35 Berrue Circle
Piscataway, NJ 08854

Tel.: (732) 445 - 2280
Fax: (732) 445 - 3138
for orders (U. S. only):
toll free (888) 999 - 6778

Table of content

Foreword

1. **INTRODUCTION**   1

PART I   9

2. **HEALTH KNOWLEDGE TODAY AND ORGANIZED SOCIAL RESPONSES TO PROMOTE HEALTH (STATE OF RESEARCH)**   10

2.1 HEALTH AND CO-DETERMINANTS OF HEALTH   12
2.1.1 INTRODUCTION   12
2.1.2 THE SEARCH FOR AN INTEGRATIVE THEORY OF HEALTH AND DISEASE   14
2.1.3 FACTORS THAT INFLUENCE OR CO-DETERMINE HEALTH - A GENERAL PICTURE   22
2.1.4 THE SOCIAL ECOLOGICAL MODEL (AND SYSTEMS PERSPECTIVE) ON HEALTH   40
2.1.5 SYNOPSIS AND DISCUSSION   43

2.2 HEALTH PROMOTION - AN ORGANIZED SOCIAL RESPONSE TO THE KNOWLEDGE OF FACTORS THAT INFLUENCE OR CO-DETERMINE HEALTH   45
2.2.1 INTRODUCTION - SOCIAL ECOLOGICAL APPROACHES TO THE PROMOTION OF HEALTH   45
2.2.2 HEALTH PROMOTION - DEFINITIONS AND KEY FEATURES   51
2.2.3 THE SETTINGS APPROACH IN HEALTH PROMOTION   60
2.2.4 HEALTH PROMOTION IN THE 21ST CENTURY - EVOLUTION, REVIEW, CHALLENGES   69
2.2.5 'NEW' APPROACHES IN HEALTH PROMOTION   81
2.2.6 LARGE SCALE EFFORTS TO DEVELOP HEALTH PROMOTING SETTINGS: PROJECTS, MOVEMENTS, NETWORKS   89
2.2.7 SEARCHING FOR 'GOOD' COLLABORATIVE PRACTICE - LESSONS LEARNED IN HEALTH PROMOTION   101

2.3 FROM UNDERSTANDING HEALTH TO HEALTH PROMOTION TO 'HEALTH PROMOTION NETWORKS' - INTERMEDIATE SYNOPSIS AND DISCUSSION   116
2.3.1 WHERE DID THE JOURNEY LEAD TO SO FAR?   116
2.3.2 HEALTH AND HEALTH PROMOTION – RELEVANT LESSONS LEARNED   118

2.4 INTERORGANISATIONAL NETWORKS -FEATURES AND DEVELOPMENT   122
2.4.1 INTRODUCTION   122
2.4.2 ORGANIZATIONAL NETWORKING AND THE 'NEW ORGANIZATION'   124
2.4.3 FEATURES AND TYPES OF NETWORKS OF ORGANIZATIONS   140
2.4.4 ACHIEVING CHANGE IN ORGANIZATIONS AND ORGANIZATIONAL SYSTEMS   160
2.4.5 FORMING AND MAINTAINING INTERORGANISATIONAL NETWORKS (IONS)   174
2.4.6 ASSESSING INTERORGANISATIONAL NETWORK (ION) PERFORMANCE   183
2.4.7 SYNTHESIS AND DISCUSSION - A CONCEPTUAL FRAMEWORK OF INTERORGANISATIONAL NETWORKS (IONS) AND BEYOND   189

3. **A FRAMEWORK FOR THE ASSESSMENT OF INTERNATIONAL NETWORKS FOR THE DEVELOPMENT OF HEALTH PROMOTING SCHOOLS (HPS)**   193

3.1 FOUNDATIONS OF AN ASSESSMENT FRAMEWORK FOR SUCH NETWORKS   193
3.1.1 INTRODUCTION   193
3.1.2 A COMPREHENSIVE ASSESSMENT FRAMEWORK FOR INTERORGANISATIONAL NETWORKS (IONS)   194
3.1.3 THE ION ASSESSMENT FRAMEWORK AND HEALTH PROMOTION: DO THEY FIT?   204

3.1.4	ASSESSMENT IN HEALTH PROMOTION - SELECTED MODELS AND IMPLICATIONS FOR THE ION ASSESSMENT FRAMEWORK	209
3.2	SYNOPSIS: THE GENERAL ASSESSMENT FRAMEWORK APPLICABLE TO INTERNATIONAL NETWORKS FOR THE DEVELOPMENT OF HEALTH PROMOTING SCHOOLS	225

4. THE 3-STEP-CASE STUDY APPROACH — 230

4.1	INTRODUCTION AND METHODS USED	230
4.1.1	RATIONAL FOR THE CASE STUDY APPROACH	231
4.1.2	CASE SELECTION AND DATA COLLECTION	232
4.2	THE STRUCTURE OF EACH CASE STUDY	236
4.2.1	THE OVERALL ANALYSIS OF EACH NETWORK CASE (STEP 1)	238
4.2.2	SYNTHESIZING ANALYSIS I OF EACH NETWORK CASE (STEP 2)	240
4.2.3	SYNTHESIZING ANALYSIS II OF ALL NETWORK CASES (STEP 3)	245

PART II — 247

5. THE "EUROPEAN NETWORK OF HEALTH PROMOTING SCHOOLS" (ENHPS) - A CASE STUDY FROM AN INTER-NATIONAL AND INTER-ORGANIZATIONAL RESEARCH PERSPECTIVE — 248

5.1	PRIMARY CASE STUDY: OVERALL ANALYSIS OF THE EUROPEAN NETWORK (ENHPS)	248
5.1.1	INTRODUCTION - THE EUROPEAN CONTEXT AND THE BIRTH OF THE ENHPS	248
5.1.2	RATIONAL, GOALS, AND CORE CONCEPTS	253
5.1.3	STRUCTURAL SET-UP AND KEY ACTORS OF THE ENHPS INITIATIVE	262
5.1.4	DEVELOPMENTS OVER TIME: THE EVOLUTION OF THE 'EUROPEAN NETWORK OF HEALTH PROMOTING SCHOOLS' (ENHPS)	273
5.1.5	INTERACTIONS AND RELATIONS OF ENHPS NETWORK MEMBERS	292
5.2	SYNTHESIZING ANALYSIS I - STRUCTURAL AND PROCESS FEATURES OF THE ENHPS	319
5.2.1	MEMBERSHIP OR BORDERS OF THE EUROPEAN NETWORK (FOR THE DEVELOPMENT) OF HEALTH PROMOTING SCHOOLS (ENHPS)	319
5.2.2	THE STRUCTURE OF THE EUROPEAN NETWORK FOR THE DEVELOPMENT OF HEALTH PROMOTING SCHOOLS	323
5.2.3	THE EUROPEAN NETWORK'S 'OPERATIONAL PROCESSES' AND 'ORGANIZATIONAL NETWORKING'	335
5.2.4	DISTANCE, ASSESSMENT CULTURE, AND SATISFACTION WITHIN THE EUROPEAN NETWORK	343
5.3	ENHPS COUNTRY CASE 1: THE "EUROPEAN NETWORK OF HEALTH PROMOTING SCHOOLS" IN GERMANY	348
5.3.1	THE GERMAN NETWORK INITIATIVE - CONTEXT AT THE OUTSET, CONCEPTS, GOALS	348
5.3.2	STRUCTURAL SET-UP AND KEY ACTORS OF THE 'MODEL EXPERIMENTS' AND NETWORK IN GERMANY	359
5.3.3	DEVELOPMENTS OVER TIME: THE EVOLUTION OF THE GERMAN NETWORK FOR THE DEVELOPMENT OF HEALTH PROMOTING SCHOOLS	364
5.3.4	INTERACTIONS AND RELATIONS OF NETWORK MEMBERS	372
5.4	SYNTHESIZING ANALYSIS I - STRUCTURAL AND PROCESS FEATURES OF THE GERMAN NETWORK	390
5.4.1	MEMBERSHIP OR BORDERS OF THE GERMAN NETWORK FOR THE DEVELOPMENT OF HEALTH PROMOTING SCHOOLS	390
5.4.2	THE STRUCTURE OF THE GERMAN NETWORK FOR THE DEVELOPMENT OF HEALTH PROMOTING SCHOOLS	393
5.4.3	THE GERMAN NETWORK'S 'OPERATIONAL PROCESSES' AND 'ORGANIZATIONAL NETWORKING'	400

5.4.4	DISTANCE, ASSESSMENT CULTURE, AND SATISFACTION WITHIN THE GERMAN NETWORK	409
5.5	**ENHPS COUNTRY CASE 2: THE "EUROPEAN NETWORK OF HEALTH PROMOTING SCHOOLS" IN SLOVENIA**	**414**
5.5.1	THE ENHPS IN SLOVENIA - CONTEXT, CONCEPTS, GOALS	415
5.5.2	STRUCTURAL SET-UP AND KEY ACTORS OF THE SLOVENIAN 'HPS PROJECT' AND 'NETWORK OF HEALTH PROMOTING SCHOOLS'	422
5.5.3	DEVELOPMENTS OVER TIME: THE EVOLUTION OF THE SLOVENIAN 'NETWORK OF HEALTH PROMOTING SCHOOLS'	425
5.5.4	INTERACTIONS AND RELATIONS OF NETWORK MEMBERS	434
5.6	**SYNTHESIZING ANALYSIS I - STRUCTURAL AND PROCESS FEATURES OF THE SLOVENIAN NETWORK**	**452**
5.6.1	MEMBERSHIP OR BORDERS OF THE SLOVENIAN NETWORK FOR THE DEVELOPMENT OF HEALTH PROMOTING SCHOOLS	453
5.6.2	THE STRUCTURE OF THE SLOVENIAN NETWORK FOR THE DEVELOPMENT OF HEALTH PROMOTING SCHOOLS	456
5.6.3	THE SLOVENIAN NETWORK'S 'OPERATIONAL PROCESSES' AND 'ORGANIZATIONAL NETWORKING'	462
5.6.4	DISTANCE, ASSESSMENT CULTURE, AND SATISFACTION WITHIN THE SLOVENIAN NETWORK	470
6.	**LINKING THEORY AND PRACTICE: THE ION ASSESSMENT FRAMEWORK AND THE EUROPEAN NETWORK FOR THE DEVELOPMENT OF HEALTH PROMOTING SCHOOLS**	**477**
6.1	**INTRODUCTION (OR TOWARDS THE JOURNEY'S END)**	**477**
6.2	**THE NETWORKS AS A WHOLE, THEIR EVOLUTION AND HEALTH PROMOTION DIMENSION (SYNTHESIZING ANALYSIS II)**	**479**
6.2.1	NETWORK STRUCTURES AND PROCESSES IN CONTEXT: THE NETWORKS AS A WHOLE AND OVER TIME	479
6.2.2	THE NETWORKS' HEALTH PROMOTION DIMENSION	509
PART III		**517**
7.	**LESSONS LEARNED, RECOMMENDATIONS, AND OUTLOOK**	**518**
7.1	**LESSONS LEARNED FROM, AND SUGGESTIONS TOWARDS MEMBERS AND SUPPORTERS OF THE "EUROPEAN NETWORK OF HEALTH PROMOTING SCHOOLS" (ENHPS)**	**518**
7.2	**CRITICAL APPRAISAL OF THE NEW ASSESSMENT FRAMEWORK FOR INTER-ORGANISATIONAL NETWORKS FOR THE DEVELOPMENT OF HEALTH PROMOTING SCHOOLS AND SIMILAR NETWORKS**	**534**
7.2.1	CRITICAL APPRAISAL OF THE MAIN ASSESSMENT CATEGORIES, ADAPTATIONS, AND RECOMMENDATIONS	536
7.2.2	CRITICAL APPRAISAL OF THE NETWORK ASSESSMENT FRAMEWORK AS A WHOLE	553
7.3	**THESES AND OUTLOOK**	**561**
REFERENCES		**569**

Foreword

"*Interorganisational* networks" are a particular and *participatory organisational form* for institutions that strive to achieve common goals. Since the 1990s, such networks are increasingly spreading, globally. However, the word "network" has also become a buzz word, and not all those collaborations called 'network' are networks in this sense. In the area of Public Health, the European field of Health Promotion under the leadership of the World Health Organisation did spearhead *a network approach to the promotion of health*. Particular attention was given to the principles of participation and empowerment, which are at the core of health promotion. Up today, a network approach has been repeatedly experimented with to implement the so called 'settings approach' to promote health. Not only in Europe a significant number of transnational and national networks have emerged, which aim at developing – on a larger scale - 'health promoting schools', '-worksites' or '-hospitals', or 'healthy cities' or '-villages'. Many of these "real world" network examples are already 5-10 years old, some even more. Nevertheless, their systematic assessment did hardly receive (research) attention, even in times of increasing pressure in the field to proof valued outcomes. Therefore, this research clarifies the concept and basic understanding of interorganisational networks as a means to achieve complex (health promotion) goals. It integrates network and health promotion research perspectives and translates existing knowledge into a practical network assessment instrument.

The work of networks for health promotion is inherently political, as is any work to effectively improve the health of populations. Health promotion is the process of enabling individuals and communities to increase control over the factors that influence health, and thereby improve their health. These factors are not only individual behaviours, but rather a range of interrelated social, economic, and environmental factors. Most of those cannot be shaped by any single organisation or person alone; and often changes of policies or even political decision making is needed to reduce harmful factors and increase resources for health. Already to create health supportive living or working conditions *locally* in most cases needs coordinated action of different organisations or sectors across levels of society. Therefore, and because of the participatory nature of the networks examined, I am pleased to publish this study as the second book in the new series on policy making and participation.

In 2003, this study was accepted by the School of Public Health at the University of Bielefeld as doctoral dissertation. I am particularly grateful to Prof. Klaus Hurrelmann for many valuable feed backs on the way and for sensibly accompanying me during the challenging process of undertaking research while continuing my work with the World Health Organisation (WHO), Geneva. I am also grateful to Prof. Ilona Kickbusch, with whom I had the privilege to work and learn from and who encouraged me to undertake this research. I am very thankful to many professionals within and around the European, German and Slovenian networks for the development of Health Promoting Schools, whose year long sharing and documenting of developments at national and international level provided the basis for the pilot testing of my new network assessment instrument. Particularly I would like to thank Mrs. Eva Sterger, national coordinator of the Slovenian HPS-network, whose provision of access to the largely unpublished documents was essential. I am also thanking Prof. Peter Paulus who served as 2nd level supervisor for this thesis.

Last but not least, I would like to thank my husband James M. Stone and my daughter Marina who over a long period of time did bear with a significant lack of time and attention due to my double commitment in research and professional life. Without my husband's back up as main child carer this book would not have been finalised.

Ursel Broesskamp-Stone
Berne, January 2004

1. Introduction

This research project strives to contribute to a better understanding, implementation and use of international and (sub)national networks to promote health considering **several perspectives**. It is undertaken from an *international perspective*, with particular emphasis on *local* actors and their needs. It is undertaken from a *Health Promotion perspective*, but in a way that those from other fields in Public Health and beyond can easily identify what applies to their collaborative or intersectoral actions, too, be they international or local. (Indeed, much of the network assessment framework may do.) Both perspectives led to an *organizational science perspective.* This unravels that the field of Health Promotion (may be intuitively) developed early on organizational forms for its large-scale interventions that today - outside the field of Public Health and increasingly within - are recognized as those most promising to achieve *complex* goals in *rapidly changing environments* in *sustainable* ways. - The international perspective originates from the researchers ten years of work in Public Health at national and international level; where aspects of organizations' working together in the pursuit of population health (within or across sectors) remain a major challenge up today. The Health Promotion perspective originates from twenty years of work in primary prevention, health education and health promotion, and the recognition of an exciting challenge inherent in the Health Promotion concept: i.e. the achievement of health supportive changes in the *combination* of factors that jointly influence health, including the social, together with the *enabling* of people to undertake, contribute and *sustain* such changes. The organizational science perspective with focus on *inter*-organizational *networks* (rather than organizational development of individual organizations) originates from the observance of and involvement in the work of WHO and others to initiate and support international networks for the development of health promoting settings, particularly of 'Health Promoting Schools', in Europe and around world. It should be noted already here that any inter-*sectoral* collaboration or action is necessarily also an inter-*organizational* one, which explains the assumption above that much of this research may be of interest for Public Health professionals outside the Health Promotion field, too.

The **spread of international networks for the development of health promoting Settings** on a larger scale since more than a decade and around the world motivated this research project. It sets out to develop a tool for organizations and people investing and engaging in such networks, that would help to analyze and assess these networks and their functioning in more systematic and where desired comparable ways. Already in the mid 1980s the World Health Organization's Regional Office for Europe (WHO/EURO) spearheaded the creation of such networks. This was motivated by the goal to initiate and support the creation of 'Settings for health' such as cities, schools, hospitals, and workplaces - and this on a *large* scale - and nevertheless by *enabling local actors* to create and sustain these health promoting Settings in mutual exchange and learning across organizational, national, and Settings- borders. The 'Healthy Cities' movement triggered in 1985 was followed by networks for the development of 'Health Promoting Schools', 'Health Promoting Hospitals' and '- Workplaces', 'Healthy Islands', '-Villages' or '- Municipalities' - not only in Europe but rapidly also in other Regions of the world. Particularly widely applied are settings and network approach to schools, i.e. the major formal settings for health supportive learning, living and working in childhood and adolescence, which is one of the reasons why networks for the development of Health Promoting Schools were chosen as cases to be studied in this research project. The "European Network of Health Promoting Schools (ENHPS)" established in 1992 as the first network of its kind was followed in the mid 1990s by networks in the Western Pacific and Latin America. Schools, national level bodies and/or international agencies are linked in one way or the other to foster the development of Health Promoting Schools (HPS) in countries. Further network initiatives have been started or established such as in Africa, South East Asia and the northern Western Pacific. Their development is *supported by recent international recommendations and policies* by international conferences, WHO and other international bodies such as UNICEF or the European Commission. (see chap. 2.2 and 5.1)

At a global level, the 'Jakarta Declaration' from 1997 identified five priorities for Health Promotion in the 21st Century, one of which is to secure an infrastructure for health promotion. Particular reference is made to '*settings* for health as the organizational base' of the infrastructure required and in light of new challenges the need of creating 'new and diverse *networks* to achieve *intersectoral* collaboration'. (WHO 1997) The cornerstones of the Health Promotion approach as outlined in the Ottawa Charter and the content of the Jakarta Declaration just mentioned were confirmed by the *World Health Assembly* when passing its Resolution 51.12 on Health Promotion (WHA 1998). With view to the school setting, the 'WHO Expert Committee on Comprehensive School Health Education and Health Promotion' 1995 referred to networks and other organizing mechanisms, too, when explaining its global level recommendations. Related health promotion actions proposed include the fostering of active *intersectoral* collaboration between health and education ministries and developing school health committees and *'networks'* across public and NGO sectors. Among the barriers to the development of comprehensive school health programs commonly identified at local, district and national level is the lack of program infrastructure that includes a lack of *'organizing mechanisms'*. (WHO 1996a, b, d) **This indicates that there is already an awareness of the need for organizational forms to support sustainable Public Health action such as Health Promotion actions that is more specific than the fairly general notion of 'intersectoral cooperation'; And that 'networks' however defined are one of the preferred forms at least in the field of Health Promotion.** Here lies the focus of this research project.

To understand the research approach taken (and as further elaborated in chapter 2.2) it should be noted that internationally one definition of **Health Promotion** is preeminent today: Health Promotion is the process of *enabling* people (individuals *and* communities) to increase control over the *'determinants'* of health, and *thereby* improve their health. It is a comprehensive approach to create and maintain health that embraces actions not only directed at skills of *individuals* but also at changing living *conditions* so as to alleviate their impact on public and individual health (WHO 1998a). Today, there is wide agreement that aims and impact of Health Promotion go beyond changing health behaviors and include changes of the social and physical *environment*. As stated already in the Ottawa Charter (1986) and supported by latest health research "health is created and lived by people within the *settings of their everyday life* (...). Health is created by caring for oneself and others, by being able to make decisions and have control over one's life circumstances, and by ensuring that the society one lives in creates conditions that allow the attainment of health by all its members." (see chap. 2.1) A 'setting' can be understood as the place or social context in which people engage in daily activities (such as schools, work sites and neighborhoods) in which many factors (personal, social, organizational, and other environmental factors) interact and affect health and well-being. The interdisciplinary and multi-professional field of Health Promotion is concerned with action and advocacy to address the full *range* of the potentially modifiable determinants of health, not only those which are related to the actions of individuals, such as health behaviors or lifestyles, but also factors such as income and social status, education, employment and working conditions, access to appropriate health relevant services, and the physical environments. In *combination* these factors create different living conditions which impact on health.

World wide the *school* setting is understood as **a key setting** for promoting health. Schools reach large portions of young and adult populations (over a billion via formal education each day). More children than ever are attending school, for increasingly longer periods, and during influential stages in their lives (e.g. when lifestyles and values are being formed). In 1995, the 'WHO Expert Committee' on school health estimated that schools have the potential to do more than perhaps any other single institution to improve the well-being and competence of children and adolescents (WHO 1996b p1). It stressed the importance of *continued development, implementation and evaluation* of school health promotion programs. Research in developing and developed countries demonstrates that school health programs can simultaneously reduce common health problems, increase the efficiency of the education system and advance public health, education and social and economic development. Recognising that schools deserve a high priority within international, national and local health promotion strategies, the World Health Organisation and its partners since the early 1990s developed *international initiatives* focusing on schools and the creation of **'Health Promoting Schools' (HPS)**. This contributes to *two global goals:* UNESCO's *Education for All* and WHO's *Health for All*. (WHO 1996d)

Basic health promotion strategies include *advocacy* for health to create the essential conditions for health and *mediating* between the different interests in society in the pursuit of health. (WHO 1986, 1998a, 1997) And the major approaches in the field of Health Promotion include a) the widely recognized health promoting 'Settings - approach'; and b) an approach widely implemented yet less discussed and as of now neglected in health promotion research: a *'network' approach* which (as introduced and elaborated in chapters 2.2 to 3) is suggested as another major approach. It is not the same as, but may effectively be used for intersectoral action or collaboration.

Against this background it is understood that the **knowledge base of Health Promotion** is twofold: It encompasses the results of studies on a) the *factors that influence or determine the health of populations* and their interrelations and distribution, as well as the distribution of health within populations; and b) the *organized social response* to these factors or determinants of health and their distribution (i.e. health promotion actions or interventions). Kickbusch (1996) did highlight this early on. In spite of remaining knowledge gaps in the first knowledge area on health determinants and their distribution (see chap. 2.1), researchers in health promotion do point out that it is nevertheless very timely to direct more efforts to intervention research instead of continuing to mainly describe health status and health risks of population groups, a major focus in Public Health (e.g. Nutbeam 1997, 1997b; Speller et al 1998). This seems to be even more important as health promotion practice in many countries and regions around the world is experimenting since a decade or more with comprehensive health promotion interventions, which are designed to respond to the complex nature of creating and maintaining health and with special attention to sustainable participatory actions and the creation of environments conducive to 'healthy' lifestyles and health - such as the above mentioned 'networks' to create health promoting settings. (see chap. 2.2) From the international perspective it can be stated that after decades of 'over-researching' of behavior change interventions (Marmot 1996; Noack 1997) it is still necessary to shift more research attention towards comprehensive interventions that address social and other environmental determinants of health and of health relevant behaviors such as those that implement the health promoting Settings approach. While 'community development' research for health has already a longer Public Health research tradition, research on health supportive '*organizational* development' such as on Health Promoting Schools, - Hospitals and - Workplaces is still fairly young. However, in comparison to the latter Public Health research on *inter-organizational networks* to promote health hardly exists. Here, this research project steps in.

The research is guided by the following three theses:

a.) The sustainable creation of 'health promoting settings' (such as Health Promoting Schools) on a *large scale* across countries is enabled and facilitated by a *network approach* for mutual benefit and learning.

b) International networks for the development of 'health promoting settings' (such as the 'European Network of Health Promoting Schools') are *inter-organizational* networks. Therefore, their assessment requires the use of *general interorganizational network indicators* besides those related to Health Promotion goals.

c) The organizational form of "interorganizational networks" matches well with Health Promotion goals, strategies and principles in general and the 'health promoting settings'- approach in particular.

Indicators are needed for both measuring effects of health promotion actions as well as planning such actions. This applies to networks such as those for the development of health promoting Settings, too. In a climate of ongoing economic recessions and scarce resources worldwide the (public and donor) interest in indicators to facilitate planning and measuring the effects of large-scale health promotion initiatives such as the fostering of the above-mentioned networks is rising. In comparison to the extensive, though not yet satisfying research base on the range of factors that *co-determine* health, research on comprehensive health promotion *interventions* that include elements of creating health supportive settings or systems (and, thus, organisational and policy changes in support of health) is in its infancy. In Health Promotion, intervention research 'lacks far behind the practice' (Nutbeam 1997b). Up today, there is a lack of Health Promotion indicators beyond the domain of behavioural change, particularly as to health supportive changes in social, organisational and policy environments. Increasingly researchers point out that the search for 'evidence' in Health Promotion should be broadened "to include studies that measure the impact of interventions on systems and organisational development as well as change in individual behaviour", which is not at all as easy as it may seem to be (Speller et al 1998 p3; see also McQueen 2001). Over the last few years some researchers have responded to this challenge by proposing comprehensive *outcome models for Health Promotion interventions,* one by a group around Rootman and the WHO Regional Office for Europe (Rootman et al 2001b), another one by Nutbeam (1999, 2000). However, while they provide some valuable orientation they are not specific enough for the assessment of *networks* for the development of health promoting Settings (see chap. 3). This leaves this research project with some conceptual and development work to do - because:

The goal of this research project is:

to develop a practical instrument for the assessment of international networks for the development of 'Health Promoting Schools' in terms of both structures and processes.

Thus, it aims to contribute to future planning, monitoring and evaluation efforts concerning *networks* of this type such as other 'health promoting settings' networks.

To reach this goal the following objectives have been defined:

1. to *develop a conceptual framework* for the collection of baseline and other data on international networks for the development of Health Promoting Schools (HPS) in terms of both *structures and processes*; as part of this, to critically review existing sets of indicators for assessing or monitoring such networks;

2. to *apply this framework* to one international network for the development of Health Promoting Schools (HPS) as well as two national networks therein, i.e. to *pilot test* the usefulness of the framework in describing these networks, identifying commonalties and differences and documented effects, and analyzing current capacities and future potentials - taking into account both the goals set by these networks and expectations and challenges towards such networks as indicated by, for example, the current scientific knowledge base for Health Promotion;

3. to *identify 'key' characteristics* of international networks for the development of Health Promoting Schools in terms of both structures and processes and *suggest a set of practical indicators* equally in terms of both - as a base for future evaluation and monitoring efforts.

When starting to work along these lines it became soon clear that the analysis of Health Promotion networks such as those for the development of Health Promoting Schools cannot be undertaken on the base of current Health Promotion research knowledge alone, i.e. health development knowledge and health promotion intervention knowledge, and that the *"network" itself* would need much more attention. Even where intervention knowledge addresses already organisational changes in support of health it is focused on changes of *individual* organisations such a schools that directly impact on health and health related lifestyles, but not on interrelations *between* such organisations such as in the form of networks *of* health relevant organisations. Therefore, the review of current research knowledge had to be broadened and more attention given to the organisational sciences. To introduce the reader to the overall work finally undertaken to achieve goal and objectives the following metaphor may be useful:

The reader is invited to join the researcher in: a) taking a swim in Public Health waters, particularly the sea of Health Promotion research and practice; then b) diving into the underlying waters of organisational sciences to discover treasures related to networks promising to be valuable if brought back to the surface of the Health Promotion sea, then c) indeed returning to the surface of this sea with the treasure found and with the help of those looking at a large colourful coral reef system called ‚European Network of Health Promoting Schools'. After having got in touch with 'real life' in the Health Promotion sea the reader may come along and step out of the water to reflect on the journey as a whole. - It will need some fitness and perseverance particularly for those that are neither familiar with Health Promotion waters nor those of the organisational sciences, but unravelling complexity and discovering simplicity therein will be rewarding.

Less metaphorical, such a journey raises many questions, for example: What types of networks did emerge as of now in Health Promotion or Public Health and how are they functioning? How can these be systematically described in a comparable way, analyzed or even assessed? What can they learn from each other? More specifically, are existing network approaches for the development of Health Promoting Schools in some regions applicable to other regions or cultural contexts? Is it worthwhile to continue to initiate and nurture such networks for the development for health promoting settings? What progress or effects can be expected? How could these and similar networks be planned, monitored and evaluated in the future? And so on… Unfortunately, at present, it is difficult to answer these questions. Research efforts to develop indicators to enhance future planning, evaluation and monitoring efforts regarding international networks for the development of Health Promoting Schools and other settings face at least two challenges: a) the lack of overviews and the different levels of quality or availability of data on existing networks, and b) the lack of appropriate models, approaches or tools to plan, evaluate and monitor such large scale health promotion actions. Therefore - and because *any* assessment, evaluation or monitoring effort of comprehensive Health Promotion actions should best be done by truly interdisciplinary *teams* rather than one researcher alone - this research project should be understood as **a pilot project** which aims at contributing to future research, evaluation and monitoring efforts regarding international networks for the development of Health Promoting Schools. How this admittedly complex pilot project was approached is further explained next.

PART I

HEALTH KNOWLEDGE TODAY AND ORGANISED SOCIAL RESPONSES TO PROMOTE HEALTH

(STATE OF RESEARCH)

- Health and co-determinants of health
- Health Promotion – an organized social response to knowledge on the above
- Interorganizational networks – features and development
- Research result I – a framework to assess interorganizational networks to promote health

2. Health knowledge today and organized social responses to promote health (State of research)

The assessment of international networks for the development of Health Promoting Schools implies to assess complex social systems that aim at achieving a complex task, the creation of educational organizations that promote health. To be able to develop an assessment framework and related indicators for such networks their key features and task need to be well understood. The bodies of knowledge need to be identified that provide the scientific base for the development of indicators for the assessments of such complex systems. This can be done in a stepwise process commencing with identifying the key concepts inherent in the term 'international networks for the development of Health Promoting Schools'. These networks have been created or emerged within the field of 'Health Promotion' that is guided by the Ottawa Charta (1986). In accordance with this latter this research builds on the following understanding (see chap. 2.2):

Health Promotion is the process of enabling individuals and communities to increase control over the factors that co-determine health and thereby improve their health. "Health Promotion not only embraces actions directed at strengthening the *skills and capabilities of individuals*, but also action directed towards changing social, environmental and economic *conditions* so as to alleviate their impact on public and individual health." (WHO 1998a, p1-2)

Against this background, the following (underlying and related) core concepts of the term 'international networks for the development of Health Promoting Schools' can be identified: '*Health*' is to be promoted through '*health promotion*' in or through '*schools*'. - '*Health Promotion*' as defined above encompasses the strategy of creating '*health promoting settings*', such as health promoting *organizations,* such as 'Health Promoting *Schools*' (HPS). - In the term 'international networks for...' the plural 'School<u>s</u>' indicates that *a number* of such Health Promoting Schools are *to be developed,* by or through '*networks*' that are 'international'. - Thus, a good understanding of *'international networks for the development of Health Promoting Schools'* will rely on the current knowledge with regard to: a) health and its development; b) health promotion, its 'settings' approach, and organizational change in support of health applicable to schools; and c) international "networks". Accordingly, **to develop a science based assessment framework for the apparently complex systems of international networks for the development of Health Promoting Schools, three bodies of knowledge are of particular relevance:**

1. health development knowledge (in the sense of "causal" knowledge as to the creation and maintaining of health);
2. intervention or action knowledge concerning the promotion of health with special attention to:
    2.1 the 'Health Promoting , particularly those that advance the dissemination of the HPS concept and its implementation by fostering the development of a number of 'Health Promoting Schools' in an international context (i.e. on a larger scale).
    2.2 This is supported by Noack (1997 p57) who in a review of "research for health promotion" concluded:

"Successful Health Promotion requires a solid scientific knowledge base related to two fundamental questions: 1) Where and how is health created ? 2) Which investments create the largest health gain and the largest reduction in inequity ?" These 'basic questions' that guide the field of health promotion up to day originate from Kickbusch (1996). The first one points to people's daily life context and the knowledge of factors that influence or co-determine health and their interactions *(health development knowledge).* The second question points to the *adequate 'social responses' to this knowledge,* i.e. the organised efforts of communities and societies and the knowledge of the conditions and dynamics of effective actions or interventions to sustain and improve people's health - with special attention to the reduction of inequities in health *(action or intervention knowledge).*

The structure of this chapter

This chapter 2 on the 'state of research' is structured according to the three bodies of knowledge identified above as providing the scientific base for developing a practical tool to *assess international networks for the development of Health Promoting Schools* (HPS) in terms of both structures and processes:

Chapter 2.1 addresses the creation and maintaining of health from a social ecological and "determinants of health" perspective - as health promotion actions such as the creation of Health Promoting Schools (HPS) aim at enabling people to increase control over the *factors that influence or co-determine health* and thereby improve their health.

Chapter 2.2 addresses the key features of the *Health Promotion* concept and main approaches for its implementation - as these currently represent both the main social responses to the breadths of knowledge on health factors or "determinants of health", and the framework for implementing the *Health Promoting Schools* concept.

Chapter 2.3 addresses the phenomenon of *"networks"*, their key features and related assessment issues from an organizational science perspective (which will complemented later from a health promotion perspective).

Together these bodies of knowledge promise to provide a good scientific basis for developing the desired assessment tool for the networks at stake.

2.1 Health and co-determinants of health

2.1.1 Introduction

Before turning to the factors that influence health, the health concept itself needs clarification. A much cited definition of health stems from the World Health Organization's (WHO) constitution:

Health is "the state of complete physical, mental and social well being and not merely the absence of disease or infirmity" (WHO Constitution 1948).

Since the 1980s, experts and health movements have brought this 'positive' and 'multidimensional' definition of health back into public and academic discussion and it has become the main reference definition for much of public health and health promotion policy and practice both in economically developing and developed countries. While criticized as being too utopian by some (*"complete…"* well-being) and as too static ("the *state of…*") this health definition has become the guiding vision for many. Nevertheless, from a scientific perspective there is a need for a new definition of health (see below).

In the 1980s, health research and debate were significantly stimulated by the work of Aaron Antonovsky (1987, 1979, 1996). He introduced the 'salutogenic model' whose basic question is "how to understand that people stay healthy and alive in spite of myriad immanent pathogens (varying from micro-biological through social) constantly confronting them" (Ben Sira 1994). Antonovsky (1979) proposed the conceptual neologism *'salutogenesis'*, the origins of health, in analogy to pathogenesis. Instead of focusing on risk factors he proposed the focus on **'salutary factors'**, which according to Antonovsky may be called also 'health promoting' factors if understood in the true sense of factors which *"actively promote health, rather than just being low on risk factors"* (Antonovsky 1996 p14).

Salutogenesis is not just the contrary of a pathogenic orientation: Pathogenic thinking is concerned with the development and treatment of diseases; salutogenesis is not the contrary in the sense of focusing on development and maintenance of health as an absolute state. **Saluto-**

genesis means to view all persons as more or less healthy and at the same time as more or less ill. The guiding question that follows is: How is a person getting more healthy and less ill? (Antonovsky 1987) This salutogenic perspective on health and its promotion is best illustrated by **a metaphor used by Antonovsky** (1987, 1996) and often referred to in full or in parts: The **pathogenic approach** of (western) curative medicine is devoted to *rescuing people that are drowning* in a dangerous river (with high investments and *without asking why* they are in there and why they cannot swim better) ('downstream' orientation). *Pathogenesis oriented prevention* is devoted to those *in danger of being pushed into the river*, asking what pushes people into the water (risk factor and 'upstream' orientation). **The salutogenic approach** to health and health promotion sees *all* human beings, by virtue of being a living system, *always* in the 'dangerous river of life', and none on the shore. The river branches off, has smaller or tricky currents, is partly polluted, etc. The assumption that all human beings are in the river means, there is no dichotomous classification health/illness but a health-disease-continuum, with each person being at a given point in time somewhere on this continuum. The **twin question** (at least for health promotion) is: How dangerous is a *particular* river? How *well* can people swim?

The effect of the salutogenic model may be described as a paradigmatic transformation in scientific thought, *from pathogenesis and risk factors to salutogenesis and factors that shape or co-determine health* (in the true sense of salutary factors). Over the last decade or two an increasing number of researchers have joined into the attempt to identify 'determinants of health'. This includes not only social epidemiologists but behavioral scientists and health psychologists, too.

Models have been created that integrate various *determinants of health relevant behaviors or actions of individuals* covering both the traditional health education focus on *intrapersonal* factors as well as *social environmental* factors (see e.g. Green, Kreuter 1991, 1999; Schwarzer 1992; Hurrelmann 2000). More recently and rapidly increasing, social epidemiologists and researchers that identify with the 'population health approach' have started to review and integrate their findings concerning the *(social) determinants of health of populations,* often directly linked to aims of (national and international) health policy and programs development in support of improving the health of entire populations and reducing inequities in health (see e.g. 'Why are some people healthy and others not?' by Evans, Barer and Marmor (1994); Marmot 1991; Marmot/ Wilkinson 1999). Also in the natural science based 'environment and health sciences' considerations of both disease *and* health have emerged (see e.g. Eis 1998).

These bodies of knowledge contribute to a better understanding of factors and processes that may help people to move on the 'health ease/dis-ease continuum' (Antonovsky) more towards health. However, the pathogenic model that searches for risk factors related to (sets of) diseases is still dominating "health" research and studies that truly focus on health development or maintenance are rare. But 'disease research' has been widened in scope beyond biological, 'intrapersonal' and individual behavioral risk factors towards the inclusion of social and broader societal influences on health and disease.

2.1.2 The search for an integrative theory of health and disease

Hurrelmann (2000) took up the challenge to develop an integrative concept and working definition of health and disease that may be acceptable for various disciplines and professionals. He reviewed, synthesized and analyzed a range of theories from the social sciences that deal with health and disease across the English and German language barrier. He identified **five main 'theoretical threads'** whose basic ideas and assumptions are summarized as follows (p 84-86): First, *'theories of learning and personality'* express that specific characteristics of personality determine the extent and profile of competencies with which a person attempts to successfully deal with or respond to environmental and physiological demands. The theories show that this process can be more or less successful. Second, *'theories of stress and coping including the salutogenic and psychosomatic theories'* also focus on individual competencies to deal or cope with internal or external strains. They underline the reciprocity of the person-environment-relationship. Health is understood as a state of balance, which has to be recreated on an ongoing basis. Third, *'socialization theories'* expand this perspective and underline the life-long process of assimilating, processing and coping with reality. They consider personal and social resources, which are understood as prerequisites for the dynamic balance between risk and protective factors. They raise awareness of the intermediate stages between 'absolute' health and 'absolute' disease. Fourth, *'interaction theories and social structure theories'* address the institutional and societal factors that are related to health and disease. Health and disease are understood as closely corresponding and partly being a reaction to socialization and power structures in society. Finally fifths, *'Public Health - theories'* focus on the analysis of interrelations between social characteristics and the health and disease status of populations.

Traditionally 'Public Health' - theories (such as the risk factor model) are being used to inform questions of specific services to be provided by medical 'health care' systems (Hurrelmann 2000). But over recent years a critical school of thought gained strengths which focuses on "determinants of health", with special attention to societal factors, and on "population health"; related social epidemiological and other research results inform about the fairly *limited* importance of medical (disease) care systems for maintaining the health of entire populations as compared to other societal sectors and systems such as economics, *education*, welfare, child care and transport (see e.g. Evans/ Stoddart 1990, 1994; Evans, Barer, Marmor 1994; Blane, Brunner, Wilkinson 1996; Wilkinson, Marmot 1998; Health Canada 2000; and chap. 2.1.3 below). Unfortunately, Hurrelmann (2000) concentrated on the former Public Health research area.

Four guiding ideas of health and disease

Hurrelmann's analyses (2000) show that the range of theories reviewed exhibit a variety of perspectives and dimensions concerning health and disease development but also have some basics in common. He elicits four guiding ideas of health and disease that are *acceptable across disciplines* while paying special attention to those ideas that may be able to guide further discussions in theory and practice: 1) the idea of health as *successful* and disease as a *unsuccessful dealing and coping* with internal and external demands; 2) the idea of health as *balance* and disease as *imbalance* of risk factors and protective factors at the physical, mental and social level; 3) the idea of *'relative'* health and *'relative"* disease according to objective and subjective criteria; and 4) the idea of health and disease as *reaction to societal conditions*.

1. Health as successful, disease as a unsuccessful dealing and coping with internal and external demands: According to the theories supporting this understanding of health and disease, the **internal demands** encompass a) a *biological* dimension (genetic disposition, physical constitution, immune, neural and hormonal systems, both their structures and dynamics) and b) a *psychological* dimension (structure of personality, temperament, and ability to take stress). These internal demands are at the same time the equipment or *resources for a person's dealing with external demands*. (see contributions of theories of learning and personality) The **external demands** encompass socio-economic status, 'ecological environment', living conditions in area of residence, factors of hygiene, educational services, working conditions, private forms of living (e.g. family), and social integration. Also the external demands are at the same time *resources needed to successfully deal with internal demands*. (see contributions of sociological theories). (see also fig. 2.1.1) - Particularly the stress- and coping theories, the salutogenic theory, and the socialization theory explicitly express this understanding of health and disease. *Competencies* are developed on the base of personal and social resources and determine the capacities for coping with internal and external demands.

According to Hurrelmann, a particular basic constellation of factors (internal and ex-

ternal resources) is needed so that health as successful coping with internal and external demands can be expected or maintained. (But which constellations this may refer to remains an open question.) If personal competencies and/or acceptable societal conditions are lacking, the risk for unsuccessful coping increases. Thus, disease can be understood as unsuccessful coping with internal and external demands.
- The author also elicits that health is possible on the base of a lifestyle that can be described as follows: it successfully integrates a (self-) conscious lifestyle (directed at work, performance, strain and rationality) and a pleasure oriented lifestyle (directed at relaxation, eating and drinking, physical activity, ties, love and sexuality). Important components of such a lifestyle are the competencies mentioned above, a positive attitude to the everyday challenges, acceptance of ones own body and psychological disposition, optimistic expectations towards the social environment, and overall the belief in the possibility of shaping one's own lifestyle. This is captured in concepts such as 'self-efficacy', 'sense of coherence', and 'productive coping with reality'.

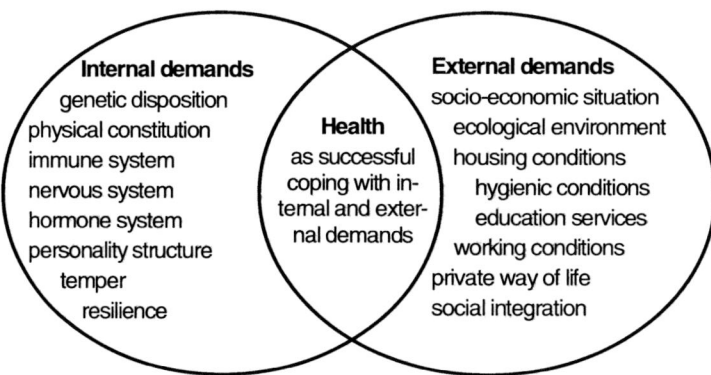

Figure 2.1.1: Health as coping with internal and external demands (Hurrelmann 2000 p88; translated by Broesskamp-Stone)

2. Health as balance, disease as imbalance of risk factors and protective factors at the physical, mental and social level:
Contradictions and tensions between demands of the various systems in life are part of normal life (not the exception in life). If health, the dynamic equilibrium between risk and protective factors breaks down, a time of relative disease begins. (Relative) health may be regained through the activation of self control ('Selbststeuerung') and external support. Such *regulatory processes are continuously needed*. To illustrate this Hurrelmann uses the concept of a regulation circle ('Regelkreis') that a person may go through several times during the life course (see fig. 2.1.2).

The regulatory processes *concern all dimensions (physical, mental and social)* of health and disease. At the same time these three dimensions are interacting, with balances or imbalances on one dimension influencing these processes on the two others. At the *physical level* both intrapersonal systems (nervous, hormone, immune systems) as well as the ability to adapt, resistance, and plasticity of the organism in its reactions to environmental demands play a role (Stock, Sachser 1998 according to Hurrelmann 2000 p90-91). At *mental level* individual needs and motivations are important, at *social level* social support and integration.

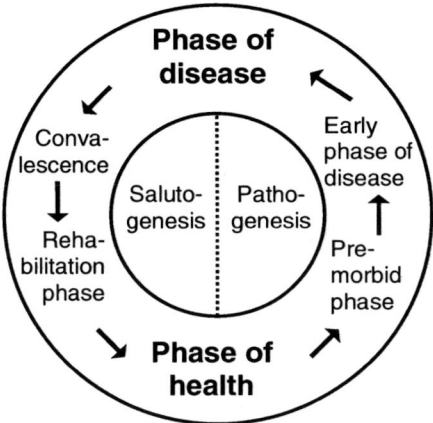

Figure 2.1.2: Regulation cycle of states of health and disease (Hurrelmann 2000 p90; translated by Broesskamp-Stone)

3. Relative health and relative disease exists and is defined considering both objective and subjective criteria: Many theories on health and disease support the understanding that a person with a chronic disease or life long handicap is not living in 'absolute' but with 'relative' disease, thus, at the same time with 'relative' health. The latter is the case when a chronically ill person succeeds in coping with its disease in a way that he or she is able to activate the remaining health potentials. Interaction and socialization theories express this most explicitly. How the physical, mental and social dimensions of health and disease 'play together' can be determined by both objective criteria (according to normative standards within professional fields) and subjective measures and perceptions. As illustrated in figure 2.1.3, both 'objective' and subjective assessments of the point on the health-disease-continuum for each of the three dimensions of health and disease (physical, mental, social) can differ at any given point in time. The figure 2.1.3 shows a practical model to document and communicate states of relative health and relative disease considering all dimensions of health and disease as well as for each the 'objective' and subjective assessments. The concept of the regulating cycle has been transformed into the model of the health-disease-continuum.

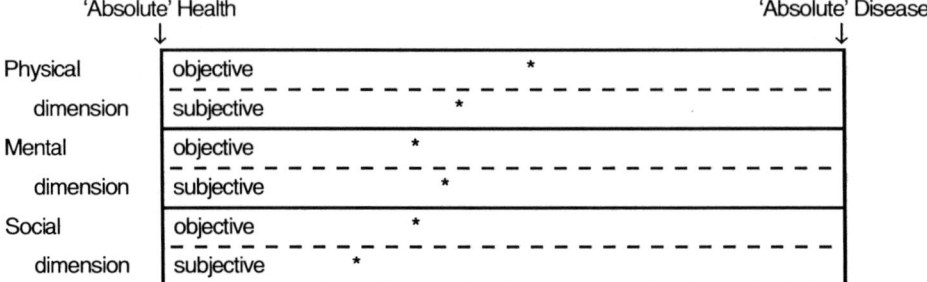

Figure 2.1.3: Health and disease as a multidimensional continuum; Hypothetical example of a person with diabetes (Hurrelmann 2000, p98)

Particularly theories of learning and personality as well as stress- and coping theories emphasize the *importance of the subjective assessment of health*. In many cases subjective assessment can predict objective disease. Hurrelmann (2000) stresses that also for ethical reasons the subjective assessment of health and disease should be clearly taken into account. He points to the right of all persons in democratic societies to maintain or regain the balance between internal and external demands in a way that matches with their own desires and ideas. With reference to interaction and role theories he underlines that assessments by (health) professionals are not 'objective' in the sense of being only based on professional standards as they are also based on normative ideas and power dimensions of society. Thus, it is not possible to provide a 'truly objective' assessment of a person's state of health or disease.

4. Health and disease as reaction to societal conditions, particularly in the areas of economics, ecology and education:
To underpin this guiding idea Hurrelmann (2000) refers to interaction and social structure theories as well as public health theories. From a macro level perspective, health and disease status of *populations* are closely linked with the structures of work and education determined by societies as well as with cultural and material living conditions. The *degree of health or disease* of individuals as well as whole populations *reflects the degree of societal development*. *Health problems* can be interpreted as the *'costs' of a country's or society's development, particularly of economic and cultural change processes* ('modernization processes').

The 'modernization' of societies is characterized by *increasing differentiation and specialization of social systems*. For example, children are decreasingly educated by their families and increasingly by educational institutions. Individuals in highly modernized societies are taking part in several differentiated and highly specialized social systems at the same time, each of which has its own dynamics, value system, and normative orientation. They have to be able to make connections among those different worlds of external, social demands, which potentially is a significant source of strain or tension, which may be expressed in mental or physical health problems. People in today's industrialized societies are always endangered to create only weak social ties and become irritated in their identity. A key feature of modernization of societies is the *individualization*. Fixed patterns of social roles in work and private life, reliable general values and norms that can guide personal action are diminishing. This gives way to a high degree of independence and freedom for each individual to shape its own life, which demands high levels of self control and self organization and this on an ongoing basis. This bears the risk of an overtaxing and overload with negative impacts on health.

Overall, this rich body of knowledge reasons Hurrelmann's **critique of the WHO definition of health** as complete state of physical, mental and social well-being and not merely the absence of disease and infirmity (WHO 1948). This is not anymore sufficient to guide research and practice today. Although it covers some of the guiding ideas (such as the multidimensional perspective on health and health as something positive with an own quality) it *overemphasizes subjective perceptions and feelings about heath* ('health is… well-being'), is too utopian ('complete… well-being') and is *unable to accommodate all four scientific sound 'guiding ideas'* of health and disease. Therefore, Hurrelmann proposes the following **alternative definition of health** which may find wide spread agreement:

"Health is the state ('Stadium') of balance between risk factors and protective factors which occurs if a person succeeds in coping with both the internal (physical and mental) and external (social and material) demands. Health is a state that conveys to a person well-being and joy of life." (Hurrelmann 2000 p94, translated from German by the author/Broesskamp-Stone)

Analogous to this definition he defines disease (differences highlighted in italics):

"Disease is the state ('Stadium') of *im*balance between risk factors and protective factors which occurs if a person *does not* succeed in coping with both the internal (physical and mental) and external (social and material) demands. Disease is a state that conveys to a person *the impairment of his or her* well-being and joy of life." (Hurrelmann 2000 p94, translated from German by the author; italics not in original)

Accordingly, Hurrelmann defines 'relative health' and 'relative disease' as "the state ('Stadium') of partially disturbed balance" (…) "which appears if a person *only partially or only for a limited time span* succeeds in (…)". They are states that allow a person "*only partial* well being and joy of life" (translated from German, italics not in original).

Health and disease - intermediate synthesis and discussion

In the field of health promotion, since long a range of intervention and change strategies with different disciplinary or theoretical roots have been integrated into one comprehensive concept, the Health Promotion concept which was first outlined in the Ottawa Charter in 1986 (see chap. 2.2). However, its theoretical underpinning with regard to the understanding of health and disease that is compatible with the many disciplines on the base of which the concept has been developed, was lacking. Here, Hurrelmann steps in from the social sciences perspective, with his suggestion of an *integration* of the various understandings of health and disease inherent in the range of social science theories and also in some theoretical frameworks from 'Public Health'. As of now, the field of Health Promotion is typically referring to the WHO definition of health as a 'state' of physical, mental and social well-being (…), - a definition which represents a widespread minimal consensus in the public (health) sectors in most countries including national Ministries of Health. But this definition does not help to answer one of the key questions guiding the field of Health Promotion: *How is health created?*

The definition of health developed by Hurrelmann does answer this question to a certain degree: health (the state of balance between risk factors and protective factors) occurs *through successful coping with both the internal (physical and mental) and external (social and material) demands*. Hurrelmann's analyses also provides hints as to the *conditions needed* for such successful coping: 'a particular basic constellation of factors' or resources (internal and external). However, this is not specified further. As will be seen in the following chapters there are good reasons for this.

International networks for the development of Health Promoting Schools follow the approach to Health Promotion as promoted by WHO: Health Promotion is understood as the process of enabling people to increase control over the factors that influence or co-determine health and thereby, improve their health (see WHO 1998a). Reference is made to actions directed at strengthening both the *skills and capabilities* of individuals and changing *social, environmental and economic conditions* so as to alleviate their impact on *public and individual* health (WHO 1998a). The consideration of 'determinants' of health, i.e. skills and capabilities of individuals as well as social, environmental and economic conditions, reminds of the consideration of 'internal (physical and mental) and external (social and material) demands' as key elements of Hurrelmann's new definition of health. Internal demands are understood as being at the same time resources for coping with external demands, and vice versa. In the field of health promotion co-'determinants' of health are often referred to as 'resources' (see e.g. Noack 1997). In addition, one of the four guiding ideas of health on the base of which Hurrelmann developed his health definition reads 'health as balance of *risk factors and protective factors* at the *physical, mental and social* level'. Against this background it seems reasonable to assume that Hurrelmann's *'demands' and 'resources' and 'risk/protective factors' refer to the same factors than the term co-'determinants of health'* used in the aforementioned definition of health promotion. This means that a) those that work in the field of health promotion as defined above and that usually refer to and/or are guided by the multidimensional but 'static' WHO definition of health, and b) those that may follow Hurrelmann's similarly multidimensional, but 'dynamic' definition of health refer to the same factors or at least categories of factors (physical, mental, social, economic and 'physical environmental'/material). – But it should be noted that this *may* or may *not* mean that the *ways or mechanisms* through which those factors influence or create and maintain health are interpreted in the same way.

Hurrelmann found that it is a '*particular* constellation of factors' that is needed to create health, i.e. the *joint* impact of *several* factors related to each other in a *specific* way, a result stemming from his cross-disciplinary analyses within the social sciences. *Which (categories of) factors* this refers to is shown in figure 2.1.1 (above) that again focuses on what is acceptable across those social sciences analyzed. With regard to the **relative importance of the various categories of factors** Hurrelmann's forth 'guiding idea' of health 'as reaction to *societal conditions,* particularly in the areas of economics, ecology and education' provides a first general answer. Chapter 2.1.3 addresses this further.

It is interesting that Hurrelmann's interdisciplinary analyses do not further address the *interplay* of these factors although there is a fast growing and much recognized body of knowledge around this issue (particularly with focus on social and societal factors and their biological pathways to influence health and disease). This may be simply due to his goal set, to develop an interdisciplinary acceptable *understanding of health and disease* (with an examination of *how* these states of health and disease are created reaching beyond that goal). This may be because there was no further consensus emerging during his cross-disciplinary analyses with regard to this issue. Or it is due to Hurrelmann's focus on *theories,* and today's models about the interplay of various health related factors or 'determinants of health' are still far from being a theory (see below). However, **health promotion practice would benefit from a better understanding of the interplay and relative importance of the range of (protective and risk) factors, demands or resources, that influence health;** this would provide guidance on how and with which foci the health promoting 'process of enabling people to gain control over the determinants of health' should be shaped. Such guidance is searched for not only in the field of Health Promotion but also in national and international health policy development in general. Particularly in the context of the latter, in recent years various models of 'determinants of health' (and disease) have been created and find much interest in research and practice. Models that attempt to explain interrelationships or show correlations stem from social epidemiologists, health economists and other social scientists. What the ensemble of such models may add to a better understanding of the factors that influence health is briefly addressed in the next section.

2.1.3 Factors that influence or co-determine health - a general picture

Introduction

In the latest WHO Health Promotion Glossary (WHO 1998a p6) the term **'determinants of health'** has been included as a new definition. 'Determinants of health' are defined as the "range of personal, social, economic and environmental factors which determine the health status of individuals and populations". Over the last years the term has become almost a buzzword in health policy, Public Health and Health Promotion. Noack (1997) stressed that **the term health 'determinant'** needs qualification because it does *not* imply a simple linear relationship between causal factors and outcome, but **implies "a non-linear interactive process involving complex pathways of factors and feed back loops. (...) Health is made possible, it is never determined in the sense of classical physics"** (Noack 1997 p64). The health impact of many single factors derives from complex interactions with many other factors within the 'causal web' of health. This is supported by an increasing number of models and conceptual frameworks of factors that influence health.

After considering a range of research internationally Noack proposed alternate terms: "*resources*" for health (such as socio-economic, physical-environmental, cultural resources) and "*predispositions*" for health (such as biological, psychological predisposing factors). Up to day, many different terms can be found in the literature such as 'factors influencing health' (e.g. Dahlgreen/Whitehead 1991), 'conditional factors' (e.g. Hurrelmann 2000), or 'protective factors' (e.g. Belz-Merkel et al 1992; Hurrelmann 2000). The term 'determinants of health' remains widely used, too (e.g. Marmot/Wilkinson 1999; WHO/EURO 1997; Evans et al 1994). For this research project it is proposed to use as the overriding term either the term "**co-determinants of health**" or **factors that jointly influence health.** The emphasis on "co"-determinants accounts for (and will keep up the awareness of the fact that) the word 'determinants' does refer to a *non*-linear *interactive* process among a *variety* of factors involving *complex* pathways and feed back loops, and that health *is never determined* in the sense of classical physics.

Where reference is made to the field of 'determinants of health' research this original term will be used.

In the 1990s, this research are has begun to shift attention away from the well known individual risk behaviors (diet, non-smoking, etc.) and particular (physical/ chemical) environmental risks, i.e. the focus of much of 'Public Health' research, towards societal factors related to 'population health' status. As such this research underpins and contributes to a more differentiated view of the category of 'social determinants' of health but from a population perspective. *The focus is on environments rather than on individual psychology and behavior* (Marmot 1999). The increased awareness of the wider range of co-determinants of health has been accompanied by a raised interest in creating **overviews of the various factors** to guide policy and practice. Overview documents that refer back to particular research results for each factor or combination of factors to proof scientific soundness are usually sizable products created in multi-disciplinary efforts that are linked to some kind of reform efforts and implementations of large-scale programs or policies for health development.

International examples include a 'core set of determinants of (urban) health' from the WHO-Kobe-Center's urban health project (WHO Kobe Center 1997/98) and the WHO/EURO Social Determinants Campaign in the context of the "Health for All"-policy renewal that resulted in publishing "The solid facts - social determinants of health" for actors in policy and practice (WHO/EURO 1997b; Tsouros, Farrington 1999). *National examples* include the second report on the health of Canadians "Toward a Healthy Future" (Federal, Provincial and Territorial Advisory Committee on Population Health 1999) and German ministerial reports on 'health and school' and 'health and general adult education', results of two co-determinants of health and Health Promotion oriented education reform projects (Broesskamp 1994; BMBF 1997).

In the scientific literature, a range of *critical reviews, analyses and syntheses* of results of largely social-epidemiological studies build the published knowledge base on co-determinants of health (and disease). This includes the Baird 1994; Berkmann, Glass 2000; Blane, Brunner, Wilkinson 1996; Dahlgreen, Whitehead 1991; Evans 1994, 1994a; Evans, Barer, Marmor 1994; Evans, Hodge, Pless 1994; Evans, Stoddart 1994, 1990; Hertzman et al 1994; Kawachi et al 1996; Marmot 1996, 1999; Mielck 2001; Mielck, Bloomfield 2001; Noack 1997; Tavlov 1996; WHO/EURO 1997b; and Wilkinson 1999, 1996, 1994; - and this list is not complete. Some of these authors or groups of authors have started to integrate various findings across disciplines in frameworks or models of 'determinants of health' or health development, which usually draw special attention to social or societal factors (e.g. Brunner, Marmot 1999; Berkmann, Glass 2000; Dahlgreen, Whitehead 1991; Evans, Stoddart

1990, 1994; Noack 1997; Tavlov 1996; Hancock 1990). In 1997, Noack concluded that, in spite of significant knowledge gaps (theoretical, conceptual, and methodological) the current knowledge on 'determinants of health' can inform and guide health promotion today.

This applies also to this research project on assessing international networks for the development of Health Promoting Schools. The concept of a Health Promoting School (HPS) builds on the concept of health promotion as the 'process of enabling people to increase control over the *factors that influence or co-determine health*. Thus, the creation of Health Promoting Schools implies enabling pupils, teachers and other members of the school community to increase their control over the co-determinants of health. A better understanding of the latter would allow to make reasoned choices with regard to the question on which determinants of health to focus here.

Co-determinants of population health - towards a common framework

This chapter aims at providing a brief overview of current knowledge and key issues of debate around co-determinants of population health. The 'determinants of health' research with a population perspective is a fairly new academic field and the vast array of particular findings is not yet integrated. Overview models that link particular (groups of) determinants with others or even try to indicate how these may interact to jointly create health or disease status have been developed created from various perspectives, but no model has yet received a particularly prominent role in the field. This has been shown by a first review of the body of literature on determinants of health already introduced and listed in the introduction above. For this research project, a selective approach has been chosen. The goal is to paint a *general* picture of what is the common understanding that emerges and to identify some of the key issues that according to researchers themselves call for modified (public) policies and practices if improving and maintaining of the health status of populations is truly the goal.

During the 1990s, the knowledge on the **'determinants of population health' and their relative importance** increased significantly. Models that are intended to be general comprehensive models, and that consider factors that influence *health* (with or without the inclusion of a disease perspective) all show three types of elements (see e.g. Noack 1997; Dahlgreen, Whitehead 1991; Brunner, Marmot 1999; Evans, Stoddart 1990, 1994; Eis 1998; Green, Kreuter 1991, 1999; Hancock 1990; Tavlov 1996; also fig. 2.1.1):

1. environmental factors:
   - social environment
   - economic environment (e.g. income distribution)
   - physical (also 'ecological') environment (includes both human made and natural environment)
   - also: health care system (pointed out by some, e.g. Evans, Stoddard 1990, 1994; Noack 1997)
2. (intra-)personal factors:
   - psychological dispositions
   - biological dispositions (include e.g. genetic dispositions)
3. an element or factors concerning the *person/ environment - interface* or -interactions:
   - coping with stress; lifestyles/health behaviors; psychological and biological learning.

Each of these categories of 'determinants of health' has rich internal structures and complex content and cannot be represented by a single homogenous variable: "single variables may capture some aspects of a particular category, but they are not the same as that category. Moreover, in specific contexts it may be the *interactions* between factors from different categories of determinants, and their *timing*, that are critical to the health of individuals and populations" (Evans, Stoddart 1994, p32 - italics not in original). Today, it is widely recognized that co-determinants of health are not only *multiple* and *complicated* but also *interact with each other in complex ways* (see e.g. Hertzman, Frank, Evans 1994; Eis 1998; Noack 1997). As determinants of health have *effects over long periods of time* the link between cause and effect is neither immediate nor direct (Hertzmann et al 1994; Eis 1998). Lately, a *'life course perspective'* is receiving increased attention in (social) epidemiology (see Kuh, Ben-Shlomo 1997; Blane 1999).

As Tavlov (1996) points out, the goal *to identify the specific contribution of each determinant* of health has been *elusive* for four main reasons: a) the high level of interaction among all health determinants; b) the lack of research on the interactions and effects among main categories of health determinants (from biological disposition and medical care to health-related behaviors and social characteristics); c) a lack of understanding of the *'sociobiological translation'*, and d) widespread insufficient measuring of the 'health' of populations by 'crude and late stage indicators' such as morbidity and mortality. Estimates of the *relative contribution of par-*

ticular categories of health determinants to gains in life expectancy, population health status or disease burden have been attempted and present a small set of incomparable information: *Genetic* inheritance may account for 5% or less of the total disease burden; *medical health care services* are estimated to have contributed about 17% to the gain in life expectancy in the twentieth century; health related *individual risk factors* accounted for between 25% and 40% to 60% of the gradient in health across social classes in the UK Whitehall Studies (Marmot 1991). Allocating a quantitative attribution to some of the many health determinants when both they all interact and the dimensions of their measurement differ is not feasible. But looking at the data generally and making *some rough assumptions* is possible and will help to review and further actions and interventions to promote health (Tavlov 1996 p75). For example:

- from a population perspective, *genetic factors* play a limited role; in most cases there is no simple connection between genetic inheritance and health effects (from a population perspective the exceptions are quantitatively not very important); (Baird 1994)

- *medical health care* is less important for achieving population health than many other factors (Evans, Barer, Marmor 1994: Blane, Brunner, Wilkinson 1996; Evans, Stoddart 1990, 1994; Marmot 1999); in addition,
    - the health care sector receives and consumes a too big proportion of the GNP in modern societies, often around 10%; it is possible "that the direct positive effects of health care on health may be outweighed by its negative effects through its competition of resources with other health-enhancing activities. *A society that spends so much on health care that it cannot or will not spend adequately on other health-enhancing activities may actually be reducing the health of its population*" (Evans, Stoddart 1994, p55 - italics as in original);

- it seems that the influence of behavioral and 'bio-medical' (biological) *risk factors for disease* (e.g. smoking, high blood pressure) is being overestimated and that - at least with view to the health of population groups and whole populations - other factors appear to be more important (Blane et al 1996; Wilkinson 1999, 1994; Marmot 1999; Marmot, Wilkinson 1999);

The role of the broad category of *'social' factors* as co-determinants of population health, also in comparison to behavioral factors, is underlined by many researchers from different perspectives and in various ways, for example:

- about half of the global burden of deaths remains unexplained by the major risk factors (malnutrition, poor water supply plus all other major risk factors (tobacco, alcohol, illicit drugs, unsafe sex, physical inactivity; hypertension; air pollution, occupational hazards;) (Murray, Lopez 1996); an increasing research base indicates that the rest is explained by 'social determinants of health' and that several of those risk factors themselves have social determinants (Marmot 1999);
- "a substantial fraction of the variation in health from one population to another, or among various strata within a single population, is unexplained by variations in genetic inheritance, medical care, and behavioral risk factors. The substantial unexplained portion probably is related to *social* characteristics" (Tavlov 1996 p75; also Berkmann, Kawachi 2000; Marmot, Wilkinson 1999; Mielck 2001)
  - recent literature reviews provide the basis for the argument that "*factors* in the social environment, *external to the health care system*, exert a major and potentially modifiable influence on the health of populations, through biological channels that are just now beginning to be understood" (Evans 1994a p23);
- whether genetic predispositions of an individual will be given expression depends on a broader range of determinants of health in the *physical and social environment* with which predispositions interact (Baird 1994);
- a *social gradient in health status* has been found (lower position on the social latter: poorer health - higher position: better health); the longitudinal Whitehall studies I and II (Marmot et al 1991, Marmot 1996; see also Syme 1994) show that there is *not only a social gradient in mortality rates and but also in the prevalence of health related behaviors and biological risk factors;* for example:
  - although the prevalence of smoking declined over the twenty years separating the two studies, the social gradient in smoking prevalence persisted, i.e. higher smoking rates in lower social grades; thus, the question is not what contributions smoking makes to generating the social gradient in ill health, but *why is there a social gradient* in smoking?
- among scientists representing the perspective on determinants of health of populations a consensus is emerging, that their are only two or three *major categories* of population health determinants; these relate to the *social and economic* environment (e.g. Blane, Brunner, Wilkinson 1996; Wilkinson 1996; Evans, Barer, Marmor 1994; Kawachi et al 1996; Tavlov 1996):

a) (absolute and relative) income/ income distribution;
   b) social cohesion/ social capital (or similar aspects of the social environment);
- with view to both 'developing' and 'developed' countries, Kawachi et al (1996) differentiate further and propose three categories of determinants of life expectancy which are postulated to be also key determinants of the health of populations, sub-populations and individuals:
   a) the *absolute level of income* (as a strong determinant in *poor countries*), which is crucial for providing prerequisites for health such as housing, food, clean water and sanitation, education and primary health care;
   b) the *distribution of income* (a strong determinant in *rich countries*), with relative income reflecting socio-economic inequality, inequity, and how people relate to each other socially;
   c) a comprehensive social factor referred to as *'social capital';*
   (Kawachi et al 1996, according to Noack 1997 p69)
- Current research studies suggest that there is a *accumulation of advantages and disadvantages throughout the life course* that determines patterns of health and disease in later life (e.g. Marmot 1996; Blane, Brunner, Wilkinson 1996), a new social epidemiological research area just being tackled by some (e.g. Kuh, Ben-Shlomo 1997; Blane 1999).

Knowledge gaps and challenges identified by several researchers concern among other issues:

- the existence of coherent *patterns of particular determinants* in a 'healthy life' (Noack 1997; Hertzmann, Frank, Evans 1994) ;
- specific *causal pathways* of health determinants (Noack 1997; Hertzmann, Frank, Evans 1994);
- the fact that much of research and policy to improve and maintain health has for long focused on *biological or individual behavioral determinants* of health or disease (Marmot 1996, p63); these areas of health determinants are *over-researched* while some of the 'important' health determinants, particularly *more complex concepts* such as 'social capital' and 'lifestyles' *still need to be further clarified and defined* (Noack 1997; Marmot 1996, p63);
- the *reasons of the social gradient* in health status and premature mortality (Marmot 1996; Wilkinson 1999).

Increasing attention is being given to **the "socio-biological translation"**, the *pathways or mechanisms between social determinants and the human biology,* as it is the body in which sooner or later health is maintained or disease is manifested, but this research is still in its infancy:

- the mechanisms by which social characteristic are received or perceived by human beings, processed into biological signals, and converted into disease or good health are far from easy to understand or being subject to clear and rigorous testing; (Tavlov 1996; Evans, Hodge, Pless 1994; Evans 1994 p.xiii; Baird 1994;)
- but "there *is* a chain that runs from the behavior of cells and moleculars, to the health of populations, and back again, a chain in which the past and present social environments of individuals, and their perceptions of those environments, constitute a key set of links. No one would pretend that the chain is fully understood, or is likely to be for a considerable time to come. But research evidence currently available no longer permits anyone to deny its existence" (Evans, Hodge, Pless 1994, p184).

Methodological problems exist in both qualitative and quantitative research related to the determinants of health (Noack 1997). This has been illustrated in various ways, for example, as follows:

- the human being is more than an accumulation of cells, the whole is more than the sum of its part that can be described by natural sciences; accordingly, it is *not nearly possible to describe the interrelationship between the environment and the health or disease of human beings through* the quantification of single agent-effect-correlations nor through the amount of all exposition-effect-relations identified by environmental toxicology; (Eis 1998)
- *the interactions of health determinants* can be compared with a set of balls all of which are in motion most of the time and having wide spheres of simultaneous influence, so that the net direction and force of the final movement have multi-factorial contributing influences of varying affinity; thus, methodologies such as multivariate analyses including regression methodologies are inadequate for deriving meaningful information for policy and program development directed at improving and sustaining health; (Tavlov 1996, p83)

Accordingly, more complex 'human-ecological' *analyses of connections* in comparison to the research on specific health determinants by single disciplines are needed (Eis 1998). A more imaginative application of qualitative approaches and methods is needed to develop and test new indicators of health determinants; and new statistical modeling techniques are to be applied to quantitatively test theoretical frameworks and indicators (Noack 1997, p70).

In light of the vast 'labyrinth' of particular findings of health relevant population studies researchers repeatedly stressed **the need for a theoretical or conceptual framework.** Several ideas have been put forward. For example, Noack (1997) urgently calls for a theoretical framework *of salutogenesis* that integrates the current knowledge on the major determinants of health, from economic and social to behavioral and psychological factors. The solely pathogenic and risk management perspective within much of Public Health research needs to be overcome and a salutogenic perspective developed (Eis 1998). Others give less emphasis to the salutogenic perspective and, for example, call for a conceptual framework or *model for investigation of heterogeneities in population health status* (Hertzmann, Frank, Evans 1994). Some researchers are critical towards the idea of developing one causal meta-theory of health development in populations: Indeed, a recent international workshop (by HEA London, CDC Atlanta and WHO Geneva) with leading social scientists and social epidemiologists on 'Theory and Action for Health' called for better 'theories of action' to guide practice, and for the creation of an overview explaining *which theories are suited best for which purposes* (London, 27-29 March 1999).

With view to **developing models on determinants of health**, Evans and Stoddart (1990, p.1348) stress the importance of distinguishing between the range of particular definitions or *concepts of health* and the range of *factors that might determine its level*, whatever the definition; different concepts of health 'are neither right nor wrong, they simply have different purposes and fields of application'. **Quality criteria** for models on health determinants have been proposed: Models should be *sufficiently comprehensive and flexible* to represent a wide range of relationships among the determinants of health. Evans and Stoddart (1990, 1994) suggest a model may be assessed as valuable and acceptable if it: a) provides *meaningful categories* in which to insert the various sorts of scientific evidence on the range of health determinants and, thus, be a good framework for further assembling such evidence (not only that from population studies but also from studies focusing on individuals; see e.g. Noack 1997, pp.64-70); b) if it allows a *definition of health that is broad enough* to encompass the dimensions that people (from health professionals to decision makers and ordinary individuals) feel to be important (see e.g. overview by Noack 1997, pp.59-63). In the light of weaknesses of current models, additional qualities have been called for such as: the *sufficient illustration of the interaction* of various factors and feed back processes ('logic models') (e.g. Eis 1998; 'WHO Ad Hoc Technical Expert Committee' held by WHO/HPR Department, Geneva, Sept.1999); and the *consideration and illustration of processes over time* (interactive and cumulative as well as adaptation processes, periods of latency), biographic dimensions (of the maintenance, creation or loss of health), as well as the 'event character' of the whole causes-effect-process (Eis 1998; Kuh, Ben-Shlomo 1997).

Social determinants versus behavioral determinants ?

Now, that a general picture of the knowledge base and remaining challenges in the area of co-determinants of *population* health has been presented it is clear: According to current knowledge there are two important, for long underestimated or neglected sets of co-determinants of population health: (absolute and relative) income and income distribution; and social cohesion, social capital, and/or similar factors. This **calls for structural or social change interventions** rather individual behavior change interventions to improve or maintain the health of populations (see e.g. Syme 1994). Another important finding is that there *are direct* pathways between social determinants and the human biology in which health manifests itself (although not yet well understood). Thus, **individual (health/ risk) behavior is a) not the only pathway and b) less important than assumed before** - an important point in the context of school related health promotion addressed by the network cases examined later. This underpins earlier calls from social scientists (such as social support researchers) for a shift in attention in public health and health promotion research and practice - away from 'health (risk) behaviors' of individuals as major determinants of health towards social or socio-structural factors. This means a significant change in focus in (public) health research and practice which (at least in the Western world) over decades presented and treated individual behaviors (particularly eating patterns, physical activity, drug use or not, etc.) either as major *causes* of health and (non-communicable) disease or at least the major *pathway* through which (social) environmental conditions influence health; (with the exception of physical environmental factors such as chemical agents). This has stirred for long most efforts to promote health into behavior change interventions, in the area of school health and beyond. However, **the latest knowledge on co-determinants of population health does not mean that health relevant behaviors - or better behavioral patterns and lifestyles - are irrelevant co-determinants of health, but they are clearly *less* relevant if one looks at the full range of factors influencing or co-determining health** that are known today. A landmark study on this issue is the Whitehall study by Marmot (1996) and colleagues which indicates their relative importance:

This study did measure a range of risk factors for cardio-vascular diseases (CVD) and also other diseases: besides biological factors such as blood pressure and height, the health relevant behaviors smoking, physical inactivity, and eating behaviors (indirectly measured via plasma cholesterol and body mass index). It was found that *a combination of all* the individual biological and behavioral *risk factors accounted only for 25 % of the social gradient* in (premature) mortality. Even when allowing for imprecision in the measurements *at least 50%* of the social gradient had to be due to factors other than the risk factors. The **50-75% of the social gradient in CVD mortality *not explained* through the measured risk factors such as smoking, physical activity and eating behaviors can presumably be explained by social and community influences and living and working conditions**. The latter exert a strong influence on biology. If they do not operate through the risk factors mentioned "there must be other *biological pathways*" through which these social determinant of health act. "The links between social and biological pathways that underlie a social patterning" of disease and health, the social gradient in health status, need still to be traced (Marmot 1996, p64). Several intervention studies such as the famous MRFIT (Syme 1996) besides the two Whitehall studies do show: As well as being difficult to change, **health related or risky behaviors seem to have less effect on health than predicted.** In the context of discussing the difficulties of using behavior change as an approach to population health, Rose (1981) calculated that the advantages to the individual of various forms of behavioral change were very small. E.g. in the Framingham study, from all those men who would modify their diets enough to reduce their cholesterol levels by 10 % up to the age of 55, 98 % would have eaten differently over 40 years without having avoided a heart attack by doing so.

If the *gains to individuals* from preventive efforts through behavior change are so small even among the most important causes of death, they are likely to be even smaller in relation to the prevention of less common causes. (Blane, Brunner, Wilkinson 1996 p6) - a strong argument for a more comprehensive approach to health promotion.

A look at the *determinants* of health relevant *behavior* and action shows that not only from a population health and overall co-determinants of health perspective but also an individual behavior change perspective social factors must receive more attention. From this angle, the general picture of 'social factors' is one of an unassembled jigsaw puzzle. As the goal of this chapter is to draw a *general picture* of co-determinants of health as before no factor is explained in detail nor is the goal to present a complete list of factors. However, according to current knowledge the general picture of the co-determinants of health would be insufficient if the category of 'behavioral' or 'lifestyle related' determinants of health would be ignored. Therefore, and as this body of knowledge has still strong influence on the field of Health Promotion and particularly school health promotion (the focus of the network cases studied in this research project), some research results will be presented. The selection made a) focuses on the *determinants* of *all* types of health relevant behavior or action and b) emphasizes that in the overall co-determinants of health picture such behaviors are factors concerning the person/environment interface (i.e. relate to *both* intrapersonal and environmental factors).

Co-determinants of health relevant behavior and action

Most conceptual and theoretical models or approaches to explain or predict health relevant behaviors or actions of individuals focus narrowly on the intrapersonal factors or 'psychological dispositions' and usually widely ignore the context in which the individual behavior or action examined takes place(see reviews by e.g. Faltermaier 1994; Schwarzer 1992, 1990; and Schwenkmetzger and Schmidt; Lohaus; and von Troschke, all 1993). A few *more advanced or comprehensive models consider both the intrapersonal and environmental dimensions of human action*. Among the most prominent examples also in the field of health promotion are the 'social-cognitive process model of health relevant action' developed by Schwarzer (1992, 1992) and the model of 'predisposing, enabling and reinforcing factors that influence health' by Green and Kreuter (1991, 1999) which both show the importance of the social environment for health supportive behaviors to occur. Most importantly, and complementary to the population health research results presented before, they show how important it is to consider the specific and daily life situation of individuals or groups of individuals.

Schwarzer identifies several intrapersonal cognitive factors which together with the subjective perception of the current situation (e.g. levels of social support) determine the volitional process. The latter together with objective barriers and resources in that current situation in turn co-determine an individual's action. This 'model of health relevant action' shows that **the social environment and also the physical environment play an important role in determining health relevant actions an individual is undertaking or refraining from in a daily life situation.** This applies not only to 'health risk behavior' but also to all actions (e.g. the participation or not of an individual in a health oriented school or community change program). In addition, social environmental factors *indirectly* influence health relevant actions of individuals; they *influence the development of important cognitions* through their influence on life experiences made by the individual *throughout its biography*. This and similar research have contributed to the today widespread awareness about the **importance of the overall daily life situation** a person needs to cope with through day-to-day behavior or action and that **in daily life the health motive is only one if any important factor to guide actions** - which obviously has consequences for interventions to promote health. These findings mirror and confirm the often quoted statement in the Ottawa Charter (1986): health is created or lost in people's every day life, where they live, love, work and play. (Schwarzer 1992; Broesskamp 1994; BMBF 1997) With view to the *various* models prevalent in health psychology Dlugosch (1994) identified three groups of determinants of health relevant behavior and health: a range of social *'environmental determinants'* (such as societal, political and cultural ones, as well as health promotion interventions and cues to action provided by the social environment); *'personal factors'* (i.e. individual characteristics relative *stabile* over time (socio-demographic, social-psychological, intra-personal variables or characteristics, learning history) as well as *situation specific* characteristics (such as emotional status)); and 'genetic dispositions'.

Green and Kreuter (1991) address behavior not only of individuals or groups of individuals but also organizations. They focus on **factors that influence 'individual and collective behavior, including organizational actions** in relation to the environment'. Each of the three 'categories' of factors identified has a different type of influence on behavior: The first category is *'predisposing factors'* that provide the rationale or motivation for the behavior, i.e. a range of cognitive factors (such as those explained in their interplay in Schwarzer's model; e.g. knowledge, values, perceived needs, self-confidence etc.). The second group is *'enabling factors'* that enable a motivation to be realized, which often refer to living or environmental conditions that facilitate or hinder the performance of an action. Reference is made to a vast array of resources and 'new' skills needed to perform a health supportive action and the organizational actions to modify the environment (e.g. availability and accessibility of community facilities, laws and regulations, priorities set at community or national level; and 'new' skills such as coalition building to achieve environmental changes in support of health). The third category is the *'reinforcing factors'* that subsequent to a behavior provide the continuing reward or incentive for the behavior and contribute to its persistence or repetition (positive or negative feed back, social recognition and support by the social environment be it family or peers, teachers or employers, health providers or community leaders). With view to the **sustainability of behavior change** in support of health addressed here, Lohaus (1993) identifies three groups of factors to be tackled: a) factors at the *individual or personal level* (emotional, cognitive, motivational situation, current behavior repertoire); b) factors at the *supra-individual level* with *direct influence* on the individual (such as parents, peers, school, media, and other institutions); and c) factors at the *supra-individual level* with *indirect influence* on the individual (such as society, subcultures, religions, ideology, rules and norms).

Throughout, authors identify a range of social factors in the closer and wider environment of individuals besides the intra-personal co-determinants of health relevant behavior. The findings above show that any given health related behavior can be explained as a function of the *collective* influence of theses types of factors (*collective causation*), with each factor potentially affecting the influence of all others. Green and Kreuter conclude: **As behavior is a multifaceted phenomenon and no single behavior is caused by just one factor, any plan to influence behavior must consider all of the sets of causal factors.** Unfortunately, as of now there is a lack of integration of results of the behavioral sciences presented above and those from population health and similar research. (Health) sociology may play an important role here. Promising research results include those on issues of personal or collective *choice* and health development (which also underpins basic strategies and principles of Health Promotion; see chap. 2.2). For example, Millio (1990) has stressed that "behavioral patterns of populations are a result of habitual selection from limited *choices*, and these habits of choice are related to: a) actual and perceived *options available*; b) beliefs and expectations developed and refined over time by *socialization, formal learning, and immediate experience*" (p.171). **Organizational behavior, decisions or policy choices made by organizations and institutions at all levels of society, set the ranges of options available to individuals for their personal choice making - including health relevant behavioral choices.** Choice making of individuals regarding health relevant selections (such as behaviors) is affected by and related to the type and amount of a) their *personal* resources and b) *societal, community and national* resources (e.g. the availability of health sustaining services and resources such as food, housing, income maintenance, physical environment protection; also penalties or rewards given for the selection or neglect of e.g. certain behaviors). (Millio 1990) However, 'choice' is not equally available to all people and choices are themselves circumscribed by material conditions; choice occurs within and is influenced by the routines of everyday life (Bunton, Macdonald 1992, p55-58).

Within this overall picture of the co-determinants of health knowledge two related factors are often directly or indirectly referred to but at the same time not clearly placed: 'education' and 'schools' as social institutions. As networks for the development of Health Promoting *Schools* are the focus of this research project this needs a brief look. Afterwards the chapter will be brought to a conclusion.

Education, schools and the determinants of health perspective

As explained earlier, much health sociology suggests an understanding of health and disease as reaction to societal conditions, particularly in the areas of economics, ecology and *education* (Hurrelmann 2000). In the area of development cooperation and from a macro perspective on population health it is known since long that levels of education in populations are clearly an important factor of health development in countries, particularly with view to girls and women (e.g. World Bank 1993; World Health Report, WHO 1995; Kuh et al 1997). Already the Ottawa Charter (1986) listed education as one of eight "prerequisites for health" (see chap. 2.2). Much of the research on social determinants of health referred to in this chapter more or less indirectly support these findings, as educational status is among those indicators commonly used when measuring socio-economic status. Wilkinson and Marmot (1998 p13) conclude that education is associated with raised health awareness and improved self-care and, therefore, people should have opportunities for educational attainment at all ages. This supports the general 'life long learning' -orientation prevalent in education systems in many countries today. In 1995, the 'WHO Expert Committee on Comprehensive School Health Education and Health Promotion' estimated that schools (the basic building blocs of education systems) have the potential to do more than perhaps any other single institution to improve the well-being and competence of children and adolescents (WHO 1996b p1). It also found that research in both developing and developed countries demonstrates that school health programs can simultaneously reduce common health problems, increase the efficiency of the education system and advance public health, education, and social and economic development. That health, economic and social development (the latter including issues of education) in countries and regions is inseparately intertwined is, today, almost common sense.

Youth health researchers, too, have since long highlighted the links between school education and the health of school aged children and adolescents, however, from a different perspective: They show that for a variety of reasons going to school is potentially *both* a health *resource* and health *hazard* (see e.g. Hurrelmann 1993, 1991, 1990; Millstein 1993). This is easy to understand when recalling form chapter 2.1.2 the understanding of health as a 'state of balance between risk and protective factors which occurs if a person succeeds in coping with both the internal and external demands'. An interdisciplinary effort to identify **school specific co-determinants of health** to guide education reform in Germany found three broad categories of such determinants (Broesskamp 1994, pp29-53): school climate and school life *outside* the classroom teaching or lessons; health supportive *style and shape* of lessons or class room teaching in *general*; and *structural* conditions within schools (with factors 'directly' influencing health and 'indirectly' influencing health and health behaviors). While 'health risk' behaviors of pupils or children have been "over-researched" (Noack 1997, Marmot 1996) social determinants of health in the school context have received only little research attention. The concept of *'school climate'* has often been used to address the **social environment** within schools (Freitag 1998 pp29-37; Broesskamp 1994 pp29-36). But only few studies addressed the impact of schools and the school climate on the social behavior or personal development of pupils and, thus, potentially on psycho-social determinants of health, and even less of such studies address explicitly the links to pupils' health. An example of the letter stems from Freitag (1998) who examined the influence of school climate on the health of pupils and teachers.

Freitag identified *six 'main dimensions'* of school climate: *individual characteristics* of: 1) teachers as well as lessons (sex/gender, age, experience, commitment, self-esteem, teaching competence, etc.); and 2) pupils (sex/gender, age, social class, social competence, self-esteem, size and composition of class, etc.); 3) *characteristics of the school as an institution* (geographical location, size, organizational structure, the latter referring to curriculum, management style of the head of school, further training of teachers, involvement of parents, openness of the school towards its environment, etc.); the dimensions 4), 5) and 6) refer to *characteristics of the interaction and relation:* between pupil and teachers (discipline, familiarity with each other, style of discussion, etc.); among pupils (cohesion, competition, discipline, etc.); and among teachers (colleagueship, respect, cooperation). In spite of many solid findings **overall, the examination of school specific environmental determinants of health is still in its infancy**.

Intermediate synopsis and discussion - with examples of current models of social factors that 'co-determine' health

All of the above shows that it is very timely that Public Health research and practice gives more emphasis on the social co-determinants of health and that models of social determinants are much needed to better guide (health promotion) research and practice. Research lacks far behind practical responses to the vast but little integrated knowledge on co-determinants of health already experimented with since long (such as the Health Promotion concept, the health promoting Settings approach and the "Health Promoting Schools" concept therein).

It seems that the 'determinants of health' research of the 1990s presents the 'reemergence of the social' in Public Health, which for decades was dominated by foci on medical care systems and services and medical approaches to prevention on the base of the 'risk factor' model with regard to specific diseases - a context in which the studies on social factors and health (whether social support research, research on inequity and health, and social epidemiology as such) did not thrive. - **Two models of social determinants of health exemplify the richness of current knowledge and thinking. At the same time, they illustrate the remaining challenges** such as the understanding of the interplay of various dimensions, from macro-social to psycho-biological processes (fig. 2.1.4 and 2.1.5). The "social determinants of health" model by Brunner and Marmot (1999) links social structure to health and disease via *material, psychosocial and behavioral pathways*. Genetic, early life development and experiences, and cultural factors are included as 'further important influences on population health'. The 'conceptual models of how social networks impact health' by Berkmann and Glass (2000) emphasizes that the well known health relevant factor *'social support'* needs to be seen together with *other* psycho-social mechanisms and within higher systems levels, particular in relation to *social network structures and the larger social and cultural contexts* that shape these structures.

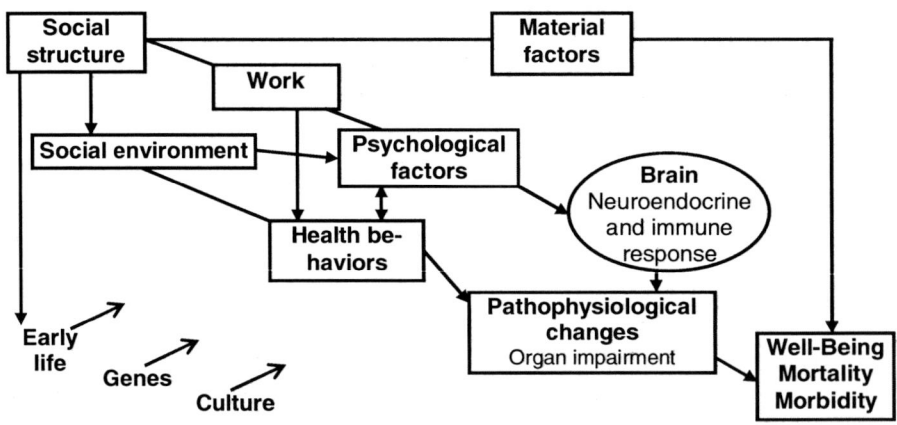

Figure 2.1.4: Social determinants of health (Brunner, Marmot 1999 p20)

The 'determinants of health' research from a population health perspective makes very explicit within Public Health research what has been shown before by work in health sociology (see e.g. Hurrelmann 2000): *individual health behavior is unlikely the only pathway through which social environments shape people's health*; there are direct links from the social environment to the biology. This is an important research result in the context of health promotion, as a tendency in the field persists to focus mainly on individual behaviors.

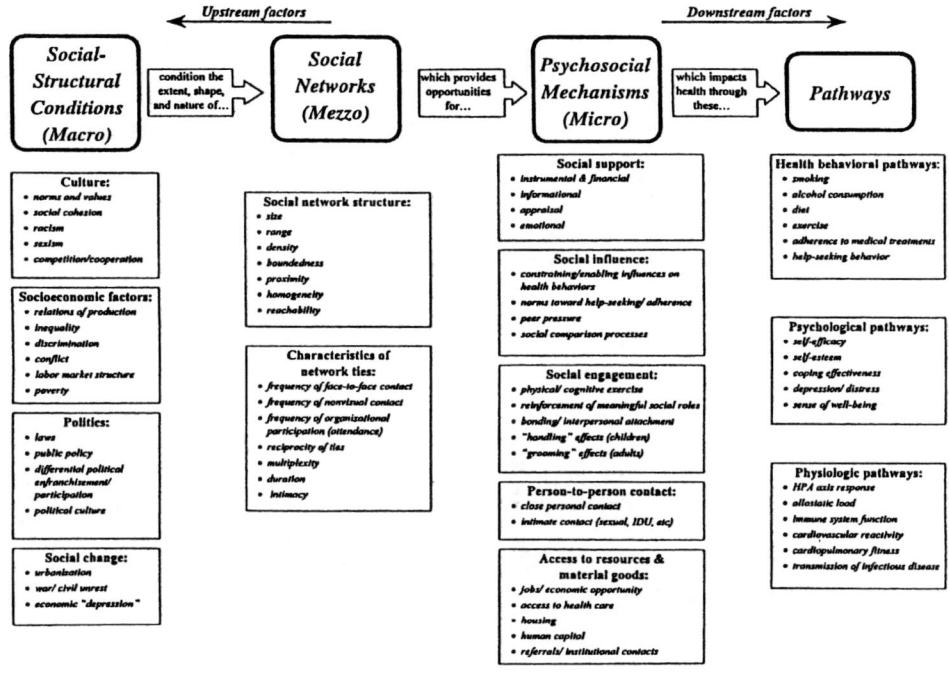

Figure 2.1.5: Conceptual models of how social networks impact health (Berkmann, Glass 2000 p143)

Social-epidemiological research has shown the powerful influences of the so called "broader determinants of health" which extend beyond the individual genetic and behavioral domains. This body of knowledge or evidence strongly supports the extension of the domains of traditional prevention efforts, a reorientation of public health and *recent developments in health promotion*. (Green, Poland, Rootman 2000) The latter is the focus of the next chapter 2.2.

Conceptual frameworks on health creation are needed to guide the 'social responses' to the current research knowledge, the focus of this chapter. They can **"organize the thousands of pieces into an orderly pattern** that is both intellectually acceptable to those who work at the frontier of change and sufficiently simple to permit a quick location, in the pattern, of any idea, problem or activity related to health" (McKay

2000 p11). The theoretical framework by Hurrelmann (2000) comes close to fulfilling this expectation, particularly if complemented by selected models of factors influencing health. The explanatory power of models of 'co-determinants of population health' may benefit from a systematic link to current population oriented theories in health sociology.

Marmot (1999) points to the **challenge** of 'unpicking' the social environment in a way that is susceptible to scientific inquiry *and* relevant to policy and practice. **"The more one attempts to unpick the environments in which people live and work and separate it into discrete analytical categories, the further we retreat from reality."** (p14) 'Social-ecological' theory or models of health have since long served as a kind of umbrella or integrating framework for attempts of *integrating knowledge* about health and its promotion, particularly where the focus is on community or local level. Due to their integrating character, and their guiding function when the Health Promotion concept was developed they are introduced now. This will also round up the picture painted in this chapter of the vast array of interrelated, predominantly social co-determinants of health.

2.1.4 The social ecological model (and systems perspective) on health

The Health Promotion concept as outlined in the Ottawa Charter rests on a social ecological model of health. The term *ecology* refers to the study of the relationships between organisms and their environment. *Human ecology* can be broadly defined as the interrelations between human beings or communities and their environments. The field of **social ecology** emphasizes more the *social, institutional and cultural contexts of people-environment relations* than did earlier versions of human ecology which focused primarily on biologic processes and geographic environments. (Stokols 1996a,b; Green, Richard, Potvin 1996). The *person-environment-interaction* has long been *at the core of human concepts of health and ill-health* and there development and maintenance, from traditional Chinese medicine and Hippocratic traditions (BC) to the social medicine of the 18th/19th century to today's social ecological model of health and ill-health (Noack 1987). Ecological schools of thought developed within a range of disciplines over time such as: human ecology and demography in sociology; social, community, environmental and health psychology; (social) learning theories and community health education in educational sciences; (social) epidemiology in public health; and human or medical geography (see Green et al 1996). The social ecological model of health is grounded in all these disciplines.

The social ecological paradigm is rooted in a set of **core principles, assumptions and themes** concerning the interrelations among environmental conditions and human behavior and health. With reference to respective studies and from a *community perspective* Stokols (1996) provides a summary:

- environmental *settings have multiple dimensions* (physical, social, cultural) that can *influence a variety of health outcomes* (e.g. physical health status, developmental maturation, emotional well-being, social cohesion); thus,
  - the health promoting capacity of such settings can be understood as the *cumulative impact* of multiple environmental conditions on the (physical, emotional, social) well-being of the people therein, over a specified time interval;
- human health is influenced both by environmental conditions and a variety of personal attributes (including genetic heritage, psychological disposition, behavioral patterns) - and this in a *dynamic interplay of environmental and personal factors*;
  - the *same* environmental conditions (e.g. change of residence, economic recession) may affect people's health *differently* - depending on their health resources or potentials (e.g. perceptions of environmental controllability, financial and intra-personal resources, health practices);
  - the level of congruence or compatibility *('fit')* between people and their environments is an important predictor of health and well being;
- to understand the dynamic relations between people and their environments, a variety of **systems theoretical concepts are incorporated into social ecology** (e.g. interdependence, homeostasis, negative feed-back);
  - people-environment relations are characterized by *cycles of mutual influence* (with features of settings influencing the people within, and concurrently, these people influence the health relevant features of the setting through individual and collective actions);
  - the health impacts of various roles and behavior patterns in organized settings are presumed to *vary* widely;
- *interdependency among environmental conditions* exists *within* a particular setting (e.g. physical and social ones) as well as *among* multiple settings and life domains (e.g. one's residence, neighborhood,

workplace, surrounding community);
- the multiple domains of human life are *nested structures* in which local settings and organizations are embedded within larger and more remote regions etc.; (therefore, efforts to promote people's health must take into account the interdependencies among immediate and more distant environments;)

- the social ecological perspective is *inherently interdisciplinary* with regard to both health *research* and the development of health promotion *programs*; this includes an integration of:
  - community wide and individual-level strategies;
  - attributing individuals and groups an *active* role in shaping their behaviors and environments;
  - multiple levels of analysis and diverse methodologies for assessing the healthfulness of settings and the health and well-being of persons and populations;

According to a systems perspective, *living systems* such as societies, social organizations and human beings form a *hierarchy of interdependent units* where the higher-level system is made up of lower-level subsystems. As documented by the research on co-determinants or resources for health and illustrated in figure 2.1.6, with regard to human health and disease it is useful to see individuals as parts of social units such as families and other primary social groups, which in turn may form subsystems of organizational or community systems, which are embedded into larger socio-cultural, economic, and political systems and again embedded into an even larger global societal and ecological system. Individuals on the other hand are made of smaller interacting sub-units such as cognitive, affective, circulatory or reproductive systems, each defined by its particular function in relation to the individual as a whole person. (Dahlgreen, Whitehead 1991; Noack 1987)

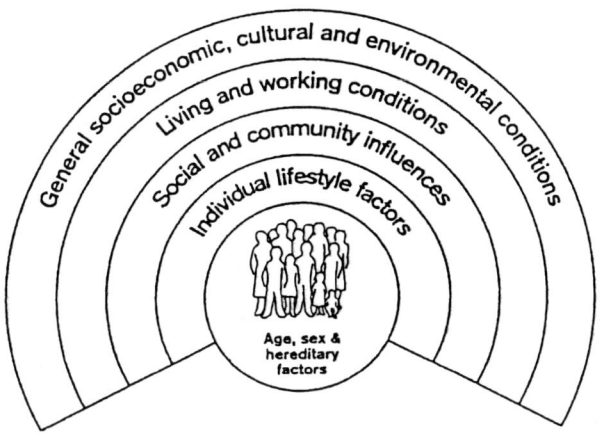

Figure 2.1.6: Factors influencing health. (Dahlgreen, Whitehead 1991)

Green, Richard and Potvin (1996) highlight *the inherent systems perspective* of the social ecological perspective on health and disease development this way: The **social ecological model of health** presents health as a product of the interdependence between the individual and subsystems of the ecosystem. - In general it can be said, the social ecological understanding of health is often referred to and widely accepted in the field of health promotion, particularly among those that focus on community level health promotion. This has specific implications for practice which will be addressed in the next chapter 2.2. The definition of health proposed by Hurrelmann (2000) reflects the social ecological model of health. In contrast to the description of health presented by Green, Richard and Potvin (1996) above, this definition highlights the active role individuals play in the creation of health: health occurs if a person *succeeds in coping* with internal and external demands. On the other hand, Green et al's definition highlights better the fact that factors at various systems levels are involved in health development, a fact that is crucial for the design of interventions.

2.1.5 Synopsis and discussion

Three overlapping and **complementary bodies of knowledge** have been presented: 1) a conceptual framework for an integrative theory of health and disease proposed by Hurrelmann (2000) that builds on the social science theories that address the health of individuals or populations; 2) lessons from modern social-epidemiology, from the new field of 'determinants of health' research with its 'population health' focus, as well as related research results; and 3) a brief outline of the social ecological perspective on health creation whose proponents often have a community perspective.

Hurrelmann offers a likely interdisciplinary acceptable and elaborate definition of health that is compatible with and may be able to guide work on the other bodies of knowledge. His theoretical frame builds on the understanding of internal and external factors that influence health. The 'population health' research highlights the need to distinguish between a focus on populations and on individuals in public health research, policy and practice. It suggests that, at least from a population perspective, there may be some co-determinants of health more important than others if health is to be maintained or improved; and it directs attention to macro level interventions that address these societal factors. The social ecological model of health appears as a more general umbrella concept of health supported by the other research results presented. It particularly highlights the importance of implementing a systems theoretical view when explaining health development. Work done under the umbrella of this model highlights important issues of health creation at community level.

All three bodies of knowledge fit with the concept of salutogenesis that is guiding the field of Health Promotion (see chap. 2.1.1), i.e. with the perspective that all people are constantly swimming in the rivers of life (and thus constantly interacting with their environment) and that the core question is how dangerous *particular* rivers are (i.e. particular living conditions at certain periods of time) and how well people can swim (i.e. can cope with their particular living conditions) during various phases in life.

The current state of research supports those approaches to health creation, maintaining or promotion that follow a systems and life course perspective and that avoid isolated actions on one or a few of the full range of factors that influence health. Today it is well understood that, for example, a focus on individual behavior change actions in support of health without considering both - the wider social context in which these behaviors occur *and,* as Hurrelmann stresses, the particular importance of that behavior as a means to cope with the daily (internal and external) demands - will not only be ineffective in most cases but bears the risk to be counterproductive. It is also well understood that there are health relevant factors that influence the social and physical environments at local level but are beyond the reach of any single community or organization such as a school and, thus, call for actions at country, inter-country and even global levels. - However, falling from a narrow individual behavior change focus into another extreme of solely focusing on most prominent social factors needs to be avoided. Corin (1994), for example, warns against an overemphasis on the today much attention receiving 'socio-economic status' as: a) this factor is only one of many social determinants of health, and b) such a narrow focus may hinder to focus on the full breadths of possible strategies to act in support of health development, and promotes an essentially passive picture of deprived people and communities for whom professionals have to act. The latter holds particularly if findings of Marmot et al (1991) regarding the social gradient in health are ignored that holds all the way up the social ladder.

In spite of remaining knowledge gaps, overall, it can be concluded that the challenge, today, is to move on from the stage of 'knowing about' to appropriate 'acting upon' this knowledge. This is the focus of the next chapter.

In spite of remaining knowledge gaps, overall, it can be concluded that the challenge, today, is to move on from the stage of 'knowing about' to appropriate 'acting upon' this knowledge. This is the focus of the next chapter.

2.2 Health Promotion - an organized social response to the knowledge of factors that influence or co-determine health

To assess a Health Promotion initiative one has to understand what "Health Promotion" is. From an *international* perspective it is apparent that the term 'health promotion' is still used in various ways. Therefore, this chapter focuses on the predominant, scientifically (and often also politically) supported understanding of health promotion.

2.2.1 Introduction - social ecological approaches to the promotion of health

In the field of public health, already in the 1980s large-scale risks to population health associated with physical as well as social and cultural environmental factors led to the reconsideration of the interdependence between human beings, their health, and their physical and social environments (Kickbusch 1989). The social ecological paradigm on health became widely recognized as a suitable framework not only for explaining the conditions and causes of health and ill health but also for guiding health-related activities as well as health and social policy (Noack 1987). Up to day, this is supported by and reflected in the work of many researchers and other experts in health promotion (see Hurrelmann 2000; Green, Poland, Rootman 2000; Green, Richard, Potvin 1996; Richard et al 1996; Stokols 1996a,b; Noack 1997; Dahlgreen, Whitehead 1991; Broesskamp 1994; WHO 1997; to name but a few). This chapter 2.2 addresses the currently main application of the social ecological (systems) perspective on the development and maintenance of people's health, the implementation of the "Health Promotion" concept. This is the guiding concept of international networks on Health Promoting Schools and other settings worldwide.

Health Promotion requires and (as shown in chapter 2.1) already rests in good part, on a solid scientific knowledge base. This builds on the truly interdisciplinary study of two areas: on the one hand, the range of *factors that influence or "co-determine" health* (that of populations or individuals), and its distribution (see above); on the other hand, the *organized social response* to these factors (Kickbusch 1997b p173; 1996), i.e. the most adequate social responses or organized efforts of communities and societies. **Maintaining and improving the health of populations requires that not only individuals but also communities and societies as a whole act on a range of interrelated factors that influence health and which are modifiable.** As will be shown, 'Health Promotion' represents the main organized social response of modern Public Health to this knowledge. Already the Ottawa Charter for Health Promotion (1986) identified *'essential prerequisites'* for health: food, shelter, peace, income, stable ecosystem, sustainable resource use, social justice, and equity (WHO 1986). Subsequent research has confirmed their relevance and importance.

Responding to the social ecological model of health

It is obvious that a response to the social ecological model of health presented in the previous chapter will not be simple but complex. Green, Richard and Potvin (1996) express this in systems theoretic terms: Health Promotion builds on the social ecological model of health (as a product of the *interdependence between individual and subsystems* such as family, community, culture, social and physical environment [see chap. 2.1.2 above]). To promote health *this ecosystem must offer social and economic conditions conducive to health and health supportive lifestyles* (including information, goods, services and opportunities to develop basic life skills so that individuals can make 'healthy choices', i.e. decisions for actions or behaviors that maintain their health); these aspects are often referred to as 'determinants of health' which also provide essential support in helping individuals modify their health relevant behaviors and reduce their exposure to risk factors.

Health Promotion Orientation	Key Determinants of health and Illness	Focus of Health Promotive Interventions	Types of Interventions Emphasized
Behavioral Change or Lifestyle Modification	Individual health behavior	Modify person's health-related attitudes, beliefs, and behavior	Active interventions (require voluntary and sustained effort by target individuals)
Environmental Enhancement and Restructuring	Quality of people's physical and social environments	Improve environmental hygiene/ safety and strengthen social supports for health	Passive interventions (require no effort by individuals exposed to them)
Social Ecological Approach	*Degree of fit* between people's biological, behavioral, and sociocultural *needs* and the environmental *resources* available to them	*Integrate* behavioral and environmentally based health promotion strategies (within a broad systems theoretical framework)	*Combination of active and passive* interventions (spanning individual, organizational, and community *levels*)

Table 2.2.1: Behavioral change, environmental enhancement, and social ecological approaches to health promotion: key emphases and differences (Stokols 1996b p287, italics not in original)

Stokols (1996b) translates the social ecological model of health into practice at community level. He distinguishes 'social ecological approaches to promote health' from 'behavioral change or lifestyle modification' and 'environmental enhancement or restructuring' approaches as shown in the self-explanatory table 2.2.1. Three **features of 'social ecological approaches to promote health'** are presented in that table, i.e. the focus on a) the *degree of fit* between people's needs and the environmental resources available to them; b) the *integration* of behavioral and environmentally based strategies within a broad *systems* theoretical framework; and c) the *combination* of active and passive interventions (spanning individual, organizational and community levels). In addition, Stokols identifies *three other* features of such approaches: d) the involvement of cross-level analyses of both health issues and related intervention strategies, e) the *implicit assumption* that regulatory (organizational and public policy) strategies and non-regulatory strategies (e.g. counseling, education) work best when they reinforce each other, and f) their 'giving rise' to broad-based social movements and *secular trends* that support public health interventions.

The inherent *strengths and limitations* of such social ecological approaches to health promotion will be discussed later. First, **a major application** of this perspective, the so called **"Health Promotion"** concept will be presented which is the *reference concept for international networks* for the development of Health Promoting Schools. After a brief look at the context in which this concept has been developed and applied its key features and approaches will be identified.

Health promotion development in context

> Box 2.2.1: Health Promotion concept development, dissemination and implementation in context - confluent forces, since the 1960s/ 1970s
> - growing emphasis on *'positive' health and improved quality of life* to overcome the widespread 'negative' definition of health as 'absence of disease';
> - recognition of the *'holistic' nature of health*, with renewed awareness of the social, mental and spiritual qualities of life
> - individuals' and communities' *desire to exercise control over their lives* (to get directly involved and actively participate…);
> - *community development and communications movements* that promoted grassroots, in contrast to top-down approaches, initiatives;
> - *self-care/self-help, women's (health), civil rights and consumer movements* in some regions that required a shift in the distribution of power from "experts" to individuals and communities;
> - recognition of the *living conditions and its social dimensions as factors that influence or "co-determine" health*, and that many health problems are related to individual *lifestyles* and that these lifestyles do not occur in a vacuum but themselves have powerful socioeconomic and cultural "co-determinants";
> - limited effectiveness of *'traditional' didactic (health) education strategies*, - together with re-orientations in prevention from individual centered to population centered approaches and from negative ("you should not…") messages to positive notions of well-being and quality of life;
> - evidence that *increased investment in medical 'health' care/ disease care* has produced *decreasing marginal returns*, as measured by improvements in health status;
> - pressure imposed on social programs and (high tech) medical care by *deteriorating economic and environmental conditions* around the world, - and public debates of an unacceptable 'explosion' of health care costs in many developed countries;
>
> *Sources: Green, Poland, Rootman 2000 p3; Broesskamp-Stone, Kickbusch, Walter 1998 p144; Kaba-Schoenstein 1996 II; Green, Raeburn 1988;*

The idea of health promotion is not new. But particularly in the 1980s, health promotion has attracted growing attention, broadened in scope and been subjected to a variety of interpretations ('Working Group on health promotion in developing countries' - WHO 1990). In the early 1980s, in a climate characterized by confluent forces (box 2.2.1), the WHO Regional Office for Europe (WHO/EURO) actively searched for new approaches to maintain and promote the health of populations to reach **'Health for All' by the year 2000**, i.e. "the attainment by all citizens of the world (…) of a level of health that will permit them to lead a socially and economically productive life' (WHA 1977). A main result of this process, the **Ottawa Charter for Health Promotion**, was adopted at the 1st International Conference on Health Promotion, Canada, 1986 (WHO 1986).

The Ottawa Charter was disseminated around the world at a remarkable pace and played a key role in the 'broadening of the scope' of health promotion. Health Promotion as outlined in this Charter was taken up quickly by a range of governmental, public, non-governmental, civil society and academic actors and organizations as the guiding framework for promoting health (Kaba-Schoenstein 1996, III) - first in Europe and 'Western' or 'developed' countries, then also in 'developing' countries world wide (see table 2.2.2). The acceptance and application of this Health Promotion concept as **the guiding framework for action** resulted from the confluence of the disparate forces and developments summarized in Box 2.2.2. These characterize *the overall context* in which international networks for the development of Health Promoting Schools have been first initiated and developed.

From a global perspective, a series of events and developments can be identified as **milestones** in development, dissemination and acceptance of the Ottawa Charter and of Health Promotion as an organized, distinct field in Public Health. Table 2.2.2 provides a short overview in this regard.

	Global development - Health policy areas	Development of 'Health Promotion'	Regional Development - Health Policy areas
1977	World Health Assembly (WHA): 'Health for All by the year 2000', adopted '79		
1978	Declaration of Alma Ata (WHO/UNICEF): Primary Health Care concept to implement 'Health for All'		
1980		WHO/EURO: New HP Program	WHO/EURO: HfA policy
1984		WHO/EURO HfA discussion document: Health Promotion concept and principles in action - a policy framework	WHO/EURO: 38 Targets for Health 2000
1986		1. Int. Conference of Health Promotion: Ottawa Charter for Health Promotion	
1988		2. Int. Conference of Health Promotion: Adelaide Recommendations on Healthy Public Policy	
1989	WHA Resolution on Health Promotion, Public Information & Education for Health	WHO Working Group: Promoting health in developing countries	
1991		3. Int. Conference of Health Promotion: Sundsvall Statement on Supportive Environments for Health	
1994		WHO/Headquarters: New HP Division	
1995	HfA Renewal process		WHO/WPRO: 'New Horizons in Health'
1997		4. Int. Conference of Health Promotion: Jakarta Declaration on Leading Health Promotion into the 21st Century	
1998	WHA: Resolution 51.12 on Health Promotion		
2000		5. Global Conference on Health Promotion: Bridging the Equity Gap (87 Health Ministers sign 'Mexico Ministerial Statement for the Promotion of Health')	

Table 2.2.2: Milestones in the development of Health Promotion as an organized, distinct field in health policy and practice from a global perspective. (HfA: Health for All; WHA: World Health Assembly)

Throughout this development, not only *health promotion* but also the field of *public health* as a whole changed. Baric (1996 p43) summarizes the change in thinking as follows: In the past, political, economic and social environments were taken as given and the health care system was supposed to enable people to lead as 'healthy' a life as possible under the circumstances (concept of 'optimal' health). The aim was to adjust people to the system and optimize their utilization of existing possibilities. *A 'new' approach looks at the system, including the environment as well as the people*, and acknowledges that *both the environment and the individuals need to undergo change* in order to create both desirable living conditions and possibilities of deriving the best advantage from them. - The term 'new approach' may mainly refer to economically developed countries of the western world as in other cultures and many developing countries holistic understandings of health and healing remain and western concepts of medicine may not yet dominate all of society. - Today, **Health Promotion is accepted as a main pillar of modern Public Health**.

After this brief outline of the recent origins and development context of health promotion, the *understanding* of health promotion will be further clarified, to continue to lay the ground for the assessment of networks such as those for the development of Health Promoting Schools.

2.2.2 Health Promotion - definitions and key features

Table 2.2.3 presents a variety of **definitions** proposed for health promotion based on a recent review undertaken by Rootman, Goodstadt, Potvin and Springett (1997). They found three components that health promotion definitions may exhibit: the declaration of Health Promotion *activities* (programs, policies, etc.) and/or *processes* (underlying mechanisms) and/or *objectives* (instrumental outcomes). Without going into details of analysis it is worth mentioning that since the 1980s the objectives are usually expressed in terms of health influencing factors or 'determinants of health', often explicitly listed (at least indicating both behavioral and environmental factors, often even listing the full range of factors known today). (see also chap. 2.1) The work around the development of the Ottawa Charter for Health Promotion and of the WHO have led to a specification or explicit mentioning of *processes* of health promotion action within definitions. The definitions mirror the general consensus within the field of Public Health and health promotion that a *range* of activities need to be combined to reach health improvements (see e.g. Jakarta Declaration 1997).

The definition of Health Promotion as ratified in the Ottawa Charter (1986) has passed the test of time:

"Health Promotion is the process of enabling people to increase control over, and to improve their health" (Ottawa Charter - WHO 1986).

A thoughtful review of recent definitions of HP and current HP practice undertaken by the WHO/EURO 'International Working Group on Evaluating Health Promotion' has shown that *this definition has a pre-eminence in the field that is not likely to disappear* in the foreseeable future. Therefore, for further work towards a common understanding of terms such as evaluation, evidence, impact, effectiveness and so forth, *the above Working Group uses, and recommends to others to use, this definition or its derivatives* as the starting point. (Ziglio 1996) This research project follows this recommendation and will use a slightly advanced version of the definition of Health Promotion provided in the Ottawa Charter:

Health Promotion is the process of enabling individuals and communities to increase control over the factors that jointly influence health, and thereby improve their health. (adapted from Nutbeam 1986 and WHO 1998a)

Source and date	Activities (programmes, polices, etc.)	Processes (underlying mechanisms)	Objectives (instrumental outcomes)	Goals (ultimate outcomes)
Winslow, 1920 (2)	"Organized community effort for the education of the individual in personal health, and the development of the social machinery"		"... to ensure everyone a standard of living"	"... the maintenance or improvement of health"
Sigerist, 1946 (1)			"... by providing a decent standard of living, good labor conditions, education, physical culture, means of rest and recreation"	"Health is promoted"
Lalonde. 1974 (3)	"... informing, influencing and assisting both individuals and organizations"	"... so that they (individuals and organizations] will accept more responsibility and be more active in matters affecting mental and physical health"		
US Department of Health, 1979 (19): "A combination of health education and Education, and Welfare,	related organizational, political and economic programs"		"...designed to support (changes in behaviour and in the environment"	that will improve health"

Source and date	Activities (programmes, polices, etc.)	Processes (underlying mechanisms)	Objectives (instrumental outcomes)	Goals (ultimate outcomes)
Green, 1980 (20)	"Any combination of health education and related organizational, political and economic interventions"		"... designed to facilitate behavioral and environmental changes"	"... that will improve health"
Green & Iverson, 1982 (21	"Any combination of health education and related organizational, political and economic supports		„...for behavior"	conducive to health"
Perry & Jessor, 1985 (22)	„The implementation of efforts"			"... to taster improved health and well-being in all tour domains of health (physical. social. psychological and personal)"
Nutbeam, 1985 (23)		"The process of enabling people to increase control"	"... over the determinants of health"	"… and thereby improve their health"
WHO, 1984 (24), 1986 (4) Epp, 1986 (25)		"The process of enabling people to increase control over (their health)"		pie to increase control" health" health"
Goodstadt et al., 1987 (26	"... through the implementation of effective programs, services, and policies"			"The maintenance and enhancement of existing levels of health"
Kar, 1989 (27)			"... and the avoidance of health risks by achieving optimal levels of the behavioural, societal, environmental, and biomedical determinants of health"	"The advancement of well-being"
O'Donnell, 1989 (28)	"The science and art of helping people choose their lifestyles"			"... to move toward a state of optimal health"
Green & Kreuter, 1991 (7)	"The combination of educational and environmental supports for actions and conditions of living"			"...conducive to health"

Table 2.2.3: Health Promotion definitions deconstructed (adapted from Rootman, Goodstadt, Potvin and Springett 1997 in Green et al 2000 pp5-6)

Defining Health Promotion - intermediate synthesis and discussion

This definition adapted from the WHO definition and the one first introduced by Don Nutbeam in 1986, has several *advantages*: *First*, it distinguishes between individuals and communities and, thus, points to different levels of complexity that Health Promotion practitioners and researchers may face when working with 'people'. The work with communities, i.e. social systems, represents a higher level of complexity than the work with an individual in support of that person's health. *Second*, it makes explicit reference to the vast body of research knowledge on factors that influence (or "co-determine") health while maintaining the original core message regarding the process by which Health Promotion will achieve its objectives: by 'enabling' (or empowering) people. The definition shows clearly that **Health Promotion was conceptualized as and remains to be a social response to the current state of research knowledge on the range of factors that influence of "co-determine" health** as outlined in chapter 2.1. As Green, Poland, Rootman (2000 p7) phrase it, this definition explicitly refers to a *"causal" mechanism or process* of Health Promotion, namely *"increas(ing) control over the determinants of health"*. - As discussed in chapter 2.1.3 today there is both much use and criticism of the term 'determinants of health' and in this research project the terminology used will be either the 'factors that influence health' or 'that *co*-determine health'. The syllable "co-" should remind the reader that health is never 'determined' in the sense of classical physics and that it is not possible to pick out just one or a few 'key determinants of health', adjust them for all people, and their health will follow.

The Health Promotion definition above also captures the *common ground* among conceptualizations of health promotion, which Green et al (2000 p7) recently summarized as follows:

"Health promotion involves a diverse set of actions, focused on individuals and their environments, which increases control over, and ultimately improves, health and well-being". Health Promotion "represents a comprehensive *social and political process*, it not only embraces actions directed at strengthening the skills and capabilities of individuals, but also action directed towards social, environmental and economic conditions so as to alleviate their impact on public and individual health" (WHO Health Promotion Glossary 1998a p1). Kickbusch (1994 p13) stresses the change processes at several levels when referring to Health Promotion as "*a process for initiating, managing, and implementing change (...) a process of personal, organizational, and policy development*". The issues of organizational development will be taken up later again.

It is important to distinguish between the general goal of promoting health - often referred to as health promotion - and the specific concept or field of Health Promotion as defined above. For this research project on assessing networks for Health Promotion such as those on *health promoting* schools it is essential to avoid any confusion of meanings under the same heading 'health promotion'. Therefore, for the reminder of the text, the writing of <u>H</u>ealth <u>P</u>romotion *with capital letters* will indicate that reference is made to the Health Promotion approach with the nature of the expected outcomes (goals and objectives) and strategies (processes and activities) as defined in the above 'WHO/Nutbeam'-definition. If this is not particularly intended, <u>h</u>ealth <u>p</u>romotion will be written in small letters.

Principles and key features of Health Promotion

In the definition of Health Promotion the notion of peoples' *level of control* over matters that influence their health captures a key element of health promotion as understood and accepted not only by many people working in the field but increasingly also decision makers (see e.g. Green, Poland, Rootman 2000; Poland, Green, Rootman 2000a WHO 1997). It embodies a **cardinal principle of Health Promotion: empowerment**. In the field of Health Promotion, empowerment means that Health Promotion is directed at ensuring that individuals and communities *gain greater control over and can exercise their rightful power* in making decisions and related to actions that can improve or damage their health (WHO 1998a; Green et al 2000). The principle of empowerment is a primary feature, though not the only one, that distinguishes Health Promotion from other health promoting activities or approaches (Green et al 2000; Raeburn, Rootman 1998). The key features suggested in the literature are summarized in Box 2.2.2.

> Box 2.2.2: Key features of Health Promotion
> - focus on enhancing health, not just on preventing problems (*salutogenic perspective*);
> - building on a *social ecological, multi-dimensional model of health* (including physical, mental, social and also spiritual dimensions); emphasis on health as *a resource for everyday life* and not as a as a goal in itself;
> - emphasis on *equity in health and social justice* ('gesundheitliche Chancengleichheit');
> - orientation toward *competencies and resources, protective factors, or "co-determinants" of health at all levels* of society (not just toward risk factors and deficits);
> - orientation toward the *general population* including 'healthy' people, and not only toward specific risk groups;
> - orientation toward *people in their everyday environment or daily life context* (as opposed to a narrow 'patient in clinical setting' perspective)
> - strong emphasis on the process of *empowerment;* inclusion of empowering activities that e.g. equalize the balance of power between professionals and people and support 'self help';
> - encouragement and support of effective and concrete public *participation* (of individuals and communities, and of stakeholders in general);
> - active fostering of *intersectoral collaboration* with or among sectors outside the health sector;
> - combination of *several complementary strategies and methods;*
> - support of *life long learning.*
>
> Health promotion in this sense is a *social ecological (systems oriented) approach to action* on health issues and the knowledge of factors that influence or "co-determine" health.
>
> (WHO/EURO 1984a,b; Kaba-Schoenstein 1996; Downie, Fyfe, Tannahill 1990; Green, Poland, Rootman 2000; Broesskamp 1994, 1992; Broesskamp-Stone, Kickbusch, Walter 1998; Ziglio 1996; Blaettner 1994; WHO 1997, 1998a; WHO 1986; Green, Raeburn 1988)

Health Promotion practice *combines* diverse complementary strategies and methods which range from information and education to organizational and community development to policy development as well as legislative and fiscal (tax) measures (Broesskamp-Stone, Kickbusch, Walter 1998 p144; Kaba-Schoenstein 1996 II p45). Its focus on effective and concrete participation requires the further development of *life skills*, both individually and collectively, and the promotion of effective *participation mechanisms*. "Life skills are abilities for adaptive and positive behavior, that enable individuals to deal effectively with the demands and challenges of everyday life" (WHO 1993).

Health Promotion is often referred to as being 'comprehensive', 'complex' and 'multi-dimensional'. This refers to the combination of the characteristics outlined in box 2.2.2, which also bring about its *'multi-disciplinary'* nature and *'multi-level'* action orientation. WHO increasingly highlights the need of a *life course perspective* in Health Promotion and prevention.

Health Promotion is a concept that strongly *emphasizes (psycho-)social factors* that influence health. This is documented in early strategic guidelines of WHO/EURO for implementing programs to promote health, according to which programs should inherently consider and even promote the following factors (Kickbusch 1991): commence from or fully integrate the *social context*, aim to create supportive environments for health; allow for *social involvement* and commitment, for *social support*, and help develop a *sense of coherence*; allow for the development of *self-esteem* and *sense of control*, and expand personal skills and explore *meaning*; be explicitly linked to *other social policy agendas* and open the debate on *investment in health;* allow for *pride* and *sense of achievement*; allow for the fact that health is not necessarily people's main aim in life.

The value base of Health Promotion

The value base of Health Promotion (HP) has been made explicit since its conceptualization (WHO 1998a, 1997, 1986) and is closely linked to the basic values that form the ethical foundations of current global and Regional health policies, particularly of the early and most recent versions of the Health for All-policies and the 'World Health Declaration' (WHA 1998b). (see e.g. 'HEALTH 21' in Europe (WHO/EURO w.y.) and 'New Horizons in Health' in the Western Pacific (WHO/WPRO 1995)). Core values are:

- the highest attainable standard of health as a fundamental human right,
- health as an individual and social value, (however, in HP health is seen not as a goal in itself but as a resource for everyday life),
- equity in health, social justice, and solidarity in action,
- participation of stakeholders (already in decision making and priority setting processes), transparency, and accountability (i.e. democratic 'principles'; see e.g. Resolution ENHPS 1997a),
- incorporation of a gender perspective into strategies,

and in general,

- the dignity and worth of every person and

- the equal rights, equal duties and shared responsibilities of all for health (World Health declaration, WHA 1998b).

Transparency can be defined as an open and honest way of working collaboratively with no hidden agendas (Tennyson, w.y.), from priority setting and planning processes onwards.

For many people, terms often used in health promotion such as *enabling, empowerment and partnership* are more than sociological concepts. They invoke strong feelings of or ideologies that include concepts of human rights, professional privilege, distribution of resources and inequality (Green, Raeburn 1988). The *human right approach* corresponds with the demand that all people should have access to basic resources for health. Health Promotion action "aims at *reducing differences* in current health status and *ensuring equal opportunities and resources* to enable all people to achieve their fullest health potential." This includes supportive environments, access to information, life skills and opportunities for making healthy choices. (Ottawa Charter p1/ WHO 1986). It is widely recognized today that **equity at least in socio-economic terms is *not* just a value but also an important factor influencing or "co-determining" the health of populations** (see also chap. 2.1).

There is also some evidence that **participation is more than a value and important for success**; participatory approaches have been found to lead more likely to sustained and meaningful changes (WHO 1997; Ziglio 1996; Green et al 1995). As searches for complex, evidence based, multifaceted interventions that can be packaged and exported to most settings have shown, "a one-size-fits-all approach (the use of identical protocols in similar settings) is often ineffective or inappropriate" (Green, Poland, Rootman 2000, p346): Several recent reports on complex intervention trials at the community level show the demonstrated need for some local autonomy, not only in implementation and adaptation of set strategies but also in the assessment of needs and the setting of priorities and objectives. This is the rational for participatory planning approaches to the development of health promotion programs.

Key strategies and approaches in Health Promotion

The Ottawa Charter identified five **key strategies** (WHO 1986, 1998a):
- Building healthy public policies
- Creating supportive environments
- Strengthening community action
- Developing personal skills

- Reorienting health services

WHO defines their core concepts as follows:

"Healthy public policy is characterized by an *explicit concern* for health and equity in *all* areas of policy, and by an *accountability* for health impact. The main aim (…) is to create a supportive environment to enable people to lead healthy lives. Such a policy makes healthy choices possible or easier for citizens [and] (…) social and physical environments health enhancing." (WHO 1988b, 1998a)

"Supportive environments for health offer people protections from threats to health, and enable people to expand their capabilities and develop self reliance in health. They encompass where people live, their local community, their home, where they work and play, including people's access to resources for health, and opportunities for empowerment." (WHO 1998a)

"Community action for health refers to *collective efforts* by communities which are directed *towards increasing community control over the [co-]determinants of health*, and thereby improving health." (WHO 1998a)

Personal skills here mean "life skills", which are "abilities for adaptive and positive behavior, that enable individuals to deal effectively with the demands and challenges of everyday life." (WHO 1993, 1998a)

'Reorienting health services' today should be understood as "reorienting health system sand services with health promotion criteria" as a critical component of health sector reforms. (see Lopez-Acuna et al 2000)

As a practical answer to the challenge to develop projects, programs and interventions on the base of *all five* strategies and the *process* definition of Health Promotion WHO and experts developed the 'settings approach' (Kickbusch 1996).

Approaches in health promotion

However, today, three approaches are commonly being distinguished and often referred to as 'entry points' for Health Promotion: specific health issues, population groups, or settings (Nutbeam 1999; Green et al 2000; Broesskamp-Stone et al 1998). As Nutbeam (1999) underlines, each approach delineates the nature of the task to promote health and prevent ill-health in different ways, emphasizing the issue, the population or the settings as a starting point. These are not mutually exclusive.

1. *Settings approach*: Particular settings offer opportunities a) for comprehensive interventions which can be directed both at health supportive behavior change and environmental change; b) to reach specific target populations (e.g. adolescents through schools, pregnant women through health care services;) (see also below)

2. *Population group approach*: Focusing on individual population groups allows for better targeting of health problems that are more common

among such groups. For example, addressing health needs and problems among disadvantaged populations may encourage interventions which address underlying social, economic, and political factors or co- determinants of health such as (un)employment, housing, low income, social exclusion, etc.

3. *Issue approach*: Focusing on a specific health issue ensures that an intervention is more overtly outcome directed, but inevitably will rely on the identification of a specific population group and setting that will be the target of such an intervention. Prominent examples of issues include HIV/AIDS and tobacco use, but increasingly also e.g. violence.

No matter which *entry point* for Health Promotion may be chosen, Kickbusch (1994c) proposes 10 *action steps for any implementation strategy* for Health Promotion: establishing credibility for the new health agenda; developing foci for agenda setting in health policy; demonstrating clear financial commitment and developing new funding mechanisms for Health Promotion; creating and strengthening Health Promotion infrastructures; facilitating intersectoral action; creating accountability; creating high-profile centers of excellence and models of good practice; supporting innovations in Health Promotion development; facilitating community empowerment; and creating visibility for Health Promotion.

Another approach that is less **presented and discussed in the literature but documented in Health Promotion practice around the world** is what may be called a **"network approach"**. Worldwide, WHO continues to initiate networking and networks *to implement the Settings approach*. An example are the networks for the development of 'Health Promoting Schools' chosen as case examples for this research project. Therefore, the Settings approach as well as networking and network building in Health Promotion will be examined in more detail here.

2.2.3 The Settings approach in Health Promotion

In the mid 1980s, WHO, notably its Regional Office for Europe (WHO/EURO) and related experts provided considerable leadership and momentum for Health Promotion through the 'settings approach'. It represents a response to the 'natural' limits of individual- or group- centered health education and prevention activities of the time with regard to their contribution to sustaining the health of populations. It highlights the interaction of economic, social and organizational environment and personal lifestyle in the places of daily life (socio-ecological perspective). The Settings approach is based on the concept and strategies of *community development* and - new at the time - practical approaches to *or-*

ganizational change and the concept of the *learning organization*. It is assumed that there is a health development potential in practically every organization or community that can be fostered through a series of defined strategies applicable in various settings (see chap. 2.3). (WHO 1998a; WHO 1986; Broesskamp-Stone et al 1998; Kickbusch 1996, 1993; Grossmann, Scala 1996; Raeburn, Rootman 1998)

For long, settings were mainly seen as places where health education takes place, where selected audiences can be comfortably reached. Professionals and health (education) agencies organized themselves around settings (with patient education reflecting the clinical settings, school health education the educational settings, public health education the community setting, and so forth) (Green et al 2000 p11). What is practiced and discussed in the literature today as the 'Settings approach' in Health Promotion reaches far beyond and will be summarized now. Recent developments in the field of Health Promotion and large scale practice to implement the Settings approach will be considered. As will be shown the latter is closely linked with a network approach.

Settings: definitions and key features

In Health Promotion, a range of settings has been addressed on a larger scale worldwide, particularly schools, workplaces, hospitals and other clinical settings, as well as cities, communities, villages, municipalities and islands. Health Promoting Schools, Healthy Cities, etc. have been defined in practical terms. However, the published literature about the basic nature and common characteristics of such settings *across* the various types as well as implications for theory and practice in Health Promotion is somewhat limited (Green, Poland, Rootman 2000). Several interpretations, definitions and categorizations of the term 'setting' can be found:

A critical and in-depths analysis across settings was recently published by Poland, Green and Rootman (2000). They examine the *usefulness of 'the Settings' approach* as an organizational framework for conceptual thinking and strategy, research and development, theory and practice in health promotion (pp341-343). They identify two categories of settings: (a) *'total institutions'* (e.g. schools, workplaces, clinical practice settings/ hospitals) or (b) *less formalized organizational structures* (e.g. communities, homes). Both categories can be linked to particular bodies of theoretical and scientific knowledge from the social sciences, particularly with (a) organizational sciences and (b) basic social sciences on social structure and relations as well as political sciences. On this basis, the authors conclude that this basic **typology of settings** is meaningful for research and analysis of HP through the settings approach.

Other authors identify a similar typology. Goldstein (1997) from a global perspective categorizes Settings in Health Promotion as either (a) *organisations* (e.g. schools, hospitals, workplaces) or (b) *broader social structures* (e.g. cities, villages, communities, etc.). In the Western Pacific Region, the WHO Regional Office (WPRO) and regional experts in Health Promotion distinguish between (a) *elemental* settings and (b) *contextual* settings (Galea, Powis and Tamplin 2000). The latter typology occurred through observations that an *increasing range* of settings is being used to promote health and that practice shows that settings such as cities are not to be compared to marketplaces and schools not to villages. Pointing to the need of a frame of reference for analyzing settings and the need to recognize the existing hierarchy of different (system) levels, Galea et al summarize: *'Elemental' settings* are those which are *indivisible* for the purpose of meaningful health promotion and health protection programs. They have three characteristics: first, they are small enough for its *members* to identify as *belonging to that setting* and to engender a *sense of one entity*; second, they have *distinguishing* social, cultural, economic and psychological *peculiarities*; and third, they have a recognizable *formal or informal administrative structure* to which health promotion or health protection activities can link. Elemental settings directly affect the life of the people who live within them; they only affect others indirectly. - Broader *'contextual'* settings contain 'elemental settings'. For example, a city may contain important elements such as schools, a hospital and food markets. An island state is a contextual setting itself enclosing other contextual settings (e.g. cities) and elemental settings (such as schools, hospitals etc.) Public health benefits accrue when effective action is taken both at the level of elemental and contextual settings.

Poland, Green and Rootman (2000) point to **differences of settings** that are prevalent both across and within categories and even within each type of setting (such as school, city, etc.): a) *variations in stakeholder interests* (goals, concerns, aspirations, ...); and b) *variations because of the contingent nature of social relations in settings* as in society in general (unpredictability because of the unique confluence of personalities and other social, economic and political influences in time and space). After a review of a set of papers directed at 'identifying innovations in theory and practice in the application of health promotion to the settings' home, school, workplace, health care institution, clinical practice, community and 'state' Poland et al (2000) do not arrive at providing a definition of 'setting' for the context of Health Promotion. But they do identify **similarities and core features** that are considered below.

Other authors and WHO do offer **definitions or conceptualizations of settings in the context of Health Promotion.** These help to clarify what the Settings approach in Health Promotion is about. The Settings approach to promote health emphasises the *modifiable* health factors that are embedded in *local* settings and recognises that behavioural patterns of people and environmental or living conditions may not be the same in different local places or settings. The Settings approach is characterised by its:

- *local orientation, and*
- *sensitivity for locally prevailing situations or needs.*

On the one hand, a setting is understood as a *social system* that encompasses many relevant environmental factors that influence a particular group of people, on the other hand as a system *in which these factors or conditions that influence health and disease can be shaped.* (Grossmann, Scala 1996) The WHO Health Promotion Glossary provides the following definition and explanation:

A **"Setting for health"** is "the *place or social context* in which people engage in *daily activities* in which environmental, organisational and personal *factors interact to affect health* and well-being" (WHO 1998a, p19). A setting is *where people actively use and shape the environment* and thus create or solve problems relating to health. Settings have 'normally' physical boundaries, a range of people with defined roles, and an organisational structure (WHO 1998a).

Poland, Green and Rootman (2000) on the base of their review across categories and types of settings identify the following **'essential building blocks'** of settings: physical structure and layout, temporal patterning of behavior, material milieu, and social milieu. As *'additional features'* highlighted by several authors they point to the *physical and built environment* as a health factor in its own right, and the *psychosocial environment*. The latter includes the quality and intimacy of relationships, degree of participation and control (i.e. hierarchy, power relations), organizational arrangements (such as the management style in formal institutions), and history of internal politics. The authors conclude that all of these psychosocial variations make settings a useful unit of analysis and unit of planning for health promotion intervention.

Independent from the health discourse, **in the social sciences settings have been conceptualized** as both

- *"physically bounded* space-times in which *people come together to perform* specific tasks (usually oriented to goals other than health)" and

- "arenas of *sustained interaction*, with *preexisting* structures, policies, characteristics, institutional values, and both formal and informal *social sanctions on behavior*"

(Green, Poland, Rootman 2000 p23 - italics not in original). From a health promotion perspective, the authors point to earlier work by U. Fuhrer 1990 and N. Thrift 1983 when describing settings as *culturally constructed but individually mediated* 'interactional and activity microenvironments': with their own cultural *codes of conduct*; impregnated with *situational characteristics*; and subject to *temporal variations* in rhythms of social interaction (day/night, weekday/weekend) and longer terms.

Settings are more than simple locations: they are both the medium and the product of social interaction. Following a definition of 'spatial structure' by Gregory and Urry (1985 p3) settings can be understood not merely as arenas in which social life unfolds but rather as *a medium through which social relations are produced and reproduced*. (Green et al 2000)

'Settings in Health Promotion' - intermediate synthesis and discussion

For the purpose of this research it appears to be useful to distinguish between a definition of a setting (such as a school) that can be the target of Health Promotion actions or interventions ("Settings approach") and the term "health promoting setting" (e.g. Health Promoting School (HPS)) that describes the *desired result* of Health Promotion through the Settings approach. Actors in international networks for the development of Health Promoting School (HPS) need a basic understanding of settings in general (schools, communities, etc.) before being able to reflect on or define the features of a 'Health Promoting School' which is part of its surrounding community and larger social systems. The WHO definition of a 'setting for health' while being explicit regarding the features of a setting is not specific enough regarding the health promoting *qualities* of that setting. Therefore, and in the light of the research results presented above, that **definition** will be modified as follows:

A Setting is "the place or social context in which people engage in daily activities [and/or come together to perform specific tasks] in which environmental, organizational and personal factors interact [and] affect health and well-being".
(Adapted from WHO 1998a)

In some cases the settings term is also used for social systems beyond the local level (e.g. Lavis, Sullivan 2000, "The State as a setting"). This expansion of understanding of a setting to macro levels of society is counterproductive in Health Promotion, where a more precise definition of content, types, and methodologies of the Settings approach is still needed to support solutions to the assessment challenges that the Settings approach to Health Promotion still poses. In addition, it waters down the strength of a *local* orientation in Health Promotion that allows higher sensitivity for locally prevailing situations and needs that is confirmed as needed by much research in Public Health. - The confining of the term 'setting' to local systems levels (cities, communities, and organizations and other social systems therein) is preeminent in the field of Health Promotion around the world. This is not to be misunderstood as neglect of the big influence of the State and other macro-level social systems such as the European Union, UN agencies and multi-national companies in shaping important broader factors that influence or co-determine health (e.g. income-distribution). Systems at higher system levels surely provide or directly influence health relevant factors in local settings (e.g. through tax policies, advertising or its regulation, etc.). But in the context of this research the State and other *macro-level systems* will be referred to as broader 'social systems', not as 'Settings'; they are considered as *the environment in which settings are embedded.* Nevertheless, they do share the general characteristics of social systems with local communities, local governments, and locally based organizations such as schools (see chap. 2.3 below). - An interesting border line case are the small Island States in the Western Pacific Region which although sovereign States usually are less populated than most cities of the world. To those the "Settings approach" has been applied.

The methodologies of community development and organizational development on the base of which the Settings approach in Health Promotion was created are specific to lower system levels or smaller units of social systems in which individuals go in and out in daily life activities and which they can shape directly and/or over the short term collectively themselves. For macro-systems such as national governments that are beyond the immediate control of individual persons and communities (or which these can shape only over the long term), other approaches exist. To reach changes in support of health at these levels requires particularly changes in the policy realm. Several policy development theories and approaches exist and have been used in the area of Health Promotion at city and higher levels of society (see e.g. de Leeuw 2000). A related approach in the field of Health Promotion that receives increasing attention internationally is the 'Investment for Health'-approach (below). It complements the 'Settings approach'.

The **understanding of 'Settings' in Health Promotion can be summarized** as presented in box 2.2.3. Its key features have to be seen in *conjunction* with those of Health Promotion (box 2.2.2).

Box 2.2.3: Settings in Health Promotion: Key features. - Settings are:
- *locally oriented and sensitive for locally prevailing situations or needs;*
- *physically and time bounded (i.e. not static) places* ("space-times"),
    - in which people engage in daily activities and/or come together to perform specific tasks (usually oriented towards goals other than health! such as pupils' education in the case of schools),
    - which may or may not represent or be embedded in health supportive physical and built environments;
- *arenas for frequent and sustained social interaction,*
    - with *preexisting* social structures, policies, rules, characteristics, values, ...
    - with patterns of *formal and informal membership* and communication,
    - with *specific* cultural codes of conduct with both formal and informal sanctions on behavior,
    - with *permeability* for behavioral norms and values prominent in society/ in the settings larger environment,
    - in which social relations are *produced and reproduced* (whether health supportive or not),
    - they are both the *medium for* and the *product of* such social interactions (and thus *modifiable*);
- *subject to temporal variations*, day by day and over the long term (some of which may be influencing health such as changes of levels of trust and social support);
- they both *produce and exhibit environmental "co-determinants" of health as well as are influenced by such factors,*
    - *physical* environmental factors (e.g. the school building and grounds, but also the streets, meadows, surrounding air, service locations, etc.),
    - *(psycho-)social* environmental factors (e.g. the social school climate, but also the level of social equity or justice in the village, city, country).

A **typology of Settings** is emerging. As shown in table 2.2.4, the literature suggests two dimensions of relevance when applying the Settings approach in Health Promotion and undertaking scientific analyses: a) the *degree of formalization* of the settings as social systems and b) the *systems level* it represents. Accordingly, at least *four categories* of Settings can be distinguished.

increasing level of formalization → increasing system level ↓	**less formalized** social systems	**more formalized** social systems/ (conglomerates of) organizations
elemental settings (lower system level)	less / in-formal elemental settings e.g. home, market place, street corner, places for leisure, informal workplaces;	formalized elemental settings e.g. school, work site (not home), hospital, day care, (some market places);
contextual settings (higher systems level)	less/in-formal contextual settings e.g. communities, neighborhoods;	formalized contextual settings e.g. cities/ municipalities, villages, small island states;

Table 2.2.4:   A four-field matrix of categories of settings

Obviously, the selectivity of these categories is not perfect. For example, in contrast to 'developed' countries in many 'developing' countries market places are not formalized. Nevertheless, there are efforts to formalize them to a certain degree to improve food safety (introduction of certain rules, regulations, controls etc. through 'Healthy Marketplace' initiatives) (Moy 1998). Thus, market places may fall in either one sub-category of elemental settings. Such a typology of Settings is also challenged by new organizational arrangements that blur the borders between formal and informal places such as tele-work places and Internet based educational institutions. Yet, many of the Settings targeted to promote health today can be categorized as indicated above. As of now, Health Promotion through the Settings approach has been less often applied to informal elemental settings and most often to organizational settings (see below). Different types of settings will require different methods and processes to achieve sustainable change to promote and maintain health. As this research project focuses on international networks for Health Promoting Schools and similar Settings, i.e. on inter*organizational* networks, only those change strategies will be examined that relate to formal organizations and interorganizational networks (see chapter 2.4).

The Settings approach addresses areas of *daily life* such as family, place of living, school, work site or places for leisure with their specific social, organizational, environmental structures and dynamics, cultures and traditions, as they jointly influence or 'co-determine' people's health concepts, health relevant behaviors and health. It is important to note that **individuals usually belong to and are effected by several settings** at the same time. These may or may not exhibit complementary or conflicting features regarding health development.

To improve clarity, from now on the term *'Setting' will be written in capital* when referring to the understanding of a Setting as summarized above and the related 'Settings approach' in Health Promotion; when written in small letters the word setting is used in its general meaning of locality, milieu, background or place. The latter will be avoided as far as possible.

Implementing the Settings approach

Health Promotion through the Settings approach has as **strategic starting point** the logic of the Setting or social system concerned. Health Promotion actors attempt: a) to identify and develop *with the stakeholders* the health *potentials* within the Setting; b) through active *participation of all those concerned*, to use their expertise for health questions in the Setting and to strengthen their action competence for shaping and creating health supportive *living conditions* (empowerment); and c) to strengthen the *cooperation competencies* within the Setting and among the different organizations and informal groupings. - Ideally, the Settings approach integrates competence promotion, lifestyle change and change of health relevant living conditions and environments at different levels, including laws, financing and organizational structures and laws or regulations. Action to promote health through different settings can take many different forms. Often some forms of **social change strategies** are employed, particularly *community or organizational development,* which leads to changes such as modifications of the physical environment, organizational structure, administration and management. (WHO 1998a; Broesskamp-Stone, Kickbusch, Walter 1998; Nutbeam 1998a). Kickbusch (1996) summarizes that *Settings projects have in common*: the policy or strategic perspective; actions at policy and technical levels; focus on organization development and institutional change; building *alliances and collaboration between* sectors, disciplines and policy/executive decision makers; and community involvement and community empowerment.

Particularly authors working with an organizational development approach in Health Promotion point out that the Settings approach and the interventions within are directed at *social systems*, - communities, organizations and networks of organizations - and *not* at individual persons and their individual health behavior. They stress that *Health Promotion as intervention into social systems requires a good understanding of the conditions for development in social systems* (Grossmann, Scala 1996; Pelikan et al 1993). This is further examined in chapter 2.4 (below). Grossman and Scala (1994) underline that in practice, using Settings as target of Health Promotion interventions needs further precision: To decide, for example, on one or several 'communities' or 'schools' as places for Health Promotion provides only a rough frame. **In each case of a particular setting chosen, such as a school, the boundaries of this social system need to be further defined**. It is critical to answer questions such as 'which people, groupings, organizations or institutions linked to or part of the Setting should and need to be involved?' (e.g. by means of a stakeholder analysis). If important stakeholders are *left out* this can cause failure of the initiative as can the opposite, a *too* wide definition of the Setting and the range of stakeholders to be involved. The latter may, for example, inhibit the development of clear and *binding* cooperation structures. Therefore, **a Setting in Health Promotion means always a circumscribed social system that is *defined* for the *purpose* of a Health Promotion intervention and in which decisions and choices are made for concrete Health Promotion activities**. This shows limits of international networks for the development of Health Promoting Schools to *exactly* define the 'Health Promoting School' for all countries and the need to account for locally specific situations or decisions in planning, assessment and evaluation efforts.

In practice, not only the social dimension of a Setting needs to be circumscribed but also the thematic focus. *The Settings approach in Health Promotion is not necessarily contradictory to a problem or health issue orientation.* Grossmann and Scala (1996) see its strength in the combination of both. But, this *should not* be misunderstood as a call for *predefining or imposing* priority health issues by *some* (e.g. health professionals). The Health Promotion and Settings approach call for the *participation* of stakeholders such as the people most concerned already in needs assessment, priority setting and planning, as well as for empowerment as a basic position of professionals and 'leaders'.

2.2.4 Health Promotion in the 21st Century -evolution, review, challenges

Latest developments in the field

It has taken a decade or more to develop the field of Health Promotion (HP) (see chap.1) and up to day the horizons have been widened year by year. Both the tenths anniversary of the Ottawa Charter in 1996 as well as the 'end of the millennium' have triggered a range of critically reviews and future analyses concerning Health Promotion. Major products of an international scale and with a far reaching involvement of reputable experts, practitioners and decision makers are the 'Jakarta Declaration on Leading Health Promotion into the 21st Century' (WHO 1997) and the subsequent World Health Assembly Resolution on Health Promotion (WHA 1998), and the report of the technical program of the 5th Global

Conference on Health Promotion held in Mexico City 2000 (WHO 2000). In addition, important technical reviews were published: 'The evidence of health promotion effectiveness' for the European Commission and the book 'Evaluation in Health Promotion' by a European/North-American WHO working group (IUHPE 1999a, 1999b; Rootman et al 2001b).

Two **remaining challenges** are widely recognized: a) to *better demonstrate and communicate* that Health Promotion policies and practices can 'make a difference' to health and quality of life; and b) to achieve *greater equity in health* (WHO 2000). The 4th International Conference on Health Promotion (Jakarta, 1997) confirmed the core of the Ottawa Charter and the five Health Promotion strategies (see above) and identified five **priorities for Health Promotion in the 21st Century.** The latter were confirmed with one exception and expanded by the World Health Assembly in 1998 [modifications by this WHA in brackets]:

- Promote social responsibility for health;
- Increasing investments for health development;
- [to consolidate and] expand ["]partnerships for health["] [~~promotion~~];
- Increase community capacity and ["]empower["] the individual [in matters of health];
- Secure an infrastructure for health promotion
  (only in Jakarta Declaration) /

Strengthen consideration of health requirements and promotion in all policies (only in WHA Resolution);

- [to adopt an *evidence-based approach* to health promotion policy and practice, using the full range of quantitative and qualitative methodologies] (the additional priority identified by WHA). (WHO 1997; WHA 1998)

Increased attention is paid to **global trends that impact on health** (see e.g. McMichael 2000; Kickbusch 1996, 1997; WHO 1997, 2000; WHA 1998; Brundtland 2000) which represent **the global environment of international networks** for developing Health Promoting Schools and similar networks. 'New' trends in the 21st Century include the rapid increase in: absolute and relative poverty; demographic changes (ageing, urbanization); epidemiological changes ('double burden of disease'); global environmental threats to human survival; spread of new (information) technologies; biotechnological advances; globalization of trade, travel and the spread of values and ideas; - plus the evolving of cross sectoral partnerships for health (private, public, civil society) (WHO 1997c). From a Health Promotion perspective Kickbusch (1996) highlights particularly three of those changes: the globalization of markets, the massive potential of communications technology, and the extreme speed of change in the physical and social environments (in particular the rapid urbanization with enormous environmental but also tragic social consequences such as homelessness/ street children). She identifies three major industries with particular impact on health: the 'health', 'lifestyle/ leisure' and 'media/ communication' industries. - *Globalization itself*, the composite process that characterizes today's increasingly interconnected world, is identified as an important 'determinant' of population health and health inequities today (McMichael 2000) and, thus, as a new challenge also for the field of Health Promotion.

To acknowledge that **health, social and economic development are inextricable linked** is a logic consequence of a Health Promotion (and modern Public Health) approach that is based on a perspective that considers the full range of factors that influence or 'co-determine' health. Health Promotion and other Public Health actors and agencies call particularly on governments to acknowledge that investments in health are a positive contributor to social and economic development. (e.g. Brundtland 2000; WHO 1997; World Bank 1993; IUHPE 1999a; see also chap. 2.2.5 below)

In the light of these new challenges, perspectives and today's knowledge of the factors that influence and 'co-determine' health, and with view to both local and national or international levels, **new forms of action** are often called for that free the potential for Health Promotion in many sectors of society. These are usually referred to as building **intersectoral partnerships or alliances** (e.g. WHA 1998; Levin, Ziglio 1996, 1997; Ziglio et al 2000, 2000a; Brundtland 2000) but also **networks, and infrastructures** for Health Promotion (e.g. Kickbusch 1996; WHO 1997). *Intersectorality* in Health Promotion refers not only to collaboration among public sectors but across public, private and NGO sectors and the civil society.

Reviewing the Settings approach: strengths and limitations

To assure appropriateness and quality of strategies and actions, international networks for the development of health promoting Settings such as 'Health Promoting Schools' need to be aware of and responsive to changes in their relevant environment. The latter includes stakeholder opinions and new research results concerning Health Promotion and the strengths, limitations or (perceived) risks of the Settings approach. Critical reviews and acknowledgments of Health Promotion, the Settings approach and its knowledge base in the late 1990s suggest a range of factors that facilitated and continue to support the widespread interest, acceptance and continuous implementation of Health Promotion through the Settings approach (see e.g. Green et al 2000; Poland et al 2000; Nutbeam 1999; IUHPE 1999b; McQueen 2000, 2000a; Goldstein 1998; Kickbusch 1996, 1995; Broesskamp 1994; Grossman, Scala 1993).

The factors supporting Health Promotion through the Settings approach can be summarized as follows:

- the results and increased recognition of research on the *range of interrelated factors that influence or "co-determine" health* (see chap.2.1); particularly, today's recognition of organizational factors as powerful in influencing or shaping individual and group behavior and the confirmation that many of the "co-determinants" of health are Settings specific (that 'health is created where people live, learn, work and play...' Ottawa Charter/WHO 1986); - nevertheless, many *macro level* (or 'broader') factors influencing health are today also recognized as demanding Health Promotion responses beyond the Settings approach;

- the increased recognition and dissemination of *social ecological theories and perspectives* on health and health promotion, with the former reinforcing the assertion that people are not definable solely by their 'risk identities' (Kickbusch 1995);

- support through *new and more appropriate Health Promotion outcome models, positive results of effectiveness reviews and critical debates of the meaning of evidence in Health Promotion* (as distinct from evidence based medicine; see McQueen 2000a);

- *legitimacy and ongoing momentum through WHO's leadership and the support of other international organizations as well as some governments* already in the mid 1980s, as well as most recently through discussions during and outcomes of international conferences such as the 4th and 5th global conferences on Health Promotion (Jakarta 1997 and Mexico 2000) and Habitat II/'local agenda 21';

- promotion through incorporation into high level *international policy documents* such as:
  o the Jakarta Declaration (WHO 1997) and World Health Assembly (WHA) Resolution 51.12 (WHA 1998): There is now "clear evidence that: (a) comprehensive approaches that use combinations of the five [HP] strategies are the most effective; (b) certain *settings offer practical opportunities* for the implementation of comprehensive strategies, such as cities, islands, local communities, markets, schools, workplaces, and health services; (...)"/ the WHA called on WHO to enhance its capacity with that of the Member

States to foster the development of health promoting settings (WHA 1998);
- o Resolution on "Healthy Settings" of the South East Asian Health Ministers urging Member States "(a) to identify by the end of 2001, at least one district to pilot a "healthy settings" program (...), (b) to evaluate the existing technical and managerial capabilities for promoting various "healthy settings" programs, and enhance these where necessary" (WHO/SEARO 2000);
- o the 'New Horizons in Health' Policy in the Western Pacific Region (WHO/WPRO 1995);
- o the new European 'Health for All 21' policy with target number 13 "Settings for the promotion of health" published in 1998 (WHO/EURO without year);
- incorporation into *country level policies* such as in the internationally negotiated 'Mexico Ministerial Statement for the Promotion of Health' that was signed in June 2000 by 87 national Health Ministries from around the world;
- high attractiveness for practitioners through offering a concrete, practical focus insofar as *Settings represent a pragmatic and manageable scale for practitioners* at which to direct comprehensive change efforts (as opposed to e.g. national or societal levels);
- attractiveness across different schools of thought in Health Promotion through *provision of an organizational framework to combine* in a targeted way both Health Promotion interventions directed at health relevant *lifestyles* and those directed at health relevant *'living conditions'*; Settings are social structures providing channels for reaching and influencing defined populations, political and other decision makers included (Goldstein 1997).

The Settings approach has become the most visible, innovative and for many the key approach in contemporary Health Promotion.

However, there are **limitations, risks and challenges of the Settings approach**, too: Critical reviews also identify limitations or even risks as well as remaining or new challenges. Kickbusch (1997) from a social ecological perspective on health development calls on *expanding the settings approach* 'in several directions': beyond organizational settings and organizational development to *'social spaces and social development'* (such as childhood, being female, growing old); towards understanding the full *impact of the information technology revolution* as a major driving force and its effects on human development and health; towards *marginalized and excluded populations, their settings* - slum dwellings, remote regions - and their health and social needs; towards a better understanding of *'socially toxic environments'* (Garbarino 1995) *and 'social capital'*, and a revisiting of Health Promotion programs with this perspective. Social scientists in health have identified a number of challenges and issues that need critical reflection and ongoing or increased attention (e.g. Green, Poland and Rootman 2000; Kickbusch 1997, 1996, 1995; Wenzel 1997). These include:

- the fact that *Settings do not exist in a vacuum and people move in and out* of settings in the course of their every day life; (a challenge for impact measurement of 'health promoting Settings' on health and personal health actions;
- the need to address not only the environmental *"co-determinants" of health behavior* (e.g. Mullen et al 1995) but also *changes to factors in the setting that directly influence health* (see also chap. 2.1.2);
- the widespread *practice labeled 'health promotion through settings' but using Settings purely instrumentally* (as medium for reaching those who are 'contained' within it and implementation space for health education/information actions);
- *'taken-for-granted' ideas* in health promotion and how these are socially constructed, embedded into power relations, and supportive of the status quo; the *opening of new possibilities of thought and action as a prerequisite for change*; (often reference is made to the work of Paolo Freire);
- the typical *assumption of face-to-face interactions between members in Settings* while the spread of new information technologies brings into being *'virtual settings' or 'communities'* that share many of the features of bounded Settings; (what is an appropriate HP response ?)
- the increasing *blurring of spatial boundaries between settings* such as work and school that traditionally are spatially clearly separate (for examples, working from home or distance education);
- the *overestimation* by some *of the effectiveness of regulatory interventions* in Settings to promote health (such as policy and organization change) that are *implemented without sufficient participation* of all stakeholders ('top down' and/or by external professionals);
- the *power relationships within Settings*, including the *'Settings paradox'* (Green, Poland, Rootman 2000), i.e. the consequences of Health Promotion actors' aligning with management or administrative authorities in Settings as the key gatekeepers to Settings which may jeopardize their ability of gaining trust and support of those with whom they wish to work in the Setting (particularly those that are most

alienated by or resistant to authorities); (see also Labonte 1994; Laverack 1999; Laverack/ Labonte 2000; Restrepo 2000)

- the question *'who is left out'* from Health Promotion through *conventional, more formal and/or more legitimate Settings* (schools, workplaces, cities, etc.) which as of now received most attention in the field; work in Settings in which those people may be found whose chances for health are most jeopardized (such as the unemployed, the homeless, the disenfranchised youth, the lonely or isolated people);

- Health Promotion through *less conventional or less 'obvious' Settings* (e.g. meeting points of youth, of unemployed people; pubs, bingo halls, night clubs; street corners;); these may be those:

   a) in which the health adverse behaviors (the traditional concern of health educators and promoters) are perhaps most common,

   b) that are the least formal in terms of their social organization of interaction and possess fewer formal channels of power of formalized institutions (i.e. they are more fluid in structure and, thus, less amenable to formal regulation and law),

   c) that are most likely to challenge wide spread biases in HP research, policies and practice towards the middle-class, rational actor, deferred gratification, health as a major goal, professional and expertise orientation (Kickbusch 1995).

- the overemphasis on *consensus building* around common aims in much of the literature on HP through Settings and the *inherent risk* of silencing certain voices in this process; the potential merit in *dissents* and resistance to resolve contradictions;

- a better understanding of *how changes in the 'normative culture' of a Setting occur and can be brought about with minimal harm*; the reciprocal relationships between (a) persons in a Setting and the characteristics and nature of that Setting (Settings structure), and (b) social and physical space in Settings; the open questions: How make people sense of and interpret particular Settings (e.g. pupils, teachers, parents)? Why and how are some issues or changes resisted and others not? How is such resistance perceived? (Green et al 2000);

In addition, St Leger (1997) identifies some *remaining practical tasks* in improving the effectiveness and unfolding the full potential of the Settings approach in Health Promotion:

- fostering *more evaluation studies* (particularly analyzing processes and impact, reflecting and discussing the lessons learned, and disseminating them widely);
- *improving intersectoral collaboration and productive partnerships* between sectors (the creation of which is often attempted and rarely achieved); in relation to this, overcoming professional boundaries;
- achieving some *early tangible gains and affirming them to the stakeholders* (as creating health promoting Settings cannot be achieved over the short term);
- building *intersectoral teams and supporting constituencies at the outset* of any implementation effort;
- *investing in multi-disciplinary education and training* (addressing knowledge and skills of multidisciplinary planning, intersectoral implementation, agency partnerships, leadership);
- *planning sufficient time and being pragmatic when integrating* the various 'elements' of the Settings approach (a range of strategies and stakeholders, and the diversity of values, beliefs, policies and practices in a Setting).

The Settings approach and beyond - synthesis and discussion:

Health Promotion through the Settings approach (or the creation of 'Settings for Health') as outlined in chapter 2.2.3 above has been confirmed on scientific as well as pragmatic grounds and is widely accepted and recommended as a key approach to promoting health around the world. Over the last years the challenges to reduce health inequalities and inequities, which are at the core of the Health Promotion concept, have received stronger attention in Health Promotion research, policies and practices. Actors in Health Promotion are called on to promote and support the (participatory and empowering) implementation of the Settings approach not only in more formal elemental and contextual settings (organizations and their conglomerates) but also in less or in-formal Settings (see table 2.2.4). Attention needs to be given particularly to elemental settings in which less socially integrated or in some way or the other disadvantaged or vulnerable people meet or engage in daily activities.

International networks for the development of Health Promotion Schools (HPS) initiated in the early 1990s, operate today in a different and rapidly changing context. As will be explained in chapter 2.3 this needs to be taken into account when focusing on the assessment of such networks. Significant societal and global changes, advances in the understanding of 'broader', macro level factors typically called 'determinants of health', and lessons learned from Health Promotion practice show: *There is a need to targeted complement Health Promotion through the Settings approach by approaches directed at national and international structures, policies and actors in a broad range of sectors that influence health.* The health of local communities is influenced by many factors that are beyond the immediate control of individual communities. With regard to Health Promotion policies and practice it follows that the 'attention span' needs to be broadened beyond health supportive community and organizational development, i.e. developmental work in Settings, to include strategically influencing the interplay of overall social, economic and health development in societies. In the light of this and in response to this *"new" Health Promotion approaches that (have the potential to) complement the Settings approach* have emerged: the so called "Investment for Health approach" and - as argued in this research project - a 'network approach'.

But before turning to these new approaches (in chap. 2.2.5 below) it is important for this research project on assessment and indicator development for international networks for the development of Health Promoting Schools, to be aware of some 'built in' or 'natural' challenges and strengths related to the Health Promotion concept that represent challenges for any assessment effort directed at Health Promotion actions. These stem from the social-ecological perspective and the empowerment principle in Health Promotion - and many of those explain the above discussed limitations, risks or challenges as well as strengths of the Settings approach.

Challenges to the field of Health Promotion inherent in its core principle of empowerment

The concept of empowerment leaves Health Promotion actors with *many conceptual, operational and evaluation challenges* (see e.g. Rootman, Goodstadt, Potvin, Springett 2001; Laverack 1999; Laverack, Labonte 2000; Issues of 'Health Education Quarterly' 1994a, b). *Empowerment* as a core principle means that Health Promotion is directed at ensuring that individuals and communities gain greater control over and can exercise their rightful power in making decisions and related to actions that can improve or damage their health (WHO 1998a; Green et al 2000). As shown in chapter 2.1 many of the broader 'co-determinants' of health are beyond the immediate or short-term control of individuals and single communities. However, Health Promotion can help people to work *collectively* to change even those influences beyond the control of an individual, small group or specific geographic community, - through 'broader based coalitions' and 'social movements (as suggested by Green, Poland and Rootman 2000) and through 'networks' - as suggested by this research project (see below). According to Green et al, Health Promotion can - in addition - buffer the negative impacts of those broader health factors or 'co-determinants' (e.g. by supporting self-help groups or compensatory services for socio-economic disadvantaged people); it also can reinforce or enhance the positive influences of the various factors on health that are beyond an individuals' control (e.g. social support or social capital). However, health research has shown that a higher sense of 'control' in itself is a health factor (e.g. Schwarzer 1992).

Challenges to the field of Health Promotion inherent in its social-ecological perspective

As much as it is scientifically sound (see chap. 2.1), the social ecological perspective inherent in the Health Promotion concept bears particular challenges for Health Promotion research and practice. The field deals not only with the **strengths but also limitations of the 'social ecological model to promoting health'**.

Looking at the **strengths**, Green, Richard and Potvin (1996) identify some 'lessons' of relevance to health promotion policy and practice: **The social ecological approach recognizes and draws explicitly attention to**:

- *unanticipated effects* of actions for change: it cautions reforms and practitioners against tampering with change in smaller systems without considering and anticipating, before the intervention, their second- and third-order consequences;

- the understanding that the organism's functioning is mediated by *behavior-environment interaction and reciprocal determinism* and its implications for behavioral and social change:
    - that environment largely controls or sets limits on the behavior that occurs in it (avoids victim blaming), and
    - that changing environmental variables results in the modification of behavior;

- the principle that a person behaves differently when observed in different environments with *environments predisposing, enabling and reinforcing individual and collective behavior (environmental specificity),* and its implications for health promotion planning and evaluation:
    - that it is not possible to identify and define *the* health promotion method or strategy superior to all others as its effectiveness always depends on its *appropriate fit* with the people, the health issues at stake, and the environment in which it is to be applied;

- the *necessity of multilevel and multi-sectoral interventions* or actions, i.e. of addressing several levels within an organizational structure or system, and multiple sectors of a social system (such as health, education, welfare, commerce, etc.) - because of the complex interdependencies of the elements making up an 'ecological web';

This is supported by Stokols (1996) who draws attention to another point:

- the *integration of both 'problem' (or causal) theories and 'intervention' theories* on particular health issues which allows to better formulate coherent, focused and theoretically grounded interventions while *avoiding* overly inclusive and diffusely organized health promotion programs.

As Green et al (1996) point out, the **issue of environmental specificity supports the local and community focus of health promotion** (see below) which allows actions to be more adaptable and sensitive to particular traditions, cultural variations, and circumstances as if they were planned at provincial, State or national levels. - The behavior-environment interaction and reciprocal determinism is the basis for the 'inexorable recognition' that *health promotion can achieve its best results by exercising whatever control or influence it can over the environment,* as the environment predisposes, enables, and reinforces individual and collective behavior. But nevertheless behaviors of individuals, groups and organizations influence their environments. This leads to the core of the Health Promotion concept, to *empower* people by giving them control over the factors that influence or 'co-determine' their (both behavioral and environmental factors). - The social ecological thinking in health promotion forces a broader perspective on planning and practice in health promotion that might otherwise drift into a reductionism, person-centered or victim-blaming orientation. However, it has its own weaknesses or pitfalls.

Green, Richard and Potvin (1996) also identify several **limitations of the social ecological model to promoting health,** including the following:

- the *inherently limited specificity* of social ecological guidelines *in identifying the particular levels and sectors in need of attention* because of an infinite variety of interactions that might apply in each distinctive organization, community or other social system;

- the *inherent evaluation challenges* as the units of analysis of social ecological interventions (such as communities or organizations) don't lend themselves to 'traditional' evaluation approaches such as experimental and control groups; (they are *open* systems evolving in a *constantly changing* environment and it cannot be assumed that, for example, in a national Health Promoting School network initiative a

control school will remain free of influence of the activities and publicity related to the 'network pilot schools');
- their *complexity breeds despair*, particularly if the social ecological model of health is interpreted in its extreme as 'everything influences everything else'; this leaves those that wish or need to act in support of health with an infinite variety of interactions that might apply in each organization, community or other social system (Kaba-Schoenstein 1996); obviously this provides little basis for setting priorities, leaves the question open of 'how much is enough' to have a positive impact on a health issue, as well as leaves practitioners such as health educators with ongoing criticism and/or feelings of insufficiency (e.g. reproach for treatment of symptoms);
- the *built-in frustration and criticism of any analysis* in an ecosystems hierarchy, both a system as a whole and component sub-systems need to be analyzed; whatever system will be selected as the focus, it will be apparent that this is a sub-system of yet another system; analysts have to subjectively decide which systems level to include and which not and any decision may be criticized by others as too broad or too narrow.

Stokols (1996) points to the following practical limitations of social ecological interventions:
- they require the integration of knowledge from several different disciplines;
- they require close coordination among persons and groups from various sectors;
- the combined use of active and passive interventions and the incorporation of multilevel, multi-method assessments of program outcomes over extended periods can be quite expensive and logistically complex;
- they risk to be designed potentially over-inclusive (i.e. all conceivable health-relevant factors are being considered) which would significantly reduce their utility in determining where, when and how to intervene.

To *prevent the over-inclusiveness* of social ecological Health Promotion interventions Stokols suggests that strategies should be based on: a) *'middle range' theories of the specific circumstances* (e.g. intrapersonal, environmental, organizational, cultural) that account for the occurrence and prevalence of particular health issues (theories of causes); and b) *a corresponding analysis of the contextual factors* that are likely to influence the effectiveness of health promotion interventions designed to change those issues (theories of intervention).

Actors of (social ecological) Health Promotion need a range of particular competencies, knowledge and skills such as in management, cooperation, policy action, negotiation, advocacy, and mediation are needed besides the specific knowledge and skills in health related areas (e.g. on the co-determinants of health and health behavior). These are usually not part of professional or other training and, therefore, *human resource development* needs special attention in efforts to implement the Health Promotion concept and approaches. (Kaba-Schoenstein 1996 V; Broesskamp-Stone et al 1998)

The following look at 'new' approaches in Health Promotion that *complement* the Settings approach will show that these approaches strive and/or have the potential to respond to many of the genuine challenges identified above.

2.2.5 'New' approaches in Health Promotion

The "Investment for Health approach"

The "Investment for Health approach" originates from the European region but has achieved recognition at global level, for example, as one of the 'priorities for HP in the 21st Century' (Jakarta Declaration 1997) and a key theme of the 5th Global Conference on Health Promotion (Mexico, 2000). The term '*Investment for Health*' (IFH) is consciously chosen as opposed to 'investment *in* health' that in health policy discourse generally refers to investments in medical (health) care. According to WHO (1998a)

"Investment for health refers to *resources which are explicitly dedicated to the production of health and health gain*. They may be invested by public and private agencies as well as by people as individuals and groups. Investment for health strategies are based on knowledge about the co-determinants of health and seek to gain political commitment to healthy public policy." - "Health gain is a way to express improved health outcomes" and is used to reflect the relative advantage of one form of health intervention over another.

The term "Investment for Health approach" (IFH) may be summarized as follows (Ziglio, Hagard, McMahon, Harvey, Levin 2000; Ziglio, Hagard, Griffiths 2000a; Levin, Ziglio 1996, 1997; WHO/EURO 1997a). Under the leadership of WHO/EURO, the Investment for Health (IFH) approach was created against the following background:

- there is a solid knowledge base on *social and economic determinants of health of populations*;

- consensus has been achieved on the *principles and goals of the Health for All-strategy and of Health Promotion*, - now the *real challenge lies in applying them* in practice in increasingly complex societies (macro perspective on whole countries or larger sub-national systems such as States/regions);
- *societies have* invariably *immediate priorities*, such as economic competitiveness and fiscal soundness, and their social institutions are directed towards achieving those priorities;
- an *atmosphere of uncertainty and anomie* (i.e. doubt and loss of values accompanied by problems of orientation) in both developing and developed countries dampens enthusiasm for long term investments to secure health and well-being;
- many countries show *still insufficient organization and resources for Health Promotion*, although Health Promotion practice greatly developed globally and evidence of its effectiveness increased.

Health Promotion programs and policies can be better implemented when countries recognize that they are capable to both producing *health outcomes* and contributing strongly to *"healthy" social and economic results* (a lesson from European experiences). The challenge lies in: a) finding ways of deploying investment for health to reinforce the priorities of societies and, conversely, b) enhancing people's health - equitably and sustainable - through the medium of social and economic development. To tackle the *root causes* of ill health and to create opportunities for better health, **Health Promotion must be integrated effectively into mainstream social and economic development** and have its influence visible in relevant programs, regulations and wide-ranged public policies. This needs to be done while adhering to core principles of Health Promotion: a focus on *health*; *full public engagement*; genuine *intersectoral* work; *equity*; *sustainability* (investments and resource management that do not compromise the health and well being of future generations; durable IFH processes;); *a broad knowledge base* (scientific knowledge, 'community judgment and insight', practical, hands-on experience).

This requires a **strategy** involving the concerted efforts of a *variety* of actors at *all* levels of government and society including *citizen participation*. The 'successful strategy' must influence sectors such as health care, education, social services, environment, economic and social development. It needs to involve public and private partners, the media, NGOs, and all other institutional arrangements relevant to social cohesion, social justice and human rights. (Ziglio et al 2000) In practice, **intersectoral collaboration or action for health is often called for but seldom real-**

ized. Miscommunications, differences in conceptual languages, different interpretations of the same terms (e.g. health or participation) need to be overcome. 'Investment for Health' -demonstration projects have shown that tools and processes of **policy making, 'collaborative communication' and management in open systems need to be capable of**: a) *assessing the structures/ systems/ processes and* current and future *opportunities* (within and outside the health sector) with regard to their impact on health, and identifying *ways of improving* this infrastructure; b) *identifying the key elements of a strategy* that enhances the population's health through selective investment (both within and outside the health sector) while supporting key economic and social priorities; and c) *negotiating for investment for better health with policy makers and key decision takers* in leading social and economic sectors. Assessing options that benefit both health and the primary intent of a specific policy sector, as well as good planning of the political process of achieving the necessary legislative, regulatory, financial, organizational or educational changes are essential. - The *processes may take different forms depending on the circumstances* in countries or regions. Examples tested by WHO/EURO include 'Health Promotion audits' in countries on behalf of the national parliament, negotiations among key sectors following a 'bargaining framework', and developing 'health gain maps' for geopolitical areas.

'Investment for health approach' - intermediate synthesis and discussion

The Investment for Health (IFH) approach as the Settings approach is systems and development oriented. While the Settings approach is locally oriented and involves community and organizational development, the IFH approach is oriented towards higher systems levels, 'the society', overall health, social and economic development in countries, and it has a particularly strong policy development focus. The latter parallels 'Healthy Cities' types of projects (see below). The particular attention in the IFH approach to high level decision makers in both government, public and private sectors may or may not be mirrored in Settings projects. The strong orientation to private sector and national level decision makers and politicians is reflected in a new set of terms: Health Promotion as an *investment* strategy; *assets* for health (not e.g. resources); health *gain* (not e.g. outcomes); *citizen participation* in intersectoral collaboration (and not e.g. empowerment or enabling people...); etc. The orientation towards countries or societies as a whole is particularly reflected in the reference to *health development* (the process of continuous, progressive improvement of the health status of individuals and groups in a population; WHO 1998a) as well as *social and economic development*. This can be interpreted as a conscious attempt by the initiators of this approach to overcome cultural ('language') barriers between the field of Health Promotion, the 'world of economics' and high level politicians, as well as to distant themselves from a 'social movement image'. This should not be misinterpreted as a neglect of core Health Promotion principles. The Investment for Health (IFH) approach builds on the same Health Promotion definition as e.g. the Settings approach; and Investment for Health (IFH) initiatives *do* involve community and NGO participation. But they consciously target national or State level decision makers, executives of companies, as well as higher societal levels, which means an increase in complexity of the Health Promotion process.

The IFH approach has been presented as a Health Promotion 'tool' to address particularly the national or State level *(policy) environment* in which, for example, Health Promotion through the Settings approach takes place. As such it is relevant for international networks for the development of Health Promoting Schools (HPS) as they strive for a large scale dissemination and implementation of the Health Promoting Schools concept which needs high level policy support. Networks may benefit from combining the Settings approach with the use of tools from the IFH approach and/or actively participating in IFH demonstration projects or processes.

Is there a "network approach" to the development of health promoting Settings ?

In 1992, Kickbusch presents the *Settings* approach and 'a *networking* approach' as two distinct approaches used by the WHO Regional Office for Europe (WHO/EURO) in Health Promotion. She adds the 'building of strategic and innovative *alliances*' as a 'key to the settings strategy'. While the *Settings approach,* so Kickbusch, focuses on how to promote health supportive environments within the *Settings of everyday life* (schools, workplaces etc.), the **networking approach 'brings the dimensions of local and global action together'**. She refers to the example of the Healthy Cities Project where each WHO project city works for its own health but at the same time contributes actively to an international effort of health supportive and sustainable development in cities. The project cities are in turn linked to groups of national network cities and to cities in interregional networks throughout the world. She points to similar efforts for linking European schools from late 1992 on (the then yet forthcoming "European Network of Health Promoting Schools" initiative examined in this research project; see below). Referring to these approaches she calls for *sustainable* public health *projects* that build on *participation* and *trust in people and processes*. - Referring to modern management approaches, Kickbusch described **alliances** as addressing *complex* issues and problems that are not being managed adequately by one organization acting alone, as well as taking up *indivisible* problems in a *proactive* process of identifying and shaping *social issues and emergent trends*. (Kickbusch 1992)

A Health Promotion glossary from 1990 produced on behalf of WHO/EURO for the International Conference 'Investment in Health' (Bonn, 1990) defines **"intermediate structures"** in health promotion. With reference to Trojan and Hildebrandt 1990

"intermediate structures are defined as: *"connecting links in a long chain of social structures* between the individual and the highest levels of power" but also between existing 'sub-cultures and the establishment' (Conrad, Schmidt 1990 p35).

They are characterized by their *intermediate position between* 'political-administrative systems', 'markets' and 'self-help groups', not clearly belonging to any of them. They can be considered as important base for the implementation of *'new'* health actions *across the borders* of established institutions. Trojan (1996) speaks of *'mediating and networking'* when referring to the creation of local, regional or national 'Kooperations*netzwerke*' (cooperative networks). According to Catford (1999) the Health Promotion perspective brings several themes into the foreground. These include 'reaching out' by engaging, *connecting*, and *horizontal networking*, and 'cutting edge' through *innovation, risk taking, boundary riding*. As will be seen later many of these issues and concepts have indeed something to do with what in the organizational sciences is called organizational networking or interorganizational networks (see chap. 2.4).

Since the 1980s, large-scale efforts for the development of health promoting Settings have been promoted by WHO and others. They include Regional and/or national level 'projects', 'initiatives', 'programs' and 'networks'. In comparison to the widespread observable practice published information on these large-scale efforts including the networks for developing health promoting Settings is limited. Such 'networks' have received little technical or research attention as far as their *network* dimension is concerned. But the latest WHO Health Promotion Glossary from 1998 includes the term 'network' as a "new definition" which indicates that technical reflection about such organizational forms has started in the field. WHO suggests that a **network** is

"a *grouping* of individuals, organizations and agencies *organized* on a *non-hierarchical* basis around *common* issues or concerns, which are pursued *proactively and systematically*, based on *commitment and trust*" (WHO 1998a p16 - italics not in original).

Since the late 1990s, international policy documents increasingly address Settings and network approach jointly and often in the context of need of intersectoral collaboration and infrastructure development. 'Securing an infrastructure for health promotion' is one of the priorities for Health Promotion in the 21st Century (Jakarta Declaration): "(…) *"Settings for health" represent the organizational base* of the infrastructure required for health promotion. New health challenges mean that new and diverse *networks need to be created to achieve intersectoral collaborations*. Such networks should provide *mutual assistance* within and among countries and *facilitate exchange* of information on which strategies have proved effective and in which settings" (WHO 1997). In South-East Asia, the WHO Member States requested WHO (a) to provide technical support (guidelines, indicators) and (b) to promote *exchange* of experiences (…) on various *"healthy settings"* approaches and strengthen *networking* among countries (WHO/SEARO 2000). (italics not in originals)

During the 1990s, not only 'network' but also 'partnership' and 'alliance' have emerged as buzz words within and beyond public health and entered the already 'older' discourse around intersectoral action or collaboration for health. This reflects the general agreement in public health and beyond that new ways of working together are needed. Particularly in the field of Health Promotion since long the organizational form of 'network' has been used and, today, is internationally recognized. The '4th International Conference of Health Promotion' in Jakarta (above) called for the development of *collaboration and networks* for health development across sectors and on national governments to take the initiative in "fostering and sponsoring *networks* for health promotion both *within and among* their countries" (WHO 1997). In June 2000, 87 Health Ministries subscribed explicitly to the 'establishment and strengthening of *national and international networks* which promote health' when signing the 'Mexico Ministerial Statement for the Promotion of Health' (Fifth Global Conference of Health Promotion 2000). The World Health Assembly Resolution on Health Promotion (WHA 1998) calls on organizations of the United Nations system, intergovernmental and nongovernmental organization and foundations, donors and the international community as a whole "to form global, regional, and local health promotion *networks*". Such calls occurred in the light of today's knowledge of new health challenges and co-determinants of health that are not only beyond the control of any individual or individual community but also of the health sector.

The recognized need for new forms of working together across (sectoral, professional, organizational, national) boundaries and layers of society draws attention to appropriate organizational

forms. However, *terminology* used to describe organizational forms *varies widely*, is often vague, and commonly agreed definitions are lacking. A look at definitions proposed, for example, by WHO shows that relevant knowledge that could inform this research project on assessing international networks for Health Promoting Schools (i.e. assumingly interorganizational networks, may not only be found under the key word 'network' but also under other organizational forms used in Health Promotion. The WHO Health Promotion Glossary (WHO 1998a) covers not only the term 'intersectoral collaboration' but since its latest edition also 'network', 'alliance', 'partnership for health promotion', and 'infrastructures for health promotion': a) 'Intersectoral collaboration' is defined as

"a *recognized* relationship between part or parts of different sectors or society which has been *formed to take action* on an issue to achieve health outcomes or intermediate health outcomes *in a way which is more effective, efficient or sustainable* than might be achieved by the health sector acting alone."

A major goal is to achieve greater awareness of the health consequences of policy decisions and *organizational practice* in different sectors, and through this, movement towards 'healthy' public policy and practice. b) An 'alliance' has been defined as a 'partnership...'. Integrating the overlapping definitions of both, an **'alliance for Health Promotion'** can be understood as a **partnership** [i.e. a *voluntary* agreement] between two or more parties or partners that pursue a set of *agreed upon* goals in Health Promotion [and work *cooperatively* towards a set of *shared* health outcomes]. Alliances often involve some form of *mediation* between the different partners in the definition of goals, ethical ground rules, joint action areas, and agreement on the *form* of cooperation. (WHO 1998a) One form of cooperation may be to create a network. The definition of a 'network' has been provided already above.

A network approach in Health Promotion -intermediate synthesis and discussion

Obviously, the *concepts of interorganizational forms used* in Health Promotion as in Public Health are *overlapping*. They vary regarding emphases on different qualities of relationships. An intersectoral collaboration could take the form of or include an alliance or partnership. An alliance or partnership may or may not be intersectoral but in any case emphasizes *voluntary* membership, *agreement and sharing* of goals, as well as 'cooperation' (in what ever way this may be defined). A **'network'** appears here to be a more particular organizational form than an alliance or partnership: while *agreed upon, common or shared* issues or concerns are emphasized as well, in addition *relationships* among members are further specified as *non-hierarchical* and based on *commitment and trust;*

and the work process to reach goals is specified not only as 'cooperative' but as *proactive and systematic.* In contrast to partnerships, alliances and networks, the term 'intersectoral action' for health does *not* necessarily imply that tasks, goals or issues addressed are common and agreed upon by all those involved.

As will be seen in chapter 2.4 on research results from the organizational sciences, the term 'alliance' may be better used as a type of organizational form similar to the term 'network' rather than as synonym for 'partnership'. **Alliances and networks can be seen as sharing core qualities but be distinguished by number of members or participants** (with alliances being small and networks bigger). This is not contradicting the definitions provided by the WHO Health Promotion Glossary but clarifies and specifies the terms and their relationships further. Already now it seems meaningful to speak on the one hand, of a general 'partnership' approach, and on the other of a more specific 'network approach' that builds on partnership. But again, these **concepts need further clarification**.

As mentioned before, 'networks' appear to be a particularly attractive organizational form for large scale implementations of the Settings approach. In the field internationally, they are being linked to notions of *spanning multiple levels of society* (local/ global; individual/ society), of *participation, innovation, and mediating functions.* Apparently, **'networks' are understood as part of needed 'infrastructures for Health Promotion'**, i.e.

"those human and material resources, organizational and administrative structures, policies, regulations and incentives which *facilitate an organized health promotion response* to public health issues and challenges" (WHO 1998a - italics not in original).

The fact that network features often referred to are trust, mutuality and sharing bring up the idea that (certain types of) such networks may also more directly contribute to the promotion of health: by contributing to an increase in 'social capital', i.e. an improvement in a lately much discussed and referred to social co-determinants of population health (see chap. 2.1). This point will be taken up later again, once the nature of networks in general and of those for developing Health Promoting Schools in particular are clarified further, from an organizational science perspective.

Diversity and lack of clarity of terminology and concepts of organizational relationships and forms is neither unique to Health Promotion or the WHO Health Promotion Glossary nor to Public Health. On the one hand, the situation reflects the increased recognition of the importance of organizational contexts for population level health improvements. On the other hand, it reflects the gap or separation of public health research and interorganizational research, and - as will be seen later - diversity and lack of consensus on theoretical or conceptual frameworks in the organizational sciences, too, in this regard. As the organizational form of 'network' is at the core of this research project, **the following chapters are dedicated to improve the understanding of the nature and effectiveness of networks** through considering both *experiential knowledge from the field of Health Promotion* (chap. 2.2.6 below) and *experiential knowledge and theoretical frameworks from the organizational sciences* (chap. 2.4). The former will help to guide a goal oriented exploration of the latter.

2.2.6 Large scale efforts to develop health promoting Settings: projects, movements, networks

As shown above there is: a) a lack of conceptual or analytic literature on a 'networking' or 'network' approach in the field Health Promotion (including the area of Health Promoting Schools); b) an increasing use of the network term in Health Promotion policy and practice; and c) an ongoing emergence or creation of 'networks of …' or 'networks for the development of…' Health Promoting Schools and other Settings around the world. The literature on this observable practice will now be reviewed to **unravel the current understandings and key features of such 'networks' as *applied* in the field of Health Promotion** up today.

Worldwide, many actors both individuals and organizations got involved in networks or similar organizational forms when engaging in creating health promoting Settings. But even minimal sets of baseline data concerning these networks (e.g. the number of participants/members, people reached, etc.) are publicly available only in *some* cases. In the light of both the movement like spreading of Health Promotion actions to implement the Settings approach worldwide (as documented e.g. during the 4th International Conference of Health Promotion, Jakarta 1997) and the paucity of written overviews and systematic analyses on and across 'Settings networks', the WHO Department for Health Promotion in 1997 initiated and guided a stock taking effort. This had two foci: Health Promotion development by world Regions in general, and *large scale efforts for the development of particular health promoting Settings* (from healthy cities, municipalities, and island states to health promoting schools, workplaces and hospitals). Authors were requested to pay particular attention to 'networks' and 'networking'.

The review confirms that starting in the mid 1980s, 'health promoting Settings' -projects and -networks have both spontaneously spread and been actively created around the world. Today, these range from

'Healthy Cities'-types of projects and networks to those for the development of health promoting schools, -hospitals and -workplaces. The various initiatives gained legitimacy and further momentum particularly through the support of WHO and its partners as well as some national governments (Green et al 2000). It is not intended to provide an overview of these large scale efforts in their entirety here. The aim is to derive that information that helps to develop an understanding of the role and forms of networking and networks in these contexts. Where feasible European developments or examples will receive special attention as European projects, programs or networks on Healthy Cities, Health Promoting Hospitals, Workplaces, etc. provide an important part of the history and/or environment of the "European Network of Health Promoting Schools", the case example in this pilot research.

International Healthy Cities 'projects', 'programs' and 'networks'

A **"healthy city"** has been defined as one "that is continually creating and improving those physical and social *environments* and expanding those *community resources* which *enable* people to mutually support each other in performing all the functions of life and in developing to their maximum potential." (WHO 1998a; WHO/EURO 1995 - italics not in original). The **WHO Healthy Cities Program** is a *long-term development project* that seeks to place health on the agenda of cities around the world, and to build a constituency of support for *public health at the local level*. It was the first health promoting 'Settings initiative' by WHO and a path finder for initiatives that followed. When looking at the foci or core concepts of the *three key developments that influenced this global program*, its major cornerstones or general orientations become quickly apparent: besides health development many aspects of coordination and cooperation among organizations and groups, public participation, and local context sensitivity. The first influential factor was and is the Ottawa Charter for Health Promotion (1986) whose foci and core concepts have been elaborated in chapter 2.2. The second influential development was and is the global 'Health for All' -strategy (WHO, UNICEF 1978) - with its emphasis on equity in health, prevention, *intersectoral cooperation*, community *participation*, and Primary Health Care. The third was and is the emergence of *local government* as a major player in development cooperation internationally - through the 'Agenda 21' on sustainable development in 1992, the 1996 UN Summit 'HABITAT II', and the related development of the 'local Agenda 21'. Related to this, all '*participatory* local governance', *partnership* models for service provision, *coordinated efforts across sectors and layers* of society (from service users to international agencies), *decentralization* of management and planning with higher level agencies in a policy and support role, etc. are emphasized. As shown in chapter 2.4 many of these concepts or orientations are also parts of modern organizational development and interorganizational co-operation approaches.

Experiences around the world show that a convergence of all *three* influences likely results in major Healthy Cities programs in countries involving a large number of towns, cities or municipalities. Overall, the work rests on the knowledge of the *environmental* co-determinants of health and the fact that *development activities* can bring both health hazards *and* health opportunities. (Goldstein 1998 - also for the information that follows)

Key actors and (network) structures for 'Healthy Cities' - development on a larger scale

From a global perspective it is clear that the development of Healthy Cities, -Villages or -Municipalities (here briefly subsumed under 'healthy cities') is both a WHO *program or project* as well as a *movement* independent from its originator. The WHO Regional Office for Europe (EURO) in the mid 1980s started the first Healthy Cities 'Project' with initially *11 cities* from different countries that agreed to participate. Such direct work with local authorities and actors rather than with national Health Ministries *on* such work was fairly unusual for WHO. The healthy city idea spread rapidly to cities and towns across Europe and subsequently the European 'Healthy City Project' influenced the development of such projects in other regions of the world. Today over thousand cities and towns world wide are involved in healthy cities projects and often networks, most of them in Europe. Exact figures are not available (Goldstein 1998). In many countries and regions healthy cities *'networks' have emerged* over time and as shown in table 2.2.5, overall **the term 'network'** rather than the terms 'project' or 'program' became **predominantly used as label for the organizational form which links healthy cities** to a greater or lesser extent - at sub-national and national but also international levels.

Since 1995, this development was supported at *global* level, by the 'WHO Inter-Regional Program on Healthy Cities' and with WHO Regional and Country Offices increasingly involved. In some individual cases of healthy cities, other UN and development agencies cooperate or provide some funding such as in the Western Pacific Region. Today independent international (WHO) networks, programs and/or projects exist in most regions of the world (see table 2.2.5).

	Africa Francophone Countries	South East Asia	Western Pacific	American Region^ North America	Eastern Mediterranean Region	Europe
Number of Network members*	~10			US: smaller or bigger (in one case 36) Canada: 100+		"WHO HC project": ~35 in national networks: Σ>1000"
Organizational forms by level:						
sub-national level (district, regional):				Several State/ Provincial HC Networks (some with support centers)		
national level:	a WHO/CC in 1 country	HC 'programs' in several countries	at least three national HC networks	USA: Coalition for Healthier Cities and Communities	4 national networks of HC; 1 'Maghrebin HC network'	national HC networks in 27+ countries
international level / WHO Regional level:	Francophone cross-country Network of HC (with co-ordinating office); Lately regional HC conferences (also Anglophone)	networking support by WHO/ SEARO	Healthy Cities as part of Healthy Island network WHO Policy 'New Horizons in Health' (HP/ Health protection) WHO Healthy Urban Environment framework		1 'Gulf HC network'; 'general strategy on health & environment. in cities' WHO progr. (network) on HC Regional HC conference '94/ frequent events for HC coordinators;	5-year WHO 'HC Projects' (since 1987) Several 'Multi City Action Plans'
global level:	'WHO Inter-Regional Program on Healthy Cities' (1995-2000) (World Health Day 1996 on 'Healthy Cities')					

* Number of Healthy Cities, Municipalities, Villages, and/or Towns; - " Tsourso/ Farrington 1997

^ Latin America and Caribbean:: about 300 Healthy Municipalities (HM) estimated (Goldstein 1998) but *no single specific structure* for technical cooperation among them yet; at national level *functional teams* in some countries (on Health Promotion (HP), health services, and health and environment); 1st conference of majors being planned by the Pan American Health Organization (WHO/AMRO).

HC: Healthy City/ Cities   US: USA   WHO: World Health Organization
SEARO: South East Asia Region   progr.: program   WHO/CC: WHO Collaborating Center

Table 2.2.5: Networks of Healthy Cities by Region - structural information (created on the base of Goldstein 1998)

An as of now unique effort to provide a global overview on Healthy City, - Village or -Municipality development by Goldstein (1998) shows: Information on the range of both *individual* Healthy Cities projects and

'Healthy Cities projects, programs or networks' that *link* such cities by regions, countries and/or cultural or language ties, is incomplete, often not comparable, and/or not accessible. While table 2.2.5 illustrates this fact it nevertheless provides insight into the **organizational structures in support of healthy cities development** world wide.

Goldstein's data show that in some regions (such as Europe and North America) the initiation of some individual Healthy Cities 'projects' by WHO and/or others has started a kind of *'movement'* that led to the creation of Healthy Cities networks at national and/or State or Provincial levels. In other regions such as Africa, South East Asia and the Eastern Mediterranean Region, WHO (and partners) not only initiate individual Healthy Cities projects locally but serve as *active supporters support of networking or network building* among them. In again other regions such as Latin America, 'Healthy Municipalities' has become a kind of movement within overall democratization and decentralization processes without any systematic networking or network building among them. In at least one case, the Western Pacific Region, the development of Healthy Cities has been undertaken *within an existing international network structure* in the field of Health Promotion, the Healthy Islands network.

Overall, this short review shows that there is not yet the 'network' approach or the international 'project' or 'program' approach for the development of Healthy Cities, Villages etc. on a larger scale to refer to if developing an assessment framework and indicators for 'international networks' for the development of Health Promoting Schools as in this research project. But what can be seen is that **a 'network' approach however defined seems to be the preferred choice when it comes to linking health promoting Settings such as healthy cities within and across national borders**. It is also worth noting that where WHO has established a 'Regional' (i.e. European, Western Pacific, …) program or formal project on healthy cities, there, several national and also intercountry Healthy Cities networks exist. Also, from over a decade of experience in Europe it is known that Healthy Cities **networks not only may benefit the cities involved but can be strategically used** by e.g. international organizations to achieve their goals. "Extensive networking between cities" has been praised as having "developed into a formidable platform for innovation and change across Europe" (Tsouros, Farrington 1997 p276) So called 'Multi City Action Plans' (MCAPs) are among the tools that have been used in this regard: As they link Healthy Cities from different countries that wish to collaborate closely on a common health issue or topic (e.g. AIDS or occupational health) these **'Multi city action plans' likely represent international 'networks',** networks that are embedded within or even cutting across the larger and general international healthy cities' network or project structures mentioned above. Each city simultaneously starts its own program while sharing information on situation analysis, strategies, progress made, etc. with the other cities. Particularly in Europe, the 'Healthy Cities approach' and the 'Multi City Action Plans' have become an important strategy to implement European level programs on particular health issues at local level (e.g. on diabetes, accidents, AIDS) - assumingly without compromising the principle of local level priority setting as the Health Promotion concept is being applied.

Formal regulation of **membership or participation** in above mentioned international (WHO) programs, project or networks on healthy cities, villages or municipalities development seems hardly an issue. The WHO initiatives seem more or less open to all cities or villages interested to join and movement like spreading of this health promoting Settings approach is welcomed. As of now only in Europe the situation is different: The 'WHO *European* Healthy City *Project*' formally *designates* each participating city as a "Healthy City" - but only after the city makes certain commitments or fulfills certain criteria. And the number of project participants is kept small. Thus, only a small proportion of all European cities that are members of *national and/or subnational* Healthy Cities networks or programs are designated 'WHO project cities' (roughly 35); the about 1000 other cities are considered to be 'associated' cities or part of the European Healthy Cities 'movement'.

Means to facilitate linkages *among* 'Healthy Cities' and organizations supportive of healthy city development employed include regular 'inter-country meetings', newsletters and the circulation of technical reports, and an international database of Healthy Cities project coordinators. In 1999, WHO Regional 'Healthy Cities conferences' and '-workshops' were held in all regions. - Links among cities that take part in WHO's Healthy Cities programs, projects or networks are based on particular **structures and processes *within* each 'healthy city'**, particularly: one *designated* 'Healthy City project *coordinator*' and the implementation of activities often through *(intersectoral) task forces or groups* which include community members. Core strategies used to create a 'healthy city' include: a) *wide consultation processes* to develop a 'vision' of the future direction and to review strengths and qualities of the city (important to mobilize people), and b) the formulation of a *'municipal health plan'* to both raise awareness of health and environmental issues particularly among local authorities, NGOs, communities and mobilize resources for actions. Such plans may include to create elemental health promoting Settings (such as - schools or -workplaces) within the larger contextual Setting 'city'. And the preparation of such plans usually opens *new channels of communication* among stakeholders and can facilitate their ongoing cooperation, is a means to achieve *intersectoral collaboration,* and is supported by WHO through progress reviews and facilitating the exchange of technologies and models of good practice. Chapters 2.4 and 5 will explain the importance of such aspects for interorganizational work to promote health.

The European approach to the development of Healthy Cities across the region

The European 'Healthy Cities Project' inspired and influenced the creation of the 'European Network of Health Promoting Schools' (ENHPS), the network case in focus of this research project. In both initiatives WHO/EURO plays a key (initiating and guiding) role. The organizational approach taken by WHO to develop Healthy Cities is as the name 'European Healthy Cities *Project*' indicates, a *time limited project* approach to create a *limited number* of (model) Healthy Cities *throughout* Europe. Since 1997, three *subsequent, formal, 5-year 'project phases'* were implemented - with a group of 'participating' cities that underwent some changes over time. 'Phase I' (1987-1992) involved 30 designated "WHO project cities" from 16 countries; it was continued in 'phase II' (1993-1998) involving 42 designated cities from 23 countries; and currently 'phase III' is under way (1999-2004). While over the years the number of Healthy Cities designated as 'WHO project cities' remained at a scale of 30-40, large numbers of additional cities started their 'Healthy Cities projects' across Europe - according to Tsouros and Farrington (1997) until recently about thousand cities in 27 or more countries which are referred to as "associated" with the WHO bound 'Healthy City Project'. In many countries these individual cities form national networks of Healthy Cities with a *national coordinator or coordinating center* in a supportive role. (see www.who.dk) Organizational mechanisms for cross-border networking were for long limited to the small number of designated participants in the formal *'European WHO Healthy Cities Project'*. But recently, a *"network of European networks" (EURONET)* has been established with a 'coordinating center' in France. Together with a small number of 'WHO Collaborating Centers on Healthy Cities' spread in Western Europe this forms now the main infrastructure for the further development of Healthy Cities on a larger scale in Europe.

When considering the *world wide* developments sketched out above, it can be concluded that the limited data available suggest: **There is a certain pattern for the large scale dissemination of the Healthy Cities concept emerging**: Once some local examples in a region or country have been implemented, and once the Healthy City idea is being picked up by other cities (with or without the active support of an agency external to that city), *networking* among Healthy Cities is starting - 'spontaneously', i.e. independent from the initiator of the first projects, or strategically initiated and fostered by some agency (usually WHO but also others). Particularly WHO and also some of its partners appear to actively use or foster a 'network approach' in support of the creation of Healthy Cities in countries. Even in Europe, where WHO itself continues to pursue a exclusive 'Healthy Cities Project' with a small number of designated participants, *networks of cities* and lately also a *network of national Healthy Cities networks* (EURONET) have emerged. This supports the assumption that the organizational form of 'networks' is one quite suitable for implementing the health promoting Settings approach. However, there seem to be different ways of network building (e.g. more planned or formalized approaches versus a movement like emergence of networks) and some may be more suitable in some cultures and regions than in others.

International 'networks' for the development of "Health Promoting Schools"

The concept of the "Health Promoting School" (HPS) is generally accepted in many countries of the world, among professionals as well as an increasing number of high-level decision makers (WHO 1996a, p8; WHO 1997). Its history and 'rise' is elaborated in the case study in chapters 5.1 and 5.2 on the European network from which the concept originates. The general underlying purpose is to **combine education and health promotion in order to realise the potential of both.** The WHO Global School Health Initiative and WHO Health Promotion Glossary provide the following general definition:

A Health Promoting School (HPS) "can be characterised as a school constantly strengthening its capacity as a healthy setting for living, learning and working" (WHO 1998a). It "must be more than a collection of different programmes and services. It must be an organism, a living thing in which all of the parts work together" (WHO 1996d, p4).

Through this concept, the health not only of the *pupils*, but also of *school personnel and community members* are being addressed. The following set of **characteristics of a Health Promoting School** (HPS) as outlined by a WHO Expert Committee in 1995 represents a reference framework used internationally (WHO 1997c): A Health Promoting School

- fosters health *and* learning with all the measures at its disposal;
- engages health and education officials, teachers, students, parents, and community leaders in efforts to promote health;

- strives to provide a healthy environment, school health education, and school health services along with school/community projects and outreach, health promotion programmes for staff, nutrition and food safety programmes, opportunities for physical education and recreation, and opportunities for counselling, social support and mental health promotion;
- implements policies, practices and other measures that respect an individual's self-esteem, provide multiple opportunities for success, and acknowledge good efforts and intentions as well as personal achievements; and
- strives to improve the health of school personnel, families and community members as well as students, and works with community leaders to help them understand how the community contributes to health and education.

As the 'Healthy Cities' concept also the Health Promoting Schools (HPS) concept is currently being disseminated and implemented by means of **several international networks** around the world, by world 'Regions' and sub-Regions thereof. As mentioned earlier the first one, the "European Network of Health Promoting Schools (ENHPS)", was established in 1992 followed after three years by a Pacific Network for developing Health Promoting Schools and soon by one in Latin America. Further initiatives on such network building are on the way in South East Asia and sub-regions of Africa and the Western Pacific. With the exception of the first network in Europe, all networks or network initiatives are initiated and supported by the **'WHO Global School Health Initiative'**, a global level *'project'* at WHO headquarters that aims at increasing the number of schools that can truly be called 'Health Promoting Schools'. The goal is pursued by four strategies one of which is "creating *networks* and *alliances* for the development of Health Promoting Schools". Besides the 'Regional networks' just mentioned a so-called **'global alliance'** has been formed to enable teachers' representatives organizations to improve health through schools (WHO 2002). As of now this 'alliance' includes three UN organizations (UNESCO, UNICEF, WHO), the NGO 'Education International', and three national organizations from both public health and education (USA, Netherlands). This 'alliance' may be an interorganizational 'network' in itself. A second strategy, 'strengthening national capacities' to improve health through schools emphasizes as the former collaborative action, here *intersectoral collaboration* between health and education agencies. The other two strategies focus more on the improvement of school health programs as such, one on 'research', the other one on 'building capacity to advocate' for improved programs. (WHO 1996d) - The term 'network' is also used for an 'online-network of websites' created to further disseminate information on Health Promoting Schools and to strengthen existing 'partnerships'. This shows that the Global School Health Initiative as many others in Public Health uses the term 'network' in various ways and links the organizational forms of 'networks' and 'alliances' with the notion of 'partnership'. Overall, this Global Initiative seeks to mobilize and strengthen health promotion and education at *various levels* of society: local, national, 'Regional' and global, which obviously needs appropriate organizational mechanisms that link the global actor WHO with those at other levels.

The general directions for these development and activities stem from the Ottawa Charter (1986), the Jakarta Declaration (1997) and the 1995 WHO Expert Committee Recommendations on Comprehensive Schools Health Education and Promotion (WHO 1996d) which - as explained in chapter 2.2 and 1 before - support not only the basic Health Promotion and health promoting Settings approach taken by the Global School Health Initiative but also to a greater or lesser extent the organizational cooperative approach taken for large scale action. Additional insight stems from the identification of **barriers for the development of Health Promoting Schools** as identified by national, district and local education and health workers in developing and developed countries: inadequate vision and strategic *planning*; inadequate understanding and acceptance of programmes; lack of responsibility and accountability; *inadequate collaboration and co-ordination* among persons addressing health in schools; and lack of *programme infrastructure*, including financial, human and material resources as well as *organising mechanisms*. In light of these barriers the 1995 WHO Expert Committee acknowledged the importance of major strategies such as *intersectoral collaboration* and *national direction and policy ideally encouraged and assisted by* intergovernmental and a wide range of other organisations. **It is expected that coordinating mechanisms at the different levels of society form policy into action and build consensus that health is a concern for all sectors of society**. (WHO 1996b p20/22) This is mirrored in the ten recommendations of this global level Committee, particularly in recommendation number six and ten: to develop "policies, legislation, and guidelines (...) to ensure the identification, allocation, mobilisation, and co-ordination of resources at the local, national, and international levels to support health" (no.6); to further develop "international support (...) to enhance the ability of Member States, local communities, and schools to promote health and education" (no.10). This includes health promotion action such as *advocacy* towards decision makers and the general public for school health promotion, fostering *active collaboration between* health and education ministries, developing school health *committees* and *networks* that include representatives from the public and NGO sectors, developing *concerted action* by international organisations such as UN agencies and NGOs, as well as *co-ordination* among international organisations and countries "to share efforts, *reduce fragmentation and duplication* of effort, and establish a *broad vision* of comprehensive and integrated school health programmes" (WHO 1996d, p10 and 12 - italics not in original).

Unfortunately, only limited information is available or accessible on the particular 'Regional networks' for the development of Health Promoting Schools. A global overview similar to that on international Healthy Cities projects or networks is lacking and documents available focus rather on the content of the HPS concept and supportive international policies and related processes rather than the network dimension itself. (e.g. Birdthistle 1999) However, on the base of the information available and the researchers internal knowledge from her work at WHO it can be said that a general pattern is nevertheless visible: The WHO Regional networks on Health Promoting Schools involve in all cases the WHO Regional Offices in a key or *leading role*, sometimes jointly with other intergovernmental organizations. These network initiatives are all *multi-level* systems, but in this regard general information available gives the **impression that *two types of Regional networks* for the development of Health Promoting Schools have emerged**: A first type emphasizes networking only among national agencies (particularly Ministries of Health and of Education) and international organizations in a Region and, thus, represents a *two level* system spanning national and international levels. This then encourages and supports the national agencies to implement *separate additional* mechanisms *within* their countries for Health Promoting Schools development (which may take various forms including national networks of some kind). The second type of network emphasizes the direct involvement and networking of the health promoting *schools*, i.e. the local level and the Settings concerned; but it *also* involves the national/ ministerial level. The latter is thus a *three level* system spanning local, national and international levels. Whether and how the schools as local actors may be part of an international network needs further examination. But the second network type reminds of the international Healthy Cities networks or projects, which link first of all the *local* actors (the cities) across country borders. However, the little and incomparable information available leaves this idea of a network typology in the area of international networks for the development of Health Promoting Schools as a speculation. The in depths case study of one of these networks in chapter 5 will provide further insight.

International networks for the development of Health Promoting Schools and other initiatives - intermediate synopsis and discussion

Also this short review of international initiatives such as 'networks' in the specific area of *school* health promotion shows: the identification and implementation of more appropriate or 'new' *organising mechanisms* (at and across levels of societies and the education and health sectors) is the major challenge - besides (or in some cases rather than) the *content* of such efforts. The 'Health Promoting Schools' concept provides a widely recognised *common vision and goal.* This is an essential element of successful collaboration in Health Promotion and beyond, as shown in the following chapters 2.2.7 and 2.4. Also the observable practice and related policies from the school health arena support the assumption that a 'network approach' and similar organisational forms such as 'alliances' are not only attractive but appropriate organisational mechanisms for implementing the health promoting Settings approach on larger scales. And there are hints that there are several types of networks and approaches to their creation.

As of now, documents on *other international networks* to implement the Health Promotion concept do not contain much information on their 'network' dimension the analysis of which would further the understanding of the 'network approach' in Health Promotion beyond what has been already discussed above. Usually there is only information such as on actors involved, the health promotion goal pursued, and the policy environment and international recommendations that give legitimacy and explain the effort at stake. The **overall impression** is: the **field of Health Promotion is still fairly busy with explaining and further advocating for the Health Promotion concept and Settings approach as such**, and the **forms of their large scale implementation such as 'networks' are not yet the focus of documentation and assessment efforts**. However, the *'Regions for Health Network'* in Europe (RHN), an example of application of the 'network approach' in Public Health beyond the health promoting Settings approach, at its 4th Annual Conference in 1996 did reflect on the network approach chosen: The participants from various countries and networks agreed that there were *two types of 'networking'*: an *organized or formal* type such as the WHO networks, and a *more informal* type of networking largely on the basis of *personal contacts*. They felt that, generally, organized networking tends to be stronger at *higher* levels, such as the international or national level, while at the local level networks tend to be more informal, - although *both can have a place at all levels.* In any case, the *key to successful networking* identified was the 'motivation to work together' and a 'keen sense of solidarity'.

(WHO/EURO 1997 p40).

The health policy focused Regions for Health Network (RHN) shows some basic general features as the settings focused networks. *WHO initiated* the network, here *to achieve change* in the *thinking about, and action* for the protection, maintenance and promotion of health in regions. It was founded in 1992 *in response to the need for a systematic exchange* of ideas and experience in strengthening the focus of the sub-national, here regional level in countries on achieving 'Health for All' - which shows similarities to the Healthy Cities networks which focuses on the next lower (local) systems level. However, the RHN network aims to support *national* commitment to the European 'Health for All'-policy (see chap. 2.2) by developing appropriate *health policies at regional level*. As to its structural features, the network is supported by a *secretariat* at WHO/EURO. Guided by decisions of the *'Annual General Meeting'*, a *'Steering Committee'* (of six members and the secretariat) plans and monitors *joint projects* and the general functioning of the network. (WHO/EURO 1994a) It remains to be examined whether the governing structures of the networks for developing health promoting Settings such as schools differ from those of this inter-regional network.

Overall, this review of observable and documented **practice in Health Promotion** as to international networks of the development of Settings and similar networks confirms earlier judgments: that in the everyday practice of protecting and promoting health, the **term 'network'** is *often used but seldom clearly defined* and that *only lately systematic reflections on 'networks' and 'networking'* become a documented issue. While research on such networks is lacking documents available do show that **these networks have something to do with inter-organizational and intersectoral collaboration, 'partnership' and alliance building, and similar concepts and practices**. And a few systematic reviews of the effectiveness of 'intersectoral action', collaborative 'partnerships' or 'alliances' in health promotion unravels some valuable lessons learned for achieving the goal of this research project, i.e. to develop an assessment tool for international networks for developing Health Promoting Schools.

2.2.7 Searching for 'good' collaborative practice -lessons learned in Health Promotion

'Intersectoral action', 'partnerships', 'alliances' and the issue of effectiveness

The question of what are desired forms of 'intersectoral action', 'partnerships', 'alliances' and particularly what makes them successful or effective receives slowly more researchers' attention. First systematic reviews of published studies across a variety of collaborative approaches have been found to unravel the lessons learned (such as Gillies 1998 on 'alliances' and 'partnerships' for health promotion, and Roussos and Fawcett 2000 on 'collaborative partnerships' for community health improvement). Some search for an appropriate theoretical basis to guide future research and practice (such as O'Neill et al 1997 on 'intersectoral health-related interventions'); others point to the lack of theories that define the process of such action and related activities (such as coalition building) and instead pragmatically suggest a model for its understanding (e.g. Nutbeam, Harris 1999b). This situation reflects the need for and interest in identifying indicators and conditions for 'good practice' at the level of collaborative organizational forms that emerged and appear to be useful in the promotion and protection of health at the population level.

With regard to **'intersectoral health-related action'**, talked about and called for in public health since long, a review by O'Neill et al (1997) did show a striking paucity of writings informed by systematic research or theory and dominance of summaries of lessons learned by 'trial and error'. Handbooks on health education or promotion theory, research and practice show the importance of and at the same time 'weak spots' in knowledge about organizational development and interorganizational collaboration in support of health development (e.g. Glanz et al 1997; Nutbeam, Harris 1999b). At the same time, the knowledge about macro level co-determinants of health has renewed the interest of public health agencies in intersectoral action and led to several attempts to derive lessons learned about conditions for success informed through experience and research (e.g. Health Canada 2000; WHO 1997c; Harris, Wise et al 1995). However, as intersectoral action can take many forms - (Harris et al identify 13 types only one of which is 'networking' such as 'coalition' building between individuals or organizations) - a review of the various individual descriptions and 'lessons learned' does not promise to well inform this research project on interorganizational networks for Health Promotion. Thus, only systematic reviews of a range of case studies or stories and syntheses of literature have been considered, and only if undertaken by authors familiar with the Health Promotion approach.

Conditions for success or failure of intersectoral (interorganizational) action for health

Building and sustaining relationships between sectors towards common goals is a difficult task. Many of the conditions for success or failure are in place long before any specific action is taken and, therefore, it is important to not only have a *planned approach* to interorganizational action and sustainability, but also to understand the *context* in which it is being undertaken and the ability of the *infrastructure* of the organizations to deliver. Several factors of importance to understand the process by which organizations or parts of organization work together and mechanisms of success have been identified in these three areas (Harris, Wise et al 1995; Nutbeam, Harris 1999b). *Factors related to the context include*: the reasons why or necessity of organizations' working together; their openness to collaboration and change which is more likely if collaboration helps them in several ways to (a) pursue their core business, b) attract or protect resources, c) protect or gain in their areas of influence and/or d) be seen as good corporate citizens); the motivation of organizations to collaborate (as it is linked to their willingness to commit themselves and to take risks); and opportunities for interorganizational action (e.g. the fit of joint actions with immediate organization priorities such as a response to an event, crises, reform initiative, etc.). *With view to the infrastructure to undertake interorganizational actions and use opportunities relevant factors include*: the level of organizational support for an interorganizational activity (including compatibility of structures and decision-making processes); adequate levels of resources (such as time, money, infrastructures); an appropriately skilled workforce; and existing or new interorganizational relationships, formal or informal (as mechanisms within which actions can be developed and conflicts resolved). Finally, *with regard to a planned approach to action and sustainability factors of relevance include*: a clear recognition of the reasons for the interorganizational collaboration, and agreement on processes of defining goals and identifying solutions and on roles of members in the implementation; acknowledgment of the emergent and changing nature of processes and flexibility in negotiating roles and responsibilities accordingly; definition of clearly articulated and achievable goals that are understood and valued by all members; agreement on a way of working (e.g. starting 'small' to build trust and confidence before tackling bigger or more complex issues); commitment for a defined time frame and opportunities for renegotiation of tasks, roles, and relationships; commitment to joint ownership; and allocation of resources (staff, space, money, information, administrative support). Taken together these factors provide cornerstones for complex analyses of interorganizational actions (such as those across sectoral boundaries).

In light of the paucity of literature on intersectoral health-related actions O'Neill et al (1997) build on coalition theory and particularly work by Gamson when identifying five key conditions for intersectoral health-related action: a) the *initial distribution of resources* among participants (including a sense of purpose, information, prestige, contacts, authority derived from size, wealth, and so on); b) the expected *'payoffs' or 're-*

wards' that would not be obtained if members were to act alone (with *future rather than immediate* payoffs at the core, such as the expected value of future decisions); c) each member's *(non-utilitarian) preference to join with any other actor* whatever that actor's control of resources might be; d) the *'rules of the game' or 'effective decision point'* that specify the proportion and nature of resources formally necessary to control decisions (e.g. majority rules, or (often informal) agreement to aim toward consensus or unanimity in decisions, and/or to resolve conflicts in a consensual way); e) the 'organizational context' which refers here to rules defined by the organizations of the individual actors (not to the organizational environment of intersectoral collaboration). The application of this framework to three in depths case studies at local and provincial level (including coalitions among public agencies, and a public/NGO mix) indicates that the *key to whether a coalition is successful* depends on the mixture of the five parameters.

O'Neill et al highlight what often is not made explicit or only briefly mentioned: Intersectoral groups are made up of members that have co-operative and conflictual interests at the same time. To 'succeed', i.e. to emerge, maintain itself over time, and realize activities related to its goals, *co-operative interests have to dominate conflictual ones*, convergence is to dominate over divergence. The case studies indicate that for this to happen, the organizational contexts must allow that the individuals involved can work together and *relationships with authorities need to nurture convergence* within the group. Dedication to a cause (such as Health Promotion) and a *sense of purpose* as both a resource and an incentive or reward to members ensure domination of co-operation over conflict. The same applies to *strong positive ties* among members and to the *search for consensus and the use of non-authoritarian ways of restoring* it. However, the authors point to the exploratory nature of their research and methodological limitations that constrain conclusions that can be drawn.

Features of effective 'alliances' or 'partnerships' for health promotion

Gillies (1998) asks which kinds of 'alliances' or 'partnerships' for health promotion work effectively and why. Her literature review of (quasi-)experimental studies identifies two types of 'alliances' and 'partnerships' involving actors in public, private or non-governmental sectors: the majority involves 'one or more collaborators among individuals or groups or organizations' in the promotion of health but which 'do *not* seek to affect the underlying systems or structures (…) for health promotion' (but e.g. individual behavior); a few involve 'one or more collaborators among institutions, organizations or groups' which 'seek to affect the structural determinants of health'. Most studies addressed a mix of interorganizational and inter-person or inter-group alliances or partnerships and predominantly focused on 'micro level' changes (individual behaviors). Even for more narrow focused health promotion activities the review shows: The stronger the representation of the community and the greater the *community involvement* in the practical activities of health promotion, the greater the impact and the more sustainable the gains. *Durable structures which facilitate a sharing of decision-making* such as school and community coordinating councils or employee-employer-committees are key factors in successful partnerships for the promotion of health. *Mechanisms for involving local people* in planning and *providing opportunity for dissent* are important.

The complementary analysis of a set of unpublished case studies of (predominantly interorganizational) 'alliances' and 'partnerships' for health promotion collected from around the world did show that most of such practice aims at changes at community or higher systems levels, emphasizes sharing of power, responsibility and authority for change and the need to build in flexibility to allow for changes in direction needed due to structural changes in the wider (inter)national environment. Core elements of 'good partnership or alliance development' appear to be *relevant needs assessment* combined with the setting up of *committees crossing professional and lay boundaries to steer, guide and account for* the activities and programs implemented. (Gillies 1998)

These findings are well complemented by a recent comprehensive review of published studies of 'collaborative partnerships' for community health improvement by Roussos and Fawcett (2000). In contrast to Gillies' review it is a) not limited to (quasi-)experimental designs and b) focuses on partnerships that aim at population and systems level changes (not individual level change). A 'collaborative partnership' is here more clearly defined, as an alliance of *people and organizations* from *multiple* sectors working together to achieve a *common* purpose. Research in this area faces methodological challenges similarly to Health Promotion in general and various measurements of partnership effectiveness are used. Nevertheless,

"some empirical evidence and consistent reports among the reviewed studies [has been found] for seven *interconnected and modifiable factors that potentially enhance partnership ability to create environmental conditions* related to improved behavioral and population-level health outcomes" (Roussos/ Fawcett 2000 p383):

Factors enhancing partnership capacity to create systems change for health

First, having a **clear vision and mission** helps to generate *support and awareness* for the partnership, *reduces conflicting agendas*, helps identify *allies*, and *minimizes time costs and distractions* from appropriate action. A mission or goal may articulate work at a *continuum of outcomes* from categorical 'health' issues such as infant mortality to more fundamental social determinants of health such as income disparities. Aiming at, for example, 'creating a healthy community' is not specific enough. *The process used to develop* a vision and mission may be as important as the product: Full and representative participation in planning of all relevant stakeholders may help generate and sustain participation. *Periodic review and renewal* of the mission and vision may help a partnership adapt to emerging concerns.

Second, **action planning for systems change** describes the process of identifying what community and systems changes to facilitate, who will produce them and by when, and how to gain support and minimize opposition in the process of bringing about a given environmental change. *Benefits* from action planning include not only *higher rates of community change* but *increased membership* (particularly from outside the health sector), *greater sustainability* of events, and *adoption of activities by other* organizations outside the partnership. Action planning focuses attention on the way to create change, and helps develop accountability ad ownership of responsibility. However, action planning may also lead to internal *conflicts, invite potential opposition*, or contribute to the dissolution of a partnership, an underlying factor of which may be *time limitation for planning*. The latter is often imposed from outside and may force decisions and limit the use of planning to build a support *network among* initial and potential *members* of the *partnership*.

A third factor is **developing and supporting leadership**, i.e. the process of persuasion or example by means of which an individual or leadership team induces a group to pursue objectives held by the leader or shared by his or her followers. Leadership is a *most often* reported 'internal' or 'organizational' *factor for a partnership's effectiveness in creating change* at community or systems level. *Loss* of leadership may be adversely associated with rates of community change and vice versa. By using *democratic and consensus decision-making methods*, leaders my increase *member's satisfaction*, broaden community participation, and improve overall *coalition effectiveness*. Leaders can also *limit* change by surrounding themselves only with very similar others (similar professional, social, economic status).

Core competencies related to *effective leadership* include communication, meeting facilitation, negotiation, and networking. Given the variety of leadership skills needed partnerships may benefit from a *leadership team* (or core group) of people with a variety of experiences and skills, and/or from promoting (community) *'champions'* who work for desired changes in specific sectors of for specific objectives. Partnerships with *dispersed leadership* may be less vulnerable to manipulation, reduced efficacy, or dissolution than those relying on one leader only. - Different *leadership skills* may be more useful during *different stages* of partnership development: the *early* stages may require greater *facilitation and listening* skills to help engage a diverse and representative membership.; *later,* when a strong identity and community presence has been developed, *negotiation and advocacy skills* may help bring about desired changes even if these are politically less feasible.

Documentation and evaluation systems that focus on *intermediate outcomes* enhance the functioning of a partnership by helping to identify and provide **feedback** on what is and is not working. A focus on intermediate outcomes can help to document progress, celebrate accomplishments, identify barriers to progress, and redirect efforts to potentially more effective activities. The long time period required to change population level health outcomes limits the use of behavioral and community-level indicators in guiding the day-to-day activities of a partnership.

Technical assistance includes the training and *support needed to implement and sustain a collaborative partnership.* It may be provided from outside the partnership or by members with specific expertise, and in person or through Internet based support systems. It may be directed at core competencies of the partners or members (such as situation assessment, leadership development, meeting facilitation, action planning, program development and implementation, evaluation, and fundraising). It should be context-sensitive (i.e. adjust to reflect the type and level of chosen focus, available resources, the developmental stage of the collaborative partnership, and current skills and experiences). Important is that members of a partnership are able (and enabled) to identify their own needs and secure appropriate technical assistance accordingly.

Financial and other resources for work that last long enough to effect intended outcomes such as population level health improvements is crucial. The ability of a partnership to secure such resources may predict its sustainability and indicate its performance capacity. Where *staff* is hired that can facilitate systems change is hired increased rates of desired changes have been found. Financial security may depend on a partnership's *ability to demonstrate its value* to those concerned and its *contribution to desired changes* and population level outcomes.

'Making outcomes matter' to all relevant stakeholders is the last factor found to improve collaborative partnership's effectiveness, particularly with view to appropriate *intermediate* outcomes (here environmental changes) to sustain momentum, interest, and funding. Documentation and communication of success to stakeholders are important. Funding organizations can help 'make outcomes matter', for example, by using intermediate outcomes as evidence of effectiveness as well as distant outcomes.

In addition to these seven factors that enhance the effectiveness of collaborative partnerships for community health in achieving systems or environmental changes some **'broader contributors' to effectiveness** have been identified (Roussos/ Fawcett 2000 p388):

First, and as already addressed in chapter 2.1, some of the **social and economic (co-) determinants of health** are often stronger predictors of population-level health outcomes than many public health interventions. And they influence whether and how partnerships for health improvement work. Second, *civic trust* seems to influence, and be influenced by, the formation, development, and effectiveness of collaborative partnerships. **Social capital** (explained in chap. 2.1) may be both an intervening variable facilitating the relationships needed for collaboration, and a dependent variable or by product of partnerships that influence valued outcomes related to community health and development. Third, the **context or conditions that give rise** to a collaborative partnership can influence its growth and potential effect, such as: the *history* of previous collaboration on related issues; the *kind of reasons* for forming the collaboration (e.g. a felt concern and/or opportunities for external funding); and *preexisting programs and initiatives* related to or potentially affecting the collaboration or its outcomes (they are sources of partners, opposition, or effects independent of the partnership). The *primary impetus for formation* of a collaborative partnership can contribute to its effectiveness by influencing who participates and why (public funding may favor certain organizational partners; an acute health concern may first mobilize many partners and then be unsustainable). *Externally created time pressure* (e.g. through funding policies or mechanisms) may lead to rushing into action without sufficient partnership formation, planning, or competence building. A fourth broad contributor to partnership effectiveness is **community control in agenda setting**, i.e. the process of determining what concerns will be addressed and what are acceptable means of addressing them. It is a question of exercising power who identifies goals and indicators of effectiveness. (Roussos, Fawcett 2000) This last point addresses the latent challenge in Health Promotion of balancing experiential knowledge of local people and their concerns, and epidemiological data in choosing what to address and how locally.

Roussos and Fawcett (2000) develop a set of **recommendations**. **To enhance practice, collaborative partnerships should** a) *frame and communicate a clear vision and mission* that is broadly understood, defines the problem and acceptable solutions in a manor that engages (not blames) organizations or people and allows a range of strategies and environmental changes needed to the chosen concern. They should b) establish *ongoing action planning that* identifies specific systems changes to be sought to effect widespread behavior change and community level health improvements. And c), the core membership of a partnership should develop *widespread leadership*, engaging multiple (community) sectors in *facilitating change within their own peer group, organization, and context*. Collaborative partnerships should also **systematically document** their progress in facilitating environmental changes (e.g. systems change), an intermediate marker in the long process of effecting more distant population level outcomes. Evaluation should become part of an ongoing and integrated support system to guide decisions and facilitate continuous improvements. To set **conditions for success** the authors recommend:

- *Human and financial support* for the work of a collaborative partnership should be identified *early and continue throughout* the life of a partnership, support actions that *effect environmental changes* most valued by the local community and those more likely to influence population level health outcomes. Decisions on allocating resources should reflect a *sharing of risks, resources, and responsibilities* for common work among the organizations involved.

- A partnership should have *access to support and technical assistance* for enhancing competencies of its members relevant to different stages of partnership development (from needs assessment to program implementation and resource generation for sustainability).

- All those involved *including funding organizations should help make (mid and long term) outcomes matter* (through e.g. resource allocation, recognition, reward systems, etc.).

- Efforts should focus on *building capacity locally* to address issues that matter to local people in the long term (e.g. 10 years or more), across a range of health related concerns, and across generations of dispersed leadership (e.g. age range of leadership teams).

- The conditions under which efforts to improve health and well being occur and that lead to unequal outcomes, including the broader social co-determinants of health (social ties, income inequality, etc.), must be addressed and changed.

Inherent challenges for collaborative partnerships

Even the most competent collaborative partnership will face challenges such as: engaging those that experience the issue of concern (in school health promotion e.g. pupils and parents); collaboration with leaders in other sectors; sharing risks, resources, and responsibilities among partners; confronting and overcoming conflict within and outside the partnership; and maintaining adequate resources and continuity of leadership long enough to make a difference. Additional challenges include the change of the broader co-determinants of health that limit effectiveness, and, when dependent on external funding, negotiating for the time and resources needed to affect outcomes of significance.

Overall, it remains an open question what are the *intermediate indicators of partnership effectiveness* (such as systems change) that allow to better understand how partnership efforts are related to more distant population level health outcomes. What affects the capacity to promote health, the ability to bring about systems change and related outcomes (over time and across concerns) is not well understood. But a better understanding of the way partnerships create community, organizational or other systems changes and related improvement in widespread behavior and population-level health outcomes is needed to enhance practice. (Roussos, Fawcett 2000; Nutbeam, Harris 1999b; O'Neill et al 1997; Harris, Wise et al 1995)

'Good' collaborative practice - synopsis and discussion of lessons learned in Health Promotion

The review results can be summarized as presented in table 2.2.6.

Context / Environment of the collaborative
- conditions related to the formation of the collaboration: history, motivation, other programs, time;
- access to appropriate technical assistance;
- community control in agenda setting;
- social capital; broader socio-economic determinants of health that support effective action.

Its purpose
- agreed upon, clear vision / mission (periodically reviewed and renewed);
- agreed upon, clearly articulated goals and objectives.

Its processes/ relationships
- Agreed upon processes of goal definition, solution generation, ways of working, rules of the game, ...
- ongoing action planning;
- community involvement (in planning, implementation, etc.);
- continuous leadership (leadership team; use of democratic/ consensus decision making);
- dominance of cooperative over conflictual interest, through commitment at organization level, positive ties, a sense of purpose;
- sharing of risks, resources, responsibilities among all collaborators;
- systematic documentation and evaluation with focus on intermediary outcomes.

Its structures
- durable, long term resources (appropriate to achieve population level health improvements);
- availability within the collaboration of expertise / technical assistance needed;
- mechanisms of community involvement.

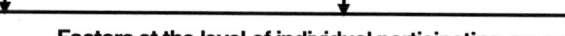

Factors at the level of individual participating organizations
- support of joint work at the level of the organization; commitment to joint ownership;
- flexibility in negotiating roles and responsibilities; a skilled workforce;
- compatibility of structures/ decision-making processes with those of the collaborative.

Table 2.2.6: Intermediary summary table: Factors enhancing the effectiveness of collaborative partnerships for the promotion of health - lessons learned from systematic reviews of interorganizational and inter-organization/ group/ community collaborations

Overall, four groups of **interrelated and modifiable factors that can enhance interorganizational collaborations** or mixed inter-organization/ inter-group collaborations for the promotion of health can be distinguished: the collaboration's environment and context, purpose, structures, and processes:

1. **Contextual and environmental factors** supporting an interorganizational collaboration's effectiveness fall into two groups:

Specific factors are:

- factors related to the formation of the collaboration: *history* of collaboration of (potential) partners, and existence of *relationships* within which joint action can be developed and conflicts resolved; *motivation or necessity* to form the collaborative partnership (a joint cause rather a funding opportunity); *preexisting programs/ initiatives* of relevance to the collaboration; absence of inadequate *time* pressure (e.g. imposed by donors);
- special *opportunities* related to one or more organizations (e.g. a reform initiative, acute reform pressure, an event, crisis)
- *access to 'adequate' technical assistance* that is needed to implement and sustain the collaboration (incl. training), with 'adequate' meaning: context-sensitivity; sensitivity to stages of development; relevance to (perceived) needs of participants and a range of health concerns (creation of basic skills); long term perspective;

More broader factors or conditions are:

- *high levels of social capital; recognition and tackling of broader social and economic determinants of health* that may limit the chance for effective interorganizational collaborative actions;
- *community control in agenda setting* (in defining the 'what' and 'how'…).

2. **Factors related to the purpose** that support interorganizational collaborations' effectiveness are:

- an agreed upon, *clear vision/ mission:* developed in an agreed upon process; clearly identifying the issue or problem, reasons for interorganizational collaboration, and acceptable solutions; acknowledging the emergent and changing nature of processes; allowing for a range of strategies to be employed; in a language broadly understood; and *periodically reviewed and renewed*;

- agreed upon, *clearly articulated goals and objectives* that are: achievable, and understood and valued by all participants and relevant stakeholders;
3. **Structural factors** supporting an interorganizational collaboration's effectiveness:
- *durable/ long-term resources* (material, financial, human, other): long enough to achieve *population* level health improvements;
- *mechanisms for community involvement*;
- *within* the collaboration availability of the *expertise and technical assistance* needed to implement and sustain the collaboration (training opportunities included);
4. **Processes / relationships** supporting an interorganizational collaboration's effectiveness are:
- *ongoing action planning,* i.e. specifying the what, who, how, by when of actions, including: identification of how to gain external support and prevent opposition, and of specific systems changes needed; agreement on roles and responsibilities; commitment for a defined time period; *opportunities for renegotiation* (of tasks, roles, relationships);
- *community involvement* (in planning, implementation, etc.);*
- *continuous leadership:* preferably widespread/ dispersed (e.g. leadership team); covering core competencies (communication, meeting facilitation, negotiation, networking); use of democratic and consensus decision making, and durable structures which facilitate such decision making (e.g. committees);
- *sharing of risks, resources, responsibilities* for the common work among all participants;
- *dominance of cooperative over conflicting interest/ of convergence over divergence* through: demonstrated commitment to the joint work at the level of the organization (not only of a committed staff member); *strong positive ties* among participating organizations and/or organizational representatives; dedication to a cause and a *sense of purpose*;
- *systematic documentation and evaluation* with focus on intermediary outcomes (as part of ongoing integrated support systems): that guide decisions and *day-to-day* activities, demonstrate the value of collaboration and contributions to desired changes, and help to identify and use appropriate (intermediary) outcome measures; complemented by activities that make the latter accepted among all relevant stakeholders.

In addition to the above 'success factors' that refer to the interorganizational collaboration for health promotion as a whole, there are **factors related to each individual (member) organization** and its capacity to be a valuable collaborator:

- *high level of organizational support to the interorganizational initiative* or activity;
- *flexibility in negotiating* roles and responsibilities;
- *commitment to joint ownership; compatibility* of the organization's *structures and decision making processes* with those of the collaborative;
- an appropriately *skilled workforce.*

In general it seems to be crucial that each participating organization or other collaborator both contributes and benefits from the joint work. O'Neill et al (1997) rightly point out that resources that may be contributed can not only take the form of financial and human resources but also a sense of purpose, information, prestige, contacts, and authority derived from size.

The identification of the above groups of factors points to an important issue: In the assessment of interorganizational networks models and indicators at two levels may be needed: first, at the level of the member organization (which refers to its features that reflect high capacity to effective interorganizational collaboration, and to processes that help a member organization to develop in this direction); second, at the level of the 'ideal', most promising or effective interorganizational network (ION). In addition and linked to this, models and indicators of most promising ways of creating, forming and maintaining such organizations and interorganizational networks (IONs) for the promotion of health are needed (and potentially even appropriate ways of dissolving a network or parts of it). These issues will be looked at from an organizational science perspective in chapter 2.4. This is necessary in light of the paucity of scientifically sound knowledge on interorganizational relationships in support of population health development within the field of Health Promotion and related areas. Nevertheless, the factors related to effective collaboration for promoting health identified so far provide a valuable first outline of a framework for interorganizational collaboration from within which base line indicators for measuring progress and success could be developed. Its particular value lies in the fact that it is derived from Health Promotion and related public health practice and as such is covering to a certain degree the knowledge gap due to the lack of systematic analyses of the network dimension of existing interorganizational networks (for the development) of health promoting Settings. However, the framework is specific neither to interorganizational relationships (several studies addressed a mix of organization/ group/ community collaborations) nor to the organizational form of networks, and it is based on a limited body of knowledge.

The findings point to *several challenges and open questions*: The factors potentially enhancing effectiveness of a collaborative for health promotion are interrelated but little is known about *how* they interplay. The processes of effective interorganizational collaboration are not well understood but it is already a progress that key areas related to effectiveness and specific factors within them have been identified. However, some factors enhancing effectiveness may be more important at particular stages of development of interorganizational collaboration but also here very little is known. Some leadership skills (e.g. facilitation, listening) are more important at early stages of development while others (e.g. negotiation, advocacy) more at later stages. Particularly technical assistance needs to be sensitive to development stages. - There are some *genuine, unavoidable challenges* in interorganizational collaboration. These include: engaging also those that experience the issue at stake (in schools e.g. pupils and parents); balancing co-operative and conflicting interests, convergence and divergence; sharing risks, resources and responsibilities; in case of dependence on external funding, negotiating the time and resources needed for long-term and complex changes at organizational and population health level; and changing the broader co-determinants of health that limit effectiveness of particular collaborative activities.

Overall, summary table 2.2.6 presents a first general draft of a framework for assessing interorganizational collaboration to promote health. It is not yet specific to interorganizational networks but indicates *core areas* for which indicators should be developed. Such indicators may turn out to be useful to collect general base line information on interorganizational networks for Health Promoting Schools (HPS) as a starting point to develop a better understanding of their nature and functioning. However, the interpretation of such information from a Health Promotion perspective will remain a challenge as long as there is no better understanding of how collaborative efforts relate to more distant population level health outcomes.

2.3 From understanding health to Health Promotion to 'Health Promotion networks' - intermediate synopsis and discussion

2.3.1 Where did the journey lead to so far?

Recalling the metaphor used in the introduction to describe this research project may help to step back for a moment and reflect on where this project led to so far - a pilot project that set out to develop a practical instrument to assess *international networks for the development of "Health Promoting Schools"* and similar 'health promoting Settings'. Up to now the reader has taken the promised swim in selected **Public Health waters and the Health Promotion sea therein**: A reflection at the outset on what is 'health' and how it is created and maintained led first and quickly **across the stream of co-determinants of health knowledge** which up today is continuously expanding. The swimmer saw that here much of the water is clearing year by year but nevertheless, many areas remain where the water is quite misty and one hardly can see. It became quite clear that: a) the *social domain* is a major if not the major domain that influences peoples health both indirectly (in the form of 'co-determinants of health behaviors') and *directly*; and b) that factors that are *beyond* the influence of *individual* actors and communities locally, and those that are not, must be considered *both*. To avoid getting lost in the currents of this "determinants of health stream" which often pull swimmers in different directions, the swim was continued in somewhat calmer waters: in **the sea of the social-ecological and systems perspective on health** where many of those currents swirl together and integrate. Although a complex environment, this swim provided orientation in the search for a better *understanding* of overall health development as to both individuals and populations, subjective and objective dimensions, and various systems levels. But also here there were challenging currents, which were felt strongly as soon as one tried to head on into **health *action* waters** where resources or co-determinants of health can be influenced.

Nevertheless the health action waters of a *social ecological* type were entered, as **the Health Promotion sea** lies therein. Here two streams are being brought together: the *'empowerment stream'* of enabling people to increase control over and *change* the factors influencing their health, and the 'co-determinants of health stream' which carries an array of *knowledge about* such factors; and while merging they create particular conditions that since long favored the creation of a range of **colorful corral reefs called 'health promoting Settings'**. Listening to reef researchers and snorkeling around the swimmer gained an understanding of their *commonalties and also differences* (e.g. that some are more 'elemental', others more 'contextual'; some more formal, others less; and many represent organizations, others composite organizational systems). In any case, the swimmer saw that 'health promoting Settings'-reefs are each *unique social systems, locally bound*, in which a variety of creatures go in and out every day for longer periods of time, shaping the reefs and being shaped by them on the way. Snorkeling through the Health Promotion sea did not only unravel corral reefs of a 'health promoting Settings' type but *other* action systems, too: Discovered were two types of systems covering larger areas than individual corral reefs. First, there are **some formations of life above and around the corral reefs called 'investment for health'**, apparently *self-organized clusters of a variety of actors* most of which significantly influence life and growth of Settings-reefs in their area. Unfortunately, the waters around these clusters are still somewhat misty and not many divers examined them more thoroughly yet. However, it was visible that the clusters are directed at *shaping the broader environment* of Settings-reefs while *pursuing particular interests* of the individual actors - with a well known actor playing a mediating and orchestrating role, WHO. Where 'investment for health'-clusters were found **'participatory waters' of the empowerment stream mixed with 'societal and economic waters' of the stream of "health determinants knowledge"** (particularly with waters of *macro* level factors shaping population health). The future behavior of the 'investment for health'-systems is hardly predictable; it may happen that existing ones dissolve and others emerge instead or in other areas. They seem to be a promising, potentially integral part of the *meso and macro environments of 'Settings'-reefs* in general and further research may unravel some lessons for other cooperative systems in the Health Promotion sea, too, such as for the second system discovered during the swim so far: **large-mesh, underwater networks directed at supporting *particular* Settings-reefs to become health promoting systems.**

Most but not all of these networks discovered in the Health Promotion sea seem to have *mainly one type of nod*, usually one particular type of Settings-reef (e.g. smaller nods such as health promoting schools or work sites, or bigger nods made of composite reef systems such as 'healthy cities' or '- villages'). Most networks were found to *spread across large areas - each linking smaller or bigger numbers of individual reefs* in the pursuit of their health promoting development. Some were already five to ten years old. As the 'investment for health'-formations also the network systems found were always connected with the well-known actor in the sea, WHO. *Some* networks (such as some of those spanning 'Health Promoting School'-reefs) appear to be connected to additional, larger reef systems such as *governments* which each have influence on particular areas of the Health Promotion sea. The swimmer saw that the large mesh network systems discovered seem to be *knitted by an elaborate, but not yet visible plan*. And as syntheses of findings of research divers did signal, they may share some features with other collaborative systems known from Health Promotion and other Public Health waters alike (e.g. with 'alliances', 'coalitions', 'intersectoral action', or 'partnerships'). However, there were hardly any results of *network* divers in the Health Promotion sea.

Against this background, it was decided: A swimmer interested in developing a practical tool to assess structure and processes of *those* network systems discovered that are related to the development of 'Health Promoting Schools'-reefs, must first of all **further examine the '*network*' dimension of these systems;** the good knowledge acquired of the networks' *goals and purpose* ('Health Promoting Schools'-development on a larger scale) is very important but not sufficient. The limited knowledge gained of *structural, process and other network features* (due to misty water around the networks only a fuzzy picture of meshes and nods emerged) reasoned to *stop the swim* across the Health Promotion sea and take a *dive* - but, in light of the yet limited general understanding of the network systems of interest - not a dive directly to the networks. Another dive was more promising to achieve the research goal: a dive into the less known waters of organizational sciences and particularly the **river of inter-organizational research** therein. This part of the journey still lying ahead aims at improving the swimmers understanding of network systems per se which - *combined* with the Health Promotion knowledge gained so far - will provide a good basis to create the desired practical network assessment tool. This tool could then be tested by using it to guide a second dive - down to one of the large-mesh networks of interest within the Health Promotion sea.

The dive into the inter-organizational sciences is the focus of the next chapter 2.4. Importantly, it will be undertaken with the Health Promotion knowledge gained so far 'in the pack'. Less metaphorical, this can be summarized as follows:

2.3.2 Health and Health Promotion – relevant lessons learned

There is wide agreement in Public Health that sustainable levels of **'health' cannot easily 'be created'** by one or a few actors alone, neither by one individual nor an individual community or a single sector of society. This applies to individual pupils, teachers, parents and schools, too. Collective action, both interorganisational (such as intersectoral) as well as interorganisational/inter-group cooperation (such as between schools and communities) is needed to sustain and improve health.

There is a wide **range of interrelated health relevant factors or 'co-determinants' of health:** intrapersonal, and environmental factors, and factors at the person-environment interface such as lifestyle factors. Environmental factors include both physical or ecological factors and the for long underestimated or neglected social and socio-economic factors. Some are modifiable locally, others at higher systems levels only (national, international, or global). Individual behavioral factors are over researched, social factors in general under-researched. The *daily-life-*situations are most important as to people's health relevant actions. First models about the range and interplay of largely social co-determinants of health are emerging and promise to guide practice in the future. Overall, current knowledge supports intervention approaches that focus on health supportive changes of *local Settings* in which various factors in dynamic combinations are influencing the inhabitants' health day by day; there is hardly support for isolated individual behavior change interventions focusing on single health relevant behaviors. In any case, sustainable behavior change is only possible if the various social determinants of such behaviors themselves are taken into account. Overall evidence suggests that interventions directly focusing on the *social and societal conditions* are more promising to achieve greatest population level health gains. While these findings much support the locally focused *Settings approach* in Health Promotion (such as a 'Health Promoting Schools' approach), it also shows that this approach alone is not sufficient.

In the field of Health Promotion today there are several complementary approaches of relevance: The *Settings approach* as mentioned above; a somewhat overlapping, broader 'investment for health' approach; and a *'network approach'* however defined (see chap. 2.2.5). Potentially each includes health supportive policy development. The Settings approach with its local orientation must be complemented by approaches tackling the supra-local or macro level factors that jointly influence health. The latter is the focus of the 'investment for health' approach (and also e.g. Healthy Public Policy initiatives). The 'network approach' in Health Promotion in focus in this research project appears to be locally focused in the sense of concentrating on developing health promoting Settings (such as schools); at the same time it seems to have a great potential as a mechanism to address those co-determinants of health that are *beyond* the influence of individual Settings (or schools). Observations of practice show that it is unlikely that the 'network approach' in Health Promotion ceases to exist in the near future; on the contrary, calls for 'new' forms of collaboration of this or similar types are on the rise and their need widely recognized. Thus, a better understanding of this approach is pressing.

Empowerment and participation are core principles of Health Promotion and as such are integral to the 'health promoting Settings'-approach. In the field of Health Promotion internationally, a network approach first emerged and is mainly used in the context of large-scale implementations of the Settings approach. Up today, a remarkable number of *international networks* for the development of *health promoting Settings* has been created or emerged worldwide. Exchange, mutual support and/or learning among Settings are usually emphasized. This supports two of the theses of this research project: that a) a network approach enables and facilitates the creation of sustainable, large scale 'health promoting Settings' and b) the organizational form of interorganisational networks matches well with Health Promotion goals, strategies and principles. Of course, this needs further examination that is the focus of the next chapters.

The literature review so far identified **several *types* of 'Settings'**: elemental Settings such as those of individual organizations (schools, hospitals, many work sites,...) and contextual Settings comprising not only a combination of organizations but groups, too (e.g. cities, villages, small islands,...). While the field of Health Promotion usually has focused on *formal* Settings, there are *informal* ones, too (e.g. street corners). But the health promoting change of informal Settings is not yet the focus of international networks in the field. With 'Health Promoting Schools' as example, **this research project focuses on networks related to *elemental, formal* 'health promoting Settings'.**

As of now, in Health Promotion **two *types* of networks** (related to the Settings approach) seem to exist: A first network type mainly links one type of formal Settings, i.e. *local* systems, across regional or national borders; but a few other organizations at other levels of society may be in the net, too (see e.g. Healthy Cities networks and some networks 'of' Health Promoting Schools). A second network type mainly links *national and international* organizations but for the purpose of health promoting developments in formal Settings at local level (as found among international networks or network initiatives for the 'development of' Health Promoting Schools). Most if not all of **these networks are likely interorganizational networks** (even in the case of contextual Settings such as 'Healthy Cities' which are made up of both organizations and local groups but nevertheless network with each other via formal Healthy Cities offices or similar bodies. Thus, so far the literature review supports the thesis put forward for this research project:, that "international networks for the development of Health Promoting Schools [and other formal elemental Settings] are *inter-organizational* networks. ..." (chap.1 p.6).

There is **wide international agreement about the general desired network outcome** of international networks for the development of Health Promoting Schools, i.e. of the networks in focus of this research project. The **"Health Promoting School"** (HPS) represents a quite complex desired outcome involving far reaching, multi-dimensional change in the organizational social system 'school'. This poses all the challenges to assessment efforts that are genuine to social-ecological interventions or interventions in open social systems (see chap. 2.2.4 above and 2.4). With view to the aim of international networks to create Health Promoting Schools (HPS) on a fairly *large scale* it should be recognized: Even regarding less complex interventions such as behavior change interventions it is *not* possible to identify and define the health promotion method or strategy superior to all others as its effectiveness always depends on its *appropriate fit* with the *particular* set of people, health issues at stake, and environment in which it is to be applied. Similarly, it cannot be expected that a network on HPS development is able to define the particular method or package of methods for creating Health Promoting Schools a) to be applied to *all* 'health promoting schools in the making' and b) according to which progress made by each of them could be measured in a standardized way of 'one size fits all'. This shows clear limits of outcome assessment efforts as to international (and national) networks to create health promoting schools or similar Settings. It remains to be examined whether modern Health Promotion research has come up with general outcome models that would help to tackle this challenge (see chap. 3). However, this issue is not as central to this research project as it may seem to be, as it first of all aims at developing a practical tool to assess international networks for the development of Health Promoting Schools as to their *structures and processes* (see chap.1). But of course, network structures and processes may be linked to the goals or desired outcomes defined by a network (an issue for chapter 2.4 below).

First systematic reviews of collaborative practice to promote health (of 'alliances', 'coalitions' and also 'intersectoral action' but not (interorganisational) 'networks') have identified commonalties and factors that make them successful in achieving self-set goals. Most of these 'lessons learned' (summarized in fig. 2.2.6) stem from collaborative partnerships at *community or local* level; and the empowerment and/or participation *principles of Health Promotion* have guided much of this practice. Here, **research knowledge in the areas of 'community development' and 'organizational development' has been systematically used**, and obviously found to match with the Health Promotion concept. However, the literature review has shown that - with view to the much called for 'new' approaches for intersectoral and/or interorganisational collaboration to promote health, and regarding the international 'networks' experimented with and implemented in the field of Health Promotion since long - **additional knowledge from the organizational sciences needs to be drawn upon:** knowledge that addresses less the development of individual organizations and more relations and collaborative links *between* a smaller or larger *number* of organizations in the pursuit of promoting health. Implementations of the broad 'investment for health'-approach experimented with and identified already several methods or tools that facilitate intersectoral and, thus, interorganisational cooperation among a range of organizational actors (with particular attention to public/private sector cooperation). However, as to the wide spread implementation of the 'network' approach for the large scale development of health promoting Settings (such as schools) that is at stake in this research project, a systematic consideration of **results from the area of interorganisational relations and network research** seems yet lacking. This is indicated in various ways: The term 'network' is often used as a buzz word or ill (if at all) defined; a clear set of terms on organizational forms and related definitions is lacking; and so are (comparable) documentation of the network dimension of the many 'health promoting Settings networks' in place; and the inclusion of the term 'network' and related ones on *inter-organizational* collaboration in latest Health Promotion handbooks and the main, internationally recognized Health Promotion Glossary is just emerging and yet insufficient. Therefore, the next chapter 2.4 reviews the state of research as to interorganisational relations and networks from an organization science perspective.

2.4 Interorganisational networks -features and development

2.4.1 Introduction

Networks in Health Promotion are a reality, a phenomenon that has spread from Europe around the world and continues to do so (chap. 2.2). *General features of these networks as derived from their descriptions* draw the attention of researchers who examine the creation, maintenance and/or performance of such networks into particular research directions. One characteristic of international networks for the development of Health Promoting Schools (HPS) and similar networks is that they *connect social systems* (not or not only individuals), and that they strive to *change social systems*, - and this around a *common purpose:* the promotion of health. Networking among 'Healthy Cities' includes networking among various subsystems of cities, its informal and formal organizations. Networking for the development of Health Promoting Schools (HPS) includes inter-ministerial links as well as 'inter-country' networking however defined. It also includes *changing existing organizations*, here the schools, so that they become "Health Promoting Schools (HPS)", which means to implement innovations in all schools over time. Thus, networking in Health Promotion in general and for the development of Health Promoting Schools (HPS) in particular has much to do with *organizational* networking or *inter-organizational* relationships and networks, with *organizational change* and *innovation dissemination* within multi-organization systems. Given the fact that international, national and/or local levels of society are linked in such networks, it has also to do with political processes that reach across layers of societies.

The strong organizational dimensions of international networks for the development of Health Promoting Schools (HPS) and similar networks does not mean that networking between individuals has no relevance. But **this research project focuses on understanding such international networks from an *international/ macro and interorganisational* perspective and does not concentrate on inter*personal* networking for health** (such as social support networks). The latter are considered only as part of the range of co-determinants of health. With regard to the goal of developing a practical instrument for the assessment of international networks for HPS development, the inter-*organizational* network dimensions will be the primary focus; relations between individuals or groups will be addressed as far as they concern an organization's function and performance within that context.

Social network theory and practice addressing inter-*personal* relationships is since long an established research area - also in relation to health (see e.g. Berkmann/ Glass 2000; Paulus 1997; Badura/ Kickbusch 1991). In contrast to this, scientific literature and analyses of inter-*organizational* networks or networking and mechanisms for their development or change is rare – and not only in relation to health but other fields, too. The exception are computer networks, the 'hard ware' of communication networks within and among organizations. Particularly theorists and analysts of management or organizational practices point out that the 'new' information technologies (IT) have a strong influence on quality and quantity of network creation and networking in societies today. *In the information age, the critical organizational form is networking* (Castells 1998; Hastings 1993). Castells' analyses (1996, 1998) of the spread of information technology, globalization and social development indicate 'the rise of the network society'. While the field of Health

Promotion demonstrates this since long, systematic analyses of the *network* (ION) dimension of networks in that and related fields remain rare. Therefore, this chapter turns to research *outside* the public health sciences but also there ION research is still in its infancy. Relevant knowledge to improve the understanding of the networks of interest and their assessment had to be searched for like a pathfinder. A variety of overall scarce sources was found, particularly analyses and theoretical frameworks from the management, organization and other social sciences. **The goal is now to identify important characteristics of interorganisational networks that are applicable to international networks for the development of Health Promoting Schools (HPS) and indicators in terms of both their structures and processes.** Ideally, a conceptual framework for the assessment of such networks will be developed, too.

The current knowledge from 'non-health' (organization and network) research will later need to be brought together with that from public health and Health Promotion research (elaborated in chapters 2.1 and 2.2). The 'match' or potential contradictions of the two bodies of knowledge will need analysis before building upon them to draft a conceptual framework for the *collection of (baseline) data* on structures and processes of the international networks in focus and for *assessing* such networks (see chap. 3). The pilot testing of the instrument will follow (chap. 5 and 6).

2.4.2 Organizational networking and the 'New Organization'

Much of the published literature on networks and networking in an organizational context is based on case studies from the management and business world. But first theoretical models are emerging. The few books directly or solely focusing on networking and inter-organizational networks (indicated e.g. by the use of the term 'network(ing)' in the title) stem from the management literature and analysis of organizational practice. These include 'Systematic Networking. A guide for personal and corporate success' by Hayes (1996) who addresses both interpersonal and interorganisational networking. Hastings (1993) concentrates on 'the new organization' and the 'culture of organizational networking'. Alter and Hage (1993) developed an interorganisational relations theory with special emphasis on interorganisational *networks*, an 'emerging theory' increasingly referred to in health education and Health Promotion literature (e.g. by Goodman et al 1997; Nutbeam 1998; and Hurrelmann 2000).

For to assess (inter)national networks such as networks for the development of Health Promoting Schools (HPS) **a good understanding of 'organizational networking processes', organizations and net-**

works of organizations is necessary. This leads to first, the identification of their *main characteristics* and second, an examination of the *creation and change* of organizations and interorganisational networks (IONs).

Networking in an organizational context

The term '**networking**' is used by different people and in different fields in a range of different ways (see e.g. Hastings 1993; Hayes 1996; WHO/EURO 1997). Clutterback points to network-environment-interactions and processes when stating that "networking is like a spider's web. When something lands on it vibrations are sent out along it ... a whole range of processes result from people being interlinked with each other" (in Hayes 1996, pIV). However, the overall semantic confusion makes it difficult to create a coherent framework for the understanding of networking and related new organizational forms, 'organizational networking' included. – Discussions of collaborative *Public Health practice* led to the distinction of two types of networking: more *informal* networking largely on the basis of personal contacts (e.g. among experts) and more organized or *formal* networking promoted through formally established networks with *agreed rules and regulations* for their operation (such as WHO related networks). Networking has been found to be possible at *any level* of society and with *varying* degrees of formalization. (WHO/EURO 1997 p38; Working Group on Partnerships... 1997 p8-9) - Analyses of a variety of corporate and individual experiences from around the world led to more differentiated views: Hayes (1996). stresses particular qualities of relations when concluding that '**networking' is about relationships, not transactions; trust rather than trade; long term, not short term; and with people and communication at the center.** Networking is about making the connections which requires a cross-flow of information. It is about **mutuality** and referral, an investment into the future. The *underlying philosophy* of networking is **'win/win' (not 'win/lose')** - even in the competitive business world. Hayes calls for *value based networks with a sense of purpose and governance*.

'**Organizational networking**' is similarly to the term 'networking' used in various ways. For example, IT specialists may refer to the electronic exchange of information while organization theorists may refer to ways in which different organizations become more interdependent (Hastings 1993). Similar terms may have different meanings such as 'interorganizational networking' and 'organizational networking'. The former may be viewed as a specific networking process within the latter or both may be seen as synonym. According to Hastings organizational networking can be understood as the *implementation* of a range of social, cultural and technological *processes that result in a devolution of power and a breakdown of organizational boundaries*. This facilitates direct person to person connections, sharing of information and joint working (both within and between organizations) in order to pursue a common goal, solve problems or satisfy the expectations of stakeholders. It encompasses *four networking processes* as explained below.

Obviously, yet no single definition of 'networking' and 'organizational networking' has received particular widespread recognition or consensus across disciplines or in the areas of Public Health, Health Promotion and health development. Therefore, for this research an appropriate working definition needs to be chosen or developed which requires the understanding of the key features of organizations and networks of organizations. This is also important with view to the goal of the networks in focus: the creation of health promoting Settings such as schools on a large scale.

Features of Organizations

Since long Western researchers underline organizations as the prominent social institutions of our time. Although 'health' is *not* a central theme, goal or task of most organizations they all influence health concepts and related behaviors of users as well as staff. Important co-determinants of health such as social status and income are determined by rank and position in organizations. By means of their internal work organization, social structures, products and ways of providing services, expectations raised among staff and clients, and implicitly communicated values, organizations including schools influence the health at least of those that learn or work within them. In the context of Health Promotion (and referring to organizations capable of learning and successfully adapting to complex and dynamic environments) Pelikan, Krajcik and Dietscher (1999) use the metaphor 'healthy organization', and so do others but unfortunately often without further definition. As Raeburn and Rootman (1998) also this research project rejects this as an over-stretching of the concept of health. The terms 'health promoting' or 'health supportive' organization are used instead (see also chap. 2.2).

That organizations are best described as **open social systems** is generally agreed upon among organization theorists and other social scientists (see e.g. Daft 1992; Grossmann, Scala 1993; Hilderbrand, Grindle 1994; Lobnig, Nowak, Pelikan 1997; Goodman, Steckler, Kegler 1997; UNDP 1997, w.y.; Pelikan et al 1999; Eoyang, Berkas 1998). In short, **general features of organizations and, thus, members of interor-**

ganisational networks **(**such as schools or public agencies) are: their *constant interactions (resource exchange) with the environment* to survive; their need to develop their internal structures in processes of *self-organization* that are adequate to the dynamics and complexity of their relevant environments (which affects their ability to carry out tasks effectively and efficiently); an identifiable *boundary or distinct membership;* one or more purposes, usually clearly expressed as *mission, goal* and objectives; *work activities* to achieve those; several *interdependent, often layered subsystems* (units, work groups, individuals, etc.); and *deliberate structures* to coordinate and direct separate sub-systems or groups. Overall, without denying complexity two basic characteristics of organizations should be kept in mind: in Hastings words (1993) *'people and structural relationships',* and *'connective mechanisms'* to both hold the elements together and make the organization work. People, groups of people, and their roles are an organization's building blocs; and matching with basic Health Promotion principles many management approaches aim at empowering employees with greater opportunities to contribute. - **An organization's relevant environment** can be captured in four 'dimensions' (UNDP 1997, w.y.): an organization's *institutional, sociopolitical, economic and environmental* context. Environmental factors such as financing frameworks, laws and regulations, the work market, and the needs of clients or customers influence an organization's options for action (Lobnig et al 1997). This holds also for public organizations such as schools.

To understand multi-organizational systems such as networks, particularly those that aim at changes in particular organizations (such as health promoting school development), it is crucial to understand **behaviors of organizations.** Two *sets* need to be distinguished: the behaviors of the interdependent *parts* (e.g. units or individuals) and the emergent, system-wide patterns of behaviors that form the behavior of *the whole*. The interaction of a large number of factors makes it *impossible to completely understand and predict* an organizations future behavior. A single cause does not have a single effect. All this makes it difficult to manage and assess organizations: prediction and controlled performance toward a goal, assumed by traditional evaluation methods, are two behaviors that can *not* be expected from organizations (Eoyang, Berkas 1998). Nevertheless, social and natural sciences alike have shown that **systems exhibiting complex behaviors** have some **common characteristics**: they *change constantly and discontinuously*; they function *simultaneously at many different levels* of scales (individual actors act relatively independent/ groupings emerge (e.g. on 'Health Promoting Schools')/ and a system as a whole shows identifiable behaviors as compared to another one); there are both quite similar *and* different behaviors (e.g. a generally accepted code of conduct does not exclude that at certain points in time one or more members behave very different than generally expected); in their interactions sub-systems are both *being transformed* and *transforming*, and generate new behavioral patterns (*emergent, self-organizing behavior*); feedback loops produce both change and stability and new structures may emerge and old ones disappear. - **In sum, the behavior of organizations *varies* and is *not predictable.*** It may move from random to chaotic to linear patterns over time or at different levels of scale, depending on particular circumstances. This must be considered when assessing interorganisational networks and (health promoting) organizational change. Also, analyzing organizational systems needs to include analyzing their *environments* as these influence their behaviors.

Since the 1990s, times parallel with the transfer of the health promoting Settings approach from contextual to organizational Settings such as schools, organization analysts pay increased attention to the *interplay between the inner form of organizations and external influences* and demands. Influential was Senge's work (1990, 1996) on **the 'learning organization', a type of organization that actively tries to cope with its environment *and* to influence it.** It is characterized by *five principles:* 1. development of personal competencies and skills of organizational members (staff) *beyond* technical demands; 2. reflection of *implicit* or hidden views, assumption and theories; 3. development of a *joint vision*, of guiding principles about the future of the organization as a joint platform for various changes; 4. working and learning in *teams* to develop new ways of communicating and collective actions and thinking; and 5. changing of the organization with special attention to its systemic features. An organization's 'capability of learning' is an essential precondition for innovation, flexibility and customer orientation. (Lobnig et al 1997) Thus, it is crucial for organizations that form or join networks for the development of Health Promoting Settings such as schools, too. This holds even more for networks where the target Settings are network members, as these commit themselves to a *double* innovation: systematic interorganisational networking and internal organizational change in support of health.

To *actively* cope with and *influence* the *environment* is of particular importance for all 'health promoting organizations': because of both the range of interrelated factors that influence health and the obviously limited resources of any individual organization. Health Promoting Hospitals research demonstrates that organizations influence themselves and their relevant environment through *decisions*, and affect the health of people in a Setting by influencing *values, norms* and *situational* resources (material infrastructures, money, time, access to attention, etc.). By this process, they also influence *personal* resources, goals and priorities of these people. *Decisions or decision making processes* of organizations can be influenced in a health promoting direction and need special attention, as need *(dis)incentives for various types of behavior* as they influence health relevant values and norms. (Pelikan et al 1999)

This is supported by work of Grossmann, Pellert and Gotwald (1997) who studied so called **'expert' organizations in public sectors** (such as public hospitals, *schools* and universities) which more or less world wide are under ongoing reform pressures directed at cost and quality control, customer and staff orientation. There are particular features and development potentials of such expert organizations as compared to other organizations. These are exhibited to a further or lesser degree and must be considered when striving for organizational change (such as in support of organizational networking or health promotion): Most staff members are **experts** with relatively **high individual autonomy** who hold the *knowledge*, the main means of producing the organization's central services, in their hands. They deliver usually complex services in direct relationships with 'clients' with the *quality of the relationships* (e.g. teacher-pupils-relations) influencing the *quality of services*. Sufficient working conditions and levels of expert motivation are important. Addressing decreased levels of expert performance and motivation is difficult in case of high job security and little performance incentives. - Experts tend to see the organization as a means for accessing resources with **often low levels of identification with the organization and its goals**. For many, internal position and contributions to the organization's functioning are *not* the main sources for professional acknowledgment but rather progress and position within their professional community. Expert organizations show **a typical contradiction**: At the level of the *subject* of the professionals their is considerable openness to implement new information or techniques quickly; at the level of the *organization* as a whole high levels of resistance against structural changes and innovations are found. Changes of expert organizations are often just reactions to changes in their environment rather than as processes of self-organization and strategic decisions.

At the organizational level, the *specialization* of the experts (e.g. teachers, or doctors) is mirrored in different fairly *autonomous sub-systems* with varying work cultures and often resource competition. These features are **obstacles for organizational tasks that cut across traditional specialization and need high levels of cooperation and coordination** within the organization (as typically required by Health Promotion activities). Another disintegrating factor of expert organizations is often the tension between experts and. In public sectors the administration is often seen as limiting factor and prolonged arm of higher hierarchies at local, State and national levels. – In addition, there are *often deficits in overall management and organizational leadership* due to technical experts rather than professional managers in respective positions. At the same time, in many public sectors core management functions (from staffing to financing) are still *centralized* and outside the individual expert organization. Despite trends of decentralization many expert organizations (public schools included) still face **high levels of individual expert autonomy and, at the same time, low organizational autonomy with high influence of governmental levels**. Yet, *quality control* of the experts' performance is approached as *self-control*, for reasons such as difficulties in measuring processes and results and standardizing quality control.

Implications for initiatives to create 'Health Promoting Schools' - intermediate synthesis and discussion

Networks for the development of Health Promoting Schools (HPS) in public school systems in Europe have likely to deal with schools as expert organization in the above sense, i.e. with: teachers as experts (with particular socialization, ideas of professionalism and quality control, etc.); the shaping force of specialism regarding organizational sub-systems and management; typical contradictions and tensions within schools (high individual/ low organizational autonomy; experts vs. administrators; (groups of) professionals vs. the goal of the school as a whole). This indicates that the creation of a 'Health Promoting School' is a challenging and longer term task not only from a health but also organizational development perspective.

Overall, much of the features of organizations identified so far remain abstract knowledge as long as they are neither integrated nor applied to a concrete example of an organization. While the idea of the learning organization provides a guiding orientation, an integrating and more *practical* framework is needed to facilitate the *application* of the above knowledge about organizations. Hastings (1993) made a significant contribution to such an integration of knowledge by developing a *practical* organizational model called 'the new organization'.

"The New Organization" and the role of networking processes

Hastings (1993) examined organizational systems mainly from the private but also public sector (including the Healthy City network). He developed a framework for understanding the different aspects of networking in relation to dimensions of 'the new organization', a type of organization that **relies much on networking processes** - both *within* the organization and *with other* organizations. Hastings' model considers not only four types of networking processes but also different *levels* of society. These features make this organization model particularly interesting for research on multi-level networks for the development of Health Promoting Schools (HPS). - Hastings does not offer an organizational theory, but "patterns or ways of understanding that emerge from the early experiences" of organizations that moved beyond traditional or more rigid forms of organizing and managing towards the 'new organization' (p13). The so called 'pathfinder' organizations are developing new forms of organizing and managing as a combined response to dissatisfactions with old organizational forms, needs to solve current organizational problems, as well as new factors that create new opportunities or challenges for an organization. The latter include the potentials of the rapidly spreading information technologies (IT), a generally better educated workforce, and the increasing globalization in general. Hastings illustrates the dimensions of 'the new organization' in his **'radar screen model'** (fig. 2.4.1).

Hastings identifies *three organizational dimensions*. Organizations may:

- be externally or internally driven,
- be people or technology driven, and
- have a 'local', regional or global focus ('local' means here 'within a country').

The first dimension refers to **relationships** an organization may focus on. Organizations that primarily look at the relationships between its *internal* elements are 'internally driven', those that look mainly at its relationships with *external* elements, other individuals and organizations, are 'externally driven'. The internal/external dimensions are *not an either/or*, but reflect an organization's strategic rationale, starting point, emphasis or preference, or what an organization wants to be in the future. Similarly, organizations have preferred **ways of connecting** internal or external elements. They may focus on *low-tech social* processes (called 'people driven') or on *high-tech IT* solutions (called 'technology driven'). Again these dimensions are *not an either/or*, but reflect an organization's focus, starting point, preference or priority. Hastings speaks of four "strategic logics" of an organization (see below). The 'Radar Screen Model' with the two organizational dimensions (relationships and ways of connecting) on the x- and y-axes encompasses a third dimension of increasing **distance between elements** of an organization. This geographic dimension spans from the "local" (here understood as 'within a country'!) and regional (here e.g. Europe) to the global level. The geographical dimension has also a psychological component: The further the geographical distance for communication, the greater it seems are the psychological, though not necessarily technical, barriers to communication and collaboration - an important aspect for *international* networks for the development of Health Promoting Schools (HPS).

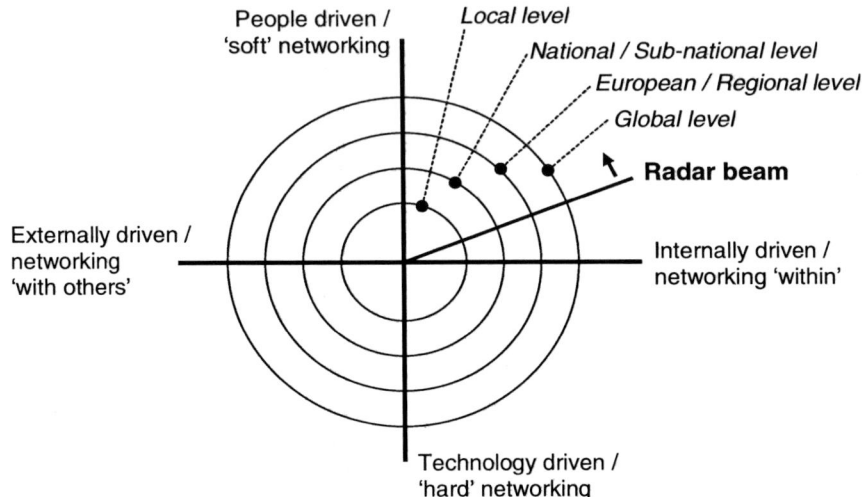

Figure 2.4.1: The radar screen model of the 'new' organization (slightly adapted from Hastings 1993, p13)

According to Hastings each strategic logic of the 'new organization' is associated with a *core networking process* (see table 2.4.1). These networking processes have a clear purpose each and are the primary means of implementing that purpose. The term **organizational networking** is used to refer to these four processes *collectively*.

Networking *within* the organization aims at breaking down boundaries and creating quick and person-to-person communications. While stimulating networking is a general strategy that sets a style and culture for an organization the creation of *specific networks or groupings of individuals* that cut across various parts of the organization (e.g. various school subjects or grades) can serve to focus activity, know-how and people with similar interest (such as staff interested in Health Promotion or school-community-links). - Breaking down boundaries within an organization aims at creating organizations that can respond rapidly and flexible, free of constraints of traditional hierarchical and functional rules of communication. This means not just *delayering* (cutting out layers of the hierarchy) but also flattening *lateral boundaries* to communication and networking (e.g. across school subject specialism). Networking processes built up over a long period of time in various ways will provide, so the premise of the 'radar screen model of the new organization', openness and elasticity of structure and communication processes of an organization. Networking *within* an organization for a particular purpose has as a starting point the awareness that a range of the resources needed are available and that their use can be maximized by breaking down of internal boundaries and high-quality communication and cooperation within and across the organization.

Strategic logic	Core networking process	Purpose
internally driven	networking *within* the organization	boundary busting
externally driven	networking *between* organizations	successful partnerships
technology driven	hard networks	connecting computers
people driven	soft networking	connecting people

Table 2.4.1: "Organizational networking": four core networking processes (Hastings 1993 p15)

Networking *between* organizations (or inter-organizational networking) may be a response to pressures or desires to cooperate (see below) that result in patterns of *partnerships*. Different forms exist (many originating from the business world such as strategic alliances). Interorganisational networking provides mechanisms for both large and small organizations, local or national ones (schools or national HPS centers), to operate beyond their local or national boundaries. In contrast to the networking *within* organizations, networking *between* organizations may have as a starting point recognizing what resources or influences the own organization not has and that others may have and can provide when entering into a partnership or cooperation. - Should an organization need or want to change **from a 'networking within' focus to a 'networking with others' focus**, its members and *the organization as a whole need a shift in mentality* from a 'having control'- mode to a 'sharing control'- mode. Perceived loss of power on the part of members of the organization in transition could provide a major obstacle to the change. - Many examples of cooperation have shown that this is not as easy in practice as it seems to be. It needs special attention in processes of organizational change. This could challenge a school that is striving to become a HPS, for example, when acting on HPS characteristics such as good school-community links in support of health promotion and education. In addition, a change in focus from solely local (e.g. school/ community) issues and actions to addressing also national or even international aspects (e.g. as part of a national network) requires changes in the mentality of people and organizations. Slogans like 'think globally, act locally' and vice versa 'think locally, act globally' illustrate this challenge.

Soft networking is the third of the four core networking processes of organizational networking identified by Hastings (1993). It includes the different ways in which people make, and are helped to make, connections with each other. A range of *soft technologies* (such as conferencing, mobility policies and travel) can be systematically used to accelerate the *creation of patterns of communication, understanding and learning* inside and outside the formal boundaries of an organization. Soft networking has been studied by organization theorists and sociologists under the heading of *the 'informal organization'*. Soft networking as conceptualized by Hastings is not referring to self-interested 'old boy networks' and using connections for private goals. Soft networking has shown to be important when individuals or groups wanted to bring about innovations and change within an organization, in *support* of the overall strategic goals and purpose of that organization. It helps to build individuals' confidence and sense of 'positive' power to make desired things happen (Moss Kanter 1983) - often without the formal exercising of traditional sources of power and authority. The fundamental *way to acquire influence without formal authority* is through the 'law of reciprocity', the almost universal belief that 'people should be paid back for what they do'. Bradford and Cohen suggest to use the metaphor of 'currencies' and exchange rates in this context. They distinguish *different types* of currencies: technical knowledge, 'inspirational currencies' such as getting involved in a task that has larger significance for the organization or society, 'position-related' currencies such as the involvement in a task that can aid promotion or advancement, and 'relationship-related' currencies such as giving personal support. (Barham 1991 quoted in Hastings 1993 p30/31). **Mutual gain or reciprocity** is at the core of cooperative behavior and soft networking. There are **two important aspects of successful soft networking**: the success in *achieving the task or goal*, and the success in *building the relationship and trust* so that the next interaction will be even more effective. - Hastings emphasizes that soft networking as compared to hard (computer) networking has to be invested in *first* to form the *infrastructure of personal contacts* throughout and between organizations; Information technologies (IT) then follow to support and enable those personal connections to expand and flourish. Soft technologies (often taken for granted) need to be better understood, more carefully and systematically developed and applied, and invested in.

Hard networking, the fourth core networking process of organizational networking as outlined by Hastings (1993) will not be addressed in detail. Important to note for this research project is that installing electronic communications will not itself create organizational networking or the 'new organization'. It is not *the* answer to organizational transformation that may be needed or desired. It is only a part of the wider 'organizational networking' approach, one that *should support and enable personal connections* (soft networking) to expand and enhance. But with increasing geographical distance among people or organizations such as in international or cross-national cooperation it is an essential and influential part of networking.

Hastings (1993) provides this **overall summary of the characteristics of 'the new organization'**:

- radical *decentralization* (of tasks, power, responsibilities - through a systematic and widespread approach; the organization consists of many types of *small, autonomous and accountable elements*, the smallest of which is the individual)
- *intense interdependence* and multidisciplinary approaches (based on the recognition that to compete and achieve goals *cooperation* is needed - e.g. by assembling coalitions and project teams)
- demanding expectations (reflected in strong simple goals and a clear sense of purpose and mission (set by leaders); *high demands* of each other among all members who have the *right to ask for cooperation*;)
- *transparent* performance standards (measured and communicated in a way that *stimulates improvement* as opposed to creating winners and losers)
- *distributed leadership* (key relationships built on very wide exercising of responsibility among people, i.e. people are prepared 'to make things happen' and share *a sense of responsibility for the whole*; requires considerable *maturity and leadership qualities* of people)
- boundary busting (awareness and *systematic elimination* of physical, personal, hierarchical, functional, cultural, psychological and practical *boundaries/ barriers to cooperation and communications*, as the base for the organization's *flexibility* and adaptiveness)
- *networking and reciprocity* (investments into facilitation of *intense* communications between people; *direct* relationships and information sharing, irrespective of considerations of role, status, level, functions, culture or location)

How can this type of a 'new' organization be created? Hastings points out that **networking is driven by a pervasive culture of reciprocity and exchange that mediates all relationships**. Organizational *networking is the means* to bring the 'new' organization into being. It means the implementation of a range of social, cultural and technological *processes to achieve organizational change* towards the concept of the 'new organization'. This entails the initiation, strengthening and maintenance of core networking processes as appropriate. Hastings points out that the **transformation of more traditional forms of organizations** (rigid bureaucracies; bureaucracies with a senior management team, or with project teams; matrix organizations; etc.) into 'the new organization' will take **many years,** for some organizations may be *even decades*. Questions of how to change organizations are further addressed below. - Overall, the culture of **the 'New Organization' versus a more traditional one** can be sketched out as follows: availability of information on a *want*-to-know (not need-to-know) basis; inclusiveness; justifying confidentiality (not communication); a *sense* of mission (not just a mission statement); individuals assume responsibility for the whole (not only for parts as in many expert organizations); *power comes from sharing* (not retaining) information; specialists *learning* from (rather than telling) others; *asking for help* is a strength (not weakness); straight talking (no hidden agendas); *tolerance for ambiguity*, and delight in difference; *self*-regulation (rather external control); and *empowerment* (rather compliance).

The 'new' organization - synthesis and discussion

Hasting's model of 'the new organization' is compatible with the understanding of organizations as social systems and of networking processes elaborated above. It provides a useful framework for the integration of the general knowledge on organizations, and significantly furthers the understanding of relationships within an organization and between an organization and the elements of its environment. The value added to the general knowledge on organizations can be summarized as follows:

The model draws attention equally to the relationships *within* an organization and relationships of the organization *with others* (organizations or individuals), thus, balancing out the overemphasis of traditional organizational models towards the former. In addition, it provides a *rational for decisions on when to focus on internal or external relationships:* If the resources needed to achieve a goal are available within the organization and their use can be maximized by improving communication and cooperation within and across the organization, 'networking within' is proposed. If some of the resources needed are <u>not</u> internally available and others have and could provide them in a cooperation, 'externally oriented networking' is suggested. The latter is usually the case when the goal of an organization includes protecting and promoting the health of its members and their families. As shown in chapter 2.1, many co-determinants or resources for health are beyond the influence of any single organization such as a school. In addition, schools are educational institutions in the first place, whose staff unlikely covers all health promotion competencies needed. - Another strengths of Hastings' model is the provision of a *consistent typology of four complementary networking processes* with clear goals or purposes identified for each (table 2.4.1). This typology is relevant not only to the analysis of organizations or networks of organizations but also for their planned change. - The model also *integrates actions of organizations at various system levels* (from local to global). This is particularly relevant to actors of international networks for the development of Health Promoting Schools (HPS) such as national HPS support centers which act at school, national and international level.

Hastings' model draws attention to additional **issues of particular relevance for international networks** for the development of Health Promoting Schools (HPS) such as:

- influences of *geographical distance between members* and its psychological and technological implications;
- the importance and *potential of the 'informal organization', of 'soft networking'* in support of an organization's goal: 'soft networking' among individuals in organizations helps to overcome or flatten lateral boundaries as well as hierarchical layers which often are embedded in formal organizational structures;
- the *relative importance of both hard (computer) networks and soft networking*, with clear emphasis on the latter which is to be supported by the former.

The model of the 'new organization' also qualifies the notions of *values, norms and cultures* in organizations: by *focusing on persons* as organizational members and less on formal organizational sub-structures, and by promoting a *culture of reciprocity and exchange* that should mediate all relationships. Overall, it matches with understandings of networking of others such as Hayes (1996) who emphasize *relationships, trust, long term perspectives* and the central roles of people and communication. Hasting's model also encompasses features of Senge's *'learning organization'*, particularly through its emphasis on reflecting and shaping organizational culture, on group and team work and learning, and the underlying systems thinking. Realizing the 'new organization' necessitates skills development, one of the corner stones of the 'learning organization'.

Most importantly, at least for this research on networks for the development of Health Promoting Schools (HPS), Hasting's presents **a model of an organization that is capable to be part of a wider network of organizations as needed.** It not only helps to better understand the organizational dimensions of *members* of such networks (such as schools or national support centers). It also indicates *when and how an organization may profit from a membership* of an inter-organizational network (ION).

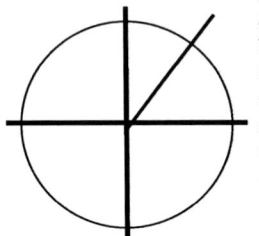

people driven (low-tech social processes)
soft networking to (help) connect people (important for innovation/change 'within' in support of overall mission/ goal);
→ patterns of communication/ learning; empowerment;

Externally driven (when resources needed are not available 'within' but through others)
interorganisational networking to create successful cooperation;
→ partnerships, synergy, resources for common goals;

internally driven (when resources needed are available 'within' but could be used better;)
networking 'within' the organization to bust vertical and lateral boundaries, and to create specific groupings across the organization around topics/ processes;
→ rapidly responding/ flexibly organization; openness and elasticity of structures/ communication processes;

technology driven (high tech IT solutions;)
hard networking to connect computers;
→ support of soft networking, particularly in national/ international contexts;

Figure 2.4.2: Hastings radar screen model of the 'New Organization': summary of the four dimensions, related networking processes, and → intended consequences. (x-axis: ways of connecting; y-axis: relationships)

Figure 2.4.2 is provides a summary of the core dimension and networking processes of the "new organization". Depending on aims, preferred directions, and context of an organization some dimensions and networking processes are more preferable than others but none of the choices excludes another. - If innovation and change 'within' the organization, patterns of communication and learning 'within' and outside, and individual self-confidence, empowerment, and 'positive power' are desired, *soft* networking should be accentuated. ('Positive power' to make desired things happen refers to power derived from a culture of *reciprocity* rather than from formal authority.) - If organizations work nationally or internationally and/or with several other organizations *hard* networking that supports soft networking is particularly important and influential. - If organizations need to be able to respond rapidly and flexibly to demands or events and/or openness and elasticity of structures and communication processes are desired, emphasis should be on networking *within* the organization, to bust vertical and lateral boundaries and to create specific interpersonal networks across the organization around selected issues.

But a sole focus on networking 'within' requires that all the resources needed to achieve a goal are available within the organization. If this is not the case or joint working would lead to a better use of resources, i.e. if partnerships are desired or needed *interorganisational* networking needs to be a focus.

In addition to an adequate combination of the strategic and networking dimensions Hastings suggests core features of the 'new' organization which match with those identified in organizational sciences and capacity development research above (chap. 2.4.2). However, Hastings explicitly proposes a **preferred direction for organizational development today:** *an organization that is capable of interorganisational networking and learning and flexible enough to adapt to and shape environmental influences.* This is quite relevant for health and educational organizations that face external demands or invitations to improve their Health Promotion potential. The boundary of this 'new organization' is more permeable. Interactions with other organizations are encouraged and common goals searched for. Mission and goal are clear, shared by all members of the organization and regularly revisited. Demanding expectations and the right for everyone to ask for cooperation are expressed. Leadership is distributed. Structures and processes reflect an *organizational culture* of reciprocity, mutual gain and exchange. This mediates all relationships. Values and underlying assumptions are reflected upon. Structures reflect decentralization with small, fairly autonomous elements or groups but which are responsible and accountable for realizing the *overall* mission and goal. Performance standards are transparent, and communicated and measured in a way that stimulates improvement. *Overall*, processes facilitate 'soft networking', intense and open communication (rather than hidden agendas), direct person-to-person relationships, information sharing, team work and team learning. Asking for help is a strength (not a weakness). Multi-disciplinary approaches are welcome. - In addition and complementary, other authors emphasize the importance of *systematic documentation and evaluation* processes.

Assessment efforts should consider four important issues: a) *Networking* positively serves the overall *organizational* goal (not individual or private ones); b) Soft networking may be 'successful' in *two* ways: for organizational goal achievement and/or building relationships and trust for *future* interactions. c) The transformation of an organization into a 'new' organization takes many *years*. d) The 'radar screen model' of the new organization is applicable to *multi*-organization systems and organizations at *all* levels of society. Thus, it will be applicable to multilevel interorganisational networks (IONs) elaborated in the next chapter, too.

While management style, incentives, and opportunities for skills development can shape the behaviors of organizations (their parts and the whole) it remains widely varying and unpredictable. Each organization is unique. Thus, **large scale efforts to help schools become 'Health Promoting Schools' (HPS) cannot work with rigid plans of organizational change** applied to all schools but **must allow and support school specific solutions**. In this situation, Hastings' dynamic and reflexive organizational **'radar screen' model offers valuable orientation**, particularly if the large scale effort of organizational change is undertaken within an interorganisational network approach. This point will be taken up in chapter 3 again. But first, the basic features of interorganisational *networks*, the focus of this research project, need examination as well as issues of how to change organizations and form and use interorganisational arrangements.

2.4.3 Features and types of networks of organizations

Introduction

So far the focus has been on features of organizations, on a better understanding of organizational *members* of international networks such as those for the development of Health Promoting Schools (HPS). Now, the *whole* that is formed by linking several organizations will be looked at more closely as it is that what is in focus of this research, i.e. *networks for* the development of HPS, not 'Health Promoting Schools'-development as such.

Interorganisational relationships have been given many names over time, in science as in popular language, and 'network' and 'networking' have become popular buzzwords during the 1990s. Most research on interorganisational relationships has a limited focus on linkages between two or three parties. But some research also addresses interorganisational relationships with four or many more members, particularly organizational research with a private sector focus and also political sciences. The many names given to such interorganisational relationships cause more confusion than improve their understanding. Terms include cartels, cooperatives, joint ventures, strategic alliances, partnerships, and networks to name but a few - and some of these terms such as 'alliances', 'partnerships' and 'networks' have increasingly been used in the field of Public Health. As Alter and Hage (1993) point out, different authors combine theses terms in different ways. Particularly the term network is increasingly used but rarely clearly defined. The academic literature is complex and disintegrated, and much of the popular literature on networking is vague and fairly vacuous.

Neither within nor across scientific disciplines such as organizational and political sciences a common understanding of interorganisational relationships and networks has been identified. What was clearly demonstrated already in the early 1990s (see e.g. reviews by Alter/ Hage 1993 and Jordan/ Schubert 1992) is true up to day. This is amazing as the praxis in various societal sectors (from business world to public health) since years shows increasingly frequent network formations. With view to the private sector this has been published already since the late 1980s (Alter, Hage 1993). But the transnational network building spearheaded by WHO/EURO since the mid 1980s among and for the development of 'Healthy Cities', 'Health Promoting Schools' and other elemental Settings received little research attention (see also chap. 2.2). Further research in this area today is more than timely as interorganisational network building is expected to spread even further and more rapidly in the near future.

Definitions and concepts of interorganisational networks

From a perspective on overall societal change Castells (1998, p5-6) describes a **'network'** as

"simply a set of inter-connected nodes. It may have a hierarchy, but it has no center. Relationships between nodes are *asymmetrical, but they are all necessary* for the functioning of the network - for the circulation of money, information, technology, images, goods, services, or people throughout the network".

Networks became powerful organizational forms due to basically technological reasons. Their 'strengths' lie in the following characteristics: flexibility, decentralizing capacity, variable geometry, and adapting to new tasks and demands without destroying their basic organizational rules or changing their overarching goals. A 'basic weakness' of networks, so Castells, is their difficulty of coordination towards a common objective or focused purpose. In this respect the concentrations of resources in space and time within vertically structured organizations have advantages. Organization and capacity development research on **interorganisational networks** also highlights issues such as flexibility, capacity to adapt, and decentralization. But they show **contradictory findings** in two points, the issues of coordination capacity and hierarchy:

First, what Castells identifies as weakness of networks is seen by others as the main reason for their existence (Alter, Hage 1993; Hastings 1993; Hilderbrand, Grindle 1994) For example, Hilderbrand and Grindle discuss networks of organizations within empirical research on 'capacity building'. The latter, part of the field of development cooperation, is usually directed at developing or transition countries. Thus, these authors share the macro perspective of Castells on societal development. The authors use the term "task networks" for networks of organizations that undertake *coordinated* activities that are *required* to accomplish a particular task. Many tasks that are important to development, the protection and promotion of population health included, require the coordinated action of several organizations. The *need for inter-organizational coordination* has been found to be the *reason* to create such networks of organizations. Second, the potential of a *hierarchy* within networks is rejected by the interorganisational relationship (IOR) researchers Alter and Hage (1993). On the base of their extensive review and synthesis of findings from theoretical and empirical work, case studies from public service and private sectors, as well as own empirical studies they postulate that networks by definition are non-hierarchical (see below).

From the organizational science perspective, Alter and Hage make a far reaching attempt to overcome the lack of integration of research results on **interorganisational relationships (IORs) and interorganisational networks (IONs)**. They build on a patchwork of IOR/ION research results from the organization sciences. In particular, they build on the concepts and distinctions of 'promotional and obligational networks' by Hollingsworth, 'equity and non-equity networks, contracts and non-contracts' by Grandori and Soda, 'competitive versus collective strategies' within organizational population-ecology theory and different types of alliances classified by Kanter (Alter, Hage 1993 p44). (Here, the term "population" refers to populations of organizations.) They describe and define organizations, networks and networking as follows: Matching with the understanding of organizations outlined in the previous section the authors stress that organizations are not autonomous entities entirely free to chose their own future. They improve the understanding of organization-environment-interactions by focusing on an organization's *organizational* environment:

- *Organizations are anchored in 'networks of interactions' with other organizations* that provide raw material or clients and/or serve as markets for products and services.

- These *interactions may* involve small or large numbers of organizations (from two to hundreds); be formally or informally established; and be ad hoc or enduring.

- These interactions are *a stabilizing force* in an organization's environment, and insuring stability reduces uncertainty.

In this sense, networking is a very necessary and successful strategy for organizations in a fast changing technological world. According to Alter and Hage:

"**Networks** constitute the *basic social form* that permits interorganisational interactions of exchange, concerted action, and joint production. Networks are *unbounded or bounded clusters* of organizations that, by definition, are *nonhierarchical* collectives of *legally separate* units." Networking is defined accordingly: "**Networking** is the *act of creating and/or maintaining* a cluster of organizations *for the purpose of* exchanging, acting, or producing among the member organizations." (Alter, Hage 1993 p46 - italics not in original)

The latter definition matches with one of the four dimensions of 'organizational networking' identified by Hastings (1993), i.e. with networking 'with others' (see previous chapter). Alter and Hage also provide a definition of **"boundary spanners"** who are important for forming and maintaining certain types of networks: These are

"individuals who engage in networking tasks and employ methods of coordination and task integration across organizational boundaries (Aldrich 1997; Katz & Kahn 1966)." (in Alter, Hage 1993 p46)

As will be seen later, within international networks on 'Health Promoting Schools' -development so called 'coordinators' are in place (at school, national and/or international levels) which fulfill 'boundary spanner' tasks. - Alter and Hage stress that their definitions of network and networking deliberately go *beyond earlier work* of theorists in their field. The latter have either focused on the purpose of exchange or on mutuality of relationships and goal setting and achievement. Alter and Hage integrate and broaden these perspectives with the explicit idea that networks can also behave as 'production systems'. An example may be the joint production of service delivery systems for promoting child and adolescent health.

The authors identify **four "normative characteristics"** common to all forms of interorganisational networks (IONs): IONs are cognitive structures, are non-hierarchical, have a division of labor, and are self-regulating (pp78-80): The notion of *cognitive structures* refers to the creation of advanced networks which requires that individuals within organizations mutually share a more or less explicit conceptual framework (e.g. on improving health through schools). They have common perceptions about the mutual technical competencies and similar judgments about useful strategies relative to their environments. Once a conceptual frame is more widely shared an area of exchange or joint action is established, based on mutually shared language, symbols, and beliefs about the effectiveness of methods. Different understandings of what works are often sources of conflict in cooperation. - In contrast to hierarchies, interorganisational networks are constituted by *lateral* linkages, thus, the authors define them as *non-hierarchical*. Nevertheless networks can vary in the degree of autonomy they possess, as they (like all organizational and interorganisational forms) are influenced by their environments. The most advanced type of interorganisational relationship, 'systemic networks' are characterized by joint decision making and problem solving (see the Alter/Hage typology below). It may happen that a network is dominated by one or a few network members, but then it is less likely to perform well. - The *division of labor* within interorganisational networks rests on the fact that each member brings a technical competency or other resource to the network. Failure of network members to demonstrate this competency or other value may terminate the relationship; successful demonstration results in mutual dependency. The division of labor protects interorganisational networks against attempts of dominant actors to control the network's functioning. - For a laterally linked cluster of autonomous organizations to act and work together, a degree of cohesion as well as giving up of sovereignty is needed. This will be achieved through democratic principles and negotiation processes with mutual adjustment of members *(self-regulation)*.

In addition to these four 'normative' characteristics of interorganisational networks (IONs), Alter and Hage (1993) identify four rather **practical dimensions**: the nature of work to be undertaken (technologies/ tasks); a range of structural properties; operational processes; and performances (levels of conflict, and interorganisational effectiveness). The authors highlight *two types* of **operational processes:** The first, *'administrative coordination'* is understood as the extent to which administrators of the various network members make decisions jointly and rely on mutual adjustment and feedback. The second, *'task integration' or 'operational coordination'* is understood as the extent to which staff of network member organizations work together interdependently across organizational boundaries. With this, Alter and Hage pay attention to the coordination at task level and the flow of 'work' (e.g. the flow of information, of products, of clients) which is lacking in much of the IOR literature. - *Methods of coordination* fall into three categories with increasing utilization of feed back: a) impersonal methods (e.g. written agreements/ contracts, rules and regulations), b) personal methods (e.g. person-to-person contact between staff members, or designation of coordinators), and c) group methods (such as face-to-face communication of several individuals planning and making decisions by consensus).

In addition to these coordination processes, five **structural properties** of interorganisational networks (IONs) are distinguished: First, the *'size'* of the network system is defines as the number of (member) organizations that participate in the work of the system. Second, a range of definitions can be found of the 'centrality' of a network; Alter and Hage side with Hickson and colleagues and define *'centrality'* in ION systems as the degree to which the total volume of work (information, clients, etc.) flows through a single or few core organizations in the network. Third, *'complexity'* (not to be confused with differentiation) of interorganisational networks is defined as the number of different service or product sectors represented by the member organizations. Fourth, *'structural differentiation'* of ION systems is defined as the degree to which there is functional and service specialization among the member organizations of the system, i.e. division of function and labor. Alter and Hage point to the positive relationship between the latter two, i.e. as networks increase the kinds of organizations involved, they are assigned limited roles. Thus, a network of mainly schools may have the tendency to low differentiation, but this must not be the case. Task scope and differentiation need to be distinguished, with task scope referring to the sophistication of *technology* (such as the use of differential diagnosis of a school's health promotion potential) and ION differentiation referring to the functional specialization among network *members*. The fifths structural property of IONs is their *'connectiveness'*, i.e. their total number of linkages between organizations in the system (the extent to which every channel is used). This can produce highly productive exchange networks. However, if such a network moves from information exchange to a chosen joint activity it may find that unity of action is very difficult given the large number of channels used. Different types or developmental stages of networks may benefit from different network structures. Alter and Hage not only identify core features of interorganisational networks (IONs), they also develop an **ION typology**, a remarkable step forward in ION research. This has been done along three dimensions: competitive versus symbiotic cooperation of network members; the number of organizations involved; and the level or extent of cooperation. But before introducing this typology it needs to be assessed how far the approach of Alter and Hage matches, complements or contradicts other ION research findings. Should these complement and confirm each other, the typology will be further examined as to its potential to serve as a guiding framework for assessing international networks for developing Health Promoting Schools and similar networks.

Hilderbrand and Grindle (1994) distinguish two 'components' of interorganisational "task"-networks: the *'organizations'* and the *'interactions among them'*. Such distinctions remind of the two general characteristics of organizations identified in previous sections: the *people and structural relationships* and the *connective mechanisms and processes*. Two basic characteristics of interorganisational networks (IONs) emerge: the *network structure or 'architecture'* (the network members and their structural relationships), the *network processes* (both 'operational processes' to make the network function and 'connective processes' to hold the network elements together). Connective processes are likely a sub-category of operational processes, as holding its elements together will be essential for the network to fulfill its purpose. Connective processes could be of particular importance in different phases of network development, for example, in the very early development phase or in time periods where some of the network members may not be in the center of network activities (see chapters 2.4.4 and 2.4.5 on changing organizations and forming networks).

Several *political scientists* have undertaken research similar to interorganisational relations (IOR) research and some have used the term network in this context. Typically, political scientists have concentrated on relationships between government or the State on the one hand and interest groups or societal actors on the other. This research draws attention to the fact that a 'government' or Ministry is not just 'another organization' in interorganisational networks (IONs). This concerns international networks for the development of Health Promoting Schools as these involve both governmental agencies such as Ministries of Education and Health and NGOs. - *'Government/interest group-relations'* researchers use the term 'network' in a variety of ways (e.g. Jordan, Schubert 1992; Cook, Whitmeyer 1992 (exchange network theory/ network analysis); Heclo 1978 (issue networks)). Not only in organizational theory and management research but also in the political sciences a clear terminology around interorganisational relations and network issues is lacking. But, as Cook and Whitmeyer point out, 'network analysis' is an area of political sciences rooted in the empirical observation that '*patterns* of interaction of many actors' can be looked at as networks (Cook, Whitmeyer 1992 p114). Jordan and Schubert (1992) criticize that the range of terms used signals a greater variety of State-interest relationships than they deliver. They review and compare ten labels or types of relations between government/State and interest groups/ societal actors developed and used in contemporary political sciences. As a consequence they propose to use the term 'policy network' as a generic label embracing different types of 'network relationship'. As a starting point they refer to the following basic definition of the term network by Hanf:

"...the term '**network**' merely denotes, in a suggestive manner, the fact that policy making includes a large number of public and private actors from different levels and functional areas of government and society." (Hanf 1978 in Jordan, Schubert 1992 p11)

The explicit inclusion of actors from *different levels* indicates that results of this type of network research may be of relevance to the conceptual work needed towards an assessment framework for multi-level networks focusing on HPS. Hanf's definition also indicates that formal or constitutional differences between State and societal actors are of less importance in policy making processes. This is confirmed by the following definition of 'policy networks' which stems from Kenis and Schneider (1989). Three policy network features are mentioned here:

"A **policy network** is described by its actors, their linkages and its boundaries. It includes a relatively stable set of mainly public and private corporate *actors*. The *linkages* between the actors serve as channels of communication and for the exchange of information, expertise, trust and other policy resources. The *boundary* of a given policy network is not in the first place determined by formal institutions but results from a process of mutual recognition dependent of functional relevance and structural embeddedness (1989: 14)." (quoted in Jordan, Schubert 1992 p12 - italics as in original)

This definition confirms network structure and processes as the two basic ION characteristics. The 'actors' are network members and address the network structure. The 'linkages' address their interactions and, thus, network processes. The dimension of 'boundary' is not a category distinct from that of network members ('actors') as it addresses the *membership selection process and criteria*. Nevertheless, the issue of boundary of a given ION points to important questions in network research such as: Do networks in general, and inter-organizational networks in particular, have or need a clear boundary ? (For organizations this is a key feature.) If yes: Who is 'in' and who is 'out'? Which criteria should be used to draw the line between network members and non-members so that their strengths such as flexibility are not compromised? This will be taken up later again.

Jordan and Schubert (1992) present results of a comparative analysis of various types of State-interest relationships or policy networks found in contemporary political sciences. Their search for an empirically useful typology of networks for policy making results in the identification of three *'main dimensions'* that describe policy networks: the *number of actors* or 'group participants' (one group; two conflicting groups; a restricted number of groups; a large number of groups with low access threshold;); the *scope of issues* discussed (sectoral or trans-sectoral); and the *type of relationships among actors* (stable or ad hoc). The authors place all review findings of interorganisational (State/interest) relationships within such a framework of 'policy networks'. But, in contrast to Alter and Hage they do not go on to propose a typology of networks. - International development cooperation research indicates that 'policy networks' and other interorganisational networks such as 'task networks' have general features in common. For example, task networks may be composed of a smaller or larger number of organizations only from one sector or of a mixture of organizations across sectors (public, private and/or NGO) (Hilderbrand/

Grindle 1994). The latter implies that sectoral or cross-sectoral issues may be addressed. In international relations research (policy) networks have been studied as well and dimensions of networks overlapping and complementary to those above have been identified. Kassim (1994) identifies the following four: *type of linkages and interactions* (degree of multiplicity), *number of actors* connected (large, small), *variety of actors* connected (wide, smaller), and *actors from which levels* of government and society (of all, some, one level). - Also Hastings (1993), from an organizational development and management perspective, points to the issue of *variety* of actors and *levels* they may represent: He found that interorganisational networks (IONs) are mechanisms for both large and small organizations, local or national ones, to operate beyond their local or national boundaries. He specifies the 'actor dimension' of networks: Networking with others requires network members *to be able to share control*, a mind-set that in practice is difficult to achieve as it is often linked to perceived loss of power.

Concepts of interorganisational networks and the Alter / Hage model - intermediate synthesis and discussion

There is clearly a paucity of interorganisational network (ION) literature. At a general level, similar or complementary sets of *general features* of interorganisational networks have been identified by various authors and across a range of research areas as outlined above. Much literature remains at a fairly general level which indicates that IONs did not receive sufficient research attention yet. However, it can be summarized that features of IONs fall into five broad categories as spelled out in table 2.4.2.

Network environment /context	
General dimensions: institutional, socio-political, economic, environmental; *(more specific by Alter and Hage (A&H) 1993 as follows)*	
Network purpose	
Mutually sharing of a conceptual framework (as a base for defining common purpose) (A&H) Goals/tasks: Scope/ complexity (lower/ higher); *(further differentiation by Alter & Hage as follows)*	
Network structure (members and their structural relationships)	**Network processes** (operational -, connective -)
Network members: By definition legally separate units *(A&H)*; Number of members (smaller/ larger; restricted or not; in flow or not;) Type of members (sector/field represented; societal level represented or focused on; individual organization/group of organizations; ...) Variety of members (smaller/ wider; one/few/many types of organizations; ...) Kind of technologies/ bodies of knowledge represented by members; Location of members (geographically dispersed/ same area)	**Relations/ interactions among members:** By definition non-hierarchical ? *(A&H)*; lateral linkages; self-regulation *(A&H)*; Informal or formal; Competitive or symbiotic *(A&H)*; Duration (stable or ad hoc) Quality criteria (often emphasized): direct person to person connections, trust, mutual benefit and reciprocity (win/win), sharing of information/resources, long term perspective;
Structural properties of the network: Network size; unbounded/ bounded ? Network centrality; by definition no center? - *Castells 1998)* Network complexity Network differentiation Network connectivity	**Umbrella concept/ core process:** Coordination: Levels or extent of cooperation (limited, moderate, broad;)
Membership criteria: mutual recognition dependent of functional relevance and structural embeddedness - *Kenis/ Schneider 1989* Threshold to enter (lower/ higher)	
Performances	
flexibility; easily adapting to new tasks/ demands (without destroying the basic organizational rules or changing overarching goals - *Castells 1998)* levels of conflict, interorganisational effectiveness *(Alter and Hage)*	

Table 2.4.2: General features of interorganisational networks (IONs) - Intermediate summary by five broad categories: a network's environment or context; purpose; structures; processes; and performances. (Where a feature was only mentioned in one source the author is mentioned.)

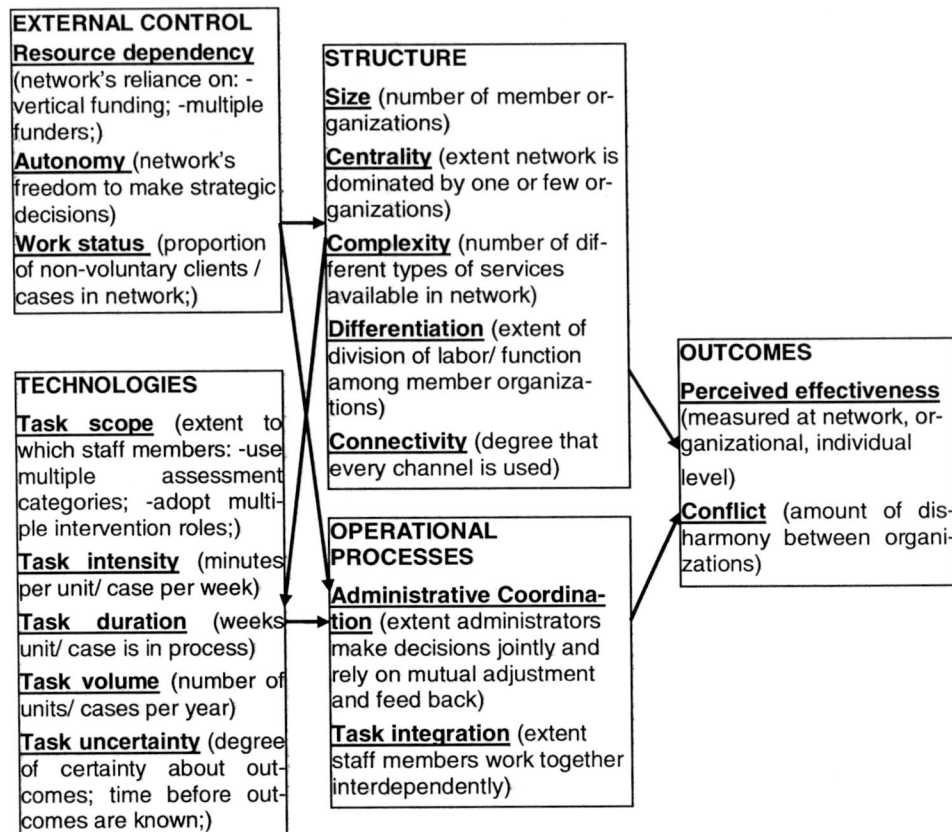

Figure 2.4.3: The conceptual framework for studying systemic interorganisational networks by Alter and Hage (1993 p103, slightly adapted)

A comparison of general features of interorganisational networks (IONs) and the Alter/Hage conceptual framework for studying IONs (table 2.4.2 and on fig. 2.4.3) shows:

- Findings of various research perspectives on interorganisational relationships can be nested *within* the Alter/Hage ION framework. This supports the assumption implemented by Alter and Hage that many research findings on coordination and relationships from studies of *single organizations* and their sub-units can be applied to *interorganisational* relationships and networks.

- The various research perspectives referred to address issues that are related to international networks for the development of Health Promoting Schools, such as international relations, public policy making, and social and economic development including health and education development in countries. This indicates that the *Alter/Hage model*, although it is heavily based on research on private sectors (in Europe, Asia and North America) as well as on (US American) public care services, *promises to serve well as guiding framework for research on international IONs in Health Promotion* such as those for developing Health Promoting Schools (HPS).

- The work by Alter and Hage on IONs is remarkable in the sense that they not only identify and clearly define *characteristics* of IONs but - on the base of this - also define particular *types* of IONs (see below) as well as address the question of what constitutes '*good performance*' of such networks (see chap. 2.4.4 below). The latter is obviously important to this research project on assessing networks for developing HPS.

Therefore, and in light of a lack of other, similarly advanced models, the research results of Alter and Hage remain an important body of knowledge also for the following chapters and its basic elements need to be explained. Structural properties (size, centrality, complexity, differentiation, connectivity) and operational processes (administrative coordination, coordination at task level/ task integration) have been already addressed above. Alter and Hage found that among the various combinations possible of structural properties (i.e. network structures) a few are more common in practice. Their illustrations in figure 2.4.4 show how significantly different structures of interorganisational systems may be and invites self-reflection on personal images of interorganisational 'networks'.

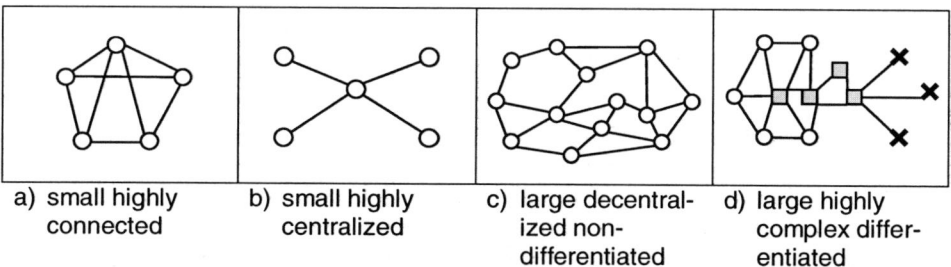

a) small highly connected   b) small highly centralized   c) large decentralized non-differentiated   d) large highly complex differentiated

Figure 2.4.4:   Graphs depicting different interorganisational 'network' structures. (Alter / Hage 1993 p150)

Particularly graph b in comparison to c points to the open question raised by the literature review regarding the dimension of *centrality* of interorganisational networks (IONs): While Alter and Hage accept both high or low centrality as a feature of an ION, for other authors (e.g. Castells

1998) a network by definition has no center. Thus, an interorganisational system such as under b would not be labeled 'network'. However, such a decision may best be made in taking not only structural characteristics into account but also process features, goals, development phase, and underlying values of network participants. At the end, the definition of what is a 'network' and what not entails both normative decisions and consideration of 'core' features of interorganisational networks (IONs) identified in research. In the following, *the decision on a network definition and conceptual framework for use in this research project will be prepared* enhancing the understanding of the ION model proposed by Alter and Hage (below) as well as of the forming and maintaining of interorganisational networks in general (chap. 2.4.4). Once, ION features, types, and development and maintenance are well understood, the ground is prepared to turn to the essential question for network assessment brought up by the work of Alter and Hage: Has it been (or is it at all) possible to identify some 'key' features or even most promising constellations of features of interorganisational networks (IONs) that lead to high levels of effectiveness, in terms of perceived effectiveness and acceptable levels of conflict or otherwise?

The interorganisational network (ION) typology by Alter and Hage

With view to interrelations among public or private organizations and a mix of both Alter and Hage (1993) follow questions that are very relevant to this research project: Which forms of networks are the most flexible and innovative, and which are most capable of producing quality and adapting efficiently? Because of this, and as the general ION features underlying this typology are supported by or complementary to those identified by other researchers, the Alter/Hage-network typology will now be presented. It promises to be a useful guiding framework for the development of an ION assessment framework needed in this research project. The authors underline that the lack of sufficient theoretical work hinders them to develop an exhaustive classification of populations of interorganisational networks. However, they advance the field of ION research significantly by suggesting a typology of interorganisational forms organized along three dimensions: 1. competitive versus symbiotic cooperation; 2. the number of organizations involved, and 3. the level or extent of cooperation.

1. Interorganisational forms fall into two basic categories: forms used for *competitive* cooperation by organizations in the *same sector*, and those used for *symbiotic* cooperation by organizations in *different sectors*. Competitors are organizations of the same kind (producing the same service or product). Symbiotic relationships occur between

organizations that may have some similarities but operate in different sectors. - Important is that directly competing organizations may less easily enter in cooperative relationships or networks than those not competing. Among the latter intense interaction is more likely and cooperative behavior more possible.

2. In the private corporate sector smaller numbers of organizations involved in cooperation have been found to increase the potential for cheating. This may be more or less relevant for interorganisational networks such as NHPS, depending on the level of competition of schools or other organizational members with regard to a selected issue.

3. Earlier work has distinguished between different levels of *exchange* among organizations, e.g. between information exchange and resource exchange or exchange linkages within different areas (technical, planning, social, economic, legal, etc.). The new idea inherent in Alter and Hage's theoretical model of interorganisational relationships and networks is the following: **Exchange is only the beginning, not the end of cooperative interorganisational behavior**. Whether among competitors or non-competing organizations, **three levels of cooperation** are being distinguished:

- 'limited' cooperation with pooling and/or exchange of information and/or resources;
- 'moderate' cooperation in accomplishing a functional purpose;
- 'broad' cooperation involving the production of a product or service.

The various facets of the Alter/ Hage typology of interorganisational linkages and networks still lack a certain degree of precision. Therefore, the following summary is to some extent *interpretative*. Table 2.4.3 provides an overview of the typology.

No. of members → *Three guiding dimensions*		Dyadic and triadic linkages		Multi-organizational / sector wide networks	
Levels of cooperation ↓	Type of Co-operation →	competitive	symbiotic	competitive	symbiotic
Limited cooperation Pooling/ exchange of:		**Obligational Linkages** e.g.: - information - resources - emotional support	e.g.: - products, services, clients - money - power - human capital	**Obligational Networks** e.g.: - information - resources - emotional support	e.g.: - products, services, clients - money - power - human capital
Moderate cooperation Joint achievement of functional objectives:		**Promotional Linkages** e.g. - technological - economic - political	e.g. - technological - economic - political	**Promotional Networks** e.g. - technological - economic - political	e.g. - technological - economic - political
Broad cooperation Joint production of:		**Systemic Production Linkages** e.g. - goods or services	e.g. - goods or services	**Systemic Production Networks** e.g. - goods or services; - joint control of production area	e.g. - goods or services

Table 2.4.3: A typology of cooperative interorganisational relationships and networks. (adapted from Alter and Hage, 1993 pp 50-61)

'Obligational networks' and linkages among organizations are characterized by *'limited'* cooperation in the sense of more or less dense reciprocal *exchange* of information and material or immaterial resources, for example, services, clients, money, power, human capital (people with valuable knowledge or skills). They are motivated by the *needs of individual organizations* rather than collective needs, i.e. each organization focuses on its own goals and likely does 'its own thing' while taking advantage of the benefits derived from the interorganisational network (ION). The exchange takes reflects and creates *mutual dependency. Members do not integrate their activities* with that of other network members. Therefore, such networks do not require high levels of mutual trust and can maintain themselves without collective governance. *'Boundary spanners'* are often prevalent.

Examples include "patterned resource exchanges" such as communication networks among researchers across organization boundaries, mutual support networks among professionals at high risk of emotional burnout, or exchanges for hidden purposes such as friendship, trust or loyalty. - In the case of a network for the development of HPS (NHPS) this may mean exchange of models of good practice, tools for evaluation or project management, or mutual support among school teams to maintain motivation and courage to work towards health supportive changes in their schools in spite of difficulties.

When obligational networks or linkages are maintained over time, and a level of interorganisational trust is established, then interorganisational forms may take on additional functions beyond exchange.

'Promotional networks' and linkages among organizations are characterized by *'moderate'* cooperation in the sense that members try to jointly achieve functional purposes. They may exchange resources as in obligational networks but, in addition, use their participation to achieve additional purposes. - Their purpose is to achieve *collective objectives that could not be achieved by a single or limited number* of organizations, or only with inappropriate levels of investments or risk taking. The achievement of these collective objectives needs to be useful or necessary for each member organization to be able to reach its individual goal or fulfill its tasks. Such objectives may be technological, economic or political in nature. The *function and activities* of these IONs have clear limits which are defined by the overlap of the interests, desires, and goals of the diverse members. They are *peripheral and segmented.* - In the case of symbiotic networks, the different technical expertise of network members may lead more likely to innovations.

Examples of cooperation at this level include collectively fundraising or financing and managing research and development tasks; joint awareness raising, marketing, advertising or purchasing; and joint lobbying or advocacy among policy and decision makers for common objectives or legislative changes. - Symbiotic promotional networks (with members from various sectors) are usually concerned with more broad based cross-cutting political decisions or legislation such as health, social security or tax issues. Examples include those seeking to solve societal problems (such as environmental degradation, gun control) or to promote causes such as human rights. - A NHPS may, for example, jointly develop and disseminate project material, fund raise and/or advocate to increase political support.

'Systemic production networks' and production linkages among organizations are characterized by *'broad'* cooperation in the sense that *essential functions* of organizations are *accomplished jointly* (broad functional integration), for example, product or service development, purchasing, (social) marketing/ advertising, dissemination/ distribution, service delivery and follow-up, and/or quality assessment/ evaluation. This results in the joint production of goods or services. The more functions are undertaken jointly, the broader the cooperation. Systemic (production) networks are complex structures. They are motivated by the desire to *produce goods or deliver services that could not be produced by any one participant alone* thus, *collectively* they are innovative. In the case of competing organizations the motive may simply be costs or financial risks too high for any one organization.

Systemic (production) networks of the symbiotic type have been found to: involve members in exchange of information, technology and other resources; require *members to arrive at goals and objectives by consensus* and to engage in joint effort to achieve them; produce products or services that typically are coordinated by one 'assembler' who connects with organizations that 'build components' of the desired product or service and who in turn connect with other organizations from other sectors. These networks have an important social element: *social bonds* develop during many meetings and via the elaborate system of joint working; these social ties are the *basis of trust and commitment* that move *beyond the mutual dependency* in exchange relationships.

The complexity and long term perspective of such IONs is illustrated by the following example on improving the situation of victims of domestic and sexual assault. In a community, over five years a women's group, police, state attorney, county hospital, legal aid and community college created and implemented an interagency protocol that a) governed the timing, scope and sequence of the network organizations' responses to crisis, and b) assigned functions, roles and tasks to each network organization. This resulted in an integrated service delivery system for victims, and the number of prosecutions for rape quadrupled and of convictions tripled. (Alter/Hage 1993).

Alter and Hage (1993) emphasize that the level of cooperation within both competing and symbiotic interorganisational networks is not only a classifying variable but also an indicator of network *evolution*. This and related issues are elaborated in chapter 2.4.5 below.

General features of interorganisational networks (IONs) - synthesis and discussion

As of now, this chapter 2.4 did focus on identifying the *general features of organizational systems* both individual organizations and interorganisational networks. This was done mainly from an organization research perspective but other social sciences were considered, too. The following summary of the general features of *interorganisational networks (IONs)* will be followed by a chapter on development, change and maintenance of such organizational systems. Afterwards, in chapter 3, a new step will be done: the vast body of research knowledge reviewed (on health, Health Promotion, and interorganisational networks) will be taken as the basis for developing a conceptual framework with practical indicators for assessing interorganisational networks (IONs) for the development of health promoting Settings such as schools, and similar networks.

Several **categories or sets of features of interorganisational networks (IONs)** have been identified that need to be taken into account in ION development, change, analyses and assessment efforts (see also fig. 2.4.3):

- network **structure**: size; centrality; complexity; differentiation; connectivity; boundaries/ membership criteria or threshold; location of members (geographically dispersed or not);

- network **processes**: level of cooperation (limited, moderate, broad - see table 2.4.3); administrative coordination (extent of joint decision making/ mutual adjustment/ feed back); operational coordination/ task integration (extent of joint interdependent working/ mutual adjustment/ feed back); self-regulation; communication processes (more or less direct/ person-to-person); methods of coordination used ('impersonal' such as contracts; 'personal' such as direct contact between individuals or designation of coordinators; 'group' methods such as meetings for joint planning and decision making);
    - → type of **relationships**: competitive or symbiotic cooperation; informal or formal links; hierarchical relations or not (?) (some authors understand the organizational form of 'networks' by definition as non-hierarchical);

- network **task, goal and purpose**: conceptual framework (as a base for defining common purpose) mutually shared or not; scope; task intensity, duration, volume; expected outcomes (types; degree of uncertainty/ long or short term);

- network **environment:** an organization's external controls (resource dependency/ autonomy/ proportion of non-voluntary clients); general dimensions (institutional/ organizational, social, political, economic, physical/natural environments);

- network **performance or outcomes**: perceived effectiveness (at individual, organization, network level); amount of conflict between member organizations; outcomes in relation to the goals set by the network;

Obviously, some relationships (within the network or with external entities) may be structurally defined. However, 'relationships' have been placed as process (rather structural) ION features as ('new') organizations capable of learning and networking as well as interorganisational networks rely much on direct and lateral communication processes across (often structural) boundaries. - The distinction between 'competitive' and 'symbiotic' interorganisational relationships or cooperation introduced by Alter and Hage (1993) is easily agreeable. But the definition of 'competing organizations' as organizations of the same kind (producing the same service or product) is not sufficient. For example, following this definition all schools within a network of Health Promoting Schools (HPS) would be defined as competitors as they offer the same basic service to communities: education. But it fairly common that they serve different sections of towns or populations groups. Thus, for the purpose of this research project, an *expanded definition of 'competing organizations'* is proposed that includes the production of the same services or products *for the same group of people* (geographically or other wise). This leaves most schools in public education systems (i.e. the core members of the network cases in focus) in symbiotic rather competitive relations.

Important **open questions** are those of **the relative importance of the various ION features identified above, how they interact to produce desired outcomes, and under which circumstances**. In this regard, the organization sciences face a problem similar to that of the public health sciences regarding the range of co-determinants of health (see chap. 2.1): While there is widespread agreement on the *range* of factors and that these are *interrelated* and interacting, it has been *yet impossible to identify <u>the</u> 'key' factors* that change interventions should focus on. The challenge is to recognize and better understand *complex dynamic interrelations and appropriately respond* to them. What Marmot pointed out with view to the social co-determinants of health applies to interorganisational networks, too: One needs to break down complex questions into manageable pieces but "not, however, focus on the manageable pieces to the exclusion of the larger picture" (Marmot 2000 p365). Simple and standard solutions are illusory whether in promoting and maintaining the health of populations or in forming and maintaining interorganisational networks.

Nevertheless, with regard to 'successful' IONs a few authors point to a *preferred* extent, degree or shape of some features or even preferred combinations of features. An examination of such information may bear answers to another set of **open questions regarding the *nature* of interorganisational networks (IONs)**: first, whether IONs have by definition no center (e.g. Castells 1998) or can exhibit different degrees of *cen-*

trality but with consequences for their outcomes (e.g. Alter/ Hage 1993); second, whether IONs are by definition 'bounded *or* unbounded' organizational forms (Alter/ Hage 1993) or do have *boundaries* as all organizations do; third, whether *relationships* are rather stable and with a long term perspective (e.g. Kenis/ Schneider 1989; Hayes 1996; Hastings 1993) or may be also ad hoc (e.g. Jordan/ Schubert 1992); and fourth, whether IONs are by definition *non-hierarchical* (Alter/ Hage 1993) or may include members that are hierarchically linked (e.g. Castells 1998) - with the former position not allowing, for example, schools and a Ministry of Education being in the same network, the latter yes. These questions are important for ION assessment and taken up in *chapter 3* which then will lead to the yet outstanding task of deciding on a definition of interorganisational networks for this research project.

The yet open issues seems not to affect another key feature of interorganisational networks (IONs): **network evolution** as unraveled by Alter and Hage with their **ION typology**. In sum, *'obligational' (or exchange) networks* engage in 'limited' cooperation with the *needs of individual member organizations* in the foreground; they exchange information or resources but joint activities are rare or ad hoc. *'Promotional' networks* engage in 'moderate' cooperation with *supra-ordinate member problems or functional purposes* in the foreground (which one member would not be able to address alone); joint activities are peripheral or segmented (e.g. joint fundraising). *'Systemic' networks* engage in 'broad' cooperation with *supra-ordinate goals* (may be societal goals) in the foreground; jointly producing services or products that could not be produced by any one member alone involves essential and enduring joint activities. (see also chap. 2.4.5). 'Exchange' is only the beginning, not the end of cooperative interorganisational behavior. - Given the multi-level character of international networks for the development of Health Promoting Schools (HPS) and their *expansion over time* a particular question arises: Could it happen that even after a longer time span an international network would consist of network sections or groups of members that remain loosely linked exchange networks while other sections or groups matured into joint action or promotional networks and again others into systemic networks? The next chapters may help to answer such questions.

Now, the attention is shifted away from questions of 'what *are*' organizations and interorganisational networks to questions of 'how to *change*' such systems: a) how to change *organizations* in a desired direction (which will be rather briefly addressed) and b) how to form or maintain interorganisational *networks* (IONs). The reasons are twofold: *First*, how to change individual organizations is a core question for international networks for the development of 'Health Promoting Schools'

(HPS), as their main purpose is to achieve the sustainable transformation of existing schools into 'Health Promoting Schools' (HPS). As ION assessment needs to take the goals set by a network into account this question has to be looked at. *Second*, the creation and maintenance of *any* interorganisational network (ION) inherently means some change at the level of the individual organizations that become network members. Indeed, becoming part of a network may be a far reaching innovation for some organizations. Thus, ION functioning cannot be understood and assessed without a certain degree of understanding of change processes of organizations. - The clarification of *processes of forming and maintaining* interorganisational networks (IONs) is done in a two step process (similarly to that of the *general features* of IONs before): first, *individual* organizations are addressed, then the larger systems of interorganisational *networks.* (chapters 2.4.4 and 2.4.5)

2.4.4 Achieving change in organizations and organizational systems

This chapter aims at clarifying the main points related to change processes in organizations but, it should be noted that **the focus is on organizations as *network* members, not on organizational change per se**. A comprehensive review of organizational change or development literature is not at stake, neither in general nor with a specific focus on school development. The **primary goal** is to create **a general understanding of current knowledge on organizational change** for two purposes: on the one hand, as a basis for a better understanding of interorganisational network functioning and processes of forming, maintaining or changing such networks; on the other hand, as a basis for assessing whether interorganisational networks for the development of Health Promoting Schools (HPS) a) have appropriate or unrealistic expectations towards their members and organizational change as such, and b) are themselves supportive of such organizational change. *Another goal* is to identify key issues or processes related those models of organizations identified before as particular relevant or promising for an interorganisational *network* context (particularly the 'new organization' and/or 'learning' organization). - Overall, relevant research knowledge falls under two broad headings: 'organizational change or development' research and 'capacity development' research.

Insights from organizational change and development research

While the interest of health promotion practitioners in organizational change continues to grow only a few systematic applications of organizational change theory in Health Promotion or health education have been published. In contrast to the many individual *behavior* change theories, organizational change theories are far less developed and analyzed and much less systematically tested. (Goodmann, Steckler, Kegler 1997; Nutbeam 1998 p56) With view to mobilizing organizations for health enhancement Goodman et al conclude: As organizations may be influenced at each of their layers (from individual to environments) *no single theory is sufficient for explaining how and why organizations change;* and, health promotion strategies directed at several systems levels *simultaneously* may be most durable in producing desired results. – Organization research itself does not propose the model to explain or guide innovation or change in organizations. Much of organizational development theory applied behavioral sciences to improve organizational effectiveness in terms of both performance and quality of work life. Up to day, the **knowledge in this area is neither integrated nor well systematized**, and typologies vary and are overlapping. For long, much attention has been given to two broad areas: the so called 'stage theory' and 'implementation theory'.

Influenced by the diffusion of innovation theory, **'stage theory'** refers to *a series of stages that organizations pass through as they innovate* new goals, programs, technologies or ideas (e.g. a new school curriculum). Various models with *different* numbers and types of stages exist (Goodman et al 1997): For example, a 'comprehensive' model by Beyer and Trice 1987 consists of seven stages; other authors use four or five innovation stages (e.g. problem definition, or alternatively awareness raising; adoption; implementation; and institutionalization). Matching with such models, Bowes (1997) decides to distinguish only **two main phases of the innovation process in organizations**: the *initiation phase that prepares a decision* to be made on an innovation, and the *implementation phase* that starts as soon as the decision is made. This draws attention to a) the fact that clear decisions need to be prepared and taken to introduce change in organizations (which needs time), and b) the question by whom decisions may be made. As will be seen later, both issues have been taken seriously by European networks for HPS development. - The umbrella term **'implementation theory'** covers more practical approaches than 'stage theory'; **sequences of action** for producing change in organizations are suggested. The most prominent implementation theories have four core steps in common: 1. diagnosis, 2. action planning, 3. organizational development interventions, and 4. evaluation.

In sum, there is **little widespread agreement but**: a) Achieving **sustainable organizational change needs time**. Even for more 'simple' innovations such as the introduction of a new curriculum element on health education authors suggest time frames of *several* organization cycles (e.g. school years). b) **Organizations that introduce an innovation pass through several stages of change.** While there is **no consensus about their optimal number and types, two major phases** are agreeable: 'initiation' and 'implementation' phase (see above). Overall, the situation maintains a lack of clarity about influential factors, how innovations move from stage to stage, and appropriate strategies for each stage of change. This makes planning for change in organizations along the lines of 'stage theory' difficult. − In the light of this, calls (e.g. by Goodman et al 1997) for further refinements of stage models beyond the institutionalization phase to include a 'renewal stage' in which established programs (the former innovations) need to evolve to meet changing demands seem questionable. The models appear to be based on more traditional organization models. Little emphasis is given to the organizations' environment. Also, evaluation is usually considered only as a final, separate step rather an integral part of a change process. The stage models seem to be more sufficient for *limited* organizational innovations (such as an introduction of a new *element* of a school curriculum) that does *not* much affect the organization as a *whole.* **For more comprehensive and fundamental changes of organizations** (such as those implied in creating a 'Health Promoting School') **other models of organizational change are needed**. Approaches to develop the 'new' organization capable of learning are more promising.

Creating the 'new' organization capable of 'learning' and organizational networking

As explained before (chap. 2.4.2) social organizations must develop their internal structures in processes of self-organization that are adequate to their relevant environments which they actively influence. Over the long run sustainable change of organizational structures and processes are achievable only from *within* the organization, not by external agents.

Lessons from work towards 'learning organizations' include that goal achievement requires *investing into a continuous process* that *integrates*: personal learning, changes of the ways of working and organizational culture, and of organizational structures. Also external conditions are modified. The overall learning processes are critically reflected. There are three central elements to success: 1. *guiding ideas* (e.g. Health Promoting Schools) which provide particular change initiatives with an overall meaning, commitment socially and as regards content, and energize development processes; 2. *theories, and practical instruments,* to assure scientifically sound problem definitions and responses and facilitate required changes; 3. *innovations at the level of infrastructures* to create sustainable organizational forms that promote learning and provide a 'place' for changes (e.g. coordination committees, interprofessional groups). (Lobnig, Nowak, Pelikan 1997; Senge 1996) – Lessons from Health Promotion practice include that neglecting one or more of the above three dimensions slow down organization development processes or leave them incomplete. And, the 'health promoting Settings' approach can well be combined with organization development and quality management. Importantly, all three strategies a) use *'open concepts'* as guiding ideas (e.g. 'health' or 'development') rather than rules and regulations which helps an organization to *maintain flexibility and at the same time stability;* they b) emphasize processes of *self-regulation* and combined bottom-up and top-own strategies with *participation* of all those concerned (as opposed to centralist 'illusions of control'). Overall, the Health Promotion concepts emphasis on positive, not deficit oriented approaches, broad participation, people's needs as starting points, and organization-environment-relations facilitates the creation of joint visions, forms of collaboration, and processes of reorganization. Establishing participation and cooperation *across* professional groups and hierarchical levels is important, and so is the promotion of reflection and organizational learning at *all* levels and in *all* organizational subsystems. Interest, acceptance, commitment and support by all those concerned maintained over a longer time span is essential. (Lobnig et al 1997)

To create Hastings' 'new' organization a culture of 'organizational networking' is needed (see chap. 2.4.2). There are several 'roots' of organizational networking (i.e. soft/ hard networking; networking within an organization/ with others) to be nurtured: *Occasions* for general information sharing, unplanned contacts and a blending of ideas (such as conferences) support innovation. 'Soft networking' can be nurtured through a range of *'soft technologies'* (from meeting space and design to mobility policies to newsletters with technical issues and contacts); *project work* (particularly in times of organizational change or the beginning of interorganisational collaboration); *sharing know-how* and an appropriate use of 'hard' (computer) networks. This all helps to create organizations capable of learning and working within interorganisational networks. (Hastings 1993)

However, it should be recalled (from chap. 2.4.2) that reform and change of 'expert organizations' (such as European schools) towards organizations capable of learning and networking pose particular challenges. **Core issues for the reform and change of 'expert organizations'** (such as many public schools) are: 1) actively addressing their inherent contradictions, particularly to get experts and sub-units relate their work to the overall goal of their organization and its development needs; 2) starting by strengthening of the core units, while using authority to balance voluntariness and compulsoriness (as experts need to 'think' the needs of the whole organization); 3) quality development at *two* performance levels: the core units and 'general' processes beyond core units (e.g. class room teaching and general school climate); 4) more resources for management and self-administration to ensure successful change management; 5) radical increase of the status of the organization's management (e.g. through management teams of experts and professional managers); and 6) stronger consideration of the needs of the 'customers' (e.g. pupils, parents) and their involvement into the quality assessment of services. (Grossmann et al 1997)

Changing organizations - intermediate synthesis and discussion

Overall, the above reviewed literature suggests some **basic general features of sustainable organizational change processes** that should be considered by international networks for the development of Health Promoting Schools (HPS): Organizational change does not occur in one step or over the short term but over the *long term (years)* and in *stages*. Consensus on type and number of stages is lacking but two broad phases are widely distinguished: an initiation phase (ending with the decision to implement) and an implementation phase (traditionally thought of to end with the institutionalization of the innovation). However, this applies more to *particular single innovations* in existing organizations (such as a new curriculum *element* in a school) rather than changes of an organization as a whole. **More recent organization models shift the focus** away form single innovations towards developing organizations that are capable of 'learning', networking, adapting to changing environments or demands, and actively modifying external conditions in relation to their mission, goals or tasks. Ideally organizations are ready and able to take up, reflect and decide on *any* innovation proposed or identified as needed at *any* point in time; **ideally openness to innovation and change is part of the organizational *culture* rather than a special effort during a limited period of time**.

At a general level, achieving organization change in this direction requires:

- *addressing organizations in relation to their environments;*
- *investments in continuous processes* that integrate learning of organizational members, changes in organizational culture, processes, and structures;

- *creating or maintaining a mission, vision or guiding idea* that allows an organization to maintain flexibility and at the same time stability, and enable responses to a variety of changes within an organization's established framework for action;
- an *appropriate knowledge base or theories* that allow sound definitions of goals and organizational responses, and an appropriate set of methods or instruments to facilitate needed changes;
- *innovations at the level of infrastructures* (such as mechanisms or bodies for coordination and team work across professional or structural boundaries);
- *accepting and supporting processes of self-regulation* of organizations and *participation* of stakeholders (rather than keeping up illusions of control);
- *investing time and other resources to establish self-observation and self-reflection* (as an integral part of the organization's culture) *as well as evaluation*; external support may be needed particularly at early stages of organizational change.

At a more practical level, organizational development and modern project management methods are valuable tools to achieve far reaching and sustainable change in complex social systems. Their use requires or implies:

- *creating interest, acceptance, commitment, and support* for an innovation *by all members or sub-systems* of the organization; (facilitating factors include involvement of reputable partners, and high levels within and external to the organization, as well as active participation of all stakeholders or their representatives throughout the process);
- *maintaining the above over a longer time span* (several years); (facilitating factors include regular communication about developments/ results and ensuring transparency);
- *directing strategies at several organizational levels simultaneously* to create desired changes in a durable and effective way;
- *implementing 'change projects'* that create *legitimate* time and space for joint reflection and change management.

Features of successful 'change projects' include: *transparency* in initiation and implementation, decision making and selection processes; *early involvement, and voluntary participation;* clarity for all stakeholders about ways of participating (such as opportunities to apply for sub-projects); *starting with the status-quo*, and developing changes *jointly with* all members of the organization.

Changing 'expert organizations' requires special attention to the relation of experts and the overall organizational goal, the organization's 'core business', performance of both core units and the organization as a whole, change management, and customer orientation.

Overall, the extent to which international networks for the development of HPS can build on established theories or models of organizational change and development is somewhat limited. For organizations that are or wish to become part of such networks two organization models promise to be of particular value. While the models of the 'learning' (Senge) and the 'new' organization (Hastings) may be valuable for any organization that plans or undergoes change, the latter seems particularly useful for *organizations as 'network members'*. It helps to better understand their role and potential benefits in a network context, and in developing or reshaping their identity as *autonomous but yet interrelated* and interdependent organizations. Both models ('learning' and 'new' organization) widen the often narrow focus on *intra*-organizational issues. They help to 'zoom out' from an individual organization towards the organization-environment interaction and beyond. As will be seen now, insights from the area of 'capacity development' in societies or societal sectors at large well complement this knowledge. They draw even more attention to multi-organizational systems.

Insights from capacity development research

The concept and approaches to 'capacity development' stem from the field of development cooperation (usually between donor countries or agencies, and 'developing' or 'transition' countries). Approaches and tools of capacity development may be applicable to research on international networks for the development of Health Promoting Schools (HPS) for several reasons: In contrast to the area of organizational theory and practice, the area of capacity and its development has a genuinely *strong macro-perspective*, i.e. organizations whose performance is looked at are seen as part of the overall society, country and even world region. At the same time the *micro level* of individuals working within or related to organizations is not overseen. This matches with both the multi-level characteristic of international networks for HPS development and the broad orientation of Health Promotion which encompasses consideration and actions on co-determinants of health at all levels of society (see chap. 2.1 and 2.2). In addition, development cooperation focuses on 'social development' which encompasses development issues in both the health and education sectors. As regards content and perspective it is close to the field of Health Promotion that guides the development of networks for HPS development and which, too, is directed at populations and ultimately at overall health development in countries and communities.

The concepts of 'capacity' to achieve a goal or task and 'capacity development' are used and defined in different ways. The focus may be on the capacity of countries, governments or the public sector at large, of an organization, individual, group, or a community. Thus, with view to international networks for the development of Health Promoting Schools (HPS) knowledge from this field can help to avoid a sole focus on individual (member) organizations (such as schools) to include 'countries' or the societal sectors concerned. The **applicability of the concept of 'capacity'** to a *range of social systems* suggests that it will be applicable also to interorganisational *networks*. The relevance of issues of capacity development for assessing international networks for HPS development can be easily illustrated: One may envision a school that is expected or wishes to transform itself into a Health Promoting School (HPS). Questions arising are: Has the school the capacity to do so? How can this be assessed? If it has not sufficient capacity, how can this be strengthened? etc. Similarly, international agencies may ask whether a Ministry of Health has the capacity to cooperate effectively with the Ministry of Education and other organizations and to take the lead in establishing a national network for HPS development.

The term 'capacity development' refers to "the efforts by actors themselves or others to enhance their ability to achieve their objectives or perform their functions more effectively, efficiently and sustainably" (UNDP 1995 p13).

Actors may be individuals, groups, communities, organizations or larger systems. The term 'capacity development' (rather '-building') draws attention to dynamic *relations between actors* and the overall policy and governing *context* for sustainable change. Capacity development can involve *formal projects or activities* with specific capacity development objectives. It takes place through a host of informal processes and activities such as *learning by doing, participation, observation* and *comparison of experience*. And it can be an important by-product or *spin-off* of the way in which development cooperation is done. - Depending on the actor in focus **different types or components of capacity development** are being applied, often in formal processes. They concern not only 'developing' countries but *any* country in which performance improvements are addressed (UNDP 1995, A/ChapII.1): Methods of 'human resource development' are directed at individuals, those of 'group or team development' at groups, 'community development' at communities, and so forth. Methods of 'organization development' apply, for example, to 'health promoting school development' and methods of 'public sector reform' and 'governance development' to public sectors and governments that are expected to support HPS developments on a large scale. Besides methods of capacity development directed at selected *actors* (above) there are complementary sets of methods directed at particular changes in the *actors' environment*. 'Policy-, infrastructure-, systems-, or technology development' are headings under which particular approaches and methods may be found. *Cross-cutting* are methods of 'leadership' and 'management' development. (UNDP 1995, 1997)

Before developing the capacity of an actor (e.g. an organization or network), the **task or objective must be specified and assessed for its appropriateness within the given context**. A key questions to ask is: *'What is required for any particular organization to achieve its purposes effectively, efficiently, and sustainably?'* This applies also to (inter)national actors that initiate health promoting processes at local level. Particular tasks appropriate for one organization or country may not or not yet be appropriate for another. A broad task or goal may require coordinated action of *several* organizations as opposed to a narrow one. And even when the capacity of one selected organization is at stake attention needs to be paid to both its *own* capacity and the coordination of its activities *with other* organizations with which it must interact to achieve its task or objective. - Capacity development and assessment of any social system (e.g. an organization or network) must consider both the *human resource requirements* for effective and efficient action and the *broader context or environment* that affects such action. Environmental factors critically influence the capacities of actors to achieve their objectives in a larger whole (e.g. in a community, partnership or society) Attention to human resources or whole organizations without a view to the context in which they are embedded has caused disappointing results in the past, for example, in countries in which schools and universities do not function well because of the lack of an 'enabling environment in the pubic sector'. (UNDP 1995, 1997; Hilderbrand/ Grindle 1994).

Capacity development has three **cornerstones**:

"It is a continuing learning and changing process. It emphasizes better use and empowerment of individuals and organizations. And it requires that systematic approaches be considered in devising capacity development strategies and programs." (UNDP 1997 p3)

The United Nations Development Program (UNDP) suggests a **'capacity development framework'** (fig. 2.4.5) that features 'four **interrelated dimensions** for sustainable capacity development': individuals; entities (organizations, groups); *interrelationships between* entities; and enabling environment (institutional, socio-political, economic, environmental contexts).

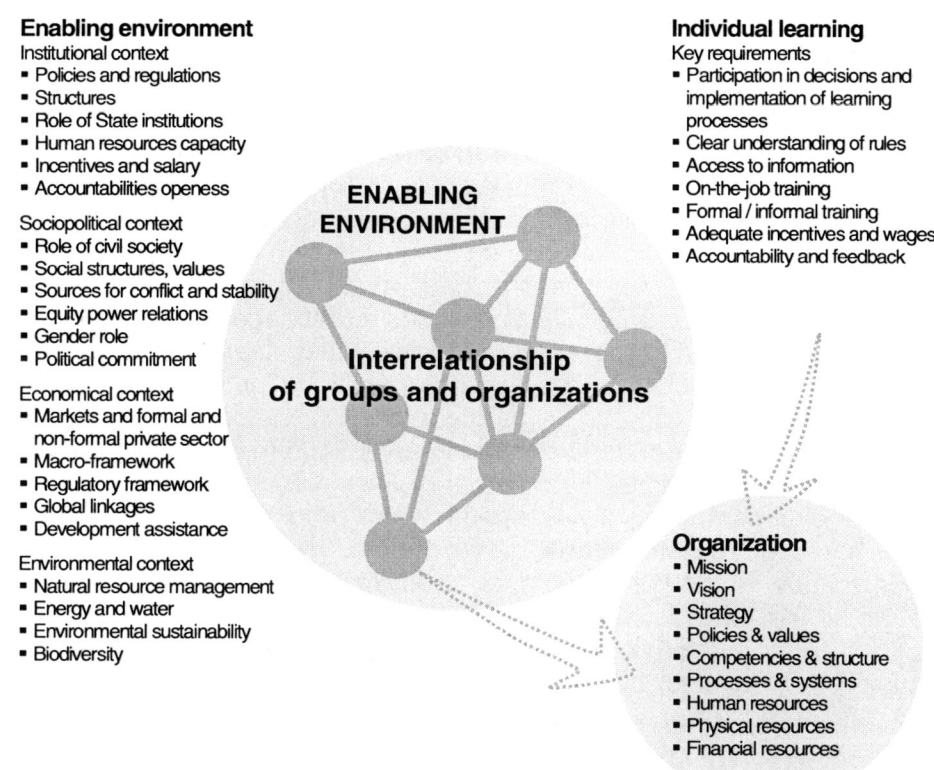

Figure 2.4.5: The UNDP capacity assessment and development framework (UNDP 1997 p11; w.y.;)

The UNDP capacity development framework emphasizes the need for *'individual learning'* including formal and informal skills development and the recognition of *values, expectations and power relationships.* However, to be productive or effective in achieving particular goals individuals need *access to various resources* (from information and money to infrastructures and work time). These are usually provided by 'their' *organizations.* In the light of complex goals (common in Health Promotion and development cooperation alike) organizations and groups establish *interrelationships* for a common purpose which can form *larger social systems* (e.g. networks). To address cross-sectoral issues individuals, groups, organizations and larger systems need an *enabling environment.* This encompasses institutional, sociopolitical, economic and environmental contexts. - The UNDP capacity development framework can be used to better understand the needs, problems and wider contextual issues *before* initiating or implementing a program for capacity development (such as for schools and their promotion of health).

According to UNDP (1997), **developing performance capacity requires** the following: First, policy and decision makers must first build *consensus on vision and goals* involving all stakeholders (including the beneficiaries) to gain their ownership and support. Second, for each task and situation strategic decisions are to be taken regarding the organizations, systems and/or groupings in society to be involved; goal specific strategic partnerships need to be developed among the latter and those and external others). Third, a focus on (usually national) *strategies to develop, sustain and properly use capacities already available* in a society is the base for the *sustainability* of any desired changes. The effectiveness of existing organizations (including schools) depends on deeper dynamics in society (such as the degree of politicization, and social trust and collaboration among people or social capital); these shape the way in which a society responds to outside interventions (e.g. a formal invitation to join an international network) and manages change. Fourth, capacity development is most *sustainable* when programs incorporate the **core characteristics of good governance:** *Responsiveness* to the *needs* of people and stakeholders; *participation* in decision making *throughout* the process of all those affected; *transparency* built on the free flow of information; *equity*, i.e. all people have equal access to opportunities and assets; *accountability* of *all* decision makers (in public, NGO, private sector and civil society) to the public as well as to institutional or organizational stakeholders; *consensus-orientation*, i.e. mediating differing interest towards what is in the best interest of the whole group; *effectiveness and efficiency*, i.e. individuals, processes and organizations produce results that meet the needs while making best use of resources; and finally, *strategic orientation*, i.e. being based on long-term (societal) vision and reflecting an analysis of the full range of existing opportunities and strengths. (UNDP 1997, w.y.) In some cases capacity development for good governance could also be an end in itself.

A fifth requirement for developing performance capacity is that people or organizations 'change the way they do things and interact'. There are several **important aspects of change** such as: the *institutionalization of participation and learning* (from intervention planning on), a facilitator of required behavioral changes; *strong political commitment and leadership,* which usually means one or more legitimate or recognized 'leaders' willing to take risks and help identify opportunities for change (and which may need resources, training and strategic technical support to bring about change); *understanding interrelations* both within an organization, its surrounding environment, and between organization and environment is another important factor; and so are *resources and their coordination* for desired actions to take place. Overall, **change means uncertainty** as various (economic, social, political, cultural and psychological) factors can affect the momentum and direction of organizational and individual change. Thus, capacity development or change programs need to take into account *degrees of risk and ambiguous outcomes* and from early on **plan for flexibility, continuous learning and feed back,** and adequate timing. - The sixths and last requirement for capacity development relates to the *role of donors or funding agencies* who need to act as *facilitators* in capacity development, in support of ownership and execution of actions by those whose capacity is addressed. Donors may advocate, network, train, provide technical support and monitor developments rather than directly involve in program implementation and management.

UNDP also proposes some *'remedies' with regard to unfavorable policy environments* which may challenge any capacity development effort: good governance (to help organizations function free from undue politicization), participation and democracy (to allow people to demand better performance and accountability from organizations that are supposed to serve them), supplementing and enhancing of existing practices (rather than their replacement), the donors' focus on partnerships, facilitation and performance, and sufficient incentives, information, resources and skills for individuals in support of desired changes. (UNDP 1997, w.y.)

From an international perspective, capacity development can be, in sum, characterized as:

"**a society-based approach**, building consensus around national goals and programs, using existing capacities, focusing on people and incorporating characteristics of good governance, while taking the larger policy-related enabling environment into account and placing technical cooperation and official development assistance in a supportive role" (UNDP 1997 p13)

This provides important orientation for international networks (for the development) of Health Promoting Schools.

Achieving change in organizational systems - synthesis and discussion

Sustainable capacity development means the sustainable improvement of the ability of an organization or larger organizational system (or network) to achieve a goal or fulfill a task. Thus, an international initiative to create and support a network for the development of Health Promoting Schools (HPS), a national HPS development effort, and individual HPS projects at school level can be understood as 'capacity development' initiatives that focus on educational organizations in countries with special emphasis on the ability of the latter to promote health. However, capacity development can involve formal projects or activities but also may take place through informal processes (learning by doing, participation, experience exchange, etc.) or as a by-product of the way development cooperation is done.

There are several key features of sustainable capacity development:
- *consideration of four basic interrelated dimensions:* individuals, organizations or groups (entities), interrelationships between entities, and the enabling environment or broader contexts;
- *consensus on a clear vision and goals;*
- *goal specific development of strategic partnerships;*
- *focus on existing capacities* (and their development/ maintenance/ proper use);
- *sustainability through incorporation of core characteristics of 'good governance'* into capacity development programs (responsiveness; participation; transparency; equity in access to opportunities/resources; accountability; consensus orientation; effectiveness/ efficiency orientation; strategic orientation with a long term perspective;)
- *consideration of important aspects of change processes* (institutionalizing participation/ continuous learning; strong political commitment/ leadership; understanding intra- and interorganisational relationships/ organization-environment-interactions; dealing with uncertainty (planning for flexibility, feed back, etc.); appropriate levels/ coordination of resources;)
- *donors as facilitators* of change, in support of ownership and actions by those concerned.

If both the earlier summary on changing individual organizations and that on developing capacities above are taken together, a general answer to the following question lies at hand:

How to achieve far reaching and sustainable change in complex social systems, whether in individual organizations such as schools or interorganisational networks?

Assessments of international networks for the development of Health Promoting Schools and similar networks must consider the related factors as these networks strive for far reaching and sustainable change in support of health development. - In general, the before mentioned interrelated dimensions must be considered (individual, organization (or group), interorganisational (or intergroup) relations, environment/ context). Organization-environment interactions can be shaped from within an organizations and outside, and in light of increasingly complex tasks or goals they must be considered. Often underestimated but of major importance for sustainable change in a desired direction is a **consensus on a clear vision and goal** of the organizational system; these should allow both maintaining flexibility and at the same time stability. A *long term perspective* needs to account for the fact that far-reaching systems changes occur neither in one step nor over the short term.

To be successful and achieve sustainable innovation or improvement, capacity development or change projects or programs must incorporate **several principles**: consensus orientation; transparency/ accountability; participation/ involvement; equity in access to opportunities and resources; building on existing capacities; and continuous learning (also at the level of organizations). These principles are *not just a matter of ideology, but of sustainable success* in implementing organizational change whether for the promotion of health, of education or other goals (such as competitiveness). The principles refer to *all* program or project phases and stages of change, and to *all* stakeholders. Most importantly they need to become an *integral part of the work or organizational culture* and some if not all can and need to be institutionalized (e.g. transparency, accountability, participation).

Essential is the establishment of **self-observation, self-reflection, evaluation,** and a general orientation towards effectiveness and efficiency - as integral part of the organizational culture and in concrete terms within programs and projects.

Equally important is the achieving *and* maintaining of **widespread 'ownership'** of the innovation or change activities (i.e. interest, understanding, acceptance, commitment and support by all members or subsystems). This does not mean that there is no need for leadership; on the contrary, **sufficient leadership in the sense of visionary guidance** has proven to be very important (which is not to be confused with good change management, the more operational side of implementing change). The involvement of 'higher levels' and/or reputable partners from within a system or outside facilitates or enables sustainable change. Donors should be facilitators and support ownership of those concerned.

When searching for a conceptual framework and indicators for assessing interorganisational networks (for the development) of Health Promoting Schools (HPS), and if it is intended that processes of organizational change be covered, then the above set of factors needs to be considered (see chap. 3). They not only underpin today's widespread emphasis on overarching concepts such as organizational culture, communication, and interpersonal and interorganisational relationships where change is at stake, but show that there will be no meaningful standard protocol that networks may use for all network schools as to their health promoting transformation. **Large scale efforts to implement the 'Health Promoting Schools' concept such as (inter)national networks need to focus on processes and mechanisms for organizational learning and change (rather than a fixed set of predefined desired 'health outcomes' for network schools).** And as each school's behavior (as that of any organization) is strictly spoken unpredictable, networks for the development of 'Health Promoting Schools'(HPS) need to be flexible.

However, it is crucial to find ways to systematically apply the current knowledge on the range of core factors or processes for sustainable improvements of the performance capacity of organization's (such as schools) or organizational systems (such as networks or sectors). In support of this, simple and practical organizational models are needed that incorporate and build on these core factors and processes. With view to this research project on international *networks* in HPS development two models are of particular relevance: The idea of the 'learning organization' (Senge) supports ideas of the 'opening up' of organizations (e.g. of 'Health Promoting Schools' towards their communities, other schools and beyond); and, as a metaphor it may be particularly attractive to the educational sector. In more concrete terms and matching with the concept of the 'learning organization', the radar screen model of the 'new' organization (Hastings/ fig. 2.4.1) represents a *visually simple* organizational framework with a *limited number of core dimensions* that nevertheless *captures the complexities and dynamics* discussed above: x- and y-axis illustrate four distinct and concrete networking processes (within/ with others; soft/ hard networking); the image of the radar beam rotating around the center illustrates the continuous self-reflection, learning, assessment, and feed back needed; the concentric circles capture the range of systems levels to be considered and potentially also the range of stakeholders to be involved. The model *has nothing to do with traditional organizational designs and yet is applicable in such organizations*. Most importantly, it is applicable to an individual school as to any organization as well as to an interorganisational network as a whole. And, it represents a mental model of an organization where *inter*organisational networking is as much an integral part as is *intra*-organizational networking. It seems that this model describes *an ideal member of interorganisational networks* (IONs). Creating such networks is the focus of the next chapter.

2.4.5 Forming and maintaining interorganisational networks (IONs)

The general characteristics of interorganisational networks (IONs) have been identified in chapter 2.4.3 above. Now, issues related to creating and bringing about change in such networks will be addressed. The question is how far network assessment can build on a good knowledge base in this regard. - Networks for the development of Health Promoting Schools (HPS) and similar networks are being developed since years. The way this is being done depends on a limited number of experienced individuals who over time developed subjective theories and assumptions about 'what works best'. But unfortunately, their knowledge has not yet been systematically derived, documented and analyzed across networks. A conceptual framework derived from scientific theories, empirical research and systematic case studies which would explain, for example, key factors influencing network development, functioning and maintenance would be quite valuable – not only for this research project on network assessment but critical self-reflection and self-assessments of networks, too. It would prepare the ground for a more systematic, science based transfer of knowledge on network building among regions and countries.

Although overall, interorganisational networks (IONs) received only limited research attention there are a few domains that address the *development* of such networks, most importantly interorganisational relations (IOR) theory (a fairly young branch of organization theory): For long, IOR researchers concentrated on factors that influence an organization's *decision to enter* a collaborative relationship with other organizations (Goodman et al 1997). Up today, little is known about how interorganizational networks can be *developed* and *maintained* but as in organization development research a few stage models exist. As shown before, interorganisational relationships or networks are a key dimension in some capacity development frameworks. 'Intersectoral action' and 'coalition' building has been studied and so has inter-organizational 'partnership building' (but this mainly with regard to private companies). The following review of research results in these areas intends to clarify whether and how far the network assessment framework to be developed in this research project (as to both network structure and processes) can or should include a) *initial* processes of network development and/or b) processes of the further development of *existing* networks over time.

Literature reviews on **reasons to enter interorganisational relationships (IORs)** identify a range of both benefits and potential costs or risks (Hastings 1993; Buechel 1996; Goodman et al 1997). To be calculated are both **potential costs or risks, versus potential benefits**, for example: loss of superiority versus opportunities to learn, adapt, and develop competencies; loss, or diversion of particular resources versus gain of particular resources (e.g. time, information, new ways of working, legitimacy, or credibility); being linked with failure versus sharing costs and risks of product or service development; loss of autonomy and control or the dilution of a position on an issue versus gain of influence over or access to a domain, audience, etc.; loss of stability or certainty versus an ability to manage uncertainty and increased effectiveness in solving complex or controversial issues; conflicts over a goals, values, or methods versus gain of mutual support, more efficient use of resources, and synergy creation; delays in action due to coordination problems or slower consensus building and decision making versus rapid responses to changing demands in the environment, or less delay in the use of new technologies. However, even if potential benefits outweigh risks or costs an organization may refrain from entering a collaboration because it fears conflict with an important third actor. This highlights once again the importance of considering environments in assessments of interorganisational collaboration.

There are yet **other factors** influencing an organization's decision to enter interorganisational relationships (IORs). A synthesis of theories of interorganisational collaboration pointed to *four main factors*: a positive attitude/ willingness to cooperate (which influences even perceptions of costs and benefits, and is linked to successful previous experiences in working together); a need for expertise; a need for financial resources and sharing of risks; and a need for 'adaptive efficiency' (i.e. the length of time needed to develop a desired new product or service, times the amount of effort) (Alter, Hage 1993 p39). Factors such as awareness of potential partners, geographic proximity, norms for collaboration, the availability of resources for maintaining a coordinated process, and demands to collaborate by powerful outside forces play a role, too. Reviews of health related collaborative partnerships point to the influence of *particular assumptions*: that a) the goal cannot be reached by any one actor or group working alone; b) participants should include a diversity of individuals and groups (representing the concern, geographic areas, etc.); c) consensus seems possible among the prospective partners (Roussos/ Fawcett 2000). - These factors need consideration if network assessment includes the initiation phase or initial creation of a network and/or explicitly addresses an existing network's strategies or actions for expansion.

From organizational development research 'stage theory' and 'contingency theory' have been used by some to study **stages of development of interorganisational relationships (IORs)**. And similarly to the stages of organizational change addressed before **different approaches exist without integration**. For example, Goodman et al (1997) point to Gray's three phases before joint action is taken and a suggestion of Florin, Mitchell and Stevenson that organization development concepts (often having 4 or 5 stages) also apply to *inter*-organizational development. Research on community coalition building in the area of health development demonstrates the complexity of the process (Roussos, Fawcett 2000) with seven stages of interorganisational collaboration development: 1) initiating mobilization (actively engaging stakeholders/ creating a diverse and representative membership); 2) establishing an organizational structure and functioning (coordinating committee/ action teams…; bylaws; mechanisms for communication/ decision making/ leadership development…); 3) building capacity for action (links among sectors/ coalitions; an 'enabling system' or intermediate organization providing (access to) information/ training/ recognition…); 4) joint planning for action (starting from a needs assessment); 5) implementing activities (with stakeholder involvement); 6) refining and/or adding activities; and 7) institutionalizing the activities. - The joint development of action plans (4) is supported if donors or other powerful agencies define deadlines that match with the sometimes slower pace of collective decision making.

With particular view to interorganisational relations of a *network* type (IONs) Alter and Hage (1993) present a **model of 'symbiotic *network* development'**. They stress that the *growth* of interorganisational collaboration is **an ongoing process**. The Alter/Hage network typology with three types of networks that represent three stages of network development (exchange or obligational networks; action or promotional networks; and systemic networks of organizations) has been introduced in chapter 2.4.3 above. The three 'stages' or better *levels of network development cover a continuum* from informal to formal links. They do not necessarily follow 'one after the next' but may time wise overlap. Table 2.4.4 summarizes the model.

	EMBRIONIC		DEVELOPED
	obligational networks	promotional networks	systemic networks
Interorganisational activities:	almost none, ad hoc; 'limited' cooperation	peripheral, segmented; 'moderate' cooperation	essential, enduring; 'broad' cooperation
Emergent properties:	boundary spanners	sharing and pooling of resources	division of labor
	rather informal, loosely linked	rather quasi-formal	rather formal
Goals:	meeting individual member organization's needs;	solving supra-ordinate member problems; accomplishing a functional purpose/ concerted action;	jointly producing a product or service in pursuit of a supra-ordinate (e.g. societal) goal;
Examples:	patterned resource exchange	Federations/coalitions of organizations	service delivery systems

Table 2.4.4: The 'model of symbiotic network development' by Alter and Hage (1993 p74)

With view to many symbiotic (not competing) organizations that form interorganisational networks (IONs) the authors state: The three types of networks or *levels of network development are distinguished by their* **increasing level of integration and interaction;** and even systemic networks may vary along these dimensions. They form a framework that describes *a continuum of institutional forms*, from informal to formal, from limited to broad cooperation, from lower to higher levels of integration and of interaction. Each institutional form has a different purpose, structure, operation and outcome. *Obligational* networks are informal, loosely linked groups of organizations having relationships of *preferred exchanges*. *Promotional* networks are quasi-formal clusters of organizations sharing and pooling resources to accomplish *concerted action*. And *systemic* networks are formal interorganisational units *jointly producing* a product or service in pursuit of a supra-organizational goal. - **The stages from obligational to promotional to systemic interorganisational networks may be difficult to notice as they overlap**. Alter and Hage stress:

"This framework is not intended to be a rigid developmental sequence; it is theoretically possible, for example, for a network to originate as a (systemic) production system, especially if mandated by law".

What table 2.4.4 does assert, however, is that "the collective tasks necessary for one form are *also necessary for each succeeding* form in order for it to be successful." (Alter, Hage 1993 p73).It is assumed that in most cases interorganisational networks (IONs) need sufficient time to first form exchange relationships to be sustainable and successful. As known from community service organizations promotional networks will not evolve toward systemic networks unless prior conditions including achieving the developmental level of an obligational network are met. **Means to increase the probability that exchange networks develop** include soft technologies such as conferences and other events, hard IT networks (phone, e-mail, electronic list serves, etc.), laws and regulations mandating exchange, as well as financial or other incentives rewarding exchange. Often, so called 'boundary spanners' are being identified, i.e. individuals who engage in networking tasks and employ methods of coordination and task integration across organizational boundaries. Organizational development techniques applied to the appropriate stage of network development can help ensure that interorganisational networks produce functional structures and processes, with minimal conflict and maximum perceived effectiveness.

Forming interorganisational relations and networks - synthesis and discussion

When the initiation or support of the creation of interorganisational relationships (IORs) such as interorganisational networks (IONs) is at stake it is important to reflect on the **'rational to join or not to join'** of potential or desired members. Both not only potential benefits and costs or risks need to be considered but **some other factors**, too. The literature suggests that **a mutually shared, clear goal** is as important for developing interorganisational collaboratives such as networks as for innovation and change in any individual organization. With regard to stages or phases of network development, some authors suggest that stage models of organization theory are applicable. But as discussed before, there is much diversity and only a minimal consensus in the field (e.g. on two broader phases: initiation and implementation phase). As illustrated in figure 2.4.6 existing 'stage models' may possibly complement the ION development theory by Alter and Hage which suggests network development as an *ongoing* process but with, nevertheless, three identifiable 'stages' or levels of network development: from obligational (exchange) networks over promotional (joint action) networks towards systemic (production) networks.

Overall, the Alter/Hage typology and development model on interorganisational networks (IONs) leads the field of interorganisational relations (or IOR) research an important step further: It allows to conceptualize (e.g. international) **networks as interorganisational systems with long term perspectives that are capable of maturing and learning:** Exchange networks are only a first step in ION development. Networks may broaden their goals sooner or later, building on previous successes or lessons learned. They may take up supra-organizational goals directed at their joint overall environment. Members of an advanced network may well remain in the network during actions or phases that do not meet fully their own interests as long as these are met during the overall course of the network's activities.

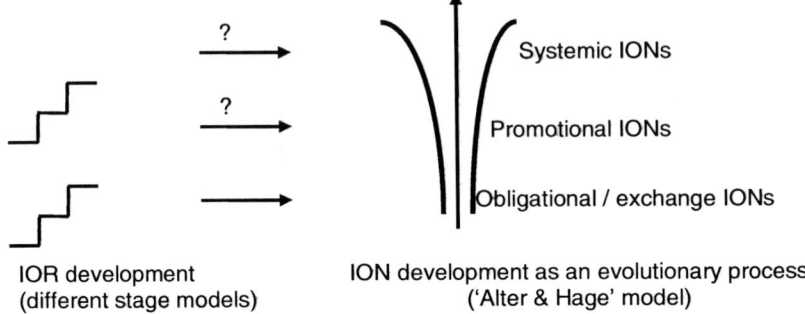

Figure 2.4.6: Illustration of stage models of interorganisational relations (IOR) development (left), the Alter/Hage model of interorganisational network (ION) development (right), and assumed relations between the two.

A *better understanding* of ION development processes may also help to **avoid or reduce conflict** among network organizations, for example, if some are willing to jointly advocate for 'Health Promotion' policies (i.e. to form a promotional network) and others are "only" interested in information exchange *about* such matters (exchange network). The latter is the first step needed before the former can occur.

Traditional 'stage models' of IOR and organization development give some orientation for the initial phase of *forming* an interorganisational network (ION), but not for their **maintenance or qualitative enhancement over time**. Here the *ION development model by Alter and Hage* (1993) provides a general, but very valuable guiding framework which clearly reflects what modern thinkers about networks express: they are investments into the future, based on a long term perspective and not obsolete if a first goal has been achieved (see chapters 2.4.2 and 2.4.3). In more concrete terms, the maintenance of IONs is guided by the current knowledge on *'cornerstones of sustainable capacity development'* of organizations and larger organizational systems elaborated in chapter 2.4.4 above.

By now, not only the general *characteristics* of interorganisational networks (IONs) have been clarified but also three broader *types* of networks and their relation to each other (in form of ION *development stages*). The existence of different network types raises the question of

which factors may lead to which ION structures and processes. *That* there are such factors has been shown already in chapter 2.4.3 ('external control', 'task or technology'). A deeper understanding would be of great value for this research project on network analysis and assessment, particularly if network structures and processes could be linked to desired outcomes. Alter and Hage (1993) explored these issues in more detail:

The search for factors that shape network structures and processes

At the end of this chapter 2.4 on current knowledge about interorganisational networks (IONs) the attention is drawn to **the interplay of various factors** of relevance identified so far. Organizational development theory focuses on structures and processes. 'Contingency theory of organizations' postulates that *organizational design reflects the degree of complexity of the environment* in which the organization is working. Alter and Hage (1993) apply this principle to interorganisational networks (IONs) as illustrated here:

'ION shaping' factors
↓
ION structures and processes
↓
ION outcomes

Network structures and processes are shaped by selected characteristics of the network's environment and the nature of the work to be undertaken. The structure and operational processes, in turn, influence the level of conflict between the organizations and the perceived effectiveness of the network in producing desired outcomes.

In more concrete terms, the authors found that **'external control'**, an environmental factor, **influences the network structure**. For example, dependency on a *single funding source* will likely result in highly centralized network structures (dominated by one or a small group of organizations), because this enhances the funding agency's ability to regulate work objectives and control costs. Also a mandated task as opposed to voluntary work will lead to higher centralized network structures to ensure accountability. Alter and Hage suggest that the higher the level of external control, the greater the amount of disharmony and *conflict* within the inter-organizational network, and the lower the *perceived effectiveness* of the network. On the other hand, where funding comes from *multiple sources* and the work is *voluntary* a network is more likely to use *group methods of coordination* such as coordinating interagency committees. These occur when networks are less regulated and have more *choice* in selecting the nature of work to be performed. - Donors that desire and promote increased coordination through group methods (an organizational development strategy) or the infusion of new resources from multiple sources can facilitate a more *intensive coordination process* that results in *less conflict and greater perceived effectiveness*.

In addition to funding patterns and mandatory/ voluntary tasks, the level of demand or *task volume* of the network appears to influence its characteristics. When the task volume is *high*, the size of the network will be larger, its structure more complex, and the degree to which member organizations connect will be low (in order to control workflow). When the task volume is *low*, group methods of coordination rather than strict adherence to rules and protocols become the norm. Moreover, the *level of conflict* will be *lower where group methods of coordination* are in place.

Factors shaping network structure and processes -synthesis and discussion

Obviously, the findings above provide only a quite **incomplete picture, but attention is drawn to three factors** that may particularly influence ION structures and processes: *patterns of funding, external mandates vs. voluntary work, and the level of demand or task volume*. - Alter and Hage (1993) suggest (and to a certain degree speculate) that *lower external control* (e.g. through multiple funding sources, freely chosen as opposed to mandated tasks, and/or donors that promote high levels of coordination within networks through group methods) likely results in less centralized network structures with interagency committees or similar groups for internal coordination. The *higher external control*, the more likely are greater levels of disharmony and conflict within networks and lower levels of perceived effectiveness. - *Bigger task volumes* tend to result in larger networks, more complex network structures, and a lower degree of connections among members. *Smaller task volumes* tend to lead to networks where group methods of coordination (rather than strict adherence to rules and protocols) predominate. And *group methods of coordination reduce the likelihood or level of conflict* within networks.

Overall, there are several **complementary entry points for plans to form or change interorganisational networks (IONs)**: organizations' reasons to enter (or not) interorganisational relationships (IORs); stage models of IOR and ION development; and factors known to influence ION structures and processes. While there is a good understanding of why and why not organizations may form interorganisational relations or collaboratives, their classification needs much improvement. With regard to interorganisational *networks* (IONs) the Alter/Hage typology appears to be sufficiently elaborated and useful. Nevertheless, as to the stages or processes of IOR and ION development **a much better understanding is still needed**; and the few existing models are yet to be integrated. **How to develop and maintain 'functional' networks is not well understood but the cornerstones of 'sustainable capacity development' of organizational systems provide valuable insight and guidance**.

A difficult question remains **how best to use interorganisational arrangements** such as networks for a particular purpose (such as the large scale development of Health Promoting Schools). Goodman et al (1997) acknowledge the Alter/Hage-network theory as one of the first to explain how external control and technology influence interorganisational relations or network structure, operational processes and outcomes. But they agree with the authors that the empirical support for this model is still limited. Further empirical research and case studies are needed to strengthen this increasingly important body of knowledge. But already now some valuable lessons can be derived as to the analysis and assessment of a network's performance:

2.4.6 Assessing interorganisational network (ION) performance

There is no general agreement about the best approach to effectiveness in interorganisational systems; several can be found. Building on Cameron 1981, Alter and Hage (1993) identify *four models of assessing interorganisational networks* (IONs). Such a network (ION) is effective to the extent that: a) it accomplishes its consensual goals ('goal model') - useful if goals are clear and measurable; and/or b) it acquires needed resources ('system-resource model') - useful if inputs can be specified and measured; and/or c) it has an absence of internal strain or exhibits smooth internal functioning (internal process model) - useful if there is a clear causal connection between internal processes and desired output; and/or d) all strategic constituencies are at least minimally satisfied ('strategic constituencies model') - useful if constituencies have powerful influences. Alter and Hage favor **a 'reasonable outcome' approach** that takes into account the *context and the barriers* to goal achievement. Considering the other models as addressing potential constraints, inter-organisational *network effectiveness is achieved when goals are met within the context of technological and resource constraints, given certain levels of internal conflicts and pressures from external constituencies* (Alter/ Hage 1993).

The conceptualization of ION effectiveness is also difficult because networks go through phases and all **assessment efforts have to be phase specific** to avoid inappropriate expectations. In addition, decisions have to be made regarding the *level of data collection*. Options are the levels of the systemic *network*, the individual *member organizations*, *individuals* such as staff members or users of the organizations, and/or the network's closer organizational *environment* (e.g. network supporters or donors). The authors stress that **there is no one best way to measuring ION effectiveness**.

Alter and Hage examined network failure in terms of **levels of conflict and perceptions of performance gap** among organizational network members and factors that are associated with network failure in this sense. Interorganisational networks (IONs) develop incrementally and their different parts may not develop at the same pace. Exchange networks do not just develop overnight into promotional network's, and the latter do not evolve into systemic networks without a certain degree of 'muddling through' and conflict. **Conflict is an inherent characteristic of developing systems** and the development process is *unlikely* coherent and rational. Conflict can be defined as disagreement, disharmony, and strife about objectives, methods, and policies between individuals and organizations in an interorganisational network. Alter and Hage conceptualize ION effectiveness at the network systems level: *Effectiveness in interorganisational systems is a perception among administrators and workers that their collective effort is achieving what it was intended to achieve, that it works smoothly, and that it is reasonable productive*. The suggested *indicator* is the 'perception of performance gap' among organizational members (i.e. the difference between the current situation and an idealized standard of 'what could be' given realistic restraints on best practice).

Refining the interorganisational network framework by Alter and Hage

On the base of literature analyses on organizations and interorganisational systems and own empirical studies Alter and Hage (1993) examined the interrelationships of the various facets of their framework for analyzing systemic networks (figure 2.4.3) and did strive to identify **key factors in the emergence of conflict and perceived effectiveness gaps in ION systems.**

With regard to environmental factors and tasks, the higher the level of *external control* and the less *autonomy* of network systems, and especially in the case of differential levels of external control among network members, the greater the amount of *conflict* among individuals and organizational members within an network. The same applies to the gap perceived between actual practice and best possible practice (*'performance gap'*) of a network, particularly with regard to vertical resource dependency. - With regard to structural properties, higher *size, complexity, and differentiation* in network systems are related to higher levels of *conflict*; the same applies to the perceived *performance gap,* which also is positively related to *centrality.* An interesting finding of the Alter/Hage study is that higher *connectivity* in network systems, in general assumed to lower the level of conflict among individuals and organizational network members, was *not* found to do so. But, higher connectivity was strongly related to smaller perceived *performance gaps.* - Technology of work per se in network systems and the amount of conflict appear not to be related to each other; but when *different actors use different technologies* and when they play different roles in the action or production process of the network, then lack of understanding and information, and disagreement over methods may occur and *conflict* is more likely. - With regard to network processes, the Alter/Hage study does *not* confirm a major assumption of the interorganisational and management literature that *coordination* reduces conflict; and also the reduction of perceived performance gaps was only weakly related to coordination, and only to higher levels of task integration or operational (not administrative) coordination.

In all interorganisational network systems conflict and perceived performance gaps are unavoidable; they are *necessary components of network development* whereby information is shared between members, roles and functions are clarified, and disagreement over objectives and methods is mediated. But levels may be extraordinary high because of the network's structure and processes. The Alter/ Hage study indicates some interesting points: The most **influential co-determinants of conflict** among network members are *autonomy and differentiation.* Vertical dependency not necessarily means loss of autonomy but when it does then conflict is generated. And it is not the size but rather the way networks are structured that generates conflict; if differentiation is necessary, this presents a functional barrier to disagreements being satisfactorily resolved. Further, the *combination of external control and functional differentiation* produces most conflict in networks. Importantly, while conflict is existential, it is the presence of *problem-solving constraints* that prevent it from being resolved. Generally and particularly in newly developing network systems, conflict, administrative coordination and task integration appear to be positively related, but there seems to be a threshold beyond which a negative relationship exists, i.e. where higher levels of task coordination reduce levels of conflict. In very *complex* systems intense coordination mechanisms such as team integration are needed and inadequate resources and experiences can prevent this from occurring.

In more practical terms the study suggests that, *to achieve low levels of conflict* those involved in network management should act *collectively* (and e.g. advocate for change of policies, rules, and regulations) if their network lacks autonomy and has high levels of differentiation which are *both barriers to conflict resolution*. If differentiation is not reducible (it may be needed to fulfill the network's task) they should seek enough resources to provide very high levels of *coordination* and integration through, for example, frequent cross-organizational in-service training, interorganisational planning groups, and teams. (Alter and Hage 1993)

Overall, the authors propose the following theoretical frame for 'systemic interorganisational networks': The *ways how systemic networks are pushed and pulled by environmental factors* (including technological ones) lead to the **suggestion of four basic forms or ideal types of systemic networks along the combinations of the two features 'resource dependency' and 'task scope'** (the latter defined as the extent to which staff uses multiple assessment categories). These basic forms or types of networks represent **directions of potential evolution** (see fig. 2.4.7).

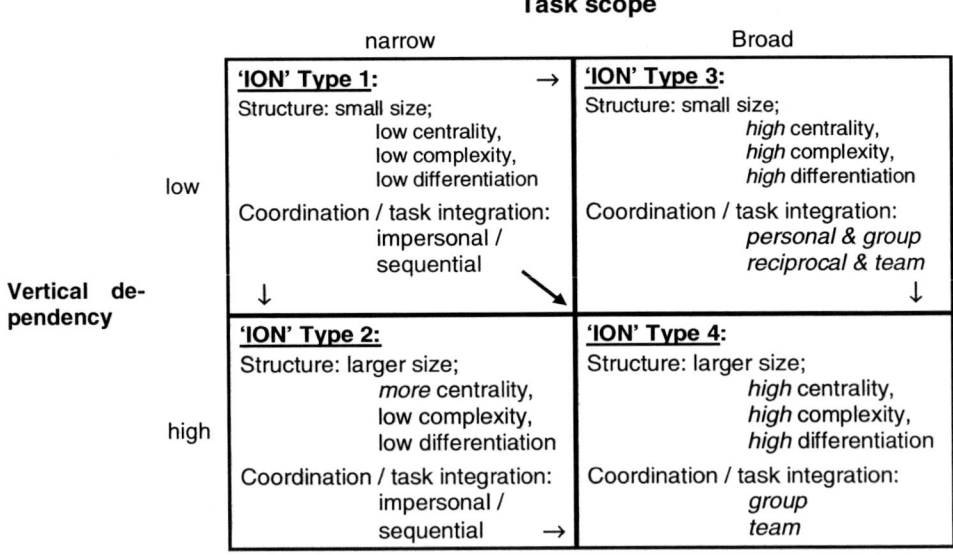

Figure 2.4.7: Core factors shaping systemic interorganisational 'networks' ('IONs'): Theoretical framework on resulting types of networks and directions of ION evolution (based on Alter & Hage 1993)

Type 1, the simplest one, is a small network with low centrality, complexity and differentiation. Type 2, still small in task scope, but highly reliant on vertical funding, is equally low in complexity and differentiation, but more centralized. Type 1 may also develop towards type 3 if there is innovation of technology, i.e. it may remain small, but become highly centralized, complex and differentiated. (The authors assume that where the level of technologies increases there is increased need for a core organization to manage the information and work flow that have become much more specialized. In turn, the very high centrality of these networks reduces the connectivity.) The most complicate network type, type 4, is large and complex. With a broadened task scope and higher reliance on vertical resource provision, it is highly centralized, complex and differentiated. Without questioning these findings an open issue should be recalled here: that other authors than Alter and Hage understand 'networks' by definition as non-centralized systems. Thus, the term 'network' used by Alter and Hage even for highly centralized interorganisational systems may be misleading and a decision on this will be made soon.

Alter and Hage postulate that certain choices of administrative coordination and task integration result from the relationship between vertical dependency and task scope in the four ideal types of systemic networks (see fig. 2.4.7). Effective network operations depend on there being a balance between environmental demands (the technology in use and the degree of dependency) and internal coordination of the network. As systemic networks move from type 1 to type 4, i.e. from low vertical dependency and narrow task to broad task scope and high vertical dependency, a) administrators in the networks must shift their coordination methods from an emphasis on impersonal methods to personal methods and then to group methods, and b) staff members should change their choice of methods from sequential 'client' handling to reciprocal to team methods. The authors also argue that *as tasks become more difficult administrators and staff must have more knowledge. To be effective, they cannot be directed by rules and plans* because pre-programming cannot anticipate all alternatives available, but *must rely on feed back from their colleagues*. This feed back is obtained *via coordination* in the form of decision-making groups and teams who focus on tasks and intervention methods. Using this set of arguments the authors derive a set of **principles** that should help those involved in managing networks **to make effective choices of coordination and integration methods**: If narrow task scope is combined with low dependency, then *impersonal* coordination and sequential task integration should be high and are quite adequate for the collaborative needs of the network system; if it is combined with high dependency, then equal amounts of impersonal *and* personal coordination as well as sequential *and* reciprocal task integration should be used to satisfy the requirements of external controls. *If a broad task scope is combined with low dependency, then personal and group coordination as well as reciprocal and team task integration should be used* to accommodate the demands of high technology; *if it is combined with high dependency, then group decision making and team task integration* must be employed to satisfy requirements imposed by both sophisticated technologies and multiple funding sources. The latter should be noted as it is obvious that networks for the development of 'Health Promoting Schools' have a *broad* task scope.

Studying networks: key factors and interrelations - synthesis and discussion

The findings of Alter and Hage give **not a complete but improved picture** of the interrelations and relevance of the various factors in their conceptual framework for studying systemic networks (fig. 2.4.3). Following their studies of 15 interorganisational networks and interpretations of findings, the following picture emerges:

1. *Increases in resource dependency and task scope* mean that systems will evolve toward *more complexly coordinated systems* - a central thesis by Alter and Hage.

2. *Perceived performance gaps and conflict at network level* (the two ION outcome measures chosen by Alter and Hage) are *unavoidable* processes in all network systems, are *necessary* components of network development and help, for example, to clarify roles and functions. But too high levels *may be dysfunctional* and can be avoided. Overall, *attention needs to be given to barriers to conflict resolution rather than to conflict alone*. The correlations found between network features and outcomes are illustrated in figure 2.4.8.

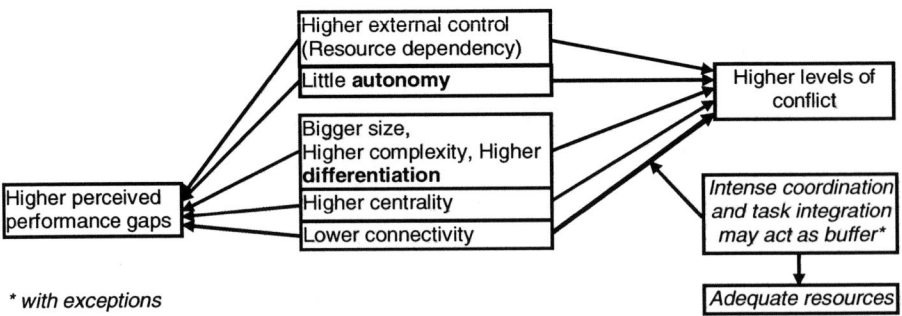

* with exceptions

Figure 2.4.8: Interorganisational network features that have been found to (indirectly or directly) impact on perceived performance and conflict levels (created on the base of Alter and Hage 1993)

Network centrality and connectivity are only associated with perceived performance gap, not with levels of conflict. Both low network autonomy and high differentiation act as strongest barrier to conflict resolution, even more so in combination. Vertical resource dependency does not necessarily worsen the situation, but can do this (if it lowers autonomy). *If high network differentiation* cannot be avoided (e.g. because of the nature of the task) intense administrative coordination and task integration can buffer unusual high levels of conflict. Overall, in *very complex systems* intense coordination is needed, too. But this needs adequate levels of resources to occur. In *newly developing network systems* (Alter and Hage call networks of 1 to 5 years of age 'young') an increase in administrative coordination and/or task integration may first raise levels of conflict and only beyond a threshold reduce its levels

2.4.7 Synthesis and discussion - A conceptual framework of inter-organisational networks (IONs) and beyond

In the light of these findings it is reasonable to simplify the Alter/Hage analysis framework for systemic networks by focusing on those features that have been confirmed as correlated to the two 'reasonable' network outcomes and/or the occurrence of different forms of networks. The *adapted* version of the framework shows figure 2.4.9. In comparison to the original frame, dimensions *external* to network structures and processes are changed: most of the proposed task dimensions have not proven to be of relevance, only task scope remains. And only two of original three 'external control' factors were confirmed, resource dependency and network autonomy to make strategic decisions. All other framework elements stayed the same.

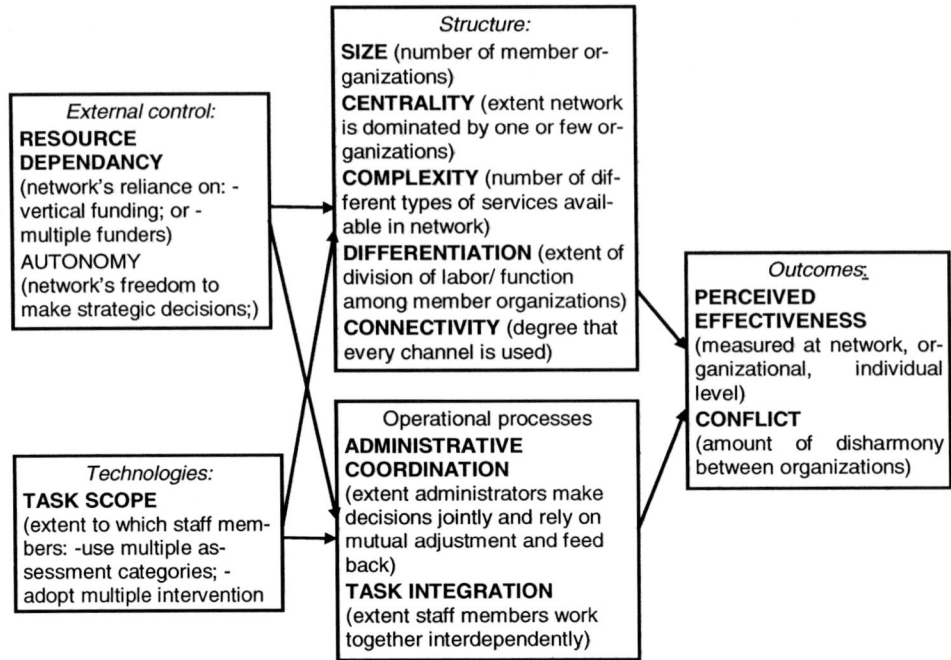

Figure 2.4.9: Conceptual framework of (systemic) interorganisational networks (adapted from Alter and Hage 1993)

As said before, the Alter/Hage framework lacks a sufficient degree of empirical underpinning yet. Nevertheless it appears to be sophisticated enough to be used in further research on interorganisational networks and serve as ION assessment framework because:

a) the framework identifies **'core' features of interorganisational networks (IONs)** (structure and process) that should be considered when starting to collect data on such networks and, in addition,

b) it allows a general understanding of **their interrelations with selected external factors and ION outcomes;**

c) the framework builds on a **'reasonable outcome' approach** that takes the context and barriers to goal achievement into account, an approach strongly supported by capacity development research (e.g. Hilderbrand/ Grindle 1994; UNDP 1995, 1997). Perceptions of 'administrators' and 'workers' (i.e. staff) of ION member organizations concerning whether the collective effort achieves the goal(s) set are measured with *two indicators*: *levels of conflict and perceived effectiveness* (each within the ION).

d) The framework is complemented by two draft theoretical 'sub-frames' which suggest additional insights at two levels: first, at the level of **interrelations between** external influences and ION features, and ION features and ION outcomes (see figure 2.4.7 and 2.4.8); second, at the level of **potential development directions** of even systemic IONs (see figure 2.4.7) in the case of changes of task scope and/or resource dependency. This will be taken up again when interpreting the case study findings (chap. 4 and 5) but caution will be needed to avoid over-interpretation in light of the yet weak empirical basis of the Alter/Hage framework.

Alter and Hage developed their framework to 'analyze' interorganisational networks (IONs), i.e. 'to examine in order to better understand' (Birley 1995). This pilot research set out to develop a practical instrument for 'assessing' structures and processes of international networks for the development of Health Promoting Schools, i.e. for their 'examination in order to decide' (e.g. on recommending or not continued support or transfer of models). More accurately, the focus that *emerged* is to develop an ION *assessment framework* that can guide future network assessment efforts in Health Promotion. *Network assessment means inherently capacity assessment, i.e. assessing the ability of the network to perform a task or achieve a goal.* As explained in chapter 2.4.4 capacity assessment (whether of an organization or larger organizational system) has to consider four interrelated dimensions (broader environment, unit of analysis [here ION], its interrelations with others, its members). If the Alter/Hage 'study' framework considers these dimensions sufficiently it can serve as ION *assessment* frame, otherwise it should be expanded to do so.

In comparison to the UNDP capacity assessment framework, the Alter/Hage network framework shows differences and similarities: a) In contrast to the UNDP framework it represents a general *'logic model'* explaining interrelationships of the different groups of factors and outcomes. b) With regard content it matches with the four basic dimensions of the capacity assessment frame (environment, interorganisational relationships, organization, individuals) but some are less elaborated than others: With view to the network *environment* it is focused on two selected factors (resource dependency and network autonomy) but the wider network environment is not specified. And while it is very specific regarding the interorganisational relationships it is less regarding the network members, i.e. *individual organizations*, and the persons therein. Member organizations are specified only as far as the 'types of services' they bring into the network are concerned (as part of network 'complexity'). But overall, network members remain 'unknown'. For example, how far member organizations are 'capable of networking' is only indirectly addressed through the 'operational process' indicators that capture the extent of administrator's joint decision making and reliance on mutual adjustment and feed back, and of interdependent working together of staff members across organizational boundaries. This may be due to the fact that the Alter/Hage framework is one on systemic networks, i.e. the most advanced network type, in which members' capabilities of networking may be assumed to be sufficient. However, as capacity research suggests *an assessment framework for interorganisational networks (IONs) should be able to guide the 'zooming in' and 'zooming out' from the unit of analysis, here the network*. Therefore, the (adapted) Alter/Hage framework should be expanded. Both the model of the new organization as well as the UNDP capacity assessment and development framework lend themselves for this purpose. The next chapter 3 addresses how.

3. A framework for the assessment of international networks for the development of Health Promoting Schools (HPS)

3.1 Foundations of an assessment framework for such networks

3.1.1 Introduction

The goal of this chapter is to develop a framework for the assessment of international networks for the development of Health Promoting Schools (HPS) by building on the state of research in the three broad domains elaborated in chapter 2: i.e. on *'interorganisational networks (IONs)'* and organizations therein in relation to *'Health Promotion'* and the Settings approach as a social response to the knowledge on *'factors that influence or co-determine health'*. At this point it is useful to recall the rough outline of **the networks in focus** of this research project, i.e. of international networks (for the development) of Health Promoting Schools (HPS) provided earlier (in chapter 2.2): They are international or cross-border and multi-level systems with a strong public sector focus (health and education). Their comprehensive goal is the *large scale development of Health Promoting Schools* which means to enhance the health promoting capacity of a large number of individual (expert) *organizations* (particularly schools) and ultimately of the whole education sector and beyond. As of now, there are **two broad remaining challenges** for this research project on developing a practical instrument for the assessment of for the networks in focus (and ideally for similar networks, too): First, integrating selected knowledge areas or models from (multi-)organizational systems research (chap. 2.4) in a way that advances the adapted Alter/Hage network framework towards a more comprehensive *assessment framework* for interorganisational networks; and second, examining the *fit* of that framework with the *Health Promotion* concept in general and latest models for Health Promotion evaluation and assessment in particular.

The comprehensive assessment framework for international networks for the development of Health Promoting Schools (HPS) - and ideally for similar interorganisational networks (IONs) to promote health, too - will be developed step by step:

1. *refinement of the adapted Alter/Hage network model* carved out in chapter 2.4 from a capacity development and HPS network perspective towards a more comprehensive ION assessment framework, i.e.:

a) *specification* at the level of the individual network *member* (because of the 'health promoting Settings' focus) and

b) *broadening* at the level of the network *environment* (because of the large scale and cross-border development focus);

2. general check of the *fit* of this ION assessment framework *with the Health Promotion concept*, and adaptation where needed;

3. more specifically, check of its *fit with Health Promotion evaluation and assessment knowledge* at two levels:

    a) general Health Promotion evaluation models or assessment approaches;

    b) particular assessment approaches by international 'health promoting Settings'-networks;

and adaptation of the comprehensive ION assessment framework where needed;

4. proposal of an assessment framework for international networks for the development of Health Promoting Schools ready for pilot testing in this research project.

3.1.2 A comprehensive assessment framework for interorganisational networks (IONs)

Advancing the ION framework adapted from Alter and Hage: "zooming in", "zooming out", and development over time

If the interorganisational *network* (ION) is the main *unit of analysis*, then - from an international and capacity development perspective - the Alter/Hage framework on systemic interorganisational networks (IONs) should be complemented to create a general 'multi-level' ION assessment framework: a) by 'zooming in' and specifying the level of the member organization, and b) by 'zooming out' into the broader network environment. This seems to be particularly meaningful for this research project as it concentrates on international networks for the development of Health Promoting Schools, with the 'European Network of Health Promotion Schools' (or ENHPS) as case example. Here not only (health promoting) capacities at the level of member organization (such as schools) are central but also the broader regional (e.g. European) context. As elaborated before, **Hastings' 'radar screen model of the new organization'** (1993) is a valuable frame that not only matches with current knowledge from organization and management research but pays special attention to interorganisational networking. Therefore, it is suggested to use this model as *guiding framework a) for that part of network assessment that looks at a network's member organizations*. As this model is even applicable to an interorganisational network as a *whole*, it should be used *b) to assess issues around a network's relationships with external others*. The **UNDP capacity assessment and development framework** provides general but valuable *guidance on elements of the broader (societal) network environment*. And it would complement potential applications of the 'Hastings-model' to a network system as a whole. How these two frames or **models complement the ION framework adapted from Alter and Hage** to form a general ION assessment framework is illustrated in table 3.1.1.

	Assessment focus	General ION assessment framework 3 modules - 3 principles	
"zooming out": ↑	broader ION environment ↑	part of UNDP capacity assessment frame ↑	* attention to development stages/ levels (ION or parts)
central unit of analysis: →	interorganisational network (ION)	adapted 'Alter/Hage'- ION framework	* 'reasonable' outcome approach
↓ "zooming in":	↓ individual member organization	↓ Hastings' radar screen model of the 'new' organization	* consideration of key factors for sustainable capacity development

Table 3.1.1: The structure of the general network assessment framework - modules and principles.

The metaphors of **zooming 'in' and 'out'** introduced by UNDP provide a good orientation for examinations of complex multilevel systems and will be used in this pilot research, too. Using the expanded assessment framework for interorganisational networks (IONs) outlined above, **"zooming out"** from a network in question leads to reflections on the *political, economic, social, and physical environments* at large (e.g. in a world Region, a country, a sub-national area). It also leads to a focus on the *institutional environment* of the network or its members. The latter is of particular importance if studying networks of public organizations (such as schools) that are integral parts of their public (education) sectors. "Zooming out" in ION assessment also draws attention to external actors such as donors who as explained before need to act as change facilitators rather external controllers if sustainable capacity development is the goal. - **"Zooming in"** draws attention to features of ION member organizations of particular relevance for their organizational networking. Core dimensions for ION assessment are the extent and combination of *four networking processes*: networking 'within' the organization, interorganisational networking ('with others'), people focused 'soft' networking, and information technology focused 'hard' networking (see chap. 2.4).

The Alter/Hage network framework and Hastings' model of the 'new' organization both take into account the fact that network assessment needs to consider the establishment of *continuous (self-) reflection, observation, evaluation processes and feed back loops* and this at both the level of the *member* organizations and of the network as a *whole* (symbolized by Hastings through the 'radar beam', figure 2.3.1). This is *essential* as the behavior of any organizational system varies and is hardly predictable. Both the behaviors of interdependent members or sub-units as well as that of an organization or network as a whole are to be considered.

Assessment principle "attention to development stages or levels"

The *time* factor is a *crucial* one in the assessment of interorganisational networks (IONs). Research from various perspectives refers to the dimensions of several *years rather than months* or weeks when processes of innovation, sustainable change or capacity development in organizational systems are addressed. Interorganisational network (ION) assessment needs to pay attention to development stages or levels in several interrelated ways (see also tables 2.4.3, 2.4.4 and figure 2.4.6):

a) with view to **network development as a continuous process** of evolving and maturing over time, with three identifiable but overlapping development stages or levels representing three network types: a) obligational (or exchange), b) promotional, and c) systemic (production) networks;

b) as to **initiating or creating interorganisational networks (IONs)** (beginning from "0");

c) with regard to **moving from one network stage, form or development level to the next** (e.g. from an exchange to a promotional network; see point a); and

d) regarding stages of **organizational change at the level of network members**, but only **if ION membership means significant organizational change** for member organizations.

In this context several points should be noted: The ION study framework adapted from Alter and Hage (1993) according to the authors refers to *systemic* interorganisational networks (IONs). The authors do not specify potential differences regarding exchange or promotional networks although they do suggest that exchange networks may not need as high levels of coordination and trust as more advanced networks. The matrix on ION development directions and basic forms (fig. 2.4.7) that is suggested as a 'sub-framework' of the overall network assessment framework being developed here supports the following interpretation: *'exchange'* of resources such as information, prestige, public attention, money etc. represents usually *a more narrow goal* or task scope that in itself *does not necessarily require personal or group methods of coordination*. But the latter may be *needed if additional goals* are being pursued or intended to be pursued in the future.

Also to be kept in mind is the fact that stages or *processes of creating interorganisational networks are not well understood*. However, the ION assessment framework outlined above includes *two main factors* that shape what network structures and processes are put in place (goal or task scope, and vertical resource dependency). In addition, *reasons to enter* a network could be a meaningful piece within the search for a better understanding, as could the *capacity for organizational networking* of (potential) network members.

Assessment principle "consideration of key factors for sustainable capacity development"

Another point is that *network development* or evolution in terms of moving from the stage of exchange network to a promotional network, and from there to a systemic network can be understood as *a process of sustainable capacity development* of the network. To assess such network development an ION assessment framework needs to cover the cornerstones of sustainable capacity development and a set of factors known to create far reaching and sustainable *change in complex social systems* (see end of chapter 2.4.4). In short these are:

- consideration of **four dimensions** (individual, organization/group, interrelationships between the latter, environment);
- **consensus on a clear vision and goal**;
- integration into the organizational culture or even institutionalization of several **principles, or characteristics of good governance** (i.e. consensus orientation, transparency and accountability, participation/ involvement, equity in access to resources, building on existing capacities, continuous learning and orientation towards evaluation and effectiveness, strategic orientation with a long term perspective) - and application of these principles to *all* stages and stakeholders;
- integration into the organizational culture and concrete projects or programs of **(self-) -reflection, -observation, -evaluation, and feed back**;

- consideration of **further aspects of change processes** (such as sufficient commitment and leadership, widespread ownership, dealing with uncertainty, understanding relationships [including organization/environment-interactions], and sufficient resources and their co-ordination).

Assessment principle "orientation towards a 'reasonable' outcome approach"

The 'reasonable outcome approach' in network assessment suggested by Alter and Hage draws attention to the basic question of "assessing interorganisational network performance in terms of what?" The network assessment framework outlined above (table 3.1.1 and fig. 2.4.9) follows Alter and Hage in focusing on two outcomes: **perceived effectiveness gaps** with view to goals set by a network, and **levels of conflict** within a network. These *are unavoidable and necessary* components of network development as an ongoing process but nevertheless need to be kept at an appropriate level to not disturb network functioning. Therefore, network assessment efforts need to pay attention to both of these factors. Particular attention needs to be paid to **barriers to conflict resolution** (such as low network autonomy and high network differentiation). This is supported by capacity researchers that stress that indicators of capacity must be sought primarily in assessments of the quality of organizational performance and constraints on it rather than of the ultimate impact of the activities undertaken. Whether assessments of interorganisational networks (IONs) in *Health Promotion* may need to go beyond this is further discussed below. In any case *there is not the one way of assessing interorganisational networks*.

An expanded conceptual framework for interorganisational network assessment

The following graph (figure 3.1.1) illustrates the general assessment framework for interorganisational networks (IONs) developed in this research project on the basis of the literature analyses in chapter 2.4. The framework's core elements are presented and where feasible also their interrelationships. It is a *'multi-level framework'* in the sense that not only the *network* under assessment is considered but also features of its *member* organization ('zooming in') as well as its wider *environment* ('zooming out'). Obviously, the broader environmental factors need further specification but this is best done in relation

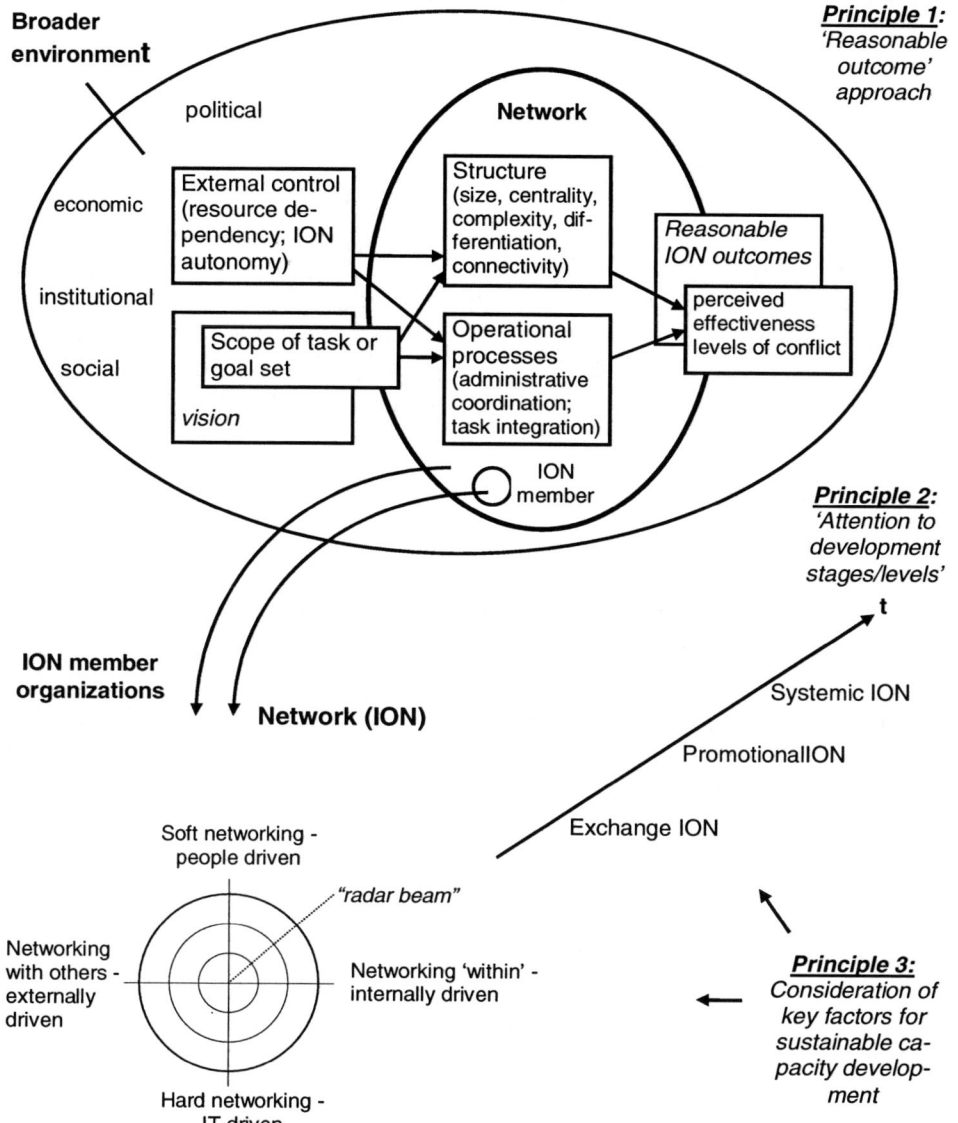

Figure 3.1.1: A comprehensive ION assessment framework - key elements and principles to assess the 'network dimension' of a network in focus (not the 'Health Promotion dimension').
Note: The radar screen model (bottom left) is applicable to both the network as a whole and its member organizations. ('Radar screen' model by Hastings 1993 / ION framework adapted from Alter and Hage 1993).

ION = interorganisational network; IT = information technology to a particular network goal (e.g. developing Health Promoting Schools (HPS)) and/or geographical area (e.g. Europe or a country therein). For example, school health promotion as a network goal points to health and education sectors as institutional context and to the broader 'co-determinants of population health'. - 'Multi-level' networks in the sense of having members from various societal levels are accommodated by the assessment framework through the network feature 'complexity'.

In short, the **three basic principles** for interorganisational network (ION) assessment identified are: a) with regard to outcome assessment a focus on *'reasonable outcomes'*; b) with regard to development sensitivity or phase specificity the consideration particularly of the ION typology and *'ION evolution* theory' by Alter and Hage (exchange, promotional, systemic networks...); and c) with regard to sustainable capacity development (an inherent element of any ION development process) the *recognition and consideration of the key factors and processes to achieve sustainable capacity development* elaborated before.

The **'radar screen model'** of an organization capable of networking visualized in figure 3.1.1 only with view to the network *member* organizations is also **applicable to the interorganisational network as a whole**. ION assessment should consider the four networking processes inherent in the 'radar screen model' in relation to *both.*

Not explicitly illustrated in figure 3.1.1 but nevertheless represented within the ION assessment framework is the essential network dimension of **relationships among member organizations**. However, particularly the structural ION features *'connectivity'* and *'centrality'* (or extent of domination of one or a few members) address these relationships, and also the factor of *'differentiation'* (or division of labor) within the network. At the level of *coordination processes*, relationships particularly at the level of administrators are spelled out (with 'coordination' referring to the extent of joint decision making, reliance on mutuality, and feed back). Regarding relationships among (other) staff members (in German the 'Arbeitsebene') the extent of working together interdependently is pointed out. - As the literature has shown, interorganisational relationships in an ION context may be *symbiotic or competitive, informal or formal, and ad hoc or enduring, but usually based on a longer term perspective* (of several years) to achieve goals or innovation. These characteristics are all supported by Alter and Hage whose ION framework is at the center of the ION assessment framework developed and suggested here.

Further specification of intra-network relationships

Other authors more than Alter and Hage particularly emphasize that interorganisational networks are based on higher levels of *trust, mutual gain,* 'win/win' philosophy or the *'law of reciprocity'*. The notion of 'trust rather than trade' indicates that other authors when using the term 'network' may think of interorganisational networks (IONs) that according to the Alter/Hage typology are more advanced forms of networks (beyond 'exchange'). Alter and Hage state that exchange networks may not need high levels of trust. However, there is no contradiction in **defining IONs as based on trustful relationships** as their development may well start as a pure exchange network which helps to *build* higher levels of trust as a base for an expansion of goals and collaboration in the future and, thus, for an evolution towards a promotional and/or systemic network.

The Alter/Hage ION typology and evolution theory also sheds light on the lack of clarity in the literature regarding **ION definitions and the issue of centrality**, i.e. the degree to which the total volume of 'work', information, clients, etc. flows through a single or few core organizations in the network, - a matter of dominance. Perspectives range from networks 'by definition having no center' over emphases on decentralizing capacities to explicit acceptance of various levels of centrality by Alter and Hage. The latter found that lower levels of centrality are related to higher levels of perceived effectiveness. Others found that IONs are the organizational form of choice if more complex goals or tasks in dynamically changing environments are to be achieved. The reference to complex goals indicates that these authors may think of networks that at least share and pool resources if not divide labor to jointly achieve the complex goal, i.e. they may have in Alter/Hage terms promotional or systemic IONs in mind. However, the *key factors of sustainable capacity development*, particularly the employing of the principles of *good governance*, are not compatible with high levels of dominance of one or a few network members or 'network centrality'. Also widespread ownership appears to be contradictory with high centrality, and the importance of (distributed) leadership does not mean dominance but visionary leadership and capabilities of leaders to convince others to support and act jointly on the common purpose. This *supports a normative decision* to define **IONs as non- or less central entities.** On the other hand, some findings of the Alter/Hage study and related hypotheses suggest that broader task scopes lead to IONs with high centrality, complexity and differentiation. Obviously, more research is needed to clarify conditions and benefits of low levels of ION centrality.

A last issue related to both relations of network members and the yet outstanding working definition of IONs is that of *'hierarchy'*. Here, a *lack of consensus* in the literature persists: perspectives range from networks being 'non-hierarchical by their very nature' (Alter/Hage) over 'striving to reduce or overcome hierarchy' to 'allowing hierarchy but no centrality'. With view to the far reaching cooperation needed across sectors and systems levels to improve and promote the health of populations (see chapters 2.1 and 2.2) and the general need for inclusiveness to achieve sustainable capacity development, for this research project it was decided to **'allow' hierarchical relationships among ION members** (such as sector immanent among schools and education authorities), **but** at the same time to demand that within the functioning of the network **members by definition are *laterally* linked and genuinely strive to avoid centrality**. The implementation of *democratic principles and negotiation processes* as essential parts of operational processes of interorganisational networks (IONs) will help to balance out and cope with the immanent tensions or dynamics; (and in any case these are desirable to achieve goals or tasks of a broader scope and sustainable capacity improvements).

With regard to **a network's relationship with 'others'** in its environment the question remained open whether an interorganisational network (ION) may be **unbounded *or* bounded** (Alter/Hage), or as an organizational system is by definition bounded with distinct membership similarly to any organization. The answer impacts on the quality of several structural network features (size, complexity, etc.). The notion of 'unbounded' networks indicates fluidity of borders over time and membership criteria that are either easy to meet and allow general inclusiveness or employed less strictly and not 'carved in stone'. Hilderbrand and Grindle (1994) distinguish two types of network members, 'primary' and 'secondary' organizations. This represents a middle way with regard to the issue of network boundary as two (or more) types of boundaries could be conceptualized: an 'inner or core network' encompassing those (primary) organizations that are more central to a *particular* goal or task or, in relation to it, are more effective than others; the second encompassing those (secondary) organizations that play a less central role for the *particular* goal or task but are nevertheless essential to it (e.g. a training provider who is more in a supportive than central role). This *'multi-boundary' network concept* allows that with regard to another network goal, or task the constellations may easily change with supporters becoming core members or vice versa. - However, for the assessment of a particular network a **reasonable decision needs to be made about the central unit of analysis** (primary and/or secondary, 'core' and or 'supporting' network). As known from policy networks a network boundary is at least co-defined if not mainly defined by the *quality* of the interorganisational *relationships* and not just formal institutional status.

These findings suggest a **modification of the network definition by Alter an Hage** (1993; chap. 2.4.3) particularly as to two points, the *relationships among members* (Alter and Hage refer only to 'non-hierarchical' collectives) and one structural feature, network *boundaries* (Alter and Hage speak of 'unbounded *or* bounded' clusters). With changes highlighted in [brackets] the modified **network definition** proposed reads as follows:

Networks constitute the basic social form that permits interorganisational interactions of exchange, concerted action, and joint production [based on *trustful* relationships]. Networks are [*bounded*] clusters of organizations that, by definition, are [*non- or less central*] collectives of *legally separate, [laterally* linked] units.

Networking remains defined accordingly: **Networking** is the act of creating and/or maintaining [*such*] a cluster of organizations for the purpose of exchanging, acting, or producing among the member organizations.

The notion of networks as 'bounded clusters' does not exclude that a network may turn out to have two boundaries and/or that its boundaries change over time or with changing goals or tasks. - **As to relationships among network members**, trustful relationships can be expected to provide the ground for process issues such as personal or team methods of coordination, joint decision making, and reliance on mutuality and feed back. If the network creation and development is understood as a process of sustainable capacity development of a) (some of) its members and/or b) the network itself, then the *sets of factors* identified above and known to create far reaching and sustainable change in complex social systems need to be considered, most of which further specify the inter-member relations, *for example*: the *integration* into the organizational culture or institutionalization of several *principles or characteristics of good governance* (consensus orientation, transparency/ accountability, participation/ involvement, equity in access to resources, etc.) and their *application to all* stages and stakeholders; plus the consideration of *further aspects of change processes* (sufficient commitment/ leadership/ ownership; dealing with uncertainty; sufficient resources and their coordination, etc.).

As of now, the intended development of a practical assessment framework for international networks for Health Promoting Schools and - as it turned out, for similar interorganisational (Settings) networks in the field of Health Promotion - has been guided by organization sciences (mainly (inter)organizational relationships research). This was a response to the challenge of assessing the '*network* dimension' of such networks. Obviously, the assessment of the '*Health Promotion* dimension' of these networks is important, too, and needs to be guided by Health Promotion (and related Public Health) research and the Health Promotion concept. Therefore, the yet *'general'* (not Health Promotion specified) *network assessment framework* developed so far will now be discussed from a *Health Promotion perspective*. This will shed first light on one theses put forward for this research project: that "the organizational form of interorganisational networks matches well with Health Promotion goals, strategies and principles in general, and the 'health promoting Settings' approach in particular" (see chap.1).

3.1.3 The ION assessment framework and Health Promotion: do they fit?

The ION assessment framework and the Health Promotion concept

At a theoretical or conceptual level, both the assessment framework for interorganisational networks (IONs) and the Health Promotion concept are based on a combined *systems theoretic and ecological perspective*. The focus on the person-environment-interaction in Health Promotion is well complemented by that on organization-environment-interactions in modern organization and management research. Today in the fields of both Health Promotion and organization development *continuous learning* is considered as a core concept and process, with complementary foci on life-long learning of individuals and ('learning') organizations as well as the active role of these entities in *shaping* their environments.

One of the five core action areas identified in the Health Promotion concept is creating supportive environments for health, which explicitly includes organizational environments. The Settings approach is being applied widely to individual organizations and also multi-organizational systems such as cities, and organization development research has informed the methods applied. The fields of organization development and Health Promotion share the features, potentials and difficulties of *multi-method interventions in social systems* and are equally challenged when it comes to calls for 'evidence of effectiveness'.

With view to basic principles and values, the concept of an interorganisational network (ION) underlying the ION assessment framework and the Health Promotion concept have a common basis. *Participation* is not only a recognized value in the field of Health Promotion (and sustainability factor as to interventions) but has proven to be a precondition for sustainable organizational change and capacity development, too. Relationships and interactions based on 'partnership' are expected and aimed at. *Empowerment* as a core principle in Health Promotion addresses imbalances of power whether between (health) professionals and 'lay' people, communities and those 'in power', or management, staff and users of 'health promoting' organizations. This matches with modern capacity development, governance, and management approaches underlying the general network assessment framework where human resources and individual staff members are highly valued, hierarchies being flattened, and self-organizing in networks takes place for mutual benefit and creating synergy. Participatory and partnership orientations imply that mutual respect, transparency, accountability and shared responsibility are highly valued.

The ION assessment framework and the knowledge of factors influencing or co-determining health

The complexity of the *interplay* of a broad **range of factors** influencing the populations' health **requires a multi-disciplinary and multi-sectoral response** to health challenges, as is Health Promotion. Intersectoral action genuinely **means interorganisational action**, and interorganisational *networks (IONs) are a specific, partnership based organizational form* used - and apparently useful - in the field of Health Promotion. In theory the network assessment framework proposed is applicable to any combination and number of organizations that may want to form a network to influence, in a coordinated and effective manor, a set of factors that influence or co-determine health. From the perspective on social 'co-determinants' of health interesting is the strong emphasis on person-to-person connections, trust and reciprocity of much of the literature on interorganisational networks. This reminds of the building blocks of **'social capital'** (see chapter 2.1.2) and raises the question whether the creation and maintenance of interorganisational networks may strengthen social capital and, thus, have the inherent potential to promote health. This will be taken up later again, after the case studies of international networks in school health promotion.

The ION assessment framework and lessons from collaborative Health Promotion practice

Interorganisational networks are a particular form of collaborative systems and, thus, confronting the ION assessment framework with lessons from Health Promotion collaboratives is reasonable. The earlier chapter 2.2.7 identified factors (potentially) enhancing effectiveness of collaboratives that fall into two *broad categories*: most of them directly refer to the collaborative itself, some to participating individual organizations (see table 2.2.6, right). The proposed ION assessment framework matches with these findings in so far as it, too, is most differentiated at the level of the interorganisational system, but also specifies features of the individual member organization (table 3.1.2, left). The **four groups of 'effectiveness factors'** identified at the level of collaborative systems in *Health Promotion* (i.e. the collaboratives' context or environment, purpose, processes and relationships, and structures) match with the respective key domains of the ION assessment framework (i.e. broader environment, scope of task or goal, structure, and operational processes of the network). Table 3.1.2 sets the factors within each of these groups side by side to facilitate a comparison.

Key features of the proposed ION assessment framework	Factors enhancing the effectiveness of collaborative partnerships - lessons from Health Promotion practice

• political, economic, institutional, social environment;
• external control:
  - resource dependency
  - network autonomy
	• conditions related to the formation of the collaboration: history, motivation, other programs, time;
	• access to appropriate technical assistance;
	• social capital; broader socio-economic 'determinants of health' that support effective action;
	• community control in agenda setting;

• vision • scope of task /of goal set	• agreed upon, clear vision/ mission (periodically reviewed and renewed); • agreed upon, clearly articulated goals and objectives.
Operational processes: • administrative coordination, i.e. at the level of administrators/ managers; • task integration, i.e. coordination at the level of technical staff/ workers;	• Agreed upon processes of goal definition, solution generation, ways of working, rules of the game,... • ongoing action planning; • community involvement (in planning, implementation, etc.); • continuous leadership (leadership team; use of democratic/ consensus decision making); • dominance of cooperative over conflictual interest, through commitment at organization level, positive ties, a sense of purpose; • sharing of risks, resources, responsibilities among all collaborators; • systematic documentation and evaluation with focus on intermediary outcomes
• size • centrality • complexity • differentiation • connectivity	• durable, long term resources (appropriate to achieve population level health improvements); • needed expertise/ technical assistance available within the collaboration; • mechanisms of community involvement.

Table 3.1.2: Presentation side by side of the features of the proposed assessment framework for interorganisational networks (IONs) (left) and success factors for collaborative practice identified by Health Promotion research (right). Each row reflects one category of factors (from top down): 1. context/ broader environment; 2. goals and purpose; 3. processes/ relationships; 4. structures.

The table shows that, with regard to the broader **environmental factors** the network assessment framework well accommodates the success factors identified regarding collaborative partnerships in Health Promotion. The more specific environmental factor 'external control' is **not negated and in parts supported** by Health Promotion experiences (with the success factor 'durable, long-term resources'). The network assessment framework's emphasis on **vision and scope of task or goal** embedded therein is **supported** by collaborative Health Promotion practice, but the latter stresses not the issue of scope but of *agreement reached* upon these points. This, however, is not contradictory.

With regard to **process factors** it is obvious that the ION assessment framework goes much less into detail than the lessons derived from reviews of collaborative practice in Health Promotion. On the one hand, this reflects the importance generally given to processes and not only outcomes in Health Promotion. On the other hand, this reflects research knowledge that network processes are dependent on the scope of network tasks or goals and, thus, can only be further specified for particular scopes. In collaborative Health Promotion, there is usually no question regarding a more narrow or wider task scope or goal: the Health Promotion concept implies (and the collaborative effort indicates) a more complex goal in the sense of influencing health relevant factors - through or while enabling people to increase control over these factors. The network model underlying the assessment framework suggests that broad task scopes or goals lead towards group and team methods of coordination and task integration. This is clearly **matching** with the processes identified in Health Promotion as potentially enhancing collaboratives' effectiveness (such as team leadership, consensus or democratic orientation, and sharing of risks and responsibilities).

With view to **structural factors** of a network, the network assessment framework is clearly structured and differentiated. Most of the factors are not mirrored in the list of success factors identified in collaborative Health Promotion practice. The exception is 'network complexity' which addresses the range of organizations participating and, thus, relates to the issue of availability of expertise needed within a collaborative system. But importantly, there are **no contradictions** between ION assessment frame and the review findings on collaborative systems in HP.

With view to the three assessment *principles* within the network assessment framework proposed the situation is as follows: The **first principle**, a 'reasonable outcome approach' is **supported** by two success factors for collaboratives in Health Promotion: a) 'systematic documentation and evaluation with an *intermediary* outcome-focus', and b) 'dominance of cooperative over conflictual interests'. The latter matches with the two network outcome indicators highlighted in the general network assessment framework so far: i.e. 'levels of conflict' and also 'perceived effectiveness'. The former (a) raises the question whether with view to interorganisational networks (IONs) in *Health Promotion* the two network outcomes identified in the *general* ION assessment framework should be complemented by health promotion-*specific* 'intermediate outcomes', an issue taken up below again. The **second principle**, attention to network development stages or levels, is **neither mirrored nor denied** by the lessons learned from collaborative Health Promotion practice. The **third principle**, consideration of key factors of sustainable capacity development, is **supported** by many of the success factors of collaborative Health Promotion practice such as: agreed upon vision and goals; ongoing action planning; leadership, consensus, and long term orientation; and mechanisms for (community) participation.

The *strong emphasis on 'community' control and involvement in effective collaboratives in Health Promotion is not directly mirrored in the ION assessment framework*. This is not a surprise as the latter a) concentrates on interorganisational networks of which community *organizations* may be part of but not 'a local community' in its broader sense; and as b) up to now the proposed network assessment framework is a general one, not yet specified with view to a particular action area such as Health Promotion. However, the assessment framework includes clearly a participation orientation as to all stakeholders which may include local communities.

The ION assessment framework and Health Promotion - intermediate synthesis and discussion

Overall, it can be said that the general network assessment framework proposed so far and the Health Promotion approach are compatible and have much **common ground** regarding conceptual and theoretical basis, underlying principles and values, and some practical aspects. **Most importantly, the assessment framework for interorganisational networks (IONs) in most of its facets is supported by current knowledge on factors enhancing the effectiveness of collaborative partnerships in Health Promotion, and in *no* aspects questioned or denied by them**. This supports the thesis put forward in chapter 1 that the organizational form of 'interorganisational networks' matches with the Health Promotion approach. - Unfortunately, the lessons derived from reviews of collaborative practice in Health Promotion do not improve the yet limited understanding of the stages of *development* of collaborative systems such as interorganisational networks (IONs).

Now that the *general* compatibility of the network assessment framework (and the organizational form of interorganisational networks) and Health Promotion is confirmed, the attention can be drawn to the *question whether assessing interorganisational networks for Health Promotion requires a health promotion specific adaptation of the general network assessment framework*, and if yes, in which way. The experiences with collaborative Health Promotion actions above indicate that the framework's element 'network processes' may need further specification. With view to interorganisational networks (IONs) that work within the Health Promotion concept to promote health, in short "Health Promotion networks" such as those for the development of Health Promoting Schools, one may also ask: Should the assessment framework's element 'reasonable outcomes' be expanded in a Health Promotion specific way, and if yes, which additional outcomes should be considered and how? These and other issues regarding the general network assessment framework's application to Health Promotion networks are addressed next.

3.1.4 Assessment in Health Promotion - selected models and implications for the ION assessment framework

The field of Health Promotion, since long searches for most appropriate assessment or evaluation frameworks that take into account that Health promotion programs or interventions tend to be complex, use multiple strategies, and operate at multiple levels (see chap. 2.2). Many policy and decision makers, (health) practitioners and researchers still overemphasize measuring individual behavioral change as the method of assessing evidence of effectiveness of Health Promotion interventions. But the effect of such interventions should be assessed across the *breadth* of its activities, not just by changes in individual behavior. There is general agreement that with the 'shift from (health) problems to people in settings' (Baric 1997) evaluation approaches used for health education interventions (a well researched area) are *not* appropriate to demonstrate accountability; but less agreement exists which assessment or evaluation models then *are* appropriate for complex Health Promotion interventions such as those in organizational or even multi-organizational Settings and systems. Interventions may combine activities as diverse as providing health information and advice, influencing health and social policy, advocating for social change, organizational development, creating intersectoral cooperation, and community development. But nevertheless Health Promotion interventions are rarely judged on the base of its effects in all these areas. In comparison to the extensive (though not yet satisfying) research base on the range of factors that influence or co-determine health (chap. 2.1), research on Health Promotion interventions that include elements of creating health promoting Settings or systems and, thus, organisational and policy changes in support of health, is rare. And overall intervention research in Health Promotion lacks far behind the practice. (Speller et al 1998; Nutbeam 1997, 1997b; Baric 1997) However, Health Promotion research started to respond to these challenges: with generic outcome models and work on interorganisational collaboratives.

Network or alliance focused assessment frameworks

As shown in chapter 3.1.2, interorganisational networks (IONs) that follow the Health Promotion concept while working towards network specific goals can be reasonably expected to fulfill criteria for 'good collaborative practice'. In addition, it is suggested that an assessment framework for such networks - if applied to the field of Health Promotion - should complement, be agreeable to, or even advance general assessment frameworks in that field of application. Therefore, this chapter looks briefly at selected *generic* evaluation frameworks or models from the field of Health Promotion and against that background, reflects upon needs to adapt the ION assessment framework when applied to networks in *Health Promotion*. A short look at assessment frameworks of international "Settings" networks as well as a recent general evaluation frame for interorganisational 'healthy alliances' leads into this work.

Assessment frameworks of international "Settings" networks:

The "European Network of Health Promoting Schools" (i.e. the so called "ENHPS" and subject of the case study that follows) aims to *disseminate* the concept and practice of Health Promoting Schools (HPS) and *refine* the concept in the light of the practical experience gained from implementation in a range of different national contexts (ENHPS w.y.; see chap. 4). In 1999, the network's international Technical Secretariat brought out the report "The ENHPS indicators for a health promoting school". It provides a **'ENHPS framework for the development of indicators'** that targets people at all network levels and **aims** to: a) provide a framework for *measuring progress* of the ENHPS *in establishing* the Health Promoting School as a *common practice* in Europe, supported by both the health and education sectors; b) to *assist* 'countries' at national level and schools at local level, *in assessing and monitoring the development* of Health Promoting Schools'. (ENHPS w.y. p2; ENHPS 1999a).

The framework is *an attempt to operationalize* at international, national, and school or local level the *10 principles for action* passed as a Resolution by the network's First Conference in 1997. These address democracy, equity, empowerment and action competence, school environment, curriculum, teacher training, measuring success, collaboration, communities, and sustainability (ENHPS 1997a). The framework is also underpinned by the 'factors of the Eco-holistic model of the Health Promoting School' which influence the structure and development of health promotion in schools: management, planning and allocation of roles; links with outside agencies, the family and community; formal curriculum; 'contextual' curriculum (i.e. the social and physical environment); feelings, attitudes, values, competencies and health promoting behaviors; plus four factors that reflect a school's wider environment: health and education related local initiatives, regional policies and initiatives, national legislation and provision, and international influences (Parsons et al 1996 in: ENHPS w.y.). The indicators presented can be adapted to reflect local, cultural, organizational and political considerations. (ENHPS w.y.)

The assessment framework by the European Network is *understood as far from being complete* and up to day subject to change. The framework document focuses on the **provision of *examples* of indicators** to serve as a 'starting point' for efforts to assess and communicate achievements and monitor change over time. The indicator examples are not only meant to be adapted by network countries or schools but also used as the basis from which more detailed and specific indicators may be developed - according to priorities and particular national or local circumstances. The framework document also contains examples of criteria but only to illustrate the reader what 'criteria' would look like. All *network members and the European Network itself* are called on to *always strive to improve*. (ENHPS w.y.)

The authors of the framework stress that the **selection of indicators** follows directly from objectives but is *influenced by other factors*, particularly the *network level* in focus and the *stage of network development*. Indicators for the whole European Network will differ from those at school level and, similarly, at early stages of development the aims, objectives, and hence indicators for network countries and schools will be very different from those at later stages of development. (ENHPS w.y.) Therefore, the framework suggests a series of **objectives, indicators** and criteria that are categorized in two ways: first, **by 'network levels'** ("international, national, and local") and second, within each level **by 'stages of development'** (i.e. "Dissemination, Structures, and Impact") (ENHPS w.y. p18). The framework for developing ENHPS indicators is illustrated in figure 3.1.2.

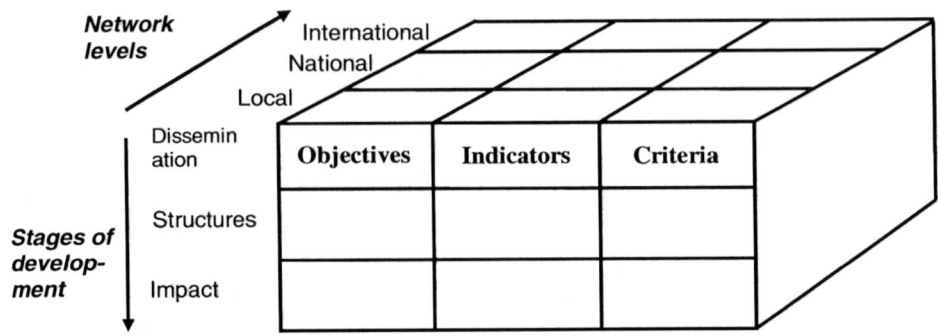

Figure 3.1.2: ENHPS Framework for identifying indicators of success (figure slightly adapted from ENHPS Technical Secretariat w.y. a, p18)

In comparison with the general assessment framework for interorganisational networks for Health Promotion developed in this chapter so far, two aspects of the above are of importance: First of all, the explicit and systematic **consideration of different network levels** within the ENHPS framework is interesting. This dimension is not made explicit in the *general* network assessment framework developed so far. The latter is 'multi-level' in the sense of considering the levels of individual network members (organizations), the network as a whole, and the network's environment, but not regarding networks as multi-level systems. The framework does, however, accommodate this dimension indirectly: A *range* of different types of services or network members (network 'complexity') is considered as is a *division of labor* among network members (network 'differentiation'). This allows - during the assessment of, for example, an international network for the development of Health Promoting Schools - to clearly distinguish a) local, national or international organizations and b) their different roles or functions within the network's overall effort to pursue its goal of creating Health Promoting Schools at a larger scale. Also, the assessment framework's 'network goal'-component may help to accommodate a multi-level network as it may be broken down into a set of objectives differentiated by levels of the network in question. Therefore, at this point the following is suggested: With view to the **general network assessment framework** drafted so far, there is **no need for an explicit additional framework component on network levels or an additional 'assessment principle' on this issue**. It is expected that the draft network assessment framework, thanks to a joint analysis of network 'complexity' and 'differentiation', sufficiently guides an examination of also 'multi-level' interorganisational networks (IONs).

Second, both the general network assessment framework developed in this research project and the indicator development framework by the

'European Network of Health Promoting Schools' (ENHPS) highlight the importance of taking into account and distinguishing **network development stages**. However, the three stages referred to in the ENHPS framework remain unclear: while it is plausible to distinguish a 'dissemination stage' (presumably of HPS concept and practice), a 'structures' stage and 'impact' stage seems questionable. In an early presentation of a draft of the framework Pattenden (1998 p40) speaks of *'key areas'* applying to all levels of the ENHPS initiative: with 'dissemination' referring to the spread of the Health Promoting Schools (HPS) concept; 'structures'/'infra-structures' to "defined working structures, including management and coordination, collaboration, resource allocation, coordinating teams, etc."; and 'impact' to "strategic planning taking place to enable the growth and implementation of the HPS concept". The case study of the European Network of Health Promoting Schools (ENHSP) presented in the next chapter will shed additional light on such issues. At this point it just needs to be noted that the **ENHPS framework** for developing indicators of success **generally supports principle 2 "attention to development stages"** of the *general ION assessment framework* developed, and **does *not* question the three network development stages proposed by Alter and Hage** (1993), i.e. exchange, promotional, and systemic networks.

According to the researcher's current knowledge the indicator development initiative of the European Network of Health Promoting Schools (ENHPS) outlined above is quite unique. Major indicator development **efforts by other international 'health promoting Settings' networks** tend to focus only on the Setting rather than the network level, too. For example, the widely recognized WHO Regional guidelines for developing Health Promoting Schools (HPS) in the Western Pacific provide a clear framework with 'components and checkpoints' for Health Promoting Schools; but networks for their development are only addressed as far as a rational for their creation is concerned (WHO/WPRO 1996 p18). A major indicator development initiative of the European 'WHO Healthy Cities Project' focused on 'indicators of determinants of health' in cities (Doyle et al 1999; WHO Healthy Cities Project 1998) and did not include indicators of intersectoral or interorganisational relations, collaboration or networking within cities. There was, however, one early study of the *national* level of *national Healthy Cities networks* that examined network participants, their activities and aspects of relationships among them (Goumans 1993). But its theoretical basis is limited and its findings give no reason to consider modifications of the general network assessment framework developed in this research project so far.

An evaluation framework for interorganisational 'healthy alliances'

Based on extensive participatory research involving a wide range of individuals involved in interorganisational 'alliances' of some kind in public health and welfare in the UK, researchers developed an *'evaluation tool for the self-assessment of healthy alliances'* (Funnel and Oldfield 1998; Speller, Rogers, Rushmere 1998b). The evaluation framework encompasses a) process measures which refer to the internal workings of an alliance, the dynamics and how the alliance functions as a working group, and b) output measures which refer to the short-term results of the activities of an alliance and not directly to health outcomes. The process of alliance-working starts long before outputs (or intermediate outcomes) can be demonstrated, according to the authors an often underestimated point. 'Good' alliance work should increase the *potential* benefits to *health outcome* in the long run. - In light of the low level of differentiation of operational processes in the general network assessment framework developed above, the **five categories of process indicators** for healthy alliances (and their main elements) may fill a gap. These are:

- *'commitment'* (whether there is commitment to an identified, *shared goal*; what commitments the alliance makes in terms of *resources* (money, people, time));
- 'community participation' (*liaison between alliance and community*; extent to which activities *empower* the community);
- 'communication' (*accessibility of the alliance* to others; *extent to which partners share* their information and *communicate* with each other);
- 'joint working' (extent to which *strategies and action plans are developed in a truly co-operative way*; *responsiveness to changing external factors*);
- 'accountability' (*mechanisms* of responsibility to each other, parent organizations, and the wider community; *evaluation* built into work and constructive *use of results*).

A **comparative look at the general network assessment framework** (figure 3.1.1) makes clear that the process categories suggested above relate to this frame but go beyond it: a) 'Commitment' to an identified, shared goal is part of the definition of interorganisational networks (IONs); but the *extent* of such commitment is *not* an explicit part of the ION assessment frame. b) All elements of the process indicator category 'communication' are more or less explicitly accommodated by the network assessment frame: an alliance's 'accessibility to external others' by the ecological approach to interorganisational networks underlying the assessment frame; the 'extent of communication among partners' by the structural network feature 'connectivity'; and the 'extent of information sharing' implicitly through the focus on joint decision in 'operational processes' as well as the 'assessment principle three' which includes issues such as transparency. The latter also includes c) 'accountability', although without specifying towards whom. d) 'Joint working' is in parts covered by the 'operational processes' dimension of the network assessment frame; but the element of *'responsiveness to changing external factors' is only indirectly accommodated* therein (through the 'broader environment' and 'external control' dimensions and the underlying ecological approach). -Thus, the **network assessment framework proposed accommodates all but one categories of process indicators of the 'healthy alliance'-evaluation framework** (above). The exception is *'community participation'*, a process specifically *demanded* - through the core principle of empowerment - *in any Health Promotion work* (be it interorganisational or not). The network assessment framework if applied to Health Promotion networks should be explicit in this regard - a hint that **Health Promotion specific indicators may need to be added**.

Besides the process indicators just discussed **six categories of 'output indicators' for 'healthy alliances'** have been identified. These (and their main elements) are:

- *'Policy changes'* within organizations that affect the target groups as a result of the alliance (level of change; quality of the policies);
- *'Service and environmental change'*, including organizational or structural change (any changes that may affect the target group as a result of the alliance activity);
- *'Skills development'* (*availability of training* and *informal skills sharing* to both alliance members and target group - both organized activities and those coming about informally as a result of the alliance process);
- *'Publicity'*, whether planned or unplanned, paid or unpaid (coverage; quality of coverage);
- *'Contact'* (how well, and with what effect the *target group* was reached - both anticipated *and* unanticipated effects);
- *'Knowledge, attitude and behavioral change'* of the target group in relation to alliance activity (may include those *'not* directly' related to health).

Another **comparative look at the general network assessment framework** (figure 3.1.1) shows that, not surprisingly the 'healthy alliance' output categories are more Health Promotion specific than the two network outcomes in the general network assessment framework: The first three output categories directly relate to three of the five Health

Promotion action areas (see chap. 2.2); the last one includes one main category of health influencing factors: health related behavior. This, too, hints into the direction that the general ION assessment framework **when applied in the field of Health Promotion may need to be made more 'Health Promotion specific'**, at the process but also outcome or output level. However, this is only possible if there are indeed a) some *general* Health Promotion outcomes or outputs and b) *general* processes or other quality indicators for Health Promotion interventions per se, and - if some or all of them could be reasonably applied to interorganisational networks for Health Promotion such as those for the development of Health Promoting Schools. *Some answers lie in existing generic evaluation or assessment models for Health Promotion initiatives or programs.* This brings up an additional point c), the question of *general* standards for evaluation or assessment efforts specific to the field of Health Promotion. These three issues (a, b and c) are addressed in the following sections.

Generic assessment models:

A general assessment framework for interorganisational networks if applied to networks in the field of Health Promotion should meet general assessment standards specific to this field of application. Although in the field of Health Promotion there is *no widely agreed set of such standards yet*, over the last few years this and related issues received more research attention. Reputable researchers and leading thinkers have put forward *first answers* which are of interest here in two ways: a) to reflect on expectations towards an interorganisational network assessment framework specific to the Health Promotion field, and b) to guide the appraisal of assessment efforts of the Health Promotion networks examined, (here the ENHPS).

Searching for generic standards for the assessment of Health Promotion initiatives

Remarkable work on evaluating Health Promotion initiatives has been undertaken since 1995 by a group of European and North-American researchers called the 'WHO European Working Group on Health Promotion Evaluation' (see Rootman, Goodstadt, Hyndman, McQueen, Potvin, Springett and Ziglio 2001b). From this extensive and multi-facetted work here only a very few aspects of particular relevance to the discussion of the general network assessment framework from a Health Promotion perspective are touched upon. Referring to features of Health Promotion initiatives such as being empowering, participatory, intersectoral, equitable, sustainable and multi-strategic (see also chap.2.2), this Working Group early on identified **four *core features* of the evaluation of Health Promotion initiatives**: first, at each stage it should *be participatory*, i.e. involving all those with a 'legitimate interest' in the initiative; second, it should *draw on a variety of disciplines*, and a *broad-range of information-gathering procedures* should be considered; third, it should *build the capacity* of individuals, communities, *organizations* and governments to address important Health Promotion concerns; fourth, it should be appropriate, designed to *accommodate the complex nature of Health Promotion interventions* and their long-term impact (Rootman 2001 p5). Some **principles** of an evaluation of Health Promotion initiatives were put forward including: the *consistency* with Health Promotion principles (particularly empowerment and participation); *applicability* to both institutional and individual, and synergistic and single outcomes; and *coverage* of all stages of the evaluation process (from agenda setting to use of results) (Rootman et al 2001b).

Potvin et al (2001), from a perspective on Health Promotion programs as open systems, identify **program features of relevance** for the evaluation of such programs:

a) *program - environment interactions,* with 'environment' meaning all aspects of the social system in which a program is implemented (for example, organizational settings such as schools, communities, a country); the two *sub-categories* distinguished are environmental conditions or relations that are the *'target of change'*, and the *'environmental conditions'* that are neither part of the program nor the target of change;

b) three broad categories of *program components*: - *objectives or expected results* (in terms of desired changes); - program *resources*, i.e. the 'raw material' to create a program (knowledge, money, staff, physical infrastructures, etc.); and - *activities or services*, i.e. the means by which objectives are pursued, which altogether form the intervention strategy;

c) program *evolution or phases* of its life cycle (an example often used is developmental phase, implementation phase, and 'phasing out' once the objectives have been achieved or the program has been transformed to address other objectives).

In the context of presenting a 'generic logic model for planning and evaluating health promotion' Goodstadt et al (2001) point out that the *evaluation* of Health Promotion initiatives is *inextricably related to and depends on*: a) a clear understanding of the conceptual framework underlying the initiative (e.g. of the HPS concept and network approach) and b) the processes and elements involved in planning the initiative. **Evaluation should examine a Health Promotion initiative as to**: a) the achievement of the *goals and objectives* identified in planning, which requires paying attention to the achievement of all levels of goals and objectives, *including the overall* Health Promotion goals, as well as the '*instrumental* objectives, processes, outcomes, products, outputs'; b) the extent of employing or reflection of the *values* identified as its *guiding principles*; c) the implementation of the core mechanism of Health Promotion: individual and community *empowerment*; d) the success in addressing the *factors that influence or co-determine health*, identified through the planning process as being *relevant* to the issue/problem of concern; and e) the *way* in which the initiative worked in one or more of the *general Health Promotion action areas* and used the *strategies identified in planning*.

Here, '*instrumental objectives, processes, and outcomes*' refer to: improved awareness, knowledge, skills, decision making, and behaviors; enhanced organizational capacity; increased community capacity and participation; enhanced health promoting policies; more equitable access to health services; and increased focus on prevention and Health Promotion in health care systems. '*Instrumental products and outputs*' refer to: programs, marketing and materials; modified organizational structures and climate; coordination of community efforts, enhanced community resources and capacities, and community coalition building; laws and regulations, and policy statements; public dialogue on decision making; and coordination of policies and activities in sectors that affect health. The '*Health Promotion action areas*' referred to are the five identified in the Ottawa Charter (see chapter 2.2) and the '*strategies*' include health education, health communication, organizational -, community -, and policy development, advocacy, and intersectoral collaboration. With view to the strategies the international Working Group points out that **evaluation can include** an assessment of the *range* of action areas and strategies employed, the *appropriateness* of the strategies included or excluded, and the *synergy or mutual support* among strategies. (Goodstadt et al 2001)

Network assessment and generic assessment standards in Health Promotion - intermediate synthesis and discussion

The above knowledge provides some orientation regarding needs to adapt the general network assessment framework when applying it to a network in the field of Health Promotion (e.g. to the ENHPS). International or national interorganisational networks (IONs) for the development of health promoting Settings can be understood as large-scale

'Health Promotion initiatives' themselves. Therefore, *an assessment framework for such networks should cover those areas of a Health Promotion initiative identified as 'to be covered' by any evaluation in Health Promotion.* If the general network assessment framework being developed here meats this standard, then it can be expected to be useful not only for the case studies within this pilot research but for future evaluations of the ENHPS and beyond. Thus, **from a Health Promotion perspective the network assessment framework should cover networks with respect to**:

- *goals and objectives* identified, including *overall* Health Promotion goals as well as 'instrumental' objectives, processes, outcomes, outputs;
- *values* and related *guiding principles*;
- the principle of *empowerment*;
- the *'relevant' factors that influence or co-determine health*; and
- the general *Health Promotion action areas* and *strategies* identified in planning.

Attention should also be paid to:

a) the *network - environment interactions* (regarding both, parts of the network environment targeted for change and other environmental components);

b) not only to objectives but also *resources* to create and maintain the network, and network *activities or services;* and

c) program or network *evolution*.

A **comparative look at the general ION assessment framework** developed so far (see figure 3.1.1) shows: First, the 'goals and objectives' set by a network are *considered; but* with view to Health Promotion the range of chosen or conceptually implied processes, outcomes or outputs need a closer look (see below). Second, by considering the 'vision' of a network the network assessment frame *can accommodate* considerations of 'values and guiding principles'. Third, as discussed in chapter 3.1.3 the network approach and assessment frame is *compatible* with an emphasis on 'empowerment'; particularly the analysis of a network's vision, goal and objectives, and operational processes *allows to examine* a network's potential to provide opportunities for empowerment to those involved - internally as well as towards its environment (customers, clients, etc.). Fourth, as explained in chapter 3.1.3 the network assessment framework is to a certain degree *capable to help examine* a network's *capability* of influencing relevant factors that influence or co-determine health; but it would need a modification of the network outcome dimension should the *extent* of this influence be assessed (see below). Sixth, a Health Promotion network's consideration of all or some of the general *Health Promotion action areas and strategies* may show in its vision, goals and objectives; but at the level of processes or outcomes the network assessment frame does *not* guide to identify such considerations.

This confirms the assumption made earlier that the general assessment framework for interorganisational networks (IONs) - when applied to networks for Health Promotion - needs to be complemented both with view to Health Promotion processes and outcomes. However, the assessment framework *does cover* the 'network-environment-interactions', *considers* the range of 'resources' to create and maintain a network (particularly through the structural ION features and the element of 'external control'), and *accommodates* (indirectly, not explicitly) network 'activities and services' to pursue objectives (within 'operational processes').

Searching for general process indicators for Health Promotion initiatives

The general network assessment framework considers network processes at the level of internal, operational processes (e.g. the extent of team or group work among network organizations), but it cannot accommodate a Health Promotion *specific* shaping of network related processes. Therefore, it is proposed to complement the general assessment framework by a specific set of process related questions, to be asked separately from the general assessment of the *network* dimensions of an interorganisational network for Health Promotion. The question of what are 'good' processes in Health Promotion initiatives that may also apply to such networks draws attention to current work and debate around 'quality' and 'best practice' in Health Promotion research. As to these very young research areas, up to now no consensus or clear direction has emerged that would help identify *Health Promotion specific* process indicators that apply to the *various* Health Promotion initiatives. (see e.g. Kahan 1998; Kahan, Goodstadt 1997; Rootman, Ziglio 1998; Speller et al 1998; Deccache, Laperche 1998; Davies, Macdonald 1998) - There is, however, a far reaching consensus in the field about general features of the Health Promotion concept as such which include process features (see chapter 2.2). Most importantly, Health Promotion initiatives are expected to be empowering or enabling individuals or communities to increase control over the factors that influence or co-determine health. Related to this initiatives are meant to be participatory. To address the range of 'co-determinants of health' and factors that shape the latter, they are also expected to usually involve intersectoral collaboration. Also continuous learning processes are usually stressed, which in a modern understanding applies not only to 'the people' or 'individuals' but to professionals, policy and decision makers, and even organizations as a whole.

Against this background and from a Health Promotion perspective the following **suggestion** is made: In the assessment of networks to promote health (such as those for developing Health Promoting Schools) the following **categories of general process indicators** be used:

- *participation* (of all those with a legitimate interest in the initiative);
- *empowerment* or processes to enable (individuals, groups, communities and organizations) to *increase control over the factors that influence or co-determine health* that are of relevance;
- *learning* (of individuals, groups, communities, organizations, and/or larger systems); and
- *intersectoral collaboration* (at whatever level of society).

A **comparative look at the general network assessment framework** (chap. 3.1.2) shows that the assessment principle 'consideration of key factors for sustainable capacity development' *covers some* of these issues, particularly the factor 'integration of principles of good governance into the organization culture'. The latter include explicitly participation and continuous learning (also of organizational systems); the principle of building on existing capacities hints at empowerment processes. Also the sustainability factor 'integration of (*self*)-reflection, -observation, and -evaluation points in that direction. And empowerment processes are generally supported by the model of the 'new' organization capable of networking which is chosen to guide network assessment at the level of member organizations and a network as a whole (see figure 3.1.1). However, *empowerment for health* or **the enabling to increase control over the factors that influence or co-determine health is not sufficiently covered** by the *general* ION assessment framework. But as said before, the framework accommodates intersectoral collaboration (through 'network complexity' and 'differentiation') even though there is no explicit call for it. - After this identification of *processes* it remains to clarify general Health Promotion *outcomes or outputs* that need to be considered when assessing networks in Health Promotion.

Searching for generic indicators of effectiveness for Health Promotion initiatives

Different types of indicators are being distinguished, and within and beyond the field of Health Promotion there is no consensus. For example,

ENHPS evaluators refer to Tones' and Tilford's classification (1994): *'outcome'* indicators can be used to identify the achievement of targets or objectives, *'intermediate'* indicators to measure progress towards targets, and *'indirect'* indicators to monitor both the process and the supplementary activities needed to support progress. The before mentioned 'generic model for planning and evaluating Health Promotion' by Goodstadt et al (2001) contains '*Health Promotion* goals' and '- objectives', '*instrumental* objectives, processes, and outcomes', and '*instrumental* activities, products and outputs'. The 'Health Promotion outcome model' by Nutbeam (1998, 1999, 2000) distinguishes '*health and social* outcomes', '*intermediate*' health outcomes, and '*Health Promotion* outcomes'.

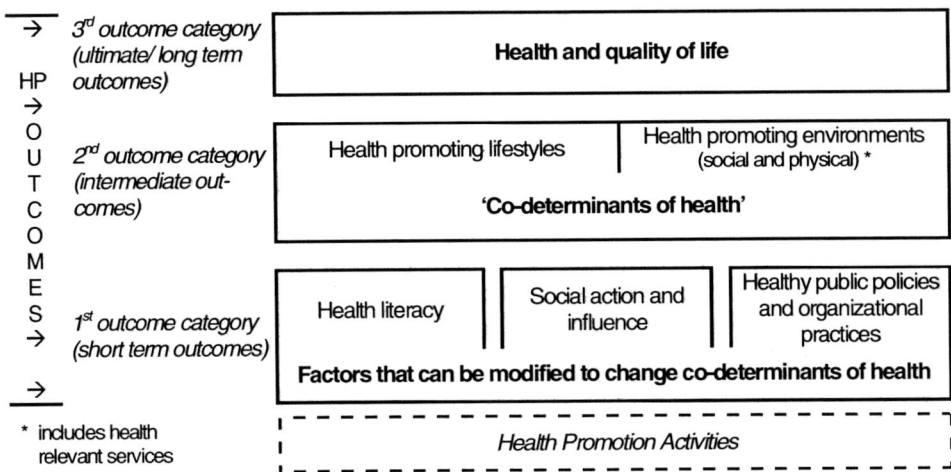

Figure 3.1.3: A model for *categorizing* Health Promotion outcomes - adapted from Nutbeam (Nutbeam 1998, 1999, 2000). (HP = Health Promotion)

The 'outcome categories' by Nutbeam (see fig. 3.1.3) appear to provide a simple and pragmatic typology of potential outcomes and found already international platforms such as in the EU funded 'evidence base of health promotion' project (IUHPE 1999a,b). While one may question one or the other sub-category, some of the examples of indicators provided, and the causality implied, the *basic elements and structure* seems to be the model's strength. This is supported by an increasing number of applications of this model (e.g. Van den Broucke 2002; Wimbush, Watson 2000; Gesundheitsfoerderung Schweiz 2002). Others are critical and used it as a starting point for further model development (e.g. Noack 2002). The model is *not* referred to by the WHO expert group around Rootman et al (2001b) whose generic model is more complex and differentiated, specifically accounting for both processes and outcomes, but not contradicting the basic *categories* of potential change in Nutbeam's model (but the implicit causality!).

Nutbeam asks which measures should be used to assess effectiveness in Health Promotion which is of particular interest for this pilot research on assessing networks for the creation of Health Promoting Schools (HPS). He suggests a 'summary' outcome *model to help define outcomes associated with Health Promotion initiatives* (see table 3.1.3). The model distinguishes three outcome categories: 1. *health and social outcomes* (i.e. the ultimate endpoints of Health Promotion interventions such as improved health status or quality of life); 2. changes in the *'determinants of health'* (such as changes regarding healthy lifestyles and health supportive environments); and 3. changes in those 'personal, social and structural *factors that can be modified in order to change the 'determinants of health'* (including policies and organizational practices). Nutbeam refers to the second outcome category as 'intermediate' health outcomes and to the third one as 'health promotion outcomes'.

'Health and social outcomes' are usually expressed in terms of mortality, morbidity, disability, dysfunction, quality of life and functional capacity. 'Intermediate outcomes' refer to the co-determinants of health highlighting two broad categories: lifestyles and environments, the complexity and interplay of which is *not visible* in this model but explained in chapter 2.1. The third outcome level refers to those 'personal, social, and structural factors' that can be modified in order to change the co-determinants of health (or intermediate health outcomes). Here, Nutbeam suggests three sub-categories: 'Health literacy' refers to the personal cognitive and social skills which determine the ability of *individuals* to gain access to, understand, and use information to promote and maintain good health. 'Social action and influence' describes the results of efforts to enhance the actions and control of *social groups* over the determinants of health. 'Healthy public policies and organizational practices' are the results of efforts to overcome structural barriers to health. (Nutbeam 1999, 2000)

Network assessment and Nutbeam's Health Promotion outcome model - intermediate discussion

With view to a *general categorization* of potential or desired outcomes of Health Promotion initiatives (such as international networks for the development of Health Promoting Schools) Nutbeam's model is attractive. In a simple way it translates the Health Promotion definition explained in chapter 2.2 (Health Promotion is the process of enabling people to gain control over the factors that influence or co-determine health and thereby, increase their health) into an outcome model. However, its implicit causality is questionable and it seems to be better to use the model as a outcome *typology*. Importantly, the model shows that expected results can refer to different 'levels' or better, broad categories - even *before* changes in co-determinants of health occur. The way Nutbeam describes the 'ultimate outcomes' it seems better to re-label that outcome category as 'health and quality of life - outcomes' (rather health and social outcomes). This helps to avoid confusion with social factors that co-determine health at the second outcome level. Another adaptation refers to the integration of the 'health services' category into the overall set of environmental co-determinants of health because services both are understood as part of the social environment and have only a limited role to play in health development of populations (see chap. 2.1).

Nutbeam avoids to visualize and at the same time implies and expresses in parts that the various outcome levels and categories are interrelated and how. His model highlights that they all have their legitimacy and role in the overall goal to improve people's health and quality of life. Health Promotion actions modify co-determinants of health, which influence ultimate health and quality of life - outcomes, and often it is necessary to first address some basic factors that influence the well known (behavioral and/or environmental) determinants of health, such as policies or organizational structures. Interorganisational network building and transforming schools into Health Promoting Schools would fall into this category. Although Nutbeam restrains himself from explicitly suggesting a logic model for Health Promotion initiatives, this is nevertheless implied. This is a often heard and major point of critique.

However, with its clear 'co-determinants of health' perspective and explicit (although not detailed) Health Promotion viewpoint, the 'Nutbeam'-outcome model as adapted above is of use in this research project: It can help to *order or classify* the often multiple objectives or expected results of Health Promotion initiatives including interorganisational networks which facilitates their systematic analysis. The 'first' outcome category seems of particular interest as it encompasses changes in organizational practices. However, in this research project this category will not be labeled '*Health Promotion* outcomes' as this is misleading: Health Promotion initiatives typically strive for outcomes in the first *and* second outcome category.

The following chapter now builds on the inputs and discussions above, summarizes the Health Promotion process and outcome issues that should complement the general network assessment framework when applied to the field of Health Promotion, and adapts the latter where needed. The case studies in chapter 5 will then pilot test the assessment framework for interorganisational networks (IONs) developed here.

3.2 Synopsis: The general assessment framework applicable to international networks for the development of Health Promoting Schools

As said before, guidance for assessing the *interorganisational network* dimension of networks for Health Promotion such as the European Network of Health Promoting Schools comes mainly from (inter-)organizational relations research (chap. 2.3). Guidance for assessing the *Health Promotion* dimension of these networks stems from two broad knowledge fields within public health sciences: knowledge on the factors that influence or *co*-determine health including their interplay (i.e. health development knowledge) on the one hand, and Health Promotion intervention knowledge on the other (chap. 2.1 and 2.2). Within both public health and organizational sciences much of the knowledge of interest here is yet to be integrated, and integrating theoretical frameworks are just being proposed or still being debated. Therefore, it is too early to try to integrate these knowledge strands when it comes to the development of a practical assessment tool for interorganisational networks to promote health. Therefore, the network assessment framework being developed here will have two parts: Part A will focus on the assessment of the *network* dimension of such networks, part B on that of their *Health Promotion* dimension.

Part A: Assessing the 'network dimension' of interorganisational networks to promote health (such as the "European Network of Health Promoting Schools")

As shown above, the general network assessment framework illustrated in figure 3.1.1 seems valid also for networks for Health Promotion. Therefore, the following is recommended:

- an examination of **network boundaries** (which may be multiple, e.g. if 'core' and 'supportive' parts exist) and in addition and related to this, a clear **decision on the unit of analysis** for each particular network study;

- the application of **the general network assessment framework** illustrated in **figure 3.1.1**, i.e. undertaking a network assessment that considers **the ensemble of key elements** of this assessment framework: the network environment (broad and specific), network goal or task, network structure (from size to connectivity), network processes, network outcomes, features of Hastings' organizational model at the level of member organizations, as well as the network as a whole, and selected 'assessment principles'.

With regard to the letter, this implies the examination also of a combination of the following factors:
- the main factors that according to the Alter/Hage -network theory (1993) shape what network structures and processes are put in place: **goal** or task scope, and **vertical resource dependency** (*see also below);
- the emphasis given to each of the **four networking processes** identified by Hastings (1993) for organizational systems capable of networking with regard to both organizational network *members* and the *network* as a whole; (with view to the *network's relationships with others* examination particularly of external funding agencies or donors and related issues of network autonomy (*see also above);
- the extent of the **network's continuous (self-)reflection, observation, evaluation processes and feed back loops** (see Hastings' radar beam metaphor);
- the **interactions and relationships among network members**, i.e. member organizations, through taking into account the following range of network features suggested by the Alter/Hage network theory and/or the organization model by Hastings:
  a) the *structural network characteristics* of 'low centrality' (refers to low levels if any of domination of one or a few), 'connectivity' (degree that every channel is used), and 'differentiation' (division of labor);
  b) the *network process characteristic* 'coordination', which refers to the extent of joint decision making, reliance on mutuality and feed back, and of working together, and related to this and more generally:
  c) the extent to which *trustful relationships, mutual gain,* and the reliance on the 'law of reciprocity' are realized and (following Hastings) this based on direct *person-to-person* connections and a *long term* perspective with an attitude to invest into the future;
  d) the extent to which *lateral linkages* (as opposed to hierarchical ones) and a striving to *avoid an evolving of centrality* are realized;
- the **development stage(s) of the network as a whole** (its emerging, evolving and maturing in general; the overlapping stages of exchange, promotional, and systemic networks);
- the **development stage(s) of member organizations** of the network (only if network membership implies significant organizational change);

- the extent of consideration of factors known to create **far reaching and sustainable change in complex social systems** (see summary in chap. 3.1.2)
- the two **selected network outcomes** in focus of the Alter/Hage - network theory, i.e. *'perceived effectiveness'* and *'levels of conflict'* within the network, and related to this **barriers to conflict resolution** (in particular low network *autonomy* and high network *differentiation*).

The order of presentation of these factors does not suggest a particular sequence of their examination. It has been explained in chapter 3.1.2 that in the organizational form of 'networks' *centrality* by definition should be low. With regard to the *relationships* among member organizations Hastings' organizational model suggests that quality relationships among actors may be facilitated by organizational networking processes that result in a devolution of power and the breaking down of organizational boundaries. As to the issue of *coordination*, and with view to *general* network assessment which is the focus of this research project, the recommendations above reflect the proposal to *not* strictly follow Alter's and Hage's distinction between features of coordination among 'administrators' on the one hand and other staff members/ 'workers' on the other. This is for two reasons:

First, it is likely that that distinction stems from the studies of networks of traditional public (health) service organizations whose member organizations were likely structured and functioning in a more traditional (also hierarchical) way with, for example, a sharp distinction between managers or administrators (who decide) and technical 'workers' (who 'work'). As shown in chapter 2.3, modern organization theory and analyses show that such organizational forms today are not the most appropriate ones anymore in many cases, particularly if organizational networking needs to take place. The model of the 'new organization' by Hastings (1993) which was integrated into the network assessment framework responds to this development, stressing the braking down of hierarchical barriers and team like working across layers and vertical structures of organizations - depending more on the task than individual staff members' hierarchical position. Second, a core principle of the Health Promotion concept is *empowerment*. Any Health Promotion initiative strives to enable people to increase control over core factors influencing their health. Thus, inter-organisational networks as alliances and other collaboratives in the field of Health Promotion *need to facilitate and support interpersonal as well as interorganisational relationships that match up with this Health Promotion principle or core mechanism.* Therefore, the network assessment framework proposed applies features of relationships among members such as 'joint decision making', and 'reliance on mutuality and feed back' to *all* of the member organizations involved and not only to decision makers.

This modification of the process feature of the Alter/Hage network frame that is at the core of the network assessment framework proposed, is not questioning the Alter/Hage theory itself: a) The authors say that for the first stage of network development (exchange networks) lower levels of trust are sufficient but higher levels are a stepping stone towards and condition for the next stages of network development, i.e. for promotional and systemic networks to evolve. b) For networks with *broad* task scopes or *complex* goals (such as those for creating health promoting Settings) group and team methods of coordination are needed and these include joint decision making.

Part B: Assessing the '*Health Promotion dimension*' of interorganisational networks to promote health (such as the "European Network of Health Promoting Schools")

As the general network assessment framework being developed is meant to be applied in the field of Health Promotion, particularly to networks for the development of Health Promoting Schools (and similar Settings), the above recommendations are complemented in three perspectives: Health Promotion values and principles, general process features of Health Promotion initiatives, and desired 'Health Promotion outcomes'.

At a general level, it is recommended to examine:

- the extent of the integration of the ecological approach (see Richard, Potvin, Kishchuk, Prlic, Green 1996);
- whether and how the network a) works in one or more of **the five Health Promotion action areas are,** and b) uses one or more of the **strategies identified in planning** (e.g. health education, organizational and policy development, advocacy, intersectoral collaboration);
- With view to network *processes* to be examined are:
- the extent to which processes allow and encourage **participation** of all those that have a legitimate interest and/or responsibility in the thematic area (in the case of Health Promoting Schools development e.g. the school communities, surrounding local communities, and health and education authorities);
- the extent to which processes of **empowerment** are supported or facilitated;
- the extent to which processes allow or encourage **continuous learning** of not only individuals or groups but organizations and larger so-

cial systems as a whole (such as individual network schools and interorganisational networks);
- the extent to which the network represents, supports, or encourages **intersectoral collaboration** at whatever level of society (e.g. among health and education sectors);

With view to network *outcomes* to be examined are:

- as far as possible, the extent of achievement of **goals and objectives set** by a network; and
- in any case of a network for Health Promotion, the way and extent to which the **relevant factors that co-determine health** (of e.g. pupils and teachers) **and their interplay** are being considered and acted upon (whether in the sense of health supportive *changes* or the maintaining of high levels of health resources or assets).

In accordance with the assessment principle of applying a 'reasonable outcome approach' in network assessment put forward in the general network assessment framework developed, many Health Promotion researchers stress that effectiveness of Health Promotion initiatives or programs have to be measured in reasonable terms. The 'Health Promotion outcome' model adapted from Nutbeam (figure 3.1.3) reflects this approach by explicitly inviting and valuing *outcome measures at the level of the co-'determinants of health' (intermediate outcomes) and at the level of activities, services or other factors that can be modified in order to change these determinants or their interplay* (direct, usually short term outcomes). Evaluators of the European Network of Health Promoting Schools, for example, state that measuring network outcomes in terms of 'health status' is unrealistic as, for example, the level of morbidity in children is influenced by many factors and a reduction of levels may take many years. But measuring, for example, the factors that influence or co-determine health supportive *behaviors* of pupils such as school satisfaction is reasonable (ENHPS/TS w.y. a). In any case, *outcome assessments of interorganisational networks (IONs) to promote health need also to take into account the network's resources* both in terms of money and knowledge, staff, physical infrastructure, etc. (Potvin et al 2001).

4. The 3-step-case study approach

4.1 Introduction and methods used

As said in chapter 1, this research and pilot project set out to not only *develop a conceptual framework for collecting baseline data* on structure and processes of 'international networks for the development of Health Promoting Schools' but also to undertake a *first pilot application* of that framework. By now, the former objective has been achieved: a **first result** of this research project is the proposed **draft assessment framework for interorganisational networks to promote health** which was developed in chapters 2 and 3 from two research perspectives: Health Promotion and interorganisational relations. The framework a) covers not only indicators of network structure and processes but also indicators regarding: network environment, reasonable outcomes, network types or levels of evolution, sustainable capacity development, and a network's 'Health Promotion compatibility'. It b) appears to be applicable not only to international networks for the development of Health Promoting *Schools* (HPS) but similar networks to promote health, too (e.g. other 'health promoting Settings' -networks). And c) the framework's 'part I' focuses on a network's 'interorganisational *network* (ION) dimension' and, thus, will apply to *any* interorganisational network; while its 'part II' allows to focus on a network's *Health Promotion* dimension.

The next step is the **pilot testing of this draft framework** for analyzing and assessing interorganisational networks to promote health - through a pilot application to examples of the network type in focus. A **case study approach** has been chosen to undertake this 'first reality check' of the assessment framework and indicators therein. As explained below one international network for the development of Health Promoting Schools has been chosen and two national networks therein. As said in chapter 1, the three pilot applications are intended to test the usefulness of the framework to guide systematic descriptions of the networks in focus, identify their commonalties and differences and documented effects, and analyze their current capacities and future potentials, - and this while considering both the *goals set* by the networks as well as *expectations towards* the networks as indicated, for example, by the current (scientific) knowledge on Health Promotion.

The pilot application of the network assessment framework will provide a basis for selecting a set of practical indicators in terms of network structures and processes - and beyond - and for achieving the overall goal to offer a practical instrument for assessing international networks for the development of Health Promoting Schools - and similar networks.

4.1.1 Rational for the case study approach

As shown in chapter 3 and figure 3.1.1 above, just for the *network* dimension of international networks to promote health about *20* indicators have been derived from the organizational sciences; and *more* indicators had to be added for the networks' *Health Promotion* dimension. This is no surprise considering that **the issue at stake** is the *assessment of international networks for the development of Health Promoting Schools* (and similar networks), i.e. of *complex social systems* with an equally *complex goal*. The scientific literature suggested a breadths of relevant knowledge for such an assessment (as reflected in the high number of indicators identified); at the same time, there was a lack of knowledge from interorganisational relations and health promotion research that would allow to right away identify a few *"key"* indicators to focus on. Thus, the draft network assessment framework remained comprehensive. And this was a *main reason to consider only one or two network case studies* as this would allow to apply and explore the *full range* of indicators identified and pilot test the draft network assessment framework as a *whole*. But even if a quite simple network study framework with a small number of indicators (e.g. five) would have been developed, a case study approach would have been the method of choice for this pilot research for the following reasons:

There is only a very **limited number of *international* networks for the development of Health Promoting Schools (HPS) worldwide.** And the same applies to other 'health promoting Settings'-networks. And of the few existing networks *several* are still in their infancy or initiating phase rather than well established. While there are a scale of five HPS related network initiatives globally (see chap. 2.2.6) the **availability, quality and/or accessibility of data** differs widely (by geographic region and also network levels) and information is *not comparable* in most cases. To focus in the light of this not only on international networks for *HPS* development but also *other* international 'health promoting Settings'-networks was not an option: The same problems of data scarcity and quality would have been faced. And in any case the total number of *established* networks to which the draft network assessment framework developed in this research project could have been meaningfully applied would not have increased much - as most of the 'other' Settings network initiatives are even younger and (with the exception of Healthy Cities networks) yet unique. (see chap. 2.2.6)

International networks for the development of 'Health Promoting *Schools*' *(HPS)* as opposed to international 'healthy cities' networks were favored as case examples for this pilot research. Two reasons spoke against the latter: a) Most documentation and evaluation efforts of the oldest healthy cities (network) project (the European project) focused on developments of the individual city *members* rather than *inter*-city *networking* on an *international* scale; (although the latter was and is practiced: since years in 'Multi City Action Plans' and lately through a new European Association of *national* Healthy City coordinating offices). b) To use - in a first research effort on *developing* an assessment tool for international, *inter*-organizational networks to promote health - such networks as case examples whose network *members* are themselves *multi*-organizational systems (such as 'healthy cities') promised to increase the already high complexity unnecessarily and potentially unproductively. In addition, one reason spoke particularly for using international network initiatives on health promoting *schools* (rather than cities) as case examples: They appeared to be of greater interest as they appeared to be multi-level systems that genuinely encompass interorganisational collaboration among national and international actors rather than local actors alone.

In sum, there were **two main reasons for the case study approach** chosen in this research project: first, the very *small number* of reasonably established and documented international networks to promote health in general, and for the development of Health Promoting Schools in particular, to which the network assessment framework under development could be applied for pilot testing; second, the complexity of that task itself, i.e. the pilot application of a comprehensive assessment framework with a large number of indicators.

4.1.2 Case selection and data collection

As Alter and Hage (1993) pointed out five year old interorganisational networks are still to be understood as 'young'. In early 2001, at the time when the case selection for this research project had to be made, there were two **international networks for the development of Health Promoting Schools** (HPS) that functioned over five years or more: the "European Network of Health Promoting Schools" (or "ENHPS") established in 1992, and the network in the southern part of the Western Pacific Region that came into being in 1995. Commonalties included the networks' formal recognition by the World Health Organization (WHO) and that both had some organizational structure and capacities at the international/ Regional level (within and beyond WHO). To decide whether one or both of these international networks could be studied, further **selection criteria** were applied:

- a sufficient *level of documentation* (in published or 'gray' literature)
- *accessibility* of documents (particularly important because a) most documents on the networks concerned represent 'gray' literature; b)

the common language barriers in international work);
- documentation in a *language* the researcher understands (English, German, or French)
- sufficient *data quality:*
  to a certain degree *comparable* levels of information and this not only as to the *international* level (Europe/ Western Pacific) but also the country level;

Through the researcher's work at the World Health Organization (WHO), the world's leading international organization in initiating and developing international 'health promoting Settings'-networks for many years, the issue of accessibility of gray literature was not much an issue, but that of information quality and comparability was. While the Western Pacific Network (the younger one of the two in question) turned out to be generally less well documented than the European Network, information gaps concerned particularly the country level. Ideas of compensating these gaps, for example, by site visits and/or a systematic approach to telephone interviews were given up for a combination of political reasons, loss of key informants, and lack of resources at the time. This meant that the case studies to pilot test the new network assessment framework developed had to rely on **document analysis**. And in this case, **the European Network was the case of choice:** a) Its overall system (structures, processes, systems levels) and developments over time were clearly better documented as those of the Western Pacific network (in parts due to its older age). b) At least a few of its member countries were documented in a way that matched the selection criteria above, a precondition for undertaking two pilot applications of the assessment framework at country level as intended.

But there were also **other reasons to limit the data gathering to document analysis**: a) From the start, the *main purpose of the case studies* in this research project was to undertake a first *pilot application* of the framework and indicators to study and assess interorganisational networks to promote health that were 'in the making'; (a comparative assessment of selected network cases was a means towards this end). b) The more it became clear that significant *conceptual work was yet needed* to reach the goal of a sound instrument for assessing interorganisational networks (IONs) to promote health, the more important became the case studies' purpose as *pilot* applications of the assessment framework. Neither the organization sciences nor Health Promotion research had sufficiently solid models directly 'at hand'. c) The main network assessment framework and set of indicators was derived from a 'non-health' domain (inter-organizational relations research) for potential integration in full or in parts into the 'health' domain, here 'Health Promotion' - a step which according to the researcher's knowledge had not yet been systematically done before. In the light of this it seemed advantageous to first pilot test the *general applicability* of the proposed network assessment framework to international networks for developing Health Promoting Schools (HPS), before considering any pilot application in the form of an assessment of and with a network 'in the field'. For the *former*, a case study approach based on document analysis applied to three well documented networks (one international and two country networks therein) was judged to be sufficient. d) This strategy was also preferred as at the time of data collection for this research project core actors and potential key informants of the networks in focus had recently been involved in larger review and evaluation efforts and many had a particularly high work load as the networks went through challenging transition times (see chap. 4). Therefore, the availability and readiness of key actors to step into a network assessment process was perceived as rather low.

Besides the above reasons to limit data collection to document analysis and the fact that there were no two international networks sufficiently documented in comparable ways, there were **other reasons to undertake a comprehensive, more in depths case study on only one international network** for the development of Health Promoting Schools (HPS) rather than on two. During the course of the literature analysis (chap. 2) covering both public health and organization sciences three issues moved into the foreground: first, the extent to which *conceptual work* was still needed for a scientifically sound network assessment in an international context and the field of Health Promotion (see chap. 3); second, the fact that current research knowledge suggests a *large number of base line indicators* on interorganisational networks (IONs) in general (a scale of 25 on goal, structure, internal processes, and closer environment alone, without considering particular Health Promotion related indicators yet); 3) the current *lack* of a good rational to identify within this large set of network indicators those that are *'key indicators'* for the assessment of the complex social system at stake, 'interorganisational network'. In the light of this, *one in depths international case study promised to be more beneficial to reach the research goals than a less detailed, more superficial but comparative study of two* international networks.

For all these reasons it was decided to concentrate on the "European Network of Health Promoting Schools" (ENHPS) as a whole, with equal emphasis on two 'country cases' therein. A wide array of gray and published literature by and on the networks was studied, in *chronological order* (rather than reading first or solely final reports and summaries), in order to grasp as far as possible developments over time within and around the networks.

Selection criteria for the 'country cases'

The network assessment framework and indicators developed and now to be tested are meant to be applicable to the *variety* of large scale networks for developing Health Promoting schools (HPS), i.e. for *national* networks or sub-systems within so called "ENHPS member countries", too. To account for this often stressed 'variety' within the "European Network of Health Promoting Schools" (ENHPS) this research project applied the following **criteria** to select national or 'country' networks: Besides the *general criteria* used for selecting the *international* network case (level/ quality/ accessibility of documentation - see above), **the two *national* networks should**:

- show *similarities* as to ENHPS *membership* (date of entry/ lengths of membership/ age);
- show *differences* as to their general *country context* (e.g. one from a big/ the other from a small country; one from a highly federalist/ the other from a more centralized state; etc.);
- together cover the main sub-Regions (i.e. here Central or Eastern *and* Western Europe).

With view to the 'country networks' within the "European Network of Health Promoting Schools" (ENHPS) *documentation* in general significantly varies and may even hardly exist. There are also problems of *accessibility* of information which are highly linked to persisting language barriers: In many Central and Eastern European countries for historical and political reasons skills to speak English (one of the main languages in international work) are not wide spread in some generations. While all ENHPS National Coordinators do speak English their key colleagues or other key actors may not. This, together with the wide spread general lack of resources for documentation (even in a network's mother tongue) and translations are barriers to international network research. In sum, as to the two ENHPS 'country cases' sought for this research project the **choices were quite limited** and a selection could not be done on the base of a literature review alone. Advice was sought from the international Technical Secretariat of the European Network whose staff is in direct contact with all 'countries' participating in the European Network since its launch and can be expected to have the best *overview* internationally about ENHPS related developments across Europe. At the time of inquiry (in early 2000) only a very few ENHPS country networks were perceived as "well functioning" and "well documented" (in English, German and/or French). Using the selection criteria above, the researcher selected the Slovenian and the German network for developing Health Promoting Schools (HPS) as the two cases to be studied.

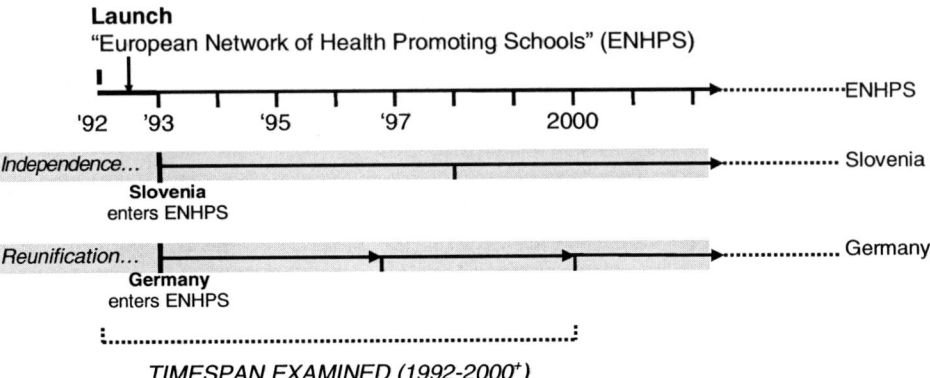

Figure 4.1.1: Illustration of time dimension and commonalties of the selected network cases: the international case "European Network of Health Promoting Schools (ENHPS)" and the two 'country cases' therein, the ENHPS in Slovenia and Germany.

As to the general *country context* the ENHPS initiatives in Germany and Slovenia show some *desired differences:* Germany is a big, highly federalist, 'older' and Western European country as compared to Slovenia, a small, more centralized, 'young' Central European country independent since 1990. Both countries have also *desired commonalties*: as illustrated in figure 4.1.1, both entered the European Network (or ENHPS) initiative in the same year (1993) and remained members up to the year 2000 and beyond; and during the 1990s (i.e. the first seven years of network development) both countries did undergo significant societal changes: Germany reunified and Slovenia achieved independence. Most importantly, in comparison to the ENHPS in other countries those selected are well documented in languages the researcher understands.

4.2 The structure of each case study

The draft interorganisational network (ION) assessment framework proposed is partly built on 'loose ground' because ION research and theory are still fairly young (see chap. 2.4). Therefore, the following **case studies** of the selected European Network and two national sub-systems **to pilot test the network assessment framework will be undertaken in three steps.** Figure 4.2.1 provides an overview.

Step 1 is a comprehensive 'primary case study' that lays the ground for more specific analyses that follow; it encompasses both interorganisational relations and Health Promotion perspectives. *Step 2 is a first 'synthesizing analysis I'* with focus on *network specific* (base line) indicators identified and at the core of the assessment framework proposed; it has a sole organization research perspective. To each network case *both* steps will be applied (see table 4.2.1), first to the European Network, then to the German, and then the Slovenian. Only after this, *step 3* will be pursued: a *'synthesizing analysis II'* that right away looks at *all three* network cases: as to *Health Promotion* specific and *remaining* network specific issues and changes over *time* - as the basis for assessing the usefulness, strengths and limitations of the network indicators and assessment framework developed and tested (chapter 6).

Chapters ↓	The 3-step-case study approach to pilot test the ION assessment framework		
	1. Primary case study The networks as a *whole*: • network (all aspects) • network environment • developments over time	**2. Synthesizing analysis I** *'Network' specific* features: • structure • operational processes; processes of organizational networking* • perceived effectiveness/ levels of conflict	**3. Synthesizing analysis II** *'Health Promotion' specific* features: • ION assessment framework, Part B The *networks as a whole*: • interplay of network features/ goals/ environment/ outcomes • network evolution; other issues;
5.1	The European Network of Health Promoting Schools (ENHPS)		
5.2	↘	Synthesizing analysis I of ENHPS	
5.3	The ENHPS in Slovenia		
5.4	↘	Synthesizing analysis I of Slovenian HPS network project	
5.5	The ENHPS in Germany		
5.6	↘	Synthesizing analysis I of German HPS network project	
6	↓ → → → →	↓	Synthesizing analysis II of ENHPS and national networks therein
	Use of ION assessment framework / research perspectives per step:		
	ION assessment framework as 'guiding matrix' = both Health Promotion and network research perspective	ION assessment framework, Part A (foci: network structure and processes) = interorganisational network research perspective only	ION assessment framework, Part A (remaining issues) and Part B = again both Health Promotion and network research perspective

*soft/ hard networking; networking within/ with others

Table 4.2.1: The 3-step-approach to the case studies for pilot testing the proposed ION assessment framework (ION = interorganisational network)

4.2.1 The overall analysis of each network case (Step 1)

The overall analysis of each of the three selected networks for the development of Health Promoting Schools (HPS) individually aims at providing **a comprehensive picture** of each network (its general features, goal, environments, developments over time, etc.). The proposed *network assessment framework* will be used as a 'guide' rather than narrowly applied; this should provide space for the *potential discovery of additional characteristics* of the 'real life' networks that may be important but not yet accommodated by the proposed network assessment framework - which would require the framework's adjustment.

As will be seen later, the 'primary case studies' of each of the selected networks (European/ Slovenian/ German) did show that one issue needed more research attention than expected - an issue that is not a distinct element of the network assessment framework but relates to several indicators therein: network border and membership. The intended pilot application of the network assessment framework at stake presupposes that the unit of analysis or assessment is defined, i.e. that a network's borders are identified. It became quickly clear that with view to the "European Network of Health promoting Schools" (ENHPS) and the two national sub-networks therein this was not as easy as it first seemed to be. Therefore, in step 1 of the overall case study, each 'primary case study' had to pay particular attention to the *overall* picture of the **interorganisational relations and interactions of key actors 'within and around' a network** in question (fig. 4.2.1) - to clarify the *roles* of these key actors *in relation to* the network in question and thereby, clarify that network's *membership or border(s)* (alongside facets of its environment). Only if a network's border(s) and thus, the unit or sub-units of analysis and assessment were reasonably clarified, the ground was prepared for the intended pilot application of the proposed network assessment framework in all its facets. Particularly some *structural* network features (size, complexity, differentiation and connectivity) as well as the extent of Hastings' four *networking* processes can only be analyzed if it is clear who is 'in' and who is 'outside' of a network system or sub-system.

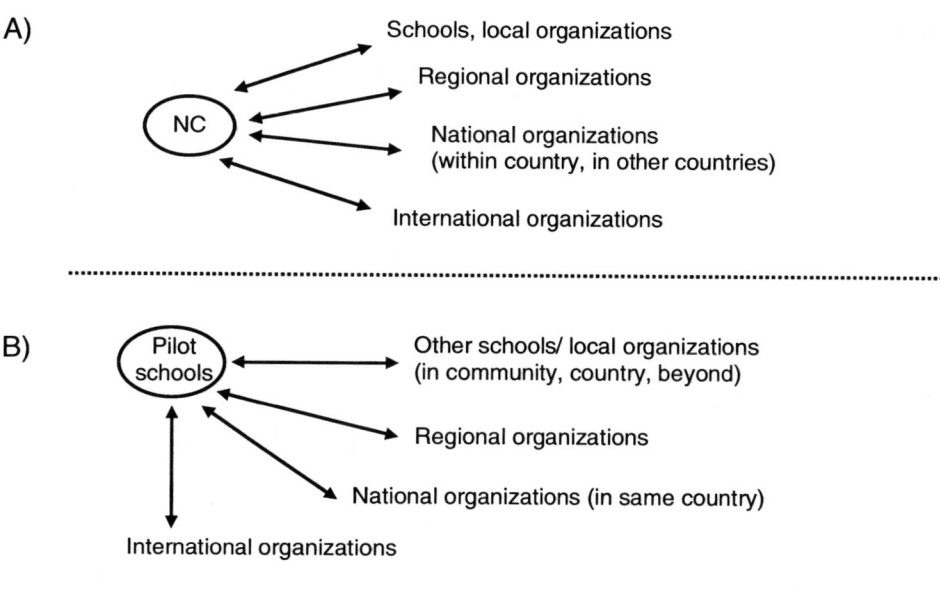

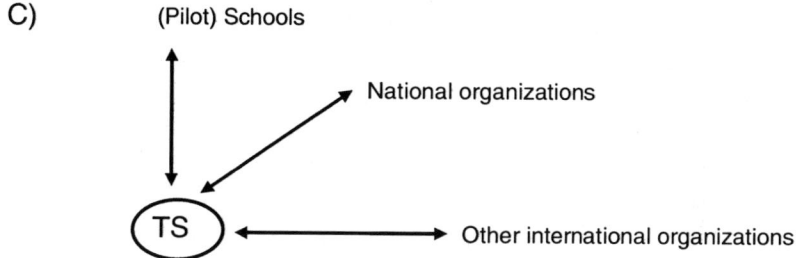

Figure 4.2.1: Possible relations and interactions of and among key organizational actors involved in the ENHPS initiative - Scheme for their analysis by systems levels (A national, B local, C international)

NC = national HPS (support/ coordinating) center
TS = international 'ENHPS Technical Secretariat'

Where in the following 'primary case studies' the analysis of the interorganisational relations and interactions of 'key actors' within *and* around a particular network is needed (due to lack of clarity about network membership or borders) this **analysis will be organized as follows**: As illustrated in figure 4.2.1 *one* key actor per *systems* level will be selected whose relationships with *all others* will be systematically examined: with view to the national level, the national HPS center or centers (NC) (which exist in all 'ENHPS countries'; as to the local level, the so called 'pilot schools' (the first generation of ENHPS network schools); and regarding the international level, the 'ENHPS Technical Secretariat' (TS). - For these analyses it needs **to be recalled and kept in mind** that, due to the very nature of interorganisational networks or by definition (see chap. 3.1.2) *inter-member relationships or interactions are* non-hierarchical or less hierarchical, show lateral linkages, and self-regulation; and are informal or formal. They exhibit qualities such as direct person-to-person-connections, trust, mutual benefit and reciprocity ('win/win'), sharing of information or resources, and a long term perspective - with people and communication put at the center of processes.

4.2.2 Synthesizing analysis I of each network case (Step 2)

The 'synthesizing analysis I' that follows *each* of the comprehensive 'primary' case studies on the European, Slovenian and German networks for the development of Health Promoting Schools, takes a pure organization research perspective: It concentrates on distinct features of Part I of the network assessment framework, i.e. on a network's *'network'* dimension as opposed to its Health Promotion dimension. However, *not all* elements of this Part I of the assessment framework (see overview fig. 3.1.1) will be in focus right away. Figure 4.2.2 illustrates the focus chosen: i.e. the set of basic and *distinct features of (and more or less 'internal' to) an interorganisational network* (rather than these features' interplay, the network as a whole, network environment and evolution).

Undertaken for each network case individually (the European/ German/ Slovenian) the 'synthesizing analysis I' will be structured as follows:

a) **network membership or borders** - as clarifying the unit of analysis is the crucial basis to identify,

b) a network's **operational processes,** i.e. in *Alter/Hage*-terms the methods of coordination used (impersonal-, personal -, group methods); and in addition and related to this,

c) the general **purpose of interactions (contacts) within a network,** according to *Alter and Hage* a main indicator not only for network types but network evolution (see below);

d) **perceived effectiveness and levels of conflict** within a network (following *Alter and Hage* captured as perceptions of *key actors* in the network).

Further aspects of 'reasonable outcomes' of the (European, Slovenian and German) networks related to both their particular 'tasks' or 'goals' and general expectations towards Health Promotion initiatives, will be addressed in the 'synthesizing analysis *II*' later on - as there are many issues that refer equally to all three networks and are better addressed en bloc. However, the 'synthesizing analysis *I*' will not only be structured around the five (sets of) *internal network features (a to e)* above that stem from the *Alter/Hage* network theory.

In addition, the 'synthesizing analysis *I*' will be structured around *five sets of indicators* that stem from *Hastings'* model of the 'new' organization and 'organizational networking' (see fig. 4.2.2 b):

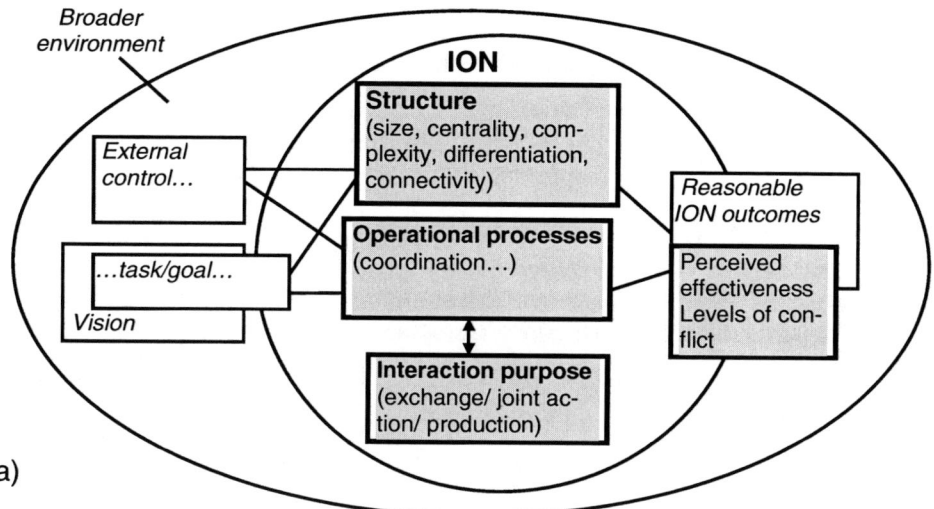

a)

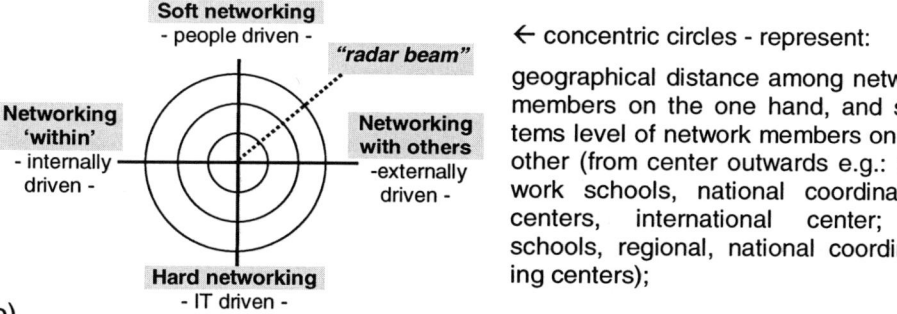

b)

← concentric circles - represent:

geographical distance among network members on the one hand, and systems level of network members on the other (from center outwards e.g.: network schools, national coordinating centers, international center; or schools, regional, national coordinating centers);

Figure 4.2.2: Step 2 of the 3-step-network case study approach - Overview of *those* elements of the ION assessment framework that are the focus of each 'synthesizing analysis I' (shaded in gray):

a) Network characteristics as in the Alter/ Hage model (1993): network structure; operational processes; purpose of interactions/contacts within the network;

b) Elements of Hastings' model of 'new' organizational systems: four networking processes; geographical distance; 'radar beam' for continuous self-reflection.

ION = interorganisational network

The additional sets of indicators from the *Hastings'* model (fig. 4.2.2.b and 2.4.1) are:

f) a **network's networking 'with external others'** and the **relation of its networking 'within' and 'with others'** - both by (groups of) network *members* and as to the network as a *whole*; (and by building on the analyses following the Alter/Hage-model (points b to d above) which cover already aspects of 'networking within' a network);

g) a **network's 'hard' networking, means of 'soft' networking,** and the **relation of 'hard' and 'soft' networking** - both by (groups of) network *members* and as to the network as a *whole*;

h) **geographical distance among network members** (Hastings' 'circles');

i) continuous **(self-)reflection, observation, evaluation processes and feed back loops within a network** (Hastings' 'radar beam');

the extent of **'organizational networking' of network members, here network *schools*** (i.e. the 'Health Promoting Schools in the making') - but *only* in the case of networks that have the *explicit* goal to improve the 'organizational networking' capacities of (some of its) network members.

Structured in this way, the 'synthesizing analysis I' that follows each individual 'basic network case study' is intended to serve as a targeted 'reality check' or pilot test of the *applicability of the range of (base line) indicators on structure and processes* of interorganisational networks to networks in Health Promotion such as the *networks for developing Health Promoting Schools* on a larger scale. Network 'structure' and 'processes' are the domains that at the outset were chosen to be the focus of this research project. However, each 'synthesizing analysis I' reaches somewhat beyond these foci by addressing also aspects of the network's *environment* (through the network's and network members' 'networking with others') and two 'reasonable' *outcome* measures (perceived effectiveness/ level of conflict). All indicators selected for the 'synthesizing analysis I' from the overall network assessment framework (chap. 3.2) stem from the *Alter/Hage network model and/or Hastings' model of the 'new' organization or multi-organizational system*, i.e. from two central 'building blocs' of the proposed assessment framework. A few issues should be noted:

First, the issue of 'organizational networking' of network *members* (point j) needs attention only if the network for Health Promoting Schools (HPS) development being studied includes the 'Health Promoting Schools' in the making as network members. This is because the implementation of the Health Promoting School (HPS) concept inherently expects schools to develop 'school-community-links', which is a matter of a school's networking 'with others' (such as organizations locally); and the school development dimension of the HPS concept requires much 'networking within' schools. (see chap. 2.2) Thus, implementing the HPS concept in schools - the overall *goal* of the network examples studied - inherently means developing the schools' organizational networking capacities as to at least two of Hastings' four networking processes: networking 'within' and 'with others'.

Second, the issue *'interaction purpose' (point d) is not an explicit element of the proposed assessment framework* for interorganisational networks (IONs) but *implicitly covered* through the assessment principle 2 'attention to network development stages/levels' (see fig. 3.1.1). However, as the purpose of interaction within a network (e.g. exchange or joint action) is one of the important indicators of network evolution to be addressed later on, it is meaningful that it be addressed in the 'synthesizing analysis I'. Thus, it is for *practical purposes* rather than for the purpose of a first adaptation of the network assessment framework, that figure 4.1.3 shows 'interaction purpose' as a distinct internal network feature (see inner ellipse).

Third, to avoid confusion it should be noted that there is an **overlap between the network features 'connectivity' and 'networking within'** (see point b and f). It reflects the overlap between the Alter/Hage network model and Hastings' organization model which has been carried forward into the proposed network assessment framework, Part I. One of the structural network features taken over from the Alter/Hage network framework, *'connectivity', addresses what Hastings calls 'networking within'* an organizational system (one of his four networking processes). - In the social sciences 'connectivity' is a common measure in network research and (as will be seen later) it has also been used by evaluators of the ENHPS in Germany. **Several dimensions of 'connectivity'** may be distinguished: In quantitative terms 'connectivity' is typically measured as a) the *number of contacts* among network members *in relation to* the maximal number of contacts possible (i.e. the extent to which 'every channel is used'); and b) the *frequency* of contacts. More qualitative aspects are c) whether there is *reciprocity* of contacts or not (whether there are truly *inter*actions); and d) issues such as whether contacts are based on relations that are: hierarchical or not; formal or informal; based or not on mutuality and trust, and/or on a long term perspective; etc.

In the **Alter/Hage**-network model and in the proposed network assessment framework accordingly, 'connectivity' refers to the first dimensions, i.e. the extent to which within a network every channel is used; this is categorized as a 'structural' network feature. Some more qualitative aspects of inter-member contacts are captured by the network feature 'operational processes' (and the indicator 'methods of coordination used'). - Other aspects of quality of contacts are exhibited by *any* "interorganisational network" (ION) *by definition*: As elaborated in chapter 2.4 and recalled above, "interorganisational networks" show a particular type of inter-member relationships or interactions (non-hierarchical or at least less hierarchical, and lateral links; direct person-to-person-connections, trust, mutual benefit and reciprocity ('win/win'); sharing of information/ resources; a long term perspective; self-regulation; informal or formal links;). People and communication are generally seen as at the center of processes. - **Hastings** model of the 'new' organization when applied to an *inter*-organizational system addresses 'connectivity' under the heading 'networking within' (as opposed to networking 'with others'). Hastings does not specify how to assess the extent of 'networking within'; he presents it as one of four interrelated networking *processes* or basic *orientations an organizational systems may focus on*, more or less, - depending on where the resources needed to achieve goals are available (within the organizational system or externally).

In the light of this, the 'synthesizing analysis I' that follows each general 'basic network case study' (the European, Slovenian, German) will address 'connectivity' and 'networking within' the network as follows: The analysis of network *structure* indicator by indicator (point b) will follow a middle way by concentrating on *the general picture* of 'connectivity' or 'networking within' the network as to *reciprocal* contacts or interactions (a defining feature of interorganisational 'networking' per se), and this only as to *groups* of network members (rather than individual members). This approach matches with and somewhat mediates between both Alter's and Hage's approach to 'connectivity' as a structural network feature and Hastings' 'networking within' as a basic organizational orientation and process. Each 'synthesizing analysis I' of a network will address also some other quality issues of inter-member contacts: under the headings 'network processes' and 'purpose of interactions' (points c and d). But the various qualities of inter-member relations and interactions that *by definition* "interorganisational networks" should show will not be addressed here one by one. These will be taken up en bloc in the 'synthesizing analysis II'.

4.2.3 Synthesizing analysis II of all network cases (Step 3)

After the basic 'network' features of the European, German and Slovenian networks for the development of Health Promoting Schools (HPS) have been examined one by one, some issues remain; and each of those will be addressed right away regarding all *three* networks: a) **'further network dimensions'** of the networks of interest, regarding: *factors that influence* network structure and processes (e.g. external control/ goals set) and their interplay; *links between* structural/ process features and selected network outcomes (perceived effectiveness/ levels of conflict) and the attention given to 'reasonable' outcomes (assessment principle 1); network *evolution* (principle 2); and issues of sustainable capacity development (principle 3);

b) **the 'Health Promotion dimension'** of the networks of interest, regarding: the integration of the *social-ecological approach* and use of a *combination* of strategies; *participation, empowerment, and continuous learning;* and valued outcomes related to goals set and desired changes in factors that 'co-determine' health. By assessing such features an even deeper understanding of interorganizational networks in general and the networks in focus in particular will arise. This last part of the overall case study will move **the networks as a *whole*** and changes over time **back into the foreground** of this study.

PART II

CASE STUDIES:

THE "EUROPEAN NETWORK OF HEALTH PROMOTING SCHOOLS" / "ENHPS" AND TWO NATIONAL SUB-NETWORKS

(PILOT TESTING OF THE ASSESSMENT FRAMEWORK)

- The "European Network of Health Promoting Schools" (ENHPS): primary case study and synthesizing analysis I
- The ENHPS in Germany: ditto
- The ENHPA in Slovenia: ditto
- Synthesizing analyses II of the European Network and the two national networks therein

5. The "European Network of Health Promoting Schools" (ENHPS) - a case study from an international and inter-organizational research perspective

5.1 Primary case study: Overall analysis of the European Network (ENHPS)

5.1.1 Introduction - the European context and the birth of the ENHPS

The 'European Network of Health Promoting Schools' or ENHPS is a tripartite project launched in 1992 by the World Health Organization's Regional Office for Europe (WHO/EURO), the European Commission (EC), and the Council of Europe (CE). This interagency partnership has been maintained up today. (IPC 1993) As any network assessment also that of the European Network must consider the wider (socio-political/ socio-economic) context in which the Network and its leading organizations operate, as well as the organizational mandates of the latter. Over a decade after the fall of the 'iron curtain' Europe sees significant social, economic and health gradients from West to East; many Central and Eastern European countries experienced heavy socio-economic crises and negative health trends. These developments have contributed to an increased general awareness of the strong and inextricable link between social, economic and health development, and they will obviously have influenced the operation of the European Network of Health Promoting Schools (ENHPS) and any other international network across Europe (heterogeneous membership in socio-economic terms; unequal fund raising opportunities; etc.). Besides these wider environmental factors some more specific factors have to be considered when assessing the European Network: *European level* public policies and infrastructures in education and health in general, and in Health Promotion and education in particular - many of them originate or relate directly to the three intergovernmental agencies (WHO/ EC/ CE) that initiated this network as a joint 'ENHPS project'. From the start this inter-agency collaboration was the international backbone of the European Network's development and, thus, not only the network's birth but its resource dependency and autonomy (important indicators in network assessment) are closely linked to these three agencies. Therefore, their mandates and policies need brief examination before turning to the network itself. To enhance the text flow also in the following the "European Network of Health Promoting Schools" will be referred to also as 'the European Network' or 'ENHPS'.

The European 'health (policy) arena' as core environment of the European Network

In Europe as elsewhere in the world, the major (public) health policy and strategy is the Regional specification of the global 'Health for All' - policy framework. With WHO as key initiator, the European Network of Health Promoting Schools has been created within **the European policy 'Health for All by the year 2000'** (HfA 2000) from 1991, and since 1999 guided by the renewed policy **'Health21'**. These policies were formally adopted by the WHO Regional Committee (i.e. by the Health Ministers of WHO Member States) which covers all member countries of the European Union and the Council of Europe, the two partners of WHO in the ENHPS project. The 'HfA 2000'-policy has allowed **WHO/EURO** to invest significant resources into the European Network of Health Promoting Schools and to influence to various degrees the network's policy environment within countries. The main link provide the five targets on 'lifestyles conducive to health' which address related *intersectoral policies; public participation*; health promoting *Settings* (including schools and neighborhoods); *education and training in health promotion; continues efforts* on healthy patterns of living; and health-harming substances - a political basis for a wide range of (school) health promotion actions in countries. This policy was revised during the European Network's second phase of development and in 1999 was replaced by the new 'Health21' policy. For the European Network it was important that this policy, too, includes reference targets on healthy living and *'Settings for the Promotion of Health'* as these and some additional targets (on young people, mental health, *multi-sectoral responsibility* for health, etc.) justify and WHO's and the public sectors' continued investments into the European Network of Health Promoting Schools. The policy's underlying *values* (equity, participation, solidarity, sustainability, accountability and sensitivity to gender issues) and the related targets match with the Health Promotion goals and principles (see chap. 2.2). As the new policy 'Health21' reflects much of the 'co-determinants of health' knowledge introduced in chapter 2.1 and clearly expresses health development as a *cross sectional task at all levels* of society and the need for strategies that initiate and support such collaboration (WHO/EURO 1998a; 1999) the European Network has also today a good policy basis (at least at European level) - a supportive factor in the network's environment even if policy adoption at international level not necessarily means its translation into policies and practices within countries.

While in the tripartite European Network 'project' it is WHO that has the main mandate, formal links and (policy) influence in the health sector it is not the only one. Since the Maastricht Treaty (1991) also the **European Community** has a mandate in public health (in general health protection and consumer protection) and the article 129 on public health explicitly states that emphasis should be given to *health promotion and disease prevention*. Against this background the **European Commission** negotiated with WHO and the Council of Europe towards the *joint launch* of the "ENHPS project" in 1992. Later, in 1996, the EU started a five year 'Community Program on Health Promotion' - a step that was, on the one hand, influenced by the perceived successes of the European Network initiative, on the other hand, an important basis for the EU's further contributions to the tripartite network project because it aimed at public awareness raising related to risk factors and health enhancing aspects of life, encouraged *pooling of ideas and experiences and sharing of know-how* between countries, and covered quality development and the three 'entry points' for Health Promotion identified in chapter 2.2: health issues (such as heart health/ physical activity/ mental health); population groups (the older and *the young*), and *work on settings*. The latter was clearly oriented towards a *network approach* and included explicitly the European Network of Health Promoting Schools and one for workplace health promotion. Training and the use of modern information technologies were addressed, too. (WHO/EURO 1998, see 'The European Commission'; Krech 1999; Theesen 1997; Parsons et al 1997) Four years after the launch of the European Network, this program offered a variety of new fundraising opportunities for network members, unfortunately at first only for those in the EU but soon and increasingly also for non-EU members.

Also the third partner in the tripartite 'ENHPS project', the **Council of Europe** (CE) is an intergovernmental actor in the field of health, but equally in various other sectors of society including education. The "Council of Europe" (CE) should not be confused with the EU and its European Council; they are quite distinct bodies but share the same flag to strengthen the development of a European identity. Created long before the EU, the Council of Europe (CE) groups 41 pluralistic democracies (the EU Members included) to harmonize policies and adopt common standards and practices across countries. Unlike its ENHPS project partners WHO and European Commission the Council of Europe operates by bringing together, at *different levels*, representatives of *national* parliaments, governments, *local and regional* authorities, international *NGOs* and youth associations to pool their knowledge and experience. Its participation and contributions to the 'European Network' initiative is up today influenced by its principle objectives: to protect and reinforce pluralistic *democracy* and human rights; to seek solutions to *social challenges* facing European society (AIDS, organized crime, discrimination...); to favor the emergence of a genuine European *cultural identity*; and to *assist central and eastern European countries* with their political, legislative and constitutional reforms. CE activities cover potentially any subject concerning the European society (except defense), from social and economic questions to health, culture, education and environment (i.e. a range of areas of co-determinants of population health). But it has been the *health* section alone that has been the partner in the ENHPS project; cross-departmental collaboration in support of this was five years after the network's launch yet to be developed (Scicluna 1997). The periodic CE conferences of specialized ministers (of education, health, youth, etc.) to analyze emerging problems offer a pathway to gain or strengthen the support of e.g. education ministers for the ENHPS in their countries. From the European Network perspective of particular importance was and is the CE's *'European Health Committee'* that is responsible for encouraging closer European cooperation on aspects of the promotion of health such as health policy, preventive measures, *education for health*, and staff training. (Council of Europe 2001; ENHPS 2000)

As of now, overall the ENHPS project is a tripartite CE-EC-WHO-project carried out by the *health* sections of these organizations (not e.g. the education sections of CE and EC). However, the **mandates of the Council of Europe and also of the European Commission in** *education* are supportive factors and, for example, have provided various channels towards funding and other support for particular ENHPS activities. As the European *health* policies and programs those on *education* are an important part of the European Network's international environment. Relevant aspects related to the *Council of Europe* have been addressed already above; those related to the *European Commission* can be sketched out as follows: The Treaties of Maastricht and Amsterdam (articles 149/150) include not only the legal mandate in public health but also a strong one for quality education - with full respect to cultural and linguistic diversity. An *overall EU education policy is lacking*, but over time *several Community activities, programs and action plans* provided opportunities for active support to the 'ENHPS project'. (European Union 2001) Examples include 'Socrates I' and 'II' and the 1996 action plan to introduce new information technologies (IT) to schools which explicitly address(ed) 'the world of education' (e.g. teachers and pupils) and funded e.g. schools and transnational projects concerned with developing *"the European dimension"* and improving the *quality of school education* - two core issues within the European Network of Health Promoting Schools as will be seen later. However, only from 1997 (i.e. five years after the launch of the European Network) all European Community programs relating to education, training and youth gradually opened up beyond EU Member States to a number of Central European countries and only since 2000, most European countries participate. Although there are no overview data on ENHPS members' use of the various EC funding opportunities there is no doubt that for the first years of network development an 'equity gap' in fundraising opportunities between EU- and non-EU network members existed impacting even on a major ENHPS evaluation efforts (see below). As to positive, the European Network potentially strengthening developments the guidelines on education, training and youth for 2000-2006 should be mentioned; 'eLearning' became one of the current EU priorities with special attention to improvements of the *IT infrastructure in schools* - an opportunity to strengthen the European Network's *network* potential. Similarly other EC program priorities such as on partnerships for knowledge acquisition between teaching establishments, and mobility and cooperation of teachers, students, etc. and the 'Socrates II' program promise support for ENHPS members and their health promoting work in a network context.

Overall it can be said that **the three initiators and core partners in the tripartite 'ENHPS project'** by or within which the "European Network of Health Promoting Schools" was launched and supported, either represent or have important influence on important sections of the Network's *international* policy and institutional *environment* covering both areas health and education: They combine important forces and resources for the implementation of the ENHPS in countries: WHO has since long the clear mandate, sole focus and leadership function in international public health and health promotion; but by the time of the launch of the ENHPS also the EU had some mandate in these areas, plus a mandate and focus in education. And the Council of Europe, as part of its overall mission towards a democratic European society, is active in *both* health and education, too - plus in many other related fields. In this set up the European Network via WHO has direct access and strong links to national *Ministries of Health*, with complementary links via the CE and EC. The Council of Europe provides channels to *Ministries of Education* and other governmental bodies as well as parliaments throughout Europe, the EU with regard to its 15 Members States.

An important factor in **successful interorganisational relations** is a *joint mission* (see chap. 2.3) which in the case of the three ENHPS initiators is that all children must be given the opportunity to achieve their maximum potential as *healthy* and *educated* adults 'who possess the energy, skills and sense of responsibility that are essential in the modern world'. The tripartite 'ENHPS project' is dedicated to reaching that goal.

From the start CE, EC and WHO/EURO recognized that to succeed the "full and sustained support of leaders at all levels in education, health, and socioeconomic development" is needed; and that *collaboration is essential to* a) *avoid duplication* of efforts, and b) provide a *coherent framework* within which to foster and sustain *innovation*, *disseminate* models of good practice, and *make opportunities* for health promotion in schools *equally available* throughout Europe. (IPC 1993)

Up to day, the *joint planning and management* of the ENHPS project is a remarkable example of long-term interorganisational collaboration at this level. The collaboration of WHO, EC and CE in school health promotion and the creation of the European Network did not come into being 'over night'. It was pre-succeeded by several years of conceptual work and discussions to bridge between health education and health promotion approaches, the latter put forward by the WHO Regional Office for Europe (WHO/EURO) as the more comprehensive one.

In the 1980s/1990s the 'Health Promoting School' (HPS) concept was developed through a series of international events and WHO/EURO prepared the ground for developing a large scale HPS project. As elaborated in chapter 2.2, during the 1980s international agreements in the understanding of health education and health promotion emerged and conceptual bridges between 'modern' health education or 'education for health' and 'Health Promotion' were built. From the late 1980s, WHO, European Commission and Council of Europe demonstrated an increasing willingness and ability to cooperate on health education and Health Promotion for school-aged children and young people. (IPC 1993, ENHPS/TS 1993b 1.1, 1997; Rasmussen et al 1996) Conceptual bridge building was followed by structural bridge building between the three intergovernmental agencies - in the form of the *joint* launch of the "European Network of Health Promoting Schools" in 1992. In the early phase, the three agencies expressed the openness of their 'project' to any other international organization that would wish to participate. However, it remained a tripartite endeavor which became recognized as a concrete example of a Health Promotion activity that has successfully incorporated the 'energies' of the three major European agencies in the joint pursuit of their goals in school health promotion. (IPC 1993 ; Burgher et al 1999; Rasmussen et al 1996)

In the following, the three ENHPS initiators and leading organizations European Commission (EC), Council of Europe (CE) and WHO/EURO will as a group be briefly referred to as 'the ENHPS initiators' or 'the three European organizations' wherever this is sufficient.

5.1.2 Rational, goals, and core concepts

Research results suggest that the type of tasks or goals of interorganisational networks influence their structures, operational processes and outcomes (see chap. 2.3). Documents on the "European Network of Health Promoting Schools" (ENHPS) published by its initiators contain *two levels of goals and purpose* which from the perspective of this research project have to be clearly distinguished:

a) goals or intentions of the ENHPS initiators related to choosing and maintaining the *organizational form* of a 'network' for their large scale effort on developing Health Promoting Schools (HPS) across Europe, - in the following referred to as the *rational for the 'network approach'* in European HPS development;

b) the purpose of that specific 'European Network'/ENHPS as an own organizational system - in the following referred to as *goals and objectives of the ENHPS*.

These two levels may not always have good selectivity. However, they do reflect different perspectives: a) that of the ENHPS *initiators*, and b) that of the network *members* and also supporters - on condition that their involvement is voluntary. Obviously, initiators are likely also supporters. At both levels (network rational and goals) changes are possible over time.

As explained in chapter 2.4, the European Network's *goals and objectives* are quite important for the assessment of its interorganisational network dimension as they will be significant reference points for perceived effectiveness and conflict or harmony among members (though unlikely the only one). The *rational* for the network approach as seen by the ENHPS initiators hints at external expectations *towards* the Network, a point to be taken up later again. This chapter focuses on the situation *at the beginning* of the ENHPS to lay the ground for examining its development over time. However, some basic changes that occurred will be already addressed to create from the start some awareness of the dynamics of the ENHPS initiative.

Rational for the network approach

The three European organizations in their first ENHPS project brochure state (IPC 1993):

The setting up of a European Network of Health Promoting Schools (ENHPS) is an effective way of *exchanging* experiences and information, and *disseminating* examples of good practice. They underpin their view by referring to repeated proposals by health and education experts, government policy-makers, researcher and teachers in various meetings and conferences. More specifically, the ENHPS has been set up to establish, *throughout* the European Region, a *group* of model schools that would (ENHPS/TS 1997):

- first demonstrate the impact of health promotion in the school setting,
- then disseminate their experience and information to the health and education sectors, influencing policy and practice in school health promotion both nationally and internationally.

Looked at from an interorganisational network (ION) perspective, these statements (short as they are) indicate an intention of the Network initiators to create an inter*organisational,* i.e. inter-school network for which two developmental stages are foreseen: An *exchange* network is aimed at first, which should be able to then develop into a 'dissemination' network directed at key actors in the Network's environment, i.e. the health and education sectors. However, the wording used remains somewhat vague. For example, is the goal a *'network'* of schools or just a *'group'*? Also the task of the 'dissemination' network is defined rather wide. One may ask how 'dissemination' is understood if schools are to disseminate information and through this influence policy and practice. Years later, an evaluation team of the ENHPS came back to this issue (Piette et al 1999) when proposing to distinguish between 'distribution' (of information) and 'dissemination' (as a process of developing good practice). The degree of openness or vagueness with regard to a second stage after a clearly defined first one is not surprising if one considers: a) the level of complexity and innovation connected already with the first stage (the creation of models of 'Health Promoting Schools' throughout Europe); and b) the fact that the organizational form chosen for the latter, an interorganisational network (ION), was at the time barely discussed or systematically analyzed and, as shown in chapter 2.3, is up today a significant organizational innovation - particularly when linked to rather bureaucratic systems such as public education sectors in Europe. This issue is an important one for this research project and will be further examined after the ENHPS has been explored in its various facets.

Goals and objectives of the "European Network of Health Promoting Schools" (ENHPS)

The *general purpose* underlying the initiation of the ENHPS is to combine education and health promotion in order to realize the potential of both.

This Network has been formed "to create within schools environments conducive to health. Working together to make their school better places in which to learn and work, pupils and school staff take action to benefit their physical, mental and social health. In the process, they gain knowledge and skills that improve the outcomes of education" (Burgher, Barnekov Rasmussen, Rivett 1999 p4).

This is the latest statement on the general goal and process rational of the ENHPS. The goal statements have undergone some changes over time and there is not the statement of goal and objectives of the European Network to be cited. At the beginning (IPC 1993), the three international initiators expressed that they support a European Network which strives to realize a set of school features which then found their way into descriptions of a 'Health Promoting School' (HPS) (see below). Thus, **from the beginning, the main goal set was to create 'Health Promoting Schools'** (HPS). For National HPS Coordinators already designated at that time, the European Network's goal was further elaborated to include **aspects beyond the individual schools**:

Through the cooperation of the 'three international partners' and other interested organizations, the ENHPS is expected to *motivate 'key players'* involved in health promotion within Europe, and to *encourage information exchange and the development of new approaches* for promoting health in the school setting. Requirements for success are commitment, creativity and perseverance from 'everyone involved', international organizations, national ministries and networks, teachers, children and parents. (NHPS/TS 1993b 1.4) Elsewhere, the goal of creating a *network of pilot schools* is implicitly expressed, as through such a network the ENHPS strives "*to introduce* the theory, methods and practices of *school health promotion to* schools, their communities and health and education services at all levels" (WHO/EURO 1998). Another time, the ultimate goal of improving and protecting the physical and emotional *health and welfare of* pupils, teachers, non-teaching staff and the wider community is highlighted (Rasmussen et al 1996).

As the name indicates, the goal or objectives of the 'European Network of Health Promoting Schools' are closely linked to the **goals of a 'Health Promoting School'**. These have been characterized by a series of action programs (ENHPS/TS w.y., 1997 p5) that aim at:

- clarifying the school's social aims and highlighting its potential for health promotion;
- promoting a sense of responsibility for the health of the individual, family and community;
- promoting pupil's self-esteem, enabling them to fulfill their physical, psychological and social potential;
- developing good relations throughout the school's internal and *external community;*
- realising the potential of specialist and other community resources to advise on and support health education and action for health promotion;
- planning a coherent health education curriculum;

- presenting a realistic and attractive range of health choices in order to encourage a healthy lifestyle; and
- providing a safe and healthy environment (meals, buildings, leisure facilities, etc.).

Obviously, goals and objectives of the European Network cover a wide range of issues and different ones have been highlighted by different actors and/or at different occasions. According to the Alter/Hage network theory a wider *scope* of an interorganisational network's *tasks or goals* calls for different network structures and operational processes than a more narrow scope. Also, network outcomes such as *'perceived effectiveness'* will depend on the goals and objectives set. Thus, network goals should be well understood if network assessment is the aim. But already the search for the rational and goal of the European Network unraveled complexity. The various statements by ENHPS initiators found represent complementary sets of goals and objectives that should be better understood. When using the Health Promotion outcome model *adapted* from Nutbeam to systematise the European Network's or 'ENHPS project's' goals (see chap. 3.1.4,/fig. 3.1.3) the following picture emerges:

- with view to the upper level of **ultimate, usually long term** outcomes, i.e. *health and quality of life outcomes*, the ENHPS aims at:

improving and protecting the health and welfare of all members of the school community and eventually also of the wider local community;

- with regard to the level of **intermediate** outcomes in terms of *'modifiable determinants of health'*, the ENHPS aims at:

the creation of health-promoting social and physical environments in schools, healthy lifestyles, and also changes related to school health services - issues captured in the set of 'goals' of a Health Promoting Schools (HPS);

- with regard to the level of **direct, usually short term** outcomes, i.e. 'intervention impact measures' the ENHPS aims at:

'changed organizational practices' within schools and beyond, such as improved information exchange, networking among pilot schools, and the introduction of the theory, methods and practices of school health promotion to schools, their communities and health and education services at all levels; the latter also indicates desired 'policy changes'; - captured in the set of 'goals' of a Health Promoting School (HPS); the ENHPS also aims at:

'social action and influence' across levels of society in the sense of achieving involvement of international and national organizations including national ministries as well as of teachers, children and parents.

This brief analysis shows that **overall, at the level of aims** put forward for or by the European Network: a) as to the ultimate/ long term outcomes, the definition of the *target group has been expanded* beyond the traditional focus on solely pupils to include *all* members of the school community (pupils *plus* school staff, and even parents) which is a distinct feature of the ENHPS; b) as to the intermediate and the direct/short term outcomes, most objectives are expressed in form of *the 'goals' of a "Health Promoting School";* and c) direct or short term outcomes include also a few objectives addressing the schools' *environment* (involvement of (inter)national actors) but these are little refined.

To be able to assess the European Network as elaborated in chapter 3, i.e. not only in its 'network' but also its *'Health Promotion* dimension' (see Part B of the network assessment framework proposed), the network's **conceptual basis** needs to be clarified. Particularly the Health Promoting Schools (HPS) concept is concerned because it a) is the European Network's major goal, and b) describes the desired 'ideal' network member at local level as perceived or defined by the network's initiators. In addition, the HPS concept and related ones (such as 'Health Promotion', 'health' and co-determinants of health') as well as the concept of a 'network' may contain explicit or implicit statements and hints as to the desired *interorganisational relations within* the European Network as well as between the Network and *external* partners; and these are important features to be considered in network assessment.

The "Health Promoting School" - concept

As shown in chapter 2.2.6 the creation of Health Promoting Schools generally means implementing a range of changes in schools. The term "Health Promoting School" (HPS) stands for *a complex concept* that in documents on the European Network (ENHPS) typically is *described rather than briefly defined*. However, National Coordinators in Europe received a short definition which later was adopted at global level: "A Health Promoting School constantly strengthens its capacity as a healthy setting for living, learning and working" (ENHPS/TS 1993b 1.2; WHO 1998a). The conceptual frame of the 'Health Promoting School' as presented by the European Network today consists of three text elements each encompassing aim, means how to achieve it, and target group. They mirror the *increased sophistication of the concept reached over time*:

"The health - promoting school aims at achieving healthy lifestyles for the total school population by developing supportive environments conducive to health. It offers opportunities for, and requires commitment to, the provision of a safe and health-enhancing social and physical environment" (IPC 1993 p1)

"A health promoting school uses its management structures, its internal and *external relationships*, its teaching and learning styles and its methods of *establishing synergy with its social environment* to create the means for pupils, teachers, and all those involved in everyday school life to take control over and improve their physical and emotional health." (ENHPS/TS w.y. and 1997 p4)

Most recently, the explicit link to educational goals has been further stressed by adding that a Health Promoting School "uses health promotion as a device to improve the whole quality of the school setting. Success here will better equip schools to enhance learning outcomes" (Burgher et al 1999 p5).

The aspects of the school's links with the local 'community' (i.e. local groups as well as organizations) and of creating synergy with the social environment suggest that **interorganisational relations are an implicit element of the Health Promoting School concept**. This is confirmed by some of the 'twelve criteria of a Health Promoting School' defined early on to spell out the type of commitment and work required from schools and countries that wish to formally participate in the European Network (WHO/EURO 1998):

- the development of good links between the school, the home and the community;
- the development of good links between associated primary and secondary schools to plan a coherent health education curriculum;
- the realization of the potential of specialist services in the community for advice and support in health education; and
- the development of the education potential of the school health services beyond routine screening towards active support for the curriculum.

According to this the 'ideal' Health Promoting School (HPS) is not only community oriented in the sense of relations and cooperation with parents and e.g. individual experts, but has *interorganisational relations* with other schools and other organizations at local level, particularly school health and other service providers. Also the Network's 'European dimension' stresses school-to-school relations (i.e. interorganisational relations). This supports the thesis of this research project that international networks for the development of Health Promoting Schools are *interorganizational* networks (see chap.1) but of course is not yet a confirmation. While the notion of HPS 'criteria' has faded over time their content has remained valid. However, *over time the description of a Health Promoting School (HPS) has become less specific, also with regard to its interorganisational dimension* which remains captured in calls for 'community'-involvement in HPS activities. (see e.g. ENHPS w.y, 1997) Overall, the holistic and **integrated (or 'whole school') approach** of the European Network (ENHPS) is stressed. 'Central to success' is the strong drive of the Health Promoting School to *integrate Health Promotion into all aspects of the school's daily routine.*

It necessitates structural change and the introduction of new ideas and methods throughout the school. These *permeate all levels* of school life: from senior management through to the classroom and links with the external community. Implementing the HPS concept considerably impacts on school life. (ENHPS 1999, 1997)

With view to the HPS concept it is interesting to note that the dimension of interorganisational relations of a Health Promoting School (HPS) is less specified in the set of 'goals' pursued than in the original set of HPS 'criteria'. This indicates, that with view to the schools interorganisational relations are seen as a means to achieve goals rather than a goal themselves. However, as will be seen later, after some years the ENHPS more or less replaced the twelve HPS criteria by '10 principles to be put in place'.

In the following briefly addressed are conceptual frames *other* than the HPS concept that may (explicitly or implicitly) be shared by and guide those closely involved in the European Network initiative. As elaborated in chapter 2, important are understandings of Health Promotion, health, and 'networks' of or within the Network, and their match with the concepts underpinned by research results and much practical experience and therefore pre-eminent in the field of Health Promotion. From interorganisational relations research it is known that shared concepts are an important basis for networks to define a common purpose.

The European Network's concepts of 'Health Promotion', 'health', and 'network'

The ENHPS in its published documents does not present a reference definition of **Health Promotion** per se but the underlying health promotion concept is expressed within the descriptions of the concept of Health Promoting Schools (HPS). For example,

the HPS concept is described as a holistic and integrated approach to health promotion. Particular reference is made to Health Promotion through the Settings approach, and to the task of creating the means for school community members '*to take control over and improve their health*'.

This shows that the modern concept of Health Promotion as elaborated in chapter 2.2 underlies the work of the European Network. (ENHPS/TS 1993b, w.y., 1997; Burgher et al 1999)

The ENHPS refers to a **Settings approach** that addresses schools as settings for 'daily life', for 'living, learning and working' and not only as places to address specific heath concerns or narrowly defined subjects within the school curriculum. Enhancing the school setting means addressing both the personal, social, physical and organizational factors that operate in this setting and the interaction between them.

This shows that the international ENHPS initiators provide technical guidance that is in accordance with the latest understanding of the Settings approach elaborated in chapter 2.2.

Applying the Settings approach to schools is seen as drawing attention to the schools' ability to enhance interorganisational working relations to the communities in which they operate, and helping schools to become accepted as 'focal points' for health promotion initiatives in their communities. (ENHPS/TS 1993b)

Without referring to a particular definition and rather indirectly the European Network of Health Promoting Schools (HPS) expresses its understanding of **health:** The HPS concept is based on a model of health that includes the 'interaction of physical, mental, social and environmental aspects'; and the improvement of both physical and emotional health is emphasized. 'Health Promoting Schools' are expected to have an innovative curriculum which takes a 'holistic view of health' and includes 'health as a positive concept' as one of the eight common themes suggested for all young people. (ENHPS/TS 1993b, w.y., 1997; Burgher et al 1999).

This and the statements on the Settings approach above indicate that the *implicit* health concept of the European Network is in accordance with a multi-dimensional understanding of health as elaborated in chapter 2.1. The emphasis on interactions of personal, social, physical and organizational factors to be addressed suggests that a *co-determinants of health-perspective is implicitly adopted*. The HPS goals or criteria above support this interpretation.

With view to **ideas of a 'Network'**, published or gray literature on the ENHPS project does not provide the definition or description of the term 'network' or networking dimensions. However, **the three initiators and leading international organizations** have developed some concrete ideas of the Network's design:

The ENHPS aims to be as *decentralized* as possible and *flexible* enough to allow for adjustments according to local and national circumstances and priorities. It is based on an *ethos of partnership*, with the participating schools 'owning' the Network and the international organizations 'supporting' it. "Partnership as both a method and goal" has become a motto. To realize its 'European dimension' the Network serves as *a platform for exchanges* and gathering of *understanding and mutual respect* across country borders. Key requirements for its 'effective *management and coordination*' at local/school, national and European level are identified (see chap. 5.1.3 below). (IPC 1993; Burgher et al 1999; Rasmussen et al 1996 p3/4; ENHPS/TS w.y., 1997) - For the *participating schools* the European Network is meant to provide a flexible framework in which they can determine their needs and work to meet them in their own ways (ENHPS 2000). - For the *health and education sectors* the network is to be a consolidating initiative which brings together existing knowledge and understanding of Health Promotion in the school setting (WHO/EURO 1998).

To achieve the goals set the ENHPS actors at international level point to commitment and perseverance required from *'everyone involved':* from international organizations, national ministries and networks, teachers, children and parents (ENHPS/TS 1993b).

When looking at the ENHPS initiators' understanding of a *"network"* presented above two important aspects of interorganisational network (ION) research come to mind: network membership and type. An important question to answer is whether only organizations (at whatever societal level) can become network members or also groups or individuals such as teachers, parents, etc. The language in ENHPS documents with view to its local level is not always clear. However, the thesis further holds that the European Network is an inter*organisational* network (ION): The Network's name 'European Network of Health Promoting *Schools*' as well as references elsewhere to a group or 'network of pilot schools' (e.g. WHO/EURO 1998) suggest that not groups of people but whole schools are network members. In the light of the *importance of the membership issue for network assessment* it will be addressed in more detail below. - Ideas about the European Network laid out by the international actors (decentralization, flexibility and adaptability, partnership approach, mutual respect, etc.) match with key characteristics of interorganisational networks (IONs) identified in the research literature (see chap. 2.3). Whether these ideas of the European Network have been realized in practice needs of course further examination and is an underlying theme of the following sections of this ENHPS case study. This will be taken up again in the synthesizing analysis II (chap. 6) later on.

The ENHPS refers clearly to *'Health Promotion'* as presented in chapter 2.2. Thus, expectations are justified that the European Network tackles necessary changes of a range of factors that influence or co-determine health. Of course this refers to the health of those people that are its main target group: pupils, teachers and other school staff, but also parents and the local community as a whole. As shown in chapter 2.1.2, many of the co-determinants of health of relevance here relate directly to each individual school, but also to each school's local environment. However, over time, Health Promoting Schools likely identify needs to change co-determinants of health that are beyond the influence of their single school or even community and which might only be modifiable in a nation wide or even international effort. This leads to the implicit if not explicit mandate of any international network on HPS development to act on changes of co-determinants of health at national or international level as far as the health of members of school communities is concerned. As explained in chapter 3 above, an assessment from an international Health Promotion perspective will consider not only the self-stated goals of the ENHPS but also this general overarching goal of Health Promotion of influencing the co-determinants of health - be it explicitly expressed as an aim by the Network or not.

As of now, this case study addressed those *aspects of the European context of the ENHPS* in more detail that are directly linked to the three European organizations that initiated and guide the Network. This was needed to better understand the core (institutional and policy) environment within which the large scale 'ENHPS initiative' was developed. The *rational and goals of the European Network* have been discussed as a main reference point for assessing the network's structures, processes and outcomes. Linked to this, the *conceptual basis* of the ENHPS as envisioned at international level has been addressed to clarify a) the concepts that those that join the European Network are expected to share, and b) whether that conceptual basis matches with latest scientific knowledge which inherently is a quality issue and linked to the likelihood that other organizations join and remain in the Network. In the European Network's overall analysis the next step needed is to examine its *structural* set up.

5.1.3 Structural set-up and key actors of the ENHPS initiative

The goal set for this research project was to develop a practical instrument for assessing international networks for the development of Health Promoting Schools as to both network *structures* and processes. The structural and process indicators within the assessment framework being pilot tested stem from the Alter/Hage network theory that, while compatible with the limited other research on interorganisational networks nevertheless lacks a strong empirical base yet. Therefore, this section of the ENHPS case study not *solely* focuses on the indicators identified but, too, follows the logic of those who initiated the European Network and documented developments over time. This allows to *unravel the true nature* of the complex ENHPS initiative and at the same time *analyze* it from a combined network and Health Promotion research perspective.

ENHPS 'project', 'network', 'initiative' ?

Documentation on the European Network of Health Promoting Schools (ENHPS) mentions both the ENHPS 'project' and the European 'Network' of Health Promoting Schools but these apparently different social systems are not clearly defined and remain fuzzy particularly when it comes to the national level. The use of the two terms indicate an issue similar to that discovered when addressing the ENHPS related goals: a rational *for the creation* of the European Network had to be distinguished from the goals *of* that network. With regard to ENHPS related organizational structures it may be similarly meaningful or necessary to clearly distinguish between (support) structures *for the creation* (and may be maintenance) of the European Network and structures *of* that Network.

As of now the impression emerged that the former is referred to as ENHPS 'project'. This issue reminds of discussions in organization research around network boundaries (chap. 2.4) and ideas of bi- or multi-boundary networks. In chapters 2.4 and 3 it was concluded that in any case for the assessment of a particular interorganisational network a reasonable decision has to be made about the central unit of analysis. In this context it was also highlighted that boundaries are co- if not *mainly* defined by the *quality of interorganisational relationships* and not just formal institutional status. To achieve clarification on borders or membership of the so called "European Network of Health Promoting Schools" in the reminder of this case study there will be a conscious distinction of terms: a) The 'tripartite **ENHPS project'** refers to the joint endeavor of the three intergovernmental agencies WHO, CE and EC (here documentation is quite clear); b) the term "**European Network** of Health Promoting Schools" will be used where the *'whole network'* and/or explicitly the ensemble of the member schools are concerned; c) the term **'ENHPS initiative'** will be *introduced as more general, overriding term*.

As long as it is not clear whether or how far ENHPS 'project' and 'network' overlap and whether, e.g., the three partner organizations in the ENHPS project are also members of the European Network or not, special attention will need to be given to the structural set-up of *both* 'ENHPS project' and 'European Network'. An improved understanding of both and of the relationships and interactions of the various actors will provide a basis for the decision to be made on the European Network's boundaries. Structures and mechanisms at all systems levels will need to be considered from European to school level and links between them, too.

From the beginning, the three initiating agencies Council of Europe (CE), European Commission (EC) and WHO/EURO outlined *key requirements for effective management and coordination* at various 'network' levels (IPC 1993): the selection of a limited number of schools in each member country (about 10); at **school level** appointment of a school project team and a school project manager; at **national level** identification of a project support center and the designation of a national coordinator; and at **international level** establishment of an international planning committee. The organization and financing of the European Network initiative at *international* level will be addressed first, which reflects the fact that the ENHPS has not emerged as a grass roots movement of, for example, many individual schools but has been initiated from outside the schools and even their countries, from the international level. The initiating intergovernmental agencies defined the cornerstones of the European Network at all its levels. As will be seen in chapter 5.4.5 below this is not to be interpreted as 'top down' network creation or management in a necessarily negative sense.

ENHPS related structures and key actors at European level

The idea of a *European* network of health promoting schools became structurally anchored when European Commission (EC), Council of Europe (CE) and the WHO Regional Office for Europe (WHO/EURO), i.e. the three 'sponsoring bodies' as they call themselves, formed the **'International Planning Committee' (IPC)** and soon after a Technical Secretariat. From the start, the self-defined role of the International Committee (IPC) was to provide a focus and to ensure the availability of links and opportunities for all parties within the network; lately, setting the 'broad course' and supplying or helping to raise funds are emphasized. The IPC comprises one *high level representative* each of the WHO, CE and EC departments on Health Promotion or (Public) Health (and none e.g. from education departments). In 1993 the Committee established the ENHPS Technical Secretariat at WHO. - Representatives of IPC and Technical Secretariat together form a European level *'technical support body'* for the European Network which over the years had not much fluctuation. Members state that the *management arrangements* (fig. 5.1.1) succeeded in *'minimizing bureaucracy while maximizing results'*. (ENHPS/TS w.y., 1997)

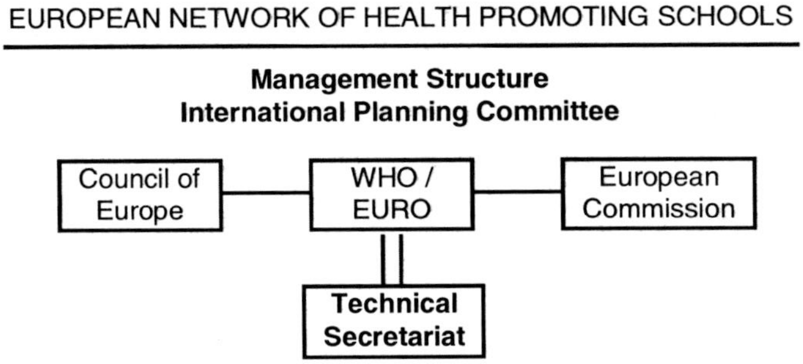

EUROPEAN NETWORK OF HEALTH PROMOTING SCHOOLS

Management Structure
International Planning Committee

Council of Europe	—	WHO / EURO	—	European Commission
		‖		
		Technical Secretariat		

Figure 5.1.1: Organization of the ENHPS project at international level - a 'technical supporting body' for the European Network of Health Promoting Schools. (ENHPS/TS 1997 p6)

The primary role and responsibility of the ENHPS **Technical Secretariat** is up today to *support the National Coordinators and their colleagues in countries* which can be seen as both a bi-lateral as well as a network undertaking. Many tasks focus on the European Network as a *whole* and the networking therein:

arranging the annual ENHPS *business meetings,* as well as international workshops etc. for National Coordinators and project teams (mainly on cross cutting issues such as communication, training of trainers, project management, and evaluation); *keeping track of developments* in network member countries and *recruiting* new ones; and producing and disseminating *information* particularly *within* the network (annual Newsletter; resource/ training materials for key actors in national networks). In addition, the Technical Secretariat has more *bi-lateral* oriented tasks such as: general advice, activity support visits, and also fund raising. - Strengthened in 1995, this Secretariat is with two professional consultants and two support staff nevertheless small in size. It provides 'invaluable support' not only to ENHPS member countries and schools but also the International Planning Committee (IPC). Importantly, the *professionals are part of the IPC*.

As such, the Technical Secretariat serves as **link between national networks and the 'ENHPS project' partners at European level**. (ENHPS/TS 1997; ENHPS Technical Secretariat 1995, 1997; Burgher et al 1999)

ENHPS related structures and key actors at national level

On the base of experiences particularly in the pilot phase the European agencies in the IPC identified **three vital organizational components of 'national HPS project networks'**: an Advisory Council or Advisory Board, a National Coordinator (NC), and a National Support Center (NSC). As to the roles and responsibilities of the latter ENHPS 'member countries' received the following guidance which shows at country level what has been noted at European level: a fuzzy differentiation between 'national HPS *projects*' and national *networks*:

A **National Advisory Board or Council** is suggested as *decision making body* with view to the 'national Health Promoting Schools (HPS) *project*'. It would need to agree on the strategy for this project and oversee its implementation; undertake regular *reviews* and be *accountable to the national Ministries* concerned (i.e. at least the Ministries of Health (MoH) and of Education (MoE)); it should *support and guide the National Coordinator*, assure adequate administrative resources from the National Support Center (NSC) for HPS development, and provide opportunities for *project consolidation and expansion*. Conceptualized as a **multi-organization body** it would comprise of interested, nominated, influential representatives from a range of organizations at *national and also local* level (from the Ministries involved and relevant national institutes to parent or teachers organizations and local education authorities). This indicates that these Boards may serve as a link between national HPS networks and their environment within their country.

The obligatory **'National Coordinator'** is responsible for coordinating the national HPS project or network and for two groups of tasks: some focused on HPS project or network development *within* their country, others on interactions with European Network members or actors *outside*. The former include: strategy development for the 'national network' in collaboration with the Advisory Board, if appropriate; setting up of an administrative office in a designated National Support Center; day-to-day management of the 'national HPS project'; and needs assessment as to their 'national HPS network' and support of corresponding actions. *Outwards oriented tasks* include: participation in international meetings to *share experiences* and lessons learnt with other ENHPS National Coordinators; and serving as their country's *focal point* both towards the European level actors and for disseminating international experiences among their country's network schools. Ideally, the National Coordinator is supported by a small team of health and education specialists or researchers. (ENHPS/TS 1993b; IPC 1993; ENHPS 1999)

The principle task of the **National Support Center** (NSC) is to *enable* the National Coordinator and the national HPS project or network as a whole to function effectively. It is responsible for offering *political support*, professional *credibility*, *access* to professional networks, and *administrative* space and support. Accordingly, a range of (national) health or education organizations could serve as such Centers in countries. (ENHPS/TS 1993b p3)

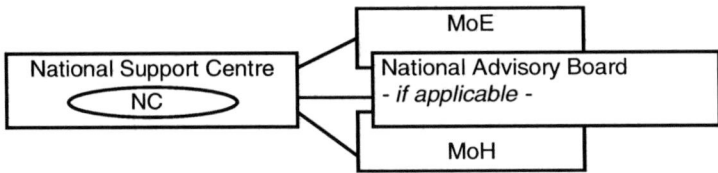

Figure 5.1.2: Structural set-up for the ENHPS initiative at national level, as recommended by the initiating European agencies (NC: National Coordinator; MoE/MoH: Ministry of Education/ of Health)

The ENHPS related **national structure** as outlined by the International Planning Committee (IPC) is illustrated in figure 5.1.2. Overall, the ENHPS membership criteria (elaborated later on) show that a) a National Advisory Board is 'recommended' but b) a National Support Center and Coordinator is a 'must' for ENHPS membership; and that c) Ministries of Education and of Health have a key role to play.

ENHPS structure and key actors at school or local level

At the European Network's local level, the schools are seen in the center.

ENHPS (pilot) schools have both an appointed 'school project manager' as well as a 'school project team' for HPS development. Within the school each **school project manager** has coordinating and leadership functions as to the school's 'HPS project' in general and the school project team in particular. As to the national and European dimensions, he/she serves as a link between the network school and both the National Coordinator as well as other ENHPS member schools. - Thus, in Hastings terms (1993) they are to be key actors in both *networking 'within' network schools and 'with others'* in the ENHPS initiative.

The role of the **'school project team'** has been defined more locally focused: to facilitate the implementation and further development of the school's 'HPS project', promote the Health Promoting Schools (HPS) approach, and maintain motivation within the school community. *Ideally it represents a school-community-link* by encompassing interested (key) people from within and outside the school (e.g. from local education departments, community NGOs, and school health services) (ENHPS/TS 1993b)

The above outline of the structural set-up of the overall ENHPS initiative has shown that *a range of organizational actors are actively involved*. As of now the question remains which are the *members* of the European Network and which have other roles. Also the relationship between the three levels of the ENHPS initiative need further clarification. A look at the European Network's defined membership and selection processes will help to clarify these issues.

The question of network membership (and of the unit of analysis of this research project)

Among the range of ENHPS *related* 'key actors' identified above network 'members' and 'others' need to be sorted out.

The **International Planning Committee (IPC)** located itself *outside* the European *Network* of Health Promoting Schools (not the 'ENHPS project') - by defining selection criteria for *two* types of members or network participants only: *'countries'* and *pilot schools,* and by usually speaking of 'their' ENHPS 'project' rather than network (ENHPS 1999; ENHPS/TS w.y, 1997; IPC w.y, 1993).

From the perspective of inter*organisational* network research the notion of **'country' membership** raises questions: Which organizations represent the 'country membership' and does the membership relate to the 'ENHPS *project'* or the "European *Network* of Health Promoting Schools" or both?

The IPC defined that 'countries' wishing to 'join' the European Network need to express their commitment to the concept of the Health Promoting School (HPS) and support the principle of cooperation between education and health authorities at the highest level. *Ministries of health <u>and</u> education* need to sign an agreement on a joint commitment towards the HPS project. Before they formally apply for their country's ENHPS membership *core infrastructures at national and local level* need to be put in place: At the *national level* this means ENHPS or HPS contact persons in the Ministries; an experienced, highly qualified National Coordinator designated by both Ministries; a designated *National Support Center*, and preferably a designated *National Advisory Board*. The European level actors stress the National Coordinator as core person in a country whose expected qualification profile reflects his/her key role in networking within both the European Network and the own country: With view to the breadths of contacts needed (politicians to school staff) good communication, motivation, coordination and negotiation skills are stressed as is strategic thinking and *creating and sustaining 'networks'* (however defined). (ENHPS/TS 1993b) - With view to the *local level*, the Ministries need to provide information on 10-20 *'pilot schools'* designated to participate in the European Network; these need to cover all levels of education, different parts of the country equally, and have one designated School Project Manager each.

Thus, **a "country's" ENHPS 'membership'** *depends* **on the Ministries of Health and Education** who need to identify and *designate the organizational core actors required* (National Support Center and pilot schools) and coordinators therein. Today, *evaluation plans and a fund raising strategy* need to be supplied, too (Burgher et al 1999).

Membership criteria and expectations towards ENHPS members

Both each participating **'country' and 'pilot school'** face particular requirements: They need to: create a 3-year 'project' *plan* and a HPS 'project' *team*; prioritize project initiatives and implement those that tackle *issues of both local and European relevance* (for use as models of good practice elsewhere); maximize the HPS project's visibility and credibility; and facilitate evaluation and dissemination of results. Activities should promote the health of young people and foster a 'spirit of collective responsibility' for personal and community health. - In addition, **each school** nominated for 'membership' in the European Network must meet the criteria set individually by its 'country', i.e. core national actors. The *general basis for nomination* is a commitment to the concept of the Health Promoting School (HPS), i.e. the schools commitment to work towards the goals and/or criteria of a HPS as originally defined at the *international* level. Qualifications required from School Project Managers relate to leadership, team work, and communication with a range of people within *and* outside the school in English, French or German. (ENHPS/TS 1993b)

When analyzing these general ENHPS nomination criteria for network schools with the help of Hastings' model of *'organizational networking'* used in the network assessment frame (chap. 3) it becomes explicit: From the start the initiators of the European Network and IPC members wanted **network schools to be able to link up or network in several directions**: a) 'within' their organization/ school and b) 'with others' - and the latter *both* 'within' the European *Network* and their local community.

In many countries ENHPS network schools were or are selected not only on the base of the above general requirements pre-defined at European level but *additional country specific criteria* (e.g. the schools' eagerness to participate and its geographical location). To ensure that the most appropriate schools are selected, a range of Health Promotion and/or organization development related issues may be addressed but this varies from country to country (see the country case studies below). The (recommended) ENHPS selection criteria include to consider existing health promotion/ education programs, physical environment, work organization, human relations programs, staff training, and perceived needs for health promotion. The ENHPS International Planning Committee stresses that it is vital that national actors ensure that pupils and school staff fully understand the implications and demands of joining the European Network and be aware of the commitment needed and time involved - the extent of which is indicated by nomination criteria such as the above.

Processes of selecting members / core actors

One of the defining criteria of interorganisational networks (IONs) is their members' working together in *mutuality* and 'win/win' philosophy which implies willful and *voluntary* participation. Research suggests that performance and sustainability of such networks rests on the voluntary participation of network members (see chap. 2.3). Therefore the *selection processes* for European Network members are briefly looked at.

The International Planning Committee (IPC) initiated a decentralized process of selecting ENHPS members or key actors: the *European* level, the IPC, selects the 'country members' by applying the above mentioned criteria; but it does not select any actor *within* a country. The national health and education *ministries* jointly select core *national* actors including the National Support Center and Coordinator. The latter organize the selection of ENHPS '*school*' members'. Two main selection processes were foreseen: a) a *competition or open invitation* approach addressing all schools in a country, with selections made at national level and b) the *initial selection* through key people in regional (i.e. sub-national) education departments. Advantages and disadvantages were communicated to 'countries' for both. *Additional* selection modes emerged in countries (e.g. random selection of pilot schools). (ENHPS/TS 1993b, 1997; WHO/EURO 1998)

The 'open invitation approach', used by the International Planning Committee (IPC) to select ENHPS 'member countries', seems to match best with the ENHPS principles of participation and democracy. From a Health Promotion perspective important is also that this approach signals potential network members (such as schools) inclusiveness rather exclusiveness and equal chances to participate. This approach guarantees *voluntary* participation which as said above is important for network performance and sustainability. 'Initial selection' of network schools by regional authorities and 'random selection' could mean either voluntary or obliged membership. But as will be seen later there are several indications that within the European Network the former is more likely. For example, pilot schools even after several years of ENHPS membership show a remarkable low drop out quote which is unusual for educational innovations (Piette et al 1999).

Financial resources of the ENHPS initiative/ external resources of the Network

As elaborated in chapter 2.3 a networks dependency from vertical or multiple sources of funding is an important factor that often influences its autonomy and its structure, operational processes and performance. The ENHPS as a whole or in parts has received *financial support* from *several* sources.

Substantial contributions came from the European Commission (EC), Council of Europe (CE) and WHO/EURO as well as from other institutions, philanthropic organizations and WHO Member States. This reflects the European Network's access to *various sources of funding* for targeted use by the ENHPS Technical Secretariat, National HPS Coordinators or even individual schools. For example: Up today, the *Technical Secretariat* receives funding from WHO/EURO and the European Commission (EC) for the coordination of project activities. The EC repeatedly provided direct *country support* to EU Member States. ENHPS countries from Central and Eastern Europe (CEE) and the Newly Independent States receive(d) funding from WHO and voluntary donations by other countries. Training initiatives in CEE countries were funded by the Council of Europe. And WHO Collaborating Centers on Health Promotion adjusted their work plans in order to support the ENHPS (Health Promotion Unit 1992). - According to those involved, this **'multiple funds strategy'** has strengthened the ENHPS. Particular priority issues in countries have been pinpointed and attracted funding. In addition, many ENHPS countries themselves set aside money from national health and education budgets in a variety of ways which frequently supports the National Support Center and Coordinator. (Barnekow Rasmussen 1996; Barnekow Rasmussen et al 1996; ENHPS Technical Secretariat 1996;) - Financial support of the *ENHPS pilot schools* takes often the form of some hours teaching reduction per week for staff that is part of the 'HPS project team', but schools may also have an own HPS project budget (WHO/EURO 1998). For particular activities some members may access EU funds as those sketched out in chapter 5.1.1 above.

The ENHPS initiative's structural set-up -intermediate synthesis and discussion

As of now, as to the structural set-up of the overall ENHPS initiative following understanding emerged: The term 'ENHPS' is often used as an umbrella term for two distinct systems. On the one hand, there is **an international ENHPS 'project'** whose key participants are at least those three European agencies that form the International Planning Committee (WHO/EURO, EC, CE). They strive to develop **the "European *Network of Health Promoting Schools*" (ENHPS)** jointly with the ENHPS Technical Secretariat, a support body created for this purpose. 'Country members' and 'school members' are distinguished. From an interorganisational network research perspective, the *notion of 'country' members needs to be broken down into organizational units*: They represent two societal levels, national and local. Key organizations at *local* level are the selected ENHPS (pilot) schools, at *national* level a) the National Support Center (including the National Coordinator), b) the National Advisory Board and c) the Ministries of Health and of Education. The terms of reference for National Coordinators indicate that similarly to the European level also at *national* level a HPS *'project'* and a HPS *'network'* are being distinguished. - It remains the question which of the key national organization are *'network'* members, which 'project' participants and which may be both - and how the two systems relate to each other. It seems that the ENHPS project or national HPS *projects* are a wider system that *initiated and continuously supports* the thriving of the national 'HPS networks' and the European Network as a whole. This **assumption of the twofold structure of the overall ENHPS initiative** is illustrated in figure 5.1.3 and will be further examined in the reminder of this case study, also with the next step of looking at ENHPS related financing mechanisms at *international* level (not within individual countries).

Regarding **the issue of resource dependency**, the *European Network as a whole*, on the one hand, is financially dependent on the 'ENHPS *project'* partners (WHO, EC, CE), i.e. on *external* resources. On the other hand, ENHPS *'sub*-networks' in *countries* are financially dependent on their Ministries of Health and of Education; and if the assumption holds that these are part of their country's 'national (EN)HPS *project*' which is to be distinguished from the country's ENHPS *network*, then the resource dependency of the European Network as a whole refers to *external* funding not only at the international but also *national* level. As external control may much influence a network's structures and processes (see chap. 2.4 and 3) this issue needs further examination in the *country* case studies (below). However, research findings addressed in chapter 2.4.6 match with observations made regarding the European Network (ENHPS): An interorganisational network's **reliance on multiple funding** tends to lead to *highly cooperative and less centralized or less hierarchical working modes*. The multiple funding strategy developed for and by the ENHPS suits its general aims and principles of partnership, interorganisational and intersectoral collaboration, decentralized working, etc. It likely strengthens the European Network's autonomy, its freedom to make strategic decisions.

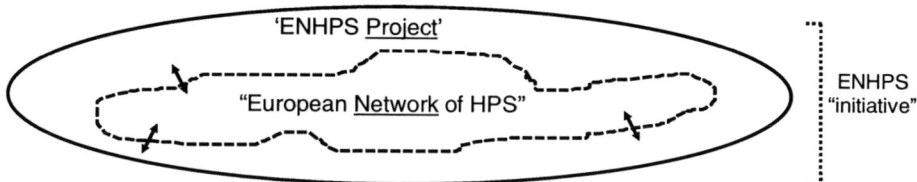

Figure 5.1.3: Assumed relation of the "European Network of Health Promoting Schools" (ENHPS) and the tripartite "ENHPS project". The ENHPS 'project' encompasses initiators and supporters of the European Network (mainly the IPC members WHO, EC, CE). The European 'Network' ENHPS is a separate social system that thrives within this supportive framework.

These and related issues will be further discussed once the ENHPS has been 'unraveled' in its entire **complexity in the *general* sense of the word** (not as defined by Alter and Hage). *Already the structural set-up of the ENHPS project and network shows as much complexity as its goals and the expectations towards it.* This complexity can be captured by key words such as: multiple goals; multiple actors, multiple systems levels; intersectorality (health/education); a large-scale and European dimension; and organizational innovations.

Initiation of **organizational innovation and change** happens at two levels at the same time: *organization (or school) development within ENHPS schools* (as genuine part of the Health Promoting Schools concept), and new ways of interorganisational collaboration in the form of and around the creation of an *international interorganisational network* (ION) involving not only pilot schools but many other organizations - with organizations often not used to collaborate with each other (e.g. Ministries of Health and of Education; schools;).

The ENHPS related financing mechanisms support the assumption that the European *Network* is surrounded by or embedded into an international (financial, political, technical) support system. Several indications and reasons have been found for such a *second ENHPS system besides the European Network itself*. And it seems to be more than appropriate to assume that a complex (innovative, large scale, long term, intersectoral, cross-level...) enterprise such as a European network for the development of Health Promoting Schools is embedded into a closer, supportive environment such as a formal multi-agency 'ENHPS project'. Therefore, from now on this study distinguishes **two systems within the overall ENHPS initiative:** the ENHPS as **a 'Network of members'** (pilot schools and 'countries' as of now), and **the supporting 'ENHPS project'** (with the IPC and may be the Technical Secretariat and even others), - while *examining the situation further*. The more network borders and membership are clarified the more the attention can be shifted towards the European *'Network'* and the analysis of its particular network structures, processes and outcomes as elaborated in chapters 2.3 and 3. While the issue of "country members" is yet to be clarified further, some specific structural aspects as to the European Network's *organizational networking* can be already addressed.

'Soft' and 'hard' networking within and around the European Network

Any interorganisational network (ION) needs the **means that encourage and allow 'soft' networking,** i.e. the linking of people from the various organizational members. Direct contact among network members and of members and other key actors is important and the international ENHPS project has created means in support of this:

With regard to its international or European dimension these include annual *business meetings* for National Coordinators; frequent international or inter-country workshops, training courses or other events; an annual ENHPS *Newsletter* 'Network News'; and a *twinning strategy* at both member country and pilot school level. Contact details of National Coordinators and ENHPS pilot schools in Newsletter and website further facilitate networking within the net and beyond. - In ENHPS *countries*, means of networking vary from case to case but face-to-face meetings of National Coordinators, other national HPS staff and school project managers, as well as national or subnational newsletters are common. (ENHPS Technical Secretariat 1995 - 2000; ENHPS/T`S 1997, 1993b; WHO/EURO 1998; Barnekow Rasmussen et al 1996b; see also country case studies below)

Particularly in an *international context* 'soft' networking among network members is often limited to annual or bi-annual meetings and as explained in chapter 2.4.2 is best supported by **'hard' networking**, the linking of the network members' computers to allow e-mail communication. Also the European Network has emphasized the use of e-mail connections mainly with view to international or inter-country networking among National Coordinators and ENHPS Technical Secretariat. As the country case studies will show, the great potential of 'hard' networking in support of overall networking and mutual learning among network schools is even in today's Europe not easy to unfold.

Overall, the *various means* of 'soft' and 'hard' networking implemented by the ENHPS provide *the basis for realizing the 'network approach'* and sustaining networking (as elaborated in chapter 2.4) among various actors in the pursuit of the common goal: creating Health Promoting Schools all over Europe. While the interactions and relations between various actors as desired or required by the European level are a structural feature addressed above, their *realization* (a process feature) remains to be further examined. Before doing so (in chap. 5.1.1 below) the *evolution* of the European Network as a whole needs attention. It is a reference frame for analyzing and assessing: a) the *qualities of interactions* of and within the European Network (to analyze and assess both whether a 'network' as defined in chap. 2.4 is truly realized and the network's operational processes); b) Hastings' four *'organizational networking processes'* that form a core part of the network assessment framework developed (chap. 3); and c) issues related to the assessment framework's principle of 'attention to *network development stages*', and at the same time, the *type* of interorganisational network the ENHPS represents (exchange/ promotional/ systemic?).

5.1.4 Developments over time: the evolution of the 'European Network of Health Promoting Schools' (ENHPS)

Obviously, considering changes over time means another increase in complexity of this case study on the 'European Network of Health Promoting Schools' (ENHPS). However, a unique part of the Alter/Hage network theory is the suggestion that different *types* of interorganisational networks (exchange, joint action, or joint production networks) represent *not just types but development stages of networks*, where the first stage (exchange) needs to be realized as a base for the second to occur and so forth (see chap. 2.4.3). In addition, Alter and Hage suggest that interorganisational networks up to five years old are 'young', and those over 10 may be considered as 'old'. This puts the overall age of the European Network launched in 1992 in context and shows that the time span examined in this case study (1992-2000) covers the 'young' European Network's and a about half of its 'middle age' - i.e. unlikely a time span in which the Network may have matured into a 'systemic network' as defined by Alter and Hage (1993). The same may apply to the interorganisational "ENHPS project", too.

Examining the European Network's development over time will provide a valuable context within which its overall assessment can take place. Attention will be paid to **various issues** such as: membership development (related to network size, complexity, etc.); activities or contributions and perceived achievements of network *members* and *actors* around it and changes over time (issues related to external control, network centrality, differentiation, etc.); *network* activities (experience exchange, joint actions, etc.); and potential changes in the network's overall direction (e.g. as to tasks or goals, priorities or strategies). Overall, the goal is to further improve the understanding of the European Network's borders and to provide a reference frame for a complementary examination of the interactions and relations of various actors (members and important others) that follows (see chap. 5.1.5 below). The latter will be the basis for final decisions as to the assumptions made regarding Network members and 'others' and network related 'projects' as supportive network environments. It also will shed light on remaining network features such as connectivity and operational processes which is needed for the Network's overall assessment.

Initiation and fast growth - the so called 'first phase' of the ENHPS initiative

The "European Network of Health Promoting Schools" (ENHPS) evolved quickly over several stages that merged into each other rather than being distinct development phases. The following examination of ENHPS development over time is based on the following references: Health Promotion Unit 1992; Macdonald et al 1992; ENHPS/TS 1993 a,b, 1997, w.y.; IPC 1993; Ziglio et al 1995; Barnekow Rasmussen et al 1996; and ENHPS 1999. Additional sources were used as mentioned in the text. The European actors usually refer to the first four years after the formal launch of the ENHPS (1992-1995) as 'the first phase'.

During the first years, the development of both the "European *Network* of Health Promoting Schools" (ENHPS) and the 'ENHPS *project*' were inseparably linked, with the 'Network' launched even *before* the formal tripartite 'project'. "Networks of Health Promoting Schools" in countries had been *an idea* pilot-tested by WHO/EURO in 1991 in four CEE countries while engaging in the far reaching negotiations with Council of Europe (CE) and European Commission (EC) directed at launching such 'HPS projects' *Europe-wide*. Already in 1992 international agreement was reached to develop this large-scale project under the auspices of all three organizations. A *first consultative meeting with* National HPS Coordinators and other representatives from overall *28 countries* was held to reach agreement on plans for the next four years, which resulted in a *draft strategy for 1992-1995* and a schedule for accepting members half-yearly from autumn 1992. The **ENHPS was formally inaugurated and**

opened for membership as the first network of this kind globally. WHO, EC and CE had already accepted 18 ENHPS 'country members' (and thus about 200 - 250 ENHPS 'pilot' schools) when they formalized their joint initiative in a written agreement. The *International Planning Committee* (IPC) was established before the *first formal 'business meeting'* with National HPS Coordinators in May 1993. Up today, the annual business meetings are the *core* mechanism for 'networking within' the European Network as far as national and international level actors are concerned (i.e. National Coordinators, IPC members, ENHPS Technical Secretariat). - The **quick growth** as to 'country members' of the European Network was facilitated by formal high-level, political and organizational back-up of the tripartite 'ENHPS project': in November 1992, both the 'Council of Ministers of Health' of the European Union and the 'Health Committee' of the Council of Europe (CE) had re-emphasized and strengthened the involvement of *CE and EC* in the ENHPS initiative; *WHO/EURO's* involvement was and remains genuine part of its technical mandate in health promotion and related areas within the Regional Health for All/Health21- policy and strategy. (see chap. 5.3.1 above) Thus, the European Network started with *strong political support from its closer environment* at international level.

There are some interesting points for discussion. According to the Alter/Hage network theory 'external control' of a network is (as a network's task or goal) a key environmental factor influencing the choice of network structures and processes being put in place (see chap. 2.3 and 3). Resource dependency (in the case of the European Network from WHO, EC and CE) *can* limit *network autonomy* but not always does. It may or may not shape a network's structures, processes and outcomes. The **main sponsors' behavior** towards the network is crucial, i.e. with view to the European Network as a whole that of the three partner agencies WHO, EC and CE. These have from the start cooperated on the base of a *high level of trust* as indicated by their joint launch of the ENHPS before any formalization of their close collaboration in writing. The *early involvement of (potential) ENHPS member countries* in developing and deciding upon a first work plan and working modes before even creating the International Planning Committee (IPC), as well as the establishing of such annual meetings as part of the overall planning and decision making process at international level indicate: From the beginning the ENHPS *initiators*, in-spite of being big intergovernmental bureaucracies and the main network sponsors, *implemented a fairly participatory and democratic approach to coordination, management and governance* within the ENHPS initiative. This view is supported by the transparency created in general financing issues and by public statements of IPC members in ENHPS Newsletters and otherwise (see e.g. Barnekow Rasmussen 1996; ENHPS Technical Secretariat 1996; Barnekow Rasmussen et al 1996). This and the International Planning Committee's (IPC's) **explicit aim to serve as a 'good example' of interorganisational cooperation for all actors** within the ENHPS initiative (Burgher et al 1999) signals - according to Alter and Hage (1993) - that the dependency on external resources of the European Network as a *whole* is unlikely limiting its autonomy in making decisions to a degree that leads to centralized network structures. This point will be taken up later again.

The work approach of the ENHPS 'project' and the structural set-up at international level have allowed the European Network's **rapid expansion** during its first four years - at least as to 'member countries'.

In its first three years alone the number of *'ENHPS member countries'* raised from 7 to 37, each with 'pilot school networks' of a manageable size. Then, in terms of 'country members' the quantitative development leveled out with four new countries in the following five years. With regard to *ENHPS school members*, data on membership development over time are less available. The ENHPS initiators had recommended countries to select only a 'manageable' number of 'pilot' schools (10-15). Matching with this, six years after its launch the ENHPS encompassed over 500 'pilot schools' in 38 countries (with over 10.000 teachers and about 500.000 pupils). But over 2000 'other' schools were linked to the European Network through national or regional arrangements, often referred to as 'associated' schools. (Burgher et al 1999; WHO/EURO 1998; ENHPS 1997) - The fact that in many ENHPS 'member countries' more schools than the small number of selected "ENHPS pilot schools" as well as other actors wished to implement the Health Promoting Schools (HPS) concept within an arrangement of support and exchange as offered by the European Network meant: The approach favored at European level to first undertake at least three years of pilot work with a clearly limited and selected number of 'ENHPS pilot schools' per country did not work out in all member countries. Several countries allowed their national ENHPS initiatives to expand earlier giving rise to some kind of *national* HPS projects or networks beyond the initial ENHPS 'pilot schools'.

That is, the **"semi-controlled" approach to ENHPS expansion** chosen at European level (i.e. no limits as to new ENHPS *'country* members' but limits as to new ENHPS *school* members per country for about three or more 'pilot years') **only partially worked out.** The ENHPS initiative developed its *own dynamics within member countries* which for a while led to the distinction of 'pilot schools' and non-pilot or 'associated' schools as to European Network activities (see e.g. the 'ENHPS Schools Data Base' - WHO/EURO 1998).

Main activities during the first three years (the so called 'first phase')

Activities of the European Network fall into two broad categories: **activities directed at the European Network as a *whole*** usually undertaken at international level, and *country specific* activities to achieve the Network's goal usually undertaken *within* individual 'ENHPS countries'. The latter vary widely and need systematic country case studies to achieve a better understanding. Information on the former stems mainly from the European actors (ENHPS Technical Secretariat and/or International Planning Committee); but views from the National Support Centers or

Coordinators and to a lesser degree ENHPS 'pilot schools' have been captured, too (via a survey to create the 'ENHPS Schools Data Base' and evaluation studies such as 'EVA 1 and 2' and the 'Canterbury study' (see WHO/EURO 1998; CE et al 1995; Piette et al 1999; Parson et al 1997).

As set out in the rational for establishing the European Network, during the first years activities focused on **establishing pilot sites at *school* level** and the needs and circumstances of each ENHPS 'pilot' school - to first demonstrate the impact of the 'health promoting Settings' approach in schools. Disseminating and *sharing* of results was a focus, too. This went hand in hand with **activities of key supporters** of the European Network (the 'ENHPS project' partners WHO, CE and EC) who focused more on the *national level* or new ENHPS *'countries'* as a whole (e.g. training seminars for National Coordinators; recruiting and support of new 'country' members). Meanwhile a German speaking sub-group of the ensemble of national ENHPS networks launched a **new international 'network within the network', an international ENHPS sub-network** with own activities (see chap. 5.1.3).

Systematic *documentation of activities at European level* started after two, three years of ENHPS development. It covered both (incomparable) case stories illustrating diversity (see Newsletter) and systematic data collection on 'pilot schools' *and* National HPS Support Centers (for the so called 'ENHPS Schools Data Base') (see ENHPS Technical Secretariat 1995; WHO/EURO 1998). Also ENHPS evaluation efforts began, with the evaluation project 'EVA' (CE et al 1995). Then, in preparation of the second work and development plan of the ENHPS initiative (1996-2000) a 'strategic review' of the European Network in 1995 and a 'first provisional appraisal' by the German speaking ENHPS sub-network were undertaken (ENHPS 1996, 1997; Sub-regional network... 1995). The results of these reviews shed not only further light on the *activities* of the European Network and/or 'ENHPS project' but also on issues of *satisfaction and perceived effectiveness* of main actors:

The **'strategic review 1995'** surveyed National HPS Coordinators on *current situation and future potential of the European Network;* results were discussed and recommendations developed jointly with them. On the base of this **the European actors concluded** (ENHPS 1996, 1997; Burgher et al 1999): Within its first three years the **ENHPS succeeded** in gaining a *good reputation* as a sound investment in health and safety of young people, and begun to 'set the *agenda* for education and Health Promotion'. At school level, it resulted in *more democratic management and teaching styles*, and provided the right framework for *addressing health needs* of staff. At European level, it helped to build *consensus and cooperation* and generated a 'sense of unity'. The international support helped facilitate vital *changes in schools*. Also **challenges and constraints** for the establishment of Health Promoting Schools (HPS) that remained to be tackled in several countries were identified: Referring to the complexity of the ENHPS, which aims at both organizational and managerial as well as behavioral changes, new and innovative *approaches to measuring the Network's impact, quality and effectiveness* were called for to consider all relevant impact areas. Some of the weaknesses identified relate to interorganisational collaboration and networking within member countries: Several of those did show *insufficient commitment* of the health and education sectors to collaborate, and some the *lack of financial and technical support* to allow the creation of effective national HPS networks. Concern arose also about *'too narrow' approaches* in many *curriculum* projects that neglect the underlying determinants of health behavior - an important point because of the European Network's health promotion goals. (ENHPS 1996, 1997; Burgher et al 1999)

These conclusions of the *European* level actors and network supporters were complemented by some recommendations from the *national* ENHPS perspective:

The **ENHPS sub-network of German-speaking national networks** (five countries) made a 'first provisional **appraisal** of the project's development' which resulted in a joint position paper called 'Cologne Recommendations' 1995. From the network research perspective important is the **particularly attention paid to both organizational innovations in support of health introduced by the ENHPS initiative** as explained before: the **Settings and network approach** of the "European Network of Health Promoting Schools" (ENHPS). The position paper shows a *differentiated* understanding of the European Network's levels and dimensions and is one of the rare documents where *others* than the International Planning Committee or Technical Secretariat write about the ENHPS as a *whole*. First, the Health Promoting Schools (HPS) concept and, thus, the *Settings approach was confirmed* as a 'workable guide' (with integrated concepts to school health promotion indeed contributing to solving problems related to health risks at schools for pupils and teachers). Cooperation beyond the realm of 'health' were justified. Attention was drawn to *training needs* of teachers (in *organization development* issues such as project management and team building) and of heads of schools as 'key' actors in HPS development. - Second, with regard to the European Network's network dimension the *links between schools*, even beyond national boundaries, were stressed. The **need to further develop several 'network levels'** was identified that to a certain degree reflect Hastings' four 'organizational networking' processes (networking 'within'/'with external others' and 'soft'/'hard' networking) and his consideration of geographic distance (Hastings 1993): 'network thinking' (in the sense of holistic attitudes); links '*within*' schools (interpersonal links, transparent decision making structures); links between *schools and their regional/local environments* (i.e. links with 'external others'); and *school-to-school links* not only across communities or regions but also nationwide and across national borders (i.e. networking over various geographic distances). *Further investments into both* 'personal encounter' (i.e. *'soft' networking*) and electronic communication and data networks (*'hard' networking*) are called for, with special emphasis on the former to reach goals and provide emotional and motivational support. This matches with Hastings' point that 'soft' networking is to be supported by 'hard' networking. - Two years later the same national HPS networks reiterated that such soft and hard networking will have an 'outstanding significance' for all ENHPS network partners in the future. ("Subregional" network of German-speaking Networks of Health Promoting Schools 1995, 1997)

Throughout the first years of ENHPS development, the three 'ENHPS project' partners and **sponsors of the European Network** (EC, CE and WHO/EURO) jointly or individually publicly expressed *satisfaction with and perceived effectiveness of the ENHPS initiative*. On the one hand, they referred to *network features* such as the European Network's size, truly European dimension, and 'complexity' (the latter not necessarily understood as by Alter and Hage 1993). They also referred to the value of the network's overall goal, the creation of 'Health Promoting Schools' that no country can afford to delay or ignore (a confirmation of the *Settings approach* in schools). On the other hand, the ENHPS initiators referred to factors in the European *Network's closer environment* (mainly their own remarkable interorganisational collaboration; and the perceptions of the 'health and education sectors' of the ENHPS as a consolidating initiative that gathers existing knowledge about 'health promotion in the school setting within a network of pilot schools').

However, *tasks to be addressed further* were recognized, too: the great differences among ENHPS member countries in 'HPS project' development due to variations in technical and financial support and the prevalence or not of reforms of the health and education sectors. (Burgher et al 1999; ENHPS/TS 1997 p5; Barnekow Rasmussen et al 1996; Theesen 1997; Scicluna 1997; and editorials in ENHPS Technical Secretariat 1995, 1996; WHO/EURO 1998)

The 'development plan 1996-2000' and beyond

The so called 'development plan 1996-2000 for the ENHPS' was a plan for the ENHPS initiative as a *whole*. It included important elements of the European Network's closer *environment* (such as the 'ENHPS project') rather than a plan for the 'European *Network'* alone. Understood at European level as having led from the 'first' into a 'second phase' of the ENHPS initiative, it - also from an interorganisational network research perspective - indeed represents a **significant shift in orientation**: with the European *'Network'* as reference point that is a clear shift **from an 'inward' orientation to an orientation towards the network's closer 'institutional environment'**. For example, stronger emphasized was to foster an increasing degree of commitment and understanding of the ENHPS related principles among not only network schools but *municipalities, Governments and others*, and the latter were called 'participants' of the ENHPS initiative. Key *policy and decision makers* were now an explicit target group of actions and the 'necessary' commitment and efforts *between international, national and local* agencies became a focus. (ENHPS 1996, 1997; Burgher et al 1999)

This and particularly the latter support the assumption that the European *Network* is not only embedded or supported by a 'ENHPS *project*' of public agencies at *international* level (WHO, EC, CE) but that such a project (potentially and desirably) also extends to the public sectors at *national and even local* levels (see fig. 5.1.4). Later, also contacts with *international* (public) agencies or initiatives were reported (Rivett 2000). – During this phase, the language of European level documents became *less inward oriented* in the sense of mainly focusing on the individual network schools and the National Coordinators as core network persons at national level; it became *more outward oriented* in the sense of looking addressing *beyond* the trio of the supporting agencies (WHO, EC and CE) towards those organizations that - in network research terms - are a crucial part of the network's 'institutional environment' *within* countries.

From the international level the attention was shifted towards the 'partnership' between the national (and may be regional) Ministries of Health and of Education and even others, and to partnerships of ENHPS 'pilot' schools and *local* organizations and groups. The whole education and health *sectors* rather than the schools only moved into focus, i.e. education and other public agencies and authorities *at all levels of society*. It were the leading *European* agencies that called for this shift: "It is not only coordinators and schools who need to take a greater lead. National, regional and local *Governments* can play a major role. Raising the status of the Health Promoting Schools project from that of HPS demonstration sites to a vehicle which effectively influences *education* policy and practice is one of the greatest challenges facing the Network over the next four years. And national government can be instrumental in achieving this." While during the first phase of ENHPS development the European agencies (WHO, CE, EC) as International Planning Committee had played the "leading role in furthering the Network's activities, it is *vital that other partners join in and assume greater responsibilities during the next phase*" (ENHPS 1997 p8 - italics not in original).

The image of the ENHPS initiative, project and network implicitly conveyed by the *plans* for 1996-2000 supports the outline derived from the first phase (see fig. 5.1.3) and shapes it even further as illustrated in figure 5.1.4.

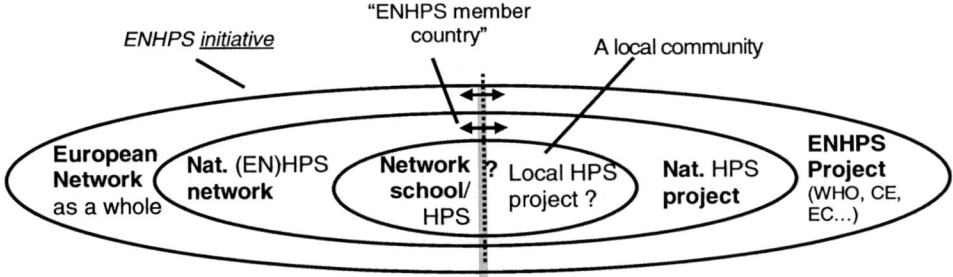

Figure 5.1.4: Direction of development of the ENHPS initiative from the perspective of interorganisational network research: The initiative encompasses *two* distinct systems with multiple layers each (European Network/ ENHPS project).

[left side: interorganisational '*network*' system/ right side: 'ENHPS *project*' system]

[outer ellipse: European ENHPS initiative as a whole/ middle ellipse: countries therein/ inner ellipse: local level]

CE:	Council of Europe	MoEs:	Ministries of Education
EC:	European Commission	MoHs:	Ministries of Health
ENHPS:	European Network of Health Promoting Schools	Nat.:	National
HPS:	Health Promoting Schools	WHO:	World Health Organization

The figure shows that all ENHPS related key actors identified so far are either ENHPS *members* (e.g. pilot schools, National Support Centers) or participants or partners in the 'ENHPS project(s)' (WHO, CE, and EC, plus (sub-)national Health and Education Ministries, plus potentially also local authorities and others). Documents refer clearly to the *international* ENHPS project and *national* 'HPS projects'; at local level the *network schools* were always the focus but later on local authorities, too.

- 280 -

Overall it can be said that three, four years after the launch of the ENHPS, the *international* organizations leading the 'ENHPS project' and likely the group of National Support Centers, too, changed foci from network 'inward' looking to looking 'outward' towards the European Network's *governmental or public sector environment* and here particularly towards the *education* sector. They started to call on the actors concerned to assume more responsibility and developed first ideas of action to realize this.

It naturally follows that the **new development objectives include several interorganisational relations and network issues** at various systems levels, i.e.:

regarding a) the network's *environment*, to strengthen the commitment from the *whole* education sector and support opportunities for collaboration with the health and other sectors; regarding b) network *members* and *local* others, to foster a greater sense of ENHPS *'project identity'* among National Coordinators, schools, parents and local communities; and regarding c) *all* those involved, to emphasize even in training on curricula issues the *change and project management*. An effective public relations campaign was planned in support of this. Also the foci of research and evaluation activities were *expanded*: As before they had to 'demonstrate the *effectiveness of HPS programs* but now those *investing* in Health Promotion at national, regional and local level were stressed as target group of results. Most interestingly, the relevance, impact and added value of the *whole 'ENHPS project'* rather than the Settings approach (or HPS) alone moved into focus.

Major activities during the transition years (or 'second phase')

Major activities at the beginning of this second phase of ENHPS development reflect this broadened view:

The before mentioned **"ENHPS Schools Data Base"** created at the time in a *joint* effort of Technical Secretariat, National Support Centers and 'pilot schools' covers not only multi-dimensional 'school portrays' (presenting the *schools'* 'HPS projects') but also **portrays of '*national* HPS projects'**. The latter consider several **aspects of interorganisational networks**: contact details on 36 National Support Centers facilitate both *networking 'within'* the European Network and the network's *accessibility for 'external others'*; the National Centers' human and financial resources hint at the network's *'resource dependency'*; official contact persons in the Ministries of Health and Education named reflect formal commitment of these *core 'external others'*; network *membership* issues are addressed ('pilot' school selection, possibilities for 'new' schools to enter, official entry criteria) and so are means of contact or '*soft' networking 'within'* national networks. Also aspects of the core business of the main 'host' or institutional environment of the European Network in countries, the education sector, are addressed (National Centers' provision of teaching materials; health education in the formal curriculum). And finally, *minimal* information on initial assessment, process and/or outcome evaluations undertaken or being planned indicates whether those involved in a 'national HPS project' or '-network' recognize their need or are able to assess and monitor their work - in other words, whether Hastings' *"radar beam" of self-reflection* and learning is installed, for example, as a basis for country specific advocacy for continued support and expansion of the European Network in that country.

Overall this indicates, that those that designed this 'ENHPS Data Base' had reached an intuitive understanding of *'national* HPS *networks'* as inter-organizational networks. The **consideration of several important features of interorganisational networks (IONs) as identified in network research** shows that *over time* at least some of the key actors in the ENHPS developed an implicit (experience based) network or ION perspective. The **'pilot school portrays'** reflect this even more:

Besides some general information (school type/ size) a range of **features of schools as** *members* **of interorganizational networks** (here the ENHPS) are addressed: their motivation to join; perceptions of membership (as to the *'European* Network', *'national* HPS project', and/or *'other* networks'); internal 'HPS project' organization (contact person, incentives for staff, etc.); *activities related to the network's goal* by network level (local/ national/ international) and/or across national borders; and minimal *information on (self-)assessment* or evaluation activities (such as 'impact planned/reached so far'; 'successful activities' and those 'carried out with difficulties'). Also a few items related to the **network schools' (local) environment** are covered: a *social description* of the school population and/or local community (which hints at social determinants of health locally); the involvement of medical health *services* in the school's HPS project; the availability of a 'local curriculum' usable for health promotion/ education purposes (a matter of the education system in place); and training and support received. In addition, the Data Bank captures the **health issues covered** by the pilot schools in their role as members of a network on *'Health Promoting Schools'*. (see WHO/EURO 1998)

The reference made to the social context locally, health related curricula, and health issues shows that the key actors within the ENHPS initiative that developed this **ENHPS Data Bank** (WHO/EURO 1998) approached this activity not only from an **implicit network perspective but explicit perspective on Health Promotion in schools**, too.

However, when looking at the ensemble of documentation by and of the ENHPS initiative it remains that **a clear concept of the (interorganisational)** *network* **dimension of the ENHPS was and is lacking**. This judgment is also supported by the fact that the need for a *broader* focus of evaluation efforts *beyond the individual network schools* has been generally recognized in recent years (and is reflected in two evaluation related activities ('EVA 2'/ Piette et al 1998, w.y.; and the 'ENHPS indicator development' effort/ ENHPS w.y.); but a clear assessment or evaluation framework for the ENHPS as a larger (network) system has not been developed, agreed upon and/or widely communicated (see also chap. 3).

Yet, the creation of the ENHPS Data Base (unfortunately never updated or further advanced as of now) proves: Within its first few years the yet 'young' European **Network as a whole matured** from - in Alter/Hage terms - an information and experience *exchange* network to a joint *action (or promotional) network*. The Data Base is a product that could not have been created by neither one of the Network members alone. This evolutionary step is also confirmed by another key activity undertaken five years after the European Network's launch: the first 'ENHPS conference' held in 1997 that produced a new guiding document:

This **"First Conference of the ENHPS"**, a mix of 400 actors within or around the ENHPS initiative from 43 countries (from education and health experts and parents and pupils to policy-makers and representatives from European agencies), created and passed a **major Resolution**. Interestingly, most of the vast range of case studies discussed fall into thematic areas that relate to *organizational development* and *interorganisational relations* in support of school health promotion: the school as a setting for Health Promotion, school policy development, and management and organization change on the one hand, and collaboration with the community, and international collaboration on the other. Nevertheless, also core topics of the education sector, curriculum development and teacher training, were a main theme. And with *'democracy'* and *'evaluation'* major political and technical challenges in sustainable health promotion throughout Europe were addressed, too. Overall, the Conference as a means of publicly taking stock of developments so far reflects a) the foci of the first years and related progress in realizing the *Settings approach* locally and a *European* level support project, and b) the lack of focus on the European Network's inherent *network approach*. (An outstanding exception, the German speaking ENHPS sub-network, has been mentioned before.)

During the Conference the overall aim and mission of the European Network and its partners were reformulated and put it into *one* sentence: 'Every child should now have the right to benefit from the HPS initiative', a simple and yet complex message.

Through its First Conference, the ENHPS took two important steps related to - in Hastings terms - its networking 'within' the net and 'with others': First, it clearly communicated to the 'outside world' what and where it is after its first five years and engaged in some dialogue with important actors in its environment. Second, it reaffirmed and strengthened among both its members and supporters several issues that are known to be core network features: the shared *conceptual base* (i.e. the 'whole school' approach or HPS concept); the joint *value base* (which here includes the improvement of equity as goal and result of the Health Promoting Schools, and democracy as a basic principle); and the *'non-prescriptive'* working mode (which here demands schools to act on a set of core values and principles but supports their choice of locally relevant work areas and activities). European Network members, supporters and others also widely agreed that the successes throughout Europe so far warrant its further implementation - which reflects a sufficiently high level of *satisfaction* within the network as a whole. - Through the Conference the ENHPS also focused its attention to some generally **agreed upon but yet less realized dimensions**:

a) the schools' role as catalysts and resource for *interorganisational collaboration* on community health and the need that outsiders recognize this role (a genuine element of the health-promoting Settings approach);

b) the crucial role of *interministerial collaboration* in health and education to move from pilot to dissemination phase (a matter of improvements within the network's closer environment in countries); and

c) the need for further improvements in the area of *evaluation* (a matter of creating or sustaining high levels of satisfaction and (perceived) effectiveness as core network outcomes).

Overall, these points indicate the increased sensibility of leading ENHPS actors to the Network's *environment* at *local and national* levels, and greater awareness of the *evaluation challenges* that come with the European Network's complexity. (Burgher et al 1999; ENHPS/TS 1998a,b; Resolution 1997)

The **Conference Resolution** was passed as the major **new policy and guidance document** for ENHPS members and supporters. It directly addresses the core *public actors* in the European Network's *environment* at international and national level: It publicly invites troika of WHO/EURO, Council of Europe and European Commission to continue their support. It calls on all European governments to adopt the Health Promoting Schools concept and consider **principles for action within 'countries'** under ten headings that cover a mix of key issues in a) modern Public Health and *Health Promotion* in general, and Health Promoting Schools development in particular; b) socio-political realities in today's Europe; and related to both c) *interorganisational* collaboration. The ten headings are: democracy, equity, empowerment, the school environment, the curriculum, teacher training, the measurement of success, *collaboration, communities,* and sustainability. Formulated on the base of five years of experience with the large scale European innovation 'ENHPS', and with involvement of the national and also school level network *members*, the Resolution replaces the guiding function of the '12 criteria of a HPS' defined at the very beginning of the ENHPS initiative (Piette et al 1999; see above).

The Resolution provides **some guidance on interorganisational collaboration for the further development of Health Promoting Schools** in countries: The *principle of 'collaboration'* refers to close intersectoral collaboration and shared responsibility in the European Network's closest *environment:* between (education and health) Ministries whose 'partnership' approach should be mirrored at *all* other levels. The *principle of 'community'* orientation in school health promotion highlights the potential for positive change not only *within* schools but of the 'partnership' *between* schools, parents, NGOs, and the local community - which reminds of Hastings' two organizational networking processes 'networking within' and 'with others' (see chap. 2.4.2).

Searching for new directions - from a transition phase into a reoriented third phase ?

In 1999, after various actions of stock taking, critical review and rethinking strategy in the second half of the 1990s some of which have been addressed above, the International Planning Committee published a new ENHPS brochure that is a kind of **'reorientation and looking forward'** document authored by staff of the ENHPS Technical Secretariat (Burgher et al 1999). With this step an earlier impression is confirmed: that the development of the **'1996-2000 development plan' lead into what may be better called a "transition phase" (rather than a clearly shaped 'second phase'**, so the original wording used). According to the new 1999 document, the "European Network of Health Promoting Schools" (initiative) strives to: prepare or make the 'transition' into an 'established long-term *project*'. This **'ringing in' of a new (third) phase** for the 'ENHPS' (network, project and/or initiative) also strives to *allow for 'different approaches to health development'* in countries, and act on the need for more 'accurate means of *measuring progress'*. Importantly, the **aims of the 'first phase'** of the European Network (initiative) are **confirmed for the new phase but expanded**:

The 'ENHPS' continues to strive for extending the implementation of the HPS concept but a *new goal* put forward is to work for the *'establishment of good practice within education and school policies* throughout Europe' (however defined). In addition, the 'ENHPS' sets out to pay *more attention to inequalities* in health and education and to carefully introduce activities aimed at vulnerable groups, and specific areas such as disadvantaged inner cities and rural districts. *To achieve these goals, the ENHPS Technical Secretariat supports National Support Centers in several areas*: as before, with 'school based' technical initiatives (from planning to evaluation); *new*, with *consultations with officials and others on a 'national strategy'* that not only increases advocacy and visibility of the country's HPS 'project' but achieves its sustainability; with the *identification of clear benefits* for schools (the 'added value' for educational processes) and of good practice; with documentation and increasing visibility via Internet, websites, etc.; and also with results of the European longitudinal WHO Survey 'Health Behavior in School-aged Children' (HBSC). (Burgher et al 1999; ENHPS/TS 1998a,b; Samdal/ Wold 1997)

From a network research perspective remarkable is that in the latest documents that present the expanded aims and new directions of the European Network (initiative) the term 'network' is hardly used in contrast to the term 'HPS project'. This may well be linked to the results of the ENHPS evaluation study called 'EVA 2' (Piette et al 1998, w.y.) undertaken directly before their publishing. This study provided some insight into the situation of the ENHPS during the transition phase (from 1996):

Earlier observations of diversity at country level were fully confirmed. Almost two thirds (21) out of the then 37 (today 41) *'national* ENHPS projects' or '-networks' were examined. - As of 1998, two thirds of these had grown in *size* through *planned* dissemination beyond the 'pilot schools' or informal *spontaneous* dissemination around 'pilot schools'. The number of network schools *varied* depending on the age of the network, resources available, dynamism of the HPS team and the type of networking (more or less formal). The drop out rate of pilot schools was close to zero. - The situation or *stage of development* of HPS projects or networks within countries *varied widely*, for example: In 1998 *some* national networks for developing Health Promoting Schools (HPS) were *well defined* with a limited number of pilot schools, without which no development of school health promotion would have occurred. Others were very *small*, not well known and fairly *isolated*. Again others saw a *flourishing of school health promotion inside and outside the network* at the same time. And in a few cases school health promotion would have occurred even without the HPS network (e.g. in form of individual school developments or local school health promotion networks).

The EVA 2 study identified **short comings in ENHPS countries** as to the planning of the *dissemination phase* (the phase of network expansion after the pilot phase with selected pilot schools only). Lacking were policy analyses to identify the 'added value' of the HPS project for the education sector, and organizational analyses to identify and build a support structure for an expansion of the HPS project or network beyond 'pilot schools' to many more schools and ultimately all those in a country. Two groups of **factors** seem to positively influence decision making **for the ENHPS expansion** to all schools in a country. The 'general factors' refer to important features of the *HPS network's environment*: educational structures and staff at regional level that could serve as Regional HPS Support Center (RSCs); a clear policy for health in schools (e.g. health as a cross-curricular topic); and good interorganisational relations between the health and education sector. The 'ENHPS specific factors' include interorganisational *network features*: first, the capacities of the National Support Center in place (to advocate and lobby, to directly communicate with decision makers, to plan and manage networks); second, a network of partners. A third supportive factor is an *evaluation approach that meets* the policy and quality requirements of the education sector, i.e. needs prevalent in the Network's *closest envirornment*. - Overall, the **main challenge** identified for national (or sub-national) HPS networks when moving from 'pilot phase' to 'dissemination phase' is to *maintain the vision and principles of the European Network of HPS while ensuring high quality work of a high number of new 'Health Promoting Schools in the making'*.

Potential actions suggested by the EVA 2 study address mainly the relation of national Health Promotion networks with their environment: an increase in visibility for the ENHPS and in communication with decision makers; collaboration with other health related networks and potentially their integration; and guidelines and recommendations for the training of teachers and school inspectors. In addition, *evaluation should cover both school and regional network levels* (an expanded focus as compared to earlier EVA 1 study). For the dissemination of the HPS concept beyond pilot schools and sustainable development of Health Promoting Schools (HPS) throughout countries it may be ideal if schools have both local curriculum time and project time to be locally defined and, thus, potentially available for the HPS project. - As to the policy environment of national HPS networks or projects, the EVA 2 study did show: In 1998 only three, but in May 1999 already 10 countries (or regions) had a *policy* in place on all schools to become Health Promoting Schools (HPS). Interestingly, in a few cases this meant a *different* scheme or awards rather than an *expansion* of the HPS *network* approach to the regional level. Regarding policy development in support of HPS development, the study identified several **counteracting factors:** With view to *features of HPS networks* and related interorganisational relations unfavorable are: a too small network size, the National Coordinator's insufficient understanding of dissemination processes, and the lack of credibility of the National Support Center from the education sector's point of view. Counteracting aspects of a *network's environment* are a too heavy bureaucracy which, for example, hinders schools to freely undertake projects, and the lack of effective intersectoral collaboration between Ministry of Health and Education. A *general factor* is insufficient differentiation between health education and Health Promotion negatively impacted, too. A **supportive factor** as to policy development for HPS development are reforms of the education system underway. (Piette et al 1998, w.y., 1999)

The development of the "European Network of Health Promoting Schools" (ENHPS) over time - intermediate synthesis and discussion

The above look across the overall development of the European Network and the 'ENHPS project' during the first seven network years provided some valuable insights for this research project as to the European Network's or ENHPS initiatives developmental phases and self-reflection: The first three years of the ENHPS initiative were **a clearly defined first phase** of development of the European Network. It focused on the desired *Network expansion* as to 'member countries' (not schools), and on *technical support* of those directly involved in transforming the limited number of 'pilot' schools per country into *'Health Promoting Schools'*. The network approach stood for *experience exchange* particularly as to the latter. At the **international level** this was realized mainly through the European Network's annual business meetings; (at the national and subnational level this varied from country to country). These first three years called 'phase 1' of the ENHPS initiative, from a network research perspective, refer to **an 'exchange network under development'** with a slowly increasing extent of information and experience exchange within the net: first there was direct exchange only annually and only among the *national* level network members (i.e. National Support Centers, not schools); later, by means of the Network Newsletter, the cross-border exchange was expanded twofold: a) as to its frequency (now at least *bi*-annually) and b) as to the type of network members involved (now also school members). To what degree this has been complemented by an exchange via e-mail among some or all National Support Centers and also the ENHPS Technical Secretariat has not been documented.

This **phase merged into a new less defined phase** of stock taking, critical review, and evaluation efforts, of reassurance as to basic principles and identification of challenges and open questions, of searching for answers and also further planning. This refers particularly to the years 1996/1997 and the year or two that followed. Mainly involved were the European Network's *national* level *members* (National Support Centers/ Coordinators), the ENHPS Technical Secretariat (as network member or supporter), and the *international* 'ENHPS project' partners WHO, CE and EC (i.e. the key actors in the European Network's closest *environment*). Network *schools* were significantly involved in only one of the activities: the creation of the 'ENHPS Schools Data Base' for which an range of base line information was collected particularly from and on the ENHPS *pilot* schools. From the interorganisational network perspective (and particularly as to the *international* level of the ENHPS initiative), this second phase may best be called **a transition phase** or phase of reflection and reorientation. On the one hand, it did provide **insight into the extent to which aims of the first phase were achieved**:

At the outset it had been stated that the network approach was chosen to effectively *exchange* experiences and information and *disseminate* "good practice" (see chap. 5.1.2). The first step was to establish *throughout* Europe a group of *model schools* (an inherent **objective 1**). These were expected to *first* demonstrate the impact of Health Promotion in the school setting (inherent **objective 2**), *before*, second, to do both: *disseminate* experiences, information, 'good' practice (inherent **objective 3**), and *influence* 'policy and practice in school health promotion nationally and internationally' (inherent **objective 4**). - Regarding the *first objective*, a network development objective, the achievement within the first three years was significant: with over 70% of European countries becoming ENHPS members with a set of pilot schools each even if the pilot schools were not yet 'a group throughout' Europe. But many schools had started to develop cross-border relations and the National Coordinators had become a European group. - As to the *second objective*, a network *performance* objective (i.e. pilot schools' 'demonstration of impact' in health promotion terms) the array of case stories published at European level indicates valuable progress made in important facets of the Health Promoting Schools concept in many pilot schools (see e.g. ENHPS Technical Secretariat 1995; WHO/EURO 1998); however, at European level more than such *indications* has not been achieved in spite of some effort of the Technical Secretariat, the tripartite 'ENHPS project' as 'leader', and the European Network as a whole: Neither during the first three years nor those that followed, the actors succeed to develop or agree upon an assessment or evaluation framework to guide and support network members to indeed demonstrate the impact of implementing the Health Promoting Schools- concept. Thus, an assessment of performance as to this ENHPS related objective needs to be done on the base of country case studies. As will be seen in chapters 5.3 to 5.6 *individual national* ENHPS networks or projects indeed *did* identify progress towards HPS development which resulted in a certain degree of satisfaction within networks and beyond.

Following the network rational set out at the very beginning of the ENHPS initiative, the inherent **objectives 3 and 4**, i.e. the *dissemination* of experiences and 'good' practice and the *influencing* of policy and practice at national and international level, were to be the goal of pilot schools only *after* a first (pilot) phase of developing model-'Health Promoting Schools'. Objectives 3 and 4 appear to be those that match with what often has been referred to as *'dissemination phase'* in ENHPS *'countries'* (not of the European Network as a whole). As to *this*, the various activities during the European Network's and/or ENHPS project's **transition phase produced mixed results** if any. While the overall goal of developing 'Health Promoting Schools' in European countries on a *large* scale was confirmed and sustained (i.e. the *dissemination* objective as to other than ENHPS 'pilot' schools), the overall picture is somewhat fuzzy with some tendencies: Those publicly reflecting on progress made and development needs to be tackled across Europe, are the *national* level network *members* (National Support Centers) and the key *international* actors (the ENHPS Technical Secretariat, and WHO, CE, and EC as 'external others'). These show a **broadened attention span and plans of action in three domains**: with regard to core *actors* in focus and *goals* of the ENHPS initiative, and *issues to be evaluated* to measure effectiveness:

First, regarding **important actors** within and around the European Network, those moved into the foreground that represent the European Network's (or national networks') closer *institutional environment within countries.* Stronger emphasis was given particularly to the public or governmental side: Ministries of Education and the education sectors as a *whole*; Health Ministries and sectors; the collaboration between these two (explicitly at all systems levels, national to local); also the National Advisory Boards or other support mechanisms in countries; and even local governments. (Before, the latter had been just an implicit or potential element within the HPS concept via its dimension of 'school-community-links', and just an issue to be tackled by individual schools rather than the ENHPS as a whole.) Unfortunately, this overall shift in attention was not embedded into a clear conceptual framework that would relate this shift to the original innovation of a European *'Network'* (for the development) of Health Promoting Schools, although this innovation was just or still being implemented in many if not most 'ENHPS countries'. Published information transmits the impression that in the European Network initiative at large (not necessarily in particular ENHPS countries) the **organizational innovation of large scale HPS development through a *network* approach lost attention - while the *public education* sectors in countries and related national policies moved particularly into the foreground**. The interorganisational network perspective and conceptual frame offered by this research project shows that this is **an unnecessary 'trade off'** and may be even counterproductive. The European *Network*, understood as an inter*organisational* network, could be seen as broadening its attention beyond network members towards core actors in its environment (Ministries, local governments, etc.). And the rightly desired policy changes in this environment in support of HPS development could become a *joint action* area of all *network members* plus its supporters (such as WHO, EC and CE).

However, major documents such as the latest ENHPS brochure (Burgher et al 1999) and the EVA 2 study report (Piette et al 1998, w.y.) do only emphasize a) the HPS concept to be implemented in all *individual* European schools and b) the need of supportive national education policies - without reflecting further on the potential inherent in the *network* approach that could support the *two* - and, in addition, key Health Promotion goals and principles in general (as discussed in chap. 3). This interpretation of the findings is supported when looking at the 'new development objectives' as well as the new guidance document, the Conference Resolution: These underline the strengthening of the commitment of the public education sectors, intersectoral collaborations between education and health sectors, and the National Centers', ENHPS schools' and local communities' greater 'project' (not network) identity - besides issues of health promoting developments *within* schools. But they do not highlight the *network* dimension of the ENHPS initiative and the impression emerging is that the *term "European Network* of Health Promoting School" (ENHPS) is *increasingly used just as a label* of an initiative or project rather than an organizational form, approach, or development direction consciously chose to achieve a complex goal.

However, on the positive side and most remarkably, the **evaluation efforts** of the ENHPS initiative undertaken **during the transition phase had clearly an expanded focus** taking into account many facets of the *overall* ENHPS or HPS projects or networks *in countries*, far beyond the former focus on health promoting developments within individual pilot schools only (see Parsons et al 1997; Piette et al 1998, w.y.; and more systematically in ENHPS w.y.). Unfortunately, the vast *array of information and recommendations derived was not systematized and integrated and only a very few made it to achieve most attention* of the European level actors: i.e. the development of *education policies* in countries in support of the HPS 'concept' and its implementation in *all* schools, - without further reflection or recognition of the *network* for the *development* of Health Promoting Schools (HPS) in *place* across Europe and in many countries. The slogan put forward 'from pilot to policy' reflects this situation (Burgher et al 1999).

Overall, this analysis supports what has been carved out step by step before: the *double-structure of the ENHPS initiative* with the *European Network* on the one hand (and national sub-networks therein), and a public-sector -'ENHPS *project*' on the other hand (as part of the network's closer supportive environment). Although the terminology used in written documents delivers a rather fuzzy picture the interorganisational network research perspective helped to unravel this sub-structure of the overall ENHPS initiative immanent from the start. When the European *Network* is the focus of attention as in this research project, the **structural framework of the ENHPS initiative visualized in figure 5.1.4 helps to systematize and better understand the various changes in emphasis on organizational actors and/or their environments that occurred over time.** This is illustrated in figure 5.1.5.

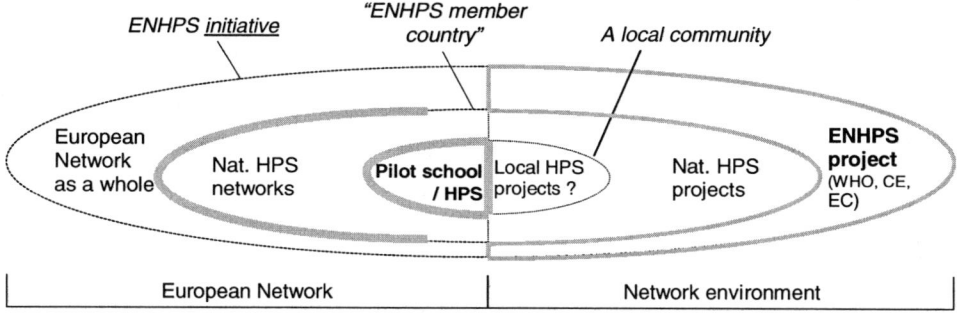

a) Foci of attention and action during the first phase of European Network development (1992-1995) – as to he European Network (left side) and the network's environment (right) (see gray zones and actors in bold).

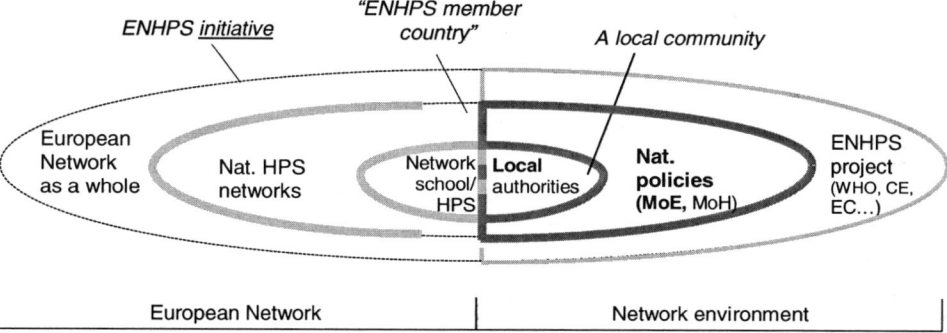

b) New foci of attention and action from 1996 on / for the 'second' phase of European Network development – as to he European Network (left side) and the network's environment (right) (new foci: see dark).

CE:	Council of Europe	ENHPS:	European Network of HPS
EC:	European Commission	HPS:	Health Promoting School(s)
MoE:	Ministry of Education	Nat.:	National
MoH:	Ministry of Health	WHO:	World Health Organization

Figure 5.1.5: From inward to outward orientation - Shifts in foci from the 'first' to the 'second' phase of European Network development (from network members to institutional or policy environments).

During the transition years that followed, i.e. roughly during years four to six of the ENHPS initiative (or a 'second phase'), the high diversity of developments in ENHPS countries mirrored the challenges inherent in the goals of the ENHPS initiative. As recalled above the ENHPS initiative did strive for some kind of 'dissemination' of the HPS concept beyond the 'pilot schools' ideally to *all* schools in a country, after the pilot schools had demonstrated the impact of Health Promotion in the school Setting; (experiences and knowledge was to be disseminated 'to the health and education sectors, influencing policy and practice' both 'nationally and internationally' - see chap. 5.1.2). However, the analysis above has shown that for long the international actors within the ENHPS initiative had no clear strategy towards this end, at least as far as documented strategies are concerned. The ENHPS went into a transition phase, following up on and initiating new reviews and evaluation projects and searching for the right way to go. Overall, at international level this led to an expansion of foci beyond network members to include *aspects* of the institutional and political environment of national HPS networks in countries: Suggested new foci were national education policies and the education sector as a whole including local education authorities. (see fig. 5.1.5 b)

In order to a) better understand how far within the ENHPS initiative an *interorganisational network* as characterized in chapter 2.4 has been realized and sustained, and b) further examine the *assumptions* made as to which group of actors are indeed European Network *members* and which rather external supporters, an important step remains to be done: the examination of the interactions and relations of the various actors identified within or close to the European Network. For example, as of now it is an open question whether the ENHPS Technical Secretariat should be considered as a network member or rather network supporter. Also, the finding that the interorganisational *network* approach may have been weakened during the European Network's transition years (from 1996) needs further examination. Once these issues have been addressed and the unit of analysis for this research project defined, the 'synthesizing analysis I' of the European Network's structures and processes can begin as elaborated in chapter 4, i.e. as a pilot application of a core part of the proposed network assessment framework (see fig. 4.2.2).

5.1.5 Interactions and relations of ENHPS network members

Although ENHPS documents usually emphasize the National Coordinators, not the National Support Centers, the ENHPS 'country' membership does rest not on a particular functionary but on national *organizations*: the Ministry of Health (MoH) and of Education (MoE), and the National

Support Center as the organization designated by the Ministries to serve the national HPS project or network. This is important for this research as the focus is on inter*organisational* (rather than interpersonal) networks. This does not mean, that professionals such as the National Coordinators - indisputable core actors at national level - are neglected. But National Coordinators act on behalf of the National Support Centers and the 'national HPS projects' or '-networks', and their professional interactions and relations with others represent those of these organizational entities. Therefore, it is appropriate to continue to focus on *organizational* ENHPS actors also in this chapter.

Introduction: Which network ? Which members ?

Examining the relations and interactions of ENHPS 'members' requires that members are clearly identified. As shown so far, **this seemingly simple question is not as easy to answer** as one may have presumed. Of course, one could take a narrow perspective and go with what the name suggests: the European Network is a network of those schools that implement the Health Promoting Schools (HPS) concept, i.e. a network of 'Health Promoting Schools in the making'. In this view all other non-school actors significantly involved in the ENHPS development are part of the European Network's environment, with some particularly close or actively supporting it. But at least two reasons speak against this narrow view: First, the three ENHPS initiators EC, CE and WHO/EURO established and use up today sophisticated criteria and mechanisms for the selection of both 'schools' *and* 'countries' that wish to join the ENHPS. EC, CE and WHO act as the 'gatekeepers' of the ENHPS and interested schools can only join the European (as opposed to a national) network if: a) their 'country' joins (i.e. MoH and MoE sign a collaborative agreement and designate a National Support Center and National Coordinator for HPS development in the country; b) the national level selects the interested school as ENHPS 'pilot school', which then is expected to work closely with the National Support Center to achieve the European Network's goals. The ENHPS is not simply a network of schools with an international supporting body that can be contacted to enter the Network, and the national level bodies are more than just 'filters' for school applications from their country. The latter have an active and ongoing role in the work and development of the ENHPS.

Second, even with view to the ENHPS *school* members a question emerges. As said before ENHPS documents distinct between ENHPS 'pilot schools' and 'other' schools linked to the ENHPS. Thus, although it is clear that the ENHPS has *school* members, the question remains *whether all or only some* of the thousands of European schools that adopted the HPS concept and started to work jointly with others towards its implementation are 'full' ENHPS members: Pilot schools may be members and the 'others' may not, or 'pilot' and 'other' schools may just represent two types of ENHPS school members in the sense of schools with different developmental status and/or tasks. The terminology used at *European level* to describe the 'other' schools - e.g. 'schools linked to the ENHPS through various national or sub-national arrangements' - indicates: The 'other' (non-pilot) schools may not be perceived as full or core members of the European Network. From an international perspective they remain in a different but rather vague status. However, there are hints that this clear distinction between 'pilot schools' and 'others' is fading: The ENHPS project in its recent years actively moves towards actions that allow its vision to be realized, i.e. the *'mainstreaming'* of the implementation of the HPS concept *throughout* European education sectors and in all schools. Thus, the concentration on 'pilot schools' may be seen as a pilot phase phenomenon.

Further complexity or an easy way of clarifying the question of ENHPS membership and borders lies in the fact that the ENHPS initiators speak of both the European *Network* of Health Promoting Schools (ENHPS) and the 'ENHPS *project'*. This opens the door to locate a range of key actors that are closely involved in the development and work of the ENHPS initiative as 'external' to the Network, but as part of the Network's *'closer'* environment. As illustrated in figure 5.1.6 **an image emerging is one of *two* environmental systems in which the European Network is operating** and apparently thriving: a more influential and (hopefully) continuously supporting one, the *'ENHPS project'*; and another one that may be called the *'wider' network environment*.

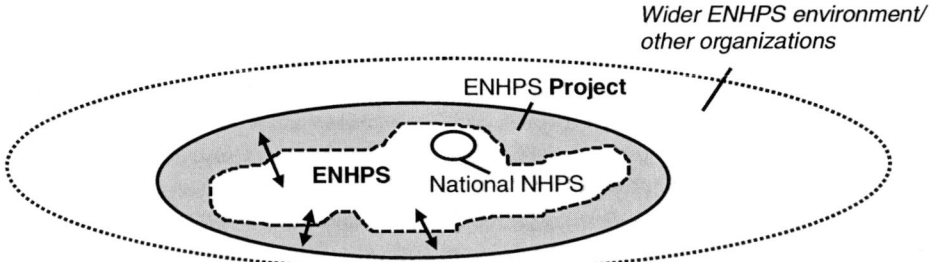

Figure 5.1.6: The European Network of Health Promoting Schools (ENHPS) and its closer and wider environments. (The ENHPS 'project' as the Networks closest environment.)

ENHPS = "European Network of Health Promoting Schools"
NHPS = National Network (for the development) of Health Promoting Schools

As suggested before the membership question is answered with view to the International Planning Committee (IPC) and the 'pilot schools'. The IPC (including EC, CE, and WHO/EURO) stated at various occasions that the European Network 'belongs to the schools', work is being done 'within a network of pilot schools', and that the three European initiators and 'sponsors' are in a 'supporting' role. Thus, the IPC and the three organizations therein are not European 'Network members' but part of the ENHPS 'project'. The initially selected 'pilot schools', limited to a number of 10-20 per ENHPS 'country', are clearly formal 'European Network members'. Remains the question whether the other key actors involved in the development of the ENHPS are *network* members or 'ENHPS *project*' participants, and whether there are only *organizational* members or participants or also others.

Obviously, from the perspective of interorganisational network (ION) research the issue of ENHPS 'country' members needs to be broken down into organizational systems that represent a 'country' with respect to the ENHPS, i.e. that act or can be seen as part of the European *Network* or ENHPS *project*. Several 'candidates' have been identified so far: the Ministries of Health and of Education (MoH and MoE); the National Advisory Board where it exists; and the National Support Centers and/or the national project offices therein. At international level the latter are represented by the National Coordinators.

With regard to those many schools that are not ENHPS 'pilot schools' but implement the HPS concept within national or sub-national arrangements linked to the European Network, the distinction of the two systems, 'European Network' and international 'ENHPS project', may not be sufficient. These 'other' schools may be seen or perceive themselves as members or participants of the *national* (or regional) HPS networks or projects in their countries. *National* HPS networks will at least overlap with the overall *European* Network - through the 'double membership' of ENHPS pilot schools. This has been considered already in figure 5.3.2 through the small circle symbolizing a national HPS network. But national networks as a *whole* may turn out to be an integral part of the European Network, if not already during the pilot years then afterwards. In the ENHPS country case studies below this issue will be further explored.

Table 5.1.1 provides **a summary** of the *key organizational actors* as well as the three *ENHPS related organizational systems* (networks or projects) that have been identified so far. It also shows the *actors' assumed membership* or participant status in relation to networks or projects. The table provides a simple framework for the further examination of the inherent assumptions about the boundaries of the so called "European Network of Health Promoting Schools" and related systems. With regard to the organizational arrangements around the ENHPS within countries (the third column) one assumption is made: the distinction proposed from an international perspective between the European *'Network'* of HPS and a related ENHPS *'project'* is already extended to the level of individual ENHPS member *countries*. That this might be reasonable or useful has been already indicated by the examination of the ENHPS related developments over time above, particularly when looking at the role of Ministries of Education and of Health in achieving 'ENHPS membership' of any actor and the shift in attention towards them after the European Network's pilot years. Nevertheless this proposal needs further examination which will be done in the two ENHPS country case studies (Slovenia and Germany) that follow later.

Organizational systems → / Key actors ↓	ENHPS project participants	European **Network** of HPS (ENHPS) members	National HPS **networks/ projects*** members/ participants*
international/ European level	IPC (EC, CE, WHO/EURO) Technical Secret. ?		
national level	MoHs ? MoEs ?	National Support Center (NSC) (or nat. project office) ? (represented by the NC)	National Advisory Boards (NABs)* MoHs ?* MoEs ?*
regional level			Regional Support Centers
local level		ENHPS pilot schools Other HPS ?	pilot schools & other HPS other local organizations* ?

Table 5.1.1: The European Network of HPS - key actors and assumed membership status as well as social systems (projects) linked to the European Network.

ENHPS: European Network of Health Promoting Schools
HPS: Health Promoting Schools
IPC: International Planning Committee
MoEs: Ministries of Education
MoHs: Ministries of Health

With regard to the *sub*-national but supra-local level of the European Network and ENHPS project some **terminology** has to be clarified to avoid confusion. Currently, a few ENHPS countries have *several* quite *separate* HPS networks due to their particular cultural and socio-political circumstances or movements for greater independence. Examples include Spain, Belgium (with two networks along the language border Flemish/ French), and the UK (with separate networks in Wales, England and Scotland but nevertheless one National Coordinator). In the context of this research project, for solely practical reasons, such independent but sub-national networks will be subsumed under the term "national" HPS networks as long as the *whole* of the European Network is concerned and not particular ENHPS countries. The term **"regional" HPS networks**, although politically appropriate for the sub-national HPS networks just mentioned, will be reserved for the various sub-national but supra-local network arrangements that have occurred as *part of the dissemination process* of the HPS concept in many 'ENHPS countries'. The International Planning Committee (IPC) and Technical Secretariat have encouraged *regional arrangements in ENHPS countries when these start to reach out to schools beyond the pilot schools*. 'Regionalisation' is seen as a dissemination strategy in several cases. Thus, "regional networks" could even occur within political areas such as Flemish Belgium or Wales. As there is no comparable information or analysis of the various regional networks as of now, the regional level cannot be addressed in this international case study on the *European* Network as a *whole*. However, the country case studies will exemplify such regional arrangements.

But now back to the clarification of the membership status of various ENHPS related key actors as to the European *Network*:

In table 5.1.1 Ministries of Health and of Education are presented as ENHPS 'project' participants and not European Network members for several reasons: a) when 'countries' join, the Ministries are required to provide the infrastructure and means *for* the ENHPS in the country, putting them into a support role; b) it is the National Support Centers (through the National Coordinators) that take part in international level networking 'within' the European Network (business meetings) and are the designated contact points for European actors at national level; c) over time, the IPC increasingly emphasized that the interagency partnership demonstrated at European level needs to be mirrored at national level and particularly points to the cooperation between Health and Education Ministries which also hints at the national Ministries' support rather than membership role. But they can be reasonably seen as part of a multi-level 'ENHPS *project*' as they a) jointly deliver to the International Planning Committee (IPC) the formal application for ENHPS membership of their 'country' and 'pilot schools' and b) are the official members or country representatives in the intergovernmental European agencies that form the IPC (i.e. WHO, Council of Europe, and eventually European Commission).

The terms of reference outlined at international level for **National Advisory Boards** in 'ENHPS countries' include its decision making function with view to the *national* HPS project, accountability towards the Ministries, securing resources from the NSC, support and guidance towards the National Coordinator, and provision of opportunities for expansion of the ENHPS *within their country*. In light of the Boards' strong national focus in HPS development, because the national HPS projects or networks are at international level represented by the National Support Center (the HPS Coordinator) and not e.g. the Presidents of these Advisory Boards, and also because the Boards do not exist in all ENHPS countries (they are optional), it is reasonable to say: National Advisory Boards or similar bodies are part of the *national* HPS projects (or may be even -networks), but are not *European Network members*.

In the light of their international role it seems appropriate to assume that the **National Support Centers** for Health Promoting Schools (HPS) development in countries (or the national HPS project offices therein) are organizational *members* of the European *Network* (represented by the National Coordinators). If this assumption holds, these National Support Centers represent the European *Networks* national level. But whether this also means that these Centers represent what is called 'ENHPS country member' is still a question. They may be the *representatives* of the 'national HPS projects' or '-networks', but the latter as a *whole*, as an own social systems may be the 'ENHPS country member'.

The International Planning Committee (IPC) generally encourages 'ENHPS countries' to develop **national and/or subnational arrangements** that foster from some point in time the expansion of the 'pilot' school network to involve a higher number of schools in the large scale implementation of the Health Promoting Schools (HPS) concept ('dissemination phase'). A variety of structures have been developed in various countries involving also *regional* organizations of some kind, but a systematic or comparative overview of these structures is lacking. However, the main reference framework for action for sub-national/ regional HPS networks or projects are the *national* HPS networks or projects rather than the *European* Network; their collaborations are usually regionally focused as country case studies illustrate.

The Health Promoting Schools (HPS) concept that pilot and associated schools commit to includes the school/community- link; this includes the collaboration with other **local organizations** in support of both the schools change process towards a Health Promoting School and its contribution to the promotion of health of the local community. Here, from the international perspective the 'local organization'/'network school'- relations cannot be addressed further due to lacking data. However, it is already suggested now to define the **schools' local partners** as *external* to the European Network (leaving the option that they may be part of '*national* HPS projects' or '-networks').

So far, the assumptions regarding the European Networks boundaries or membership and related support or sub-systems in its closer environment have been based on mainly the information available on and by the

ENHPS as a *whole;* this favors the international or European perspective in general, and - in light of their leadership role - the ideas, expectations and perspectives of International Planning Committee (IPC) and Technical Secretariat in particular. This leads to the question, what the perspectives are of, for example, the group of National Coordinators as representatives of National Support Centers or the group of 'pilot schools'. For example, do the National Support Centers (or the National Coordinators) see the national HPS project offices as member of the European Network or as some support structure around it? Do the pilot schools identify *themselves* as members of the European Network, or national HPS network or project, or may be both? At international level, only limited information is available on these aspects but a few ENHPS evaluation and documentation efforts provide some valuable insight.

Overall, ENHPS documents and statements of key representatives provide not a clear answer with regard to the European Network's boundaries but rather show a complex organizational system "of and around" the European Network (ENHPS). Within the overall ENHPS initiative, for the so called **first phase or pilot years**, some boundaries have been clearly communicated and stressed: at European level the 'ENHPS *project*' of *the three* major intergovernmental agencies; at *local* level the ENHPS 'pilot schools' (limited to 10-20 per ENHPS country). At *national* level the National Support Centers (through the National Coordinators) were in focus. During the **transition phase** that followed the European actors broadened the attention span with regard to organizational actors, not as much at European as at national and local level: At *national level*, besides the National Support Center the Health and Education Ministries and even other Ministries were brought further into focus; and at local level besides the 'pilot schools' also 'other' schools, plus the schools' organizational neighbors at community level. - This may be conceptualized as fluidity of the borders of the "European Network of Health Promoting schools", or as existence and expansion of subsystems within and/or closely related to this Network. As stressed before, for the purpose of this research project on network assessment a decision will need to be taken on the unit of analysis and proposals have just been made (see table 5.1.1). The following analysis of interactions and relations of and among all key actors will pave the way for a final decision. Special attention will also be paid to the purpose or content of these interactions and relations, for example, *exchange* of information or other resources, *concerted action*, and/or *joint production* of a service or other product. This is done in light of the network typology and network evolution theory by Alter and Hage (1993) and discussed in chapter 2.4.

Interorganisational relations and interactions within and around the ENHPS

For two reasons the relations and interactions among the various organizational actors involved in the ENHPS initiative in some way or the other are being examined here: First, it helps to clarify a step further which key organizations can be reasonably defined as *members* of the European *Network* and which as 'non-members' or external supporters but part of its closest environment (i.e. of a 'ENHPS project'). Second, it will improve the understanding of some interorganisational network features of the European Network to be assessed. As elaborated in chapter 2.4 on interorganisational networks and networking, *features of such networks that influence their performance include relationships or interactions among network members* that: are non-hierarchical or less hierarchical, show lateral linkages, and self-regulation; are informal or formal; and exhibit qualities such as direct person-to-person-connections, trust, mutual benefit and reciprocity (win/win), sharing of information and resources, and a long term perspective - with people and communication put at the center of processes. The mutual sharing of a conceptual framework is important as a base for defining common purpose.

As explained in chapter 4.2 above and illustrated in figure 4.2.1, the study of the interactions and relations at stake follows the following scheme: At each of the systems levels of the ENHPS initiative one organization has been chosen whose relationships with all others will be examined: the *National Support Center* as (assumed) ENHPS member and main link between local and international level; the *pilot schools* as confirmed ENHPS members; and the ENHPS *Technical Secretariat* as the organizational body at *international* level with the most contacts with others and as link between National Support Centers (or 'HPS projects') and International Planning Committee. The examination of the interorganisational relations and interactions within and around the "European Network of Health Promoting Schools" (ENHPS) as a whole but from an **international perspective** attempts to capture **an overall picture;** this draws attention to *patterns* across member countries rather than country specific issues; the regional level is left out (but it is considered in the country case studies below). The information available was somewhat biased with most of it stemming from the 'first phase' of the ENHPS initiative (1992-1995) and the two, three transition years that followed (e.g. Piette et al 1998, w.y., 1999; Parsons et al 1997; WHO/EURO 1998), and almost all school related information refers to the initial 'ENHPS *pilot* schools'. However, for the purpose of this case study - the *pilot testing* of the draft network assessment framework newly developed (chap. 3) - this is not a problem: Overall, from the international perspective and during the time span covered a) the structural set-up and general process features of the *European* Network (as opposed to *country* networks) did not change much; b) the bias is expected to effect the assessment of mainly *one* of the many network features in question: the potential evolutionary step of the network suggested by the Alter/Hage network theory from an exchange to a promotional or even systemic network; and c) the two ENHPS *country* case studies below are complementary and shed light on issues less visible from the international perspective and on the ENHPS as a whole.

I. Interactions and relations of National HPS Support Centers with other organizations

To derive the relevant information on this issue table 5.1.2 served as the 'search scheme'.

NATIONAL SUPPORT CENTERS' interactions and relations with:	organizations within their countries ↓		organizations outside their countries/ European Dimension ↓
'national - local' →	1. HPS: • Pilot HPS • 'other'		
'national - national' →	2. Nat. Adv. Board; Ministries of Health/ of Education;	3. other national organizations or networks	4. other ENHPS 'countries'
'national - international' →			5. IPC & TS
'the part and the whole' →	6. The 'European Network of Health Promoting Schools' as a whole		

Table 5.1.2: Schema of potential interorganisational relationships of the National HPS Support Centers with other organizations within and around the European Network/ ENHPS.

ENHPS: European Network of HPS
HPS: Health Promoting Schools
IPC: International Planning Committee
MoEs: Ministries of Education
MoHs: Ministries of Health
TS: Technical Secretariat

The 'national - local' dimension

In the following, potential links of National HPS Support Centers and local organizations other than network schools are not considered as it are usually the schools which are expected to link up with organizations in their specific communities, not the National Centers. The latter may rather work with national organizations active at local level (not individual school partners locally).

1. National Support Centers and pilot schools within their countries

The National Support Centers' relations with ENHPS 'pilot' schools and others take generally the form of hosting and supporting the National Coordinator's project office. The internationally **predefined roles and responsibilities** of the latter include close and *supportive* interactions with 'pilot' schools and others in the country (from *needs assessment* and *management* regarding the national 'HPS network' or '-project' to disseminating international experiences among network schools. While network schools may perceive themselves as being in contact with their National HPS Coordinator and team rather than a 'National Support Center' it is this Center which is the *organizational backbone and contact point* at national level for all those involved in ENHPS related activities.

The 'control' or feed back mechanisms built in into the European Network mean that *pilot schools report back to the national level* as the latter does towards the European level (annually or more frequent). Network schools have been found to have different, but usually *considerable amounts of freedom* within the overall commitment given when joining the ENHPS. **Good, trustful and empowering relations** between National Centers and pilot schools are indicated by findings of the 'Canterbury' study (Parsons et al 1997): with pilot schools perceiving National Coordinators/ teams as *most accessible and supportive* and *refraining from trying to influence* school projects, and reporting to develop their own direction according to local needs. And in some CEE countries the 'national HPS project' provided a frame for schools to pursue for the first time their own interest without requiring permission from the Ministries. - As to **'soft' networking** between National Centers and pilot schools several means are used: Among 23 ENHPS countries covered in the Data Base in more detail, *meetings* are most common as is *regular* communication via telephone and fax; and *training events* provide additional opportunities in some countries. Several (sub-)national HPS *Newsletters* support networking, too. However, three to five years after the launch of the European Network e-mail or **'hard' networking** - to use Hastings' terms - was not widely realized (with most National Centers being on-line but not pilot schools). (WHO/EURO 1998)

That most of over 200 pilot schools portrayed in the ENHPS Data Base report on 'activities' not only at local but also national level (in the form of national meetings, co-operation between schools, and work on teaching material) indicates: a) that schools engage in 'soft' networking within national ENHPS networks; and b) that *National Support Centers* (which usually organize and guide national HPS activities) are active **facilitators of interorganisational relations or networking with and among pilot schools.** As to the question from whom in their country 'pilot' schools *receive support* a look across the individual school portrays suggests: National Coordinators and thus likely National Support Centers, too, are the *number one supporters for many schools* and provide ideas, guidance, and advice. Most schools feel supported by the Coordinator in various ways, particularly often through the organization and provision of training seminars, meetings, and teaching or other materials, and also by facilitating financial support. However, the data also indicate that some schools may not receive enough support: for example, a number of schools state to receive support from others locally only (and not e.g. from their National Coordinator) and others do not state any 'support received'. (WHO/EURO 1998; Parsons et al 1997; ENHPS Technical Secretariat 1995-2000)

The 'national - national' dimension

2. National Support Centers and the National Advisory Board and/or Ministries of Health and of Education (MoH, MoE) in their countries

The relations and interactions among these key national level actors in developing the European Network are to a certain degree predefined. As said before each country's and school's ENHPS membership depends on the collaborative agreement and commitment of the respective (national) Ministries of Education and of Health, and *National Support Centers* and Coordinators are *designated* by these Ministries. A National Advisory Board, if established, is the decision making body for a 'national HPS project' but the National Center including the National HPS Coordinator may be part of that Board and, thus, *may be involved in national decision making* processes. The National Support Centers are *accountable* to the Advisory Board and/or directly to the Ministries who usually (co-)determine how much staff time and financial resources the National Support Center and/or 'national HPS project' receive. The overall structure and allocation of resources for Health Promotion at governmental levels can be a constraining or enabling factors (see e.g. Parsons et al 1997 and the country case studies below). - As the 'Canterbury study' did show the *requirement for collaboration between Education and Health Ministries* as entry criteria for a country's ENHPS membership can be a key element of success of the European Network, especially in countries where such intersectoral collaboration has not existed before. It *can empower* Support Centers' and legitimize action locally. Top-level, official commitment and ministerial guidance and legislation sympathetic to the European Network can improve the allocation of funds, documented support in government reports and the like, and supportive interdepartmental collaboration even beyond health and education. And *public esteem* in schools and local communities *can consolidate* such top level support. On the other hand, *changes of high level representatives* (such as Ministers) *can destabilize* significantly a 'national HPS project' if no national policy or other written policy documents exist to reinforce its work. (Parsons et al 1997)

Overall, the National Support Centers (and Coordinators) are understood as the main advocates for high level and ministerial support from both the health and education sectors for HPS development in countries. Within the European Network both can be found: countries with sound working relationships between Health, Education and even other Ministries and the National Center, and those where this is not sufficient. As mentioned before lately the ENHPS Technical Secretariat shifted its foci towards remaining challenges in this regard. (Parsons et al 1997; ENHPS 1996, 1997; Burgher et al 1999)

3. National Support Centers and other national organizations and networks within their countries

Several National Support Centers through the National Coordinators succeed in getting funding for specific activities from various national or international organizations such as NGOs, Charities, Foundations or the public agencies. The question whether mid or long-term collaborations have been established with some of those organizations can only be answered case by case. In several cases links exist between *individual* Health Promoting Schools and Healthy Cities, but not as links at national *network* level. Some ENHPS countries have shown that advantages result when the National Support Centers and schools associate themselves with other larger scale health education initiatives. (WHO/EURO 1998; Parsons et al 1997)

4. National Support Centers and other ENHPS member countries

The only consistent pattern of direct networking, experience exchange, discussion and joint decision making among National Support Centers across the European Network is the annual *business meeting* of National Coordinators, ENHPS Technical Secretariat and International Planning Committee. It is generally judged as very important by those involved and stimulates *information sharing and cross-national contacts*. This meeting at European level is complemented by annual information dissemination through the ENHPS Newsletter to whom *all* ENHPS members are *invited to contribute*. Additional **transnational links** among National Support Centers or 'national HPS projects' *vary widely* from few sporadic contacts to systematic and sustained networking in the German-speaking ENHPS sub-network introduced earlier. Between these extremes lie cases of one sided reception of consultations, materials and the like, single joint events, more continuous bi-lateral interactions, and joint activities among *several* ENHPS countries (such as those around the Baltic Sea). Sometimes, the degree of external funding (i.e. from outside a ENHPS country) has acted as trigger, incentive and opportunity for transnational cooperation between National Support Centers (e.g. in the cases of CEE countries). However, *language barriers* are a **counter acting factor** across Europe and so are *geographical distance and travel expenses*. (ENHPS 1996, 1997; Parsons et al 1997; ENHPS Technical Secretariat 199)

Both, twinning arrangements and networks of a limited number of 'national HPS networks' represent *cross-border interorganisational relations* that bring to life the inherent interorganisational network dimension of the European Network with regard to its *national* level. They have a *mid or long* term perspective, and are *voluntary* and *planned* forms of cooperation. They are complemented by twinning among network schools which is addressed below.

With the exception of the important and much valued annual business meetings, the cross-border interactions and relations at the European Network's *national* level appear to be a loose patch work of bilateral and a few multilateral (sometimes outstanding) cooperative links, ad hoc but also on an ongoing basis. As of now, neither an overview nor a systematic analysis of this ENHPS *network level* exists. Beyond business meetings and international training courses for all ENHPS member countries in the early years, this network dimension has not yet received much attention. One evaluation study (the 'Canterbury study'), however, has pointed out that this issue needs further examination (Parsons et al 1997). And it indeed has been reflected upon in the most recent ENHPS project on developing 'ENHPS indicators' which was introduced already in chapter 3 above (ENHPS w.y.). The emergence of the German-speaking *'network within the European Network'* (of national networks on HPS) shows that stronger and longer term relations among National Support Centers across borders are perceived as needed and can be beneficial not only for the national but also sub-national actors (network schools included).

The 'national-international' dimension

5. National Support Centers and the ENHPS Technical Secretariat and International Planning Committee (IPC)

The National Support Centers (through the National Coordinators) have the responsibility to act as contact point within their country for the European level actors (Technical Secretariat/ IPC) and external others. They meet the former at least once a year (*business meetings*) and actively participate in decision making and needs oriented planning regarding the European Network as a *whole*. (IPC 1993; Burgher et al 1999) *Further contacts and collaboration* of particular National Centers and the Technical Secretariat *vary widely*. Some Centers have a *few exchanges* of information per year only while others actively participate in *joint creations* of ENHPS products or services (e.g. pilot testing of manuals and tools) (Parsons et al 1997; see also the country case studies below). Between these extremes lie interorganisational *relations of various degrees*. All Centers have recurring opportunities to contribute to the networking within the European Network (e.g. via the annual ENHPS Newsletter) complemented by exceptional collaboration opportunities for National Center and Technical Secretariat such as around the 'First (and soon second) ENHPS Conference'.

Invitations by the Technical Secretariat to National Support Centers to publicly share experiences and case studies, the regular reports required of the National Centers by the European level, as well as other requests for information (such as for the ENHPS Schools Data Base) *may or may not* trigger or inspire bi-directional information exchange and collaboration between National Centers and Technical Secretariat. While the latter contacts the over 40 National Centers several times per year on some issue or another and the joint business meetings are a 'must', *it depends on the individual National Center to further build and maintain interactions* with the ENHPS Technical Secretariat as desired or needed.

6. National Support Centers and the "European Network of Health Promoting Schools" (ENHPS) as a whole

The National Support Centers (through the National HPS Coordinators or teams) are the organization that, in practical terms and day-to-day operations of their national HPS networks, represent the 'country' members of the European Network. In spite of country specific variations it seems that within the European Network as a whole (at least during the pilot years) the National Centers have a central role: They sustained *interorganisational interactions and relations* with the recognized ENHPS school members, the *'pilot schools'*. In several cases this applies also to 'non-pilot' schools that joined a national network later. National Centers have *lateral* links amongst each other (business meetings) and, thus, form an interorganisational international information *'exchange network'* to say the least. As to the European level of the ENHPS initiative, National Support Centers critical reflected upon and 'softened' guidance provided in some cases (such as the '12 criteria of a Health Promoting Schools' predefined by the ENHPS initiators). With *all* those involved, they jointly created a new guidance document for the European Network, the "10 principles" laid out in the ENHPS Resolution 1997. In addition, several National Centers have established bilateral, a few also *multi*-lateral interorganisational relations, and some have even formed an interorganisational network with each other (as part of their initiative to network the 'national HPS networks'. The sophisticated example is the network of German-speaking 'HPS networks' which is not only a loose information *exchange* but a joint *action* network that started to co-produce, for example, a preliminary assessment and position paper on the ENHPS (Sub-regional network... 1995).

The National Support Centers and the European Network - intermediate synthesis and discussion

Against this background, it is reasonable to confirm the assumption made earlier, that also the *National Support Centers* and not only pilot schools are organizational *'members'* of the European *Network* on Health Promoting Schools (ENHPS). In general, they share and act on the common goal of creating Health Promoting Schools (HPS), seem to have trustful relations and regularly interact with the ENHPS Technical Secretariat as well as the pilot schools, engage in joint decision making as to the European Network as a whole, and have exchange relations with each other. - In comparison to this, the *Ministries* of Health and of Education are key participants in national ENHPS or HPS *'projects'* (not the European and/or national HPS networks). They are core actors in the networks' closer *environment:* they commit themselves to its goals (for three years at least); the European Network in countries is resource dependent on them; and they do not regularly interact in mutuality with ENHPS Technical Secretariat, schools and each other across borders. Thus, it seems reasonable to understand the National Support Centers as *members* of the overall European *Network* (for the development) of HPS, and the national *Ministries* as participants of the overall 'ENHPS *project'*. As illustrated in figure 5.1.6, the picture emerging is one of a **European Network with *two* types of members: National HPS Support Centers and Health Promoting (pilot) Schools**. The ENHPS 'project' is not a mono- but *multi*-level system encompassing not only the international actors (IPC/ ENHPS Secretariat) but also national level actors (Health/ Education Ministries) - and possibly sooner or later even local level authorities.

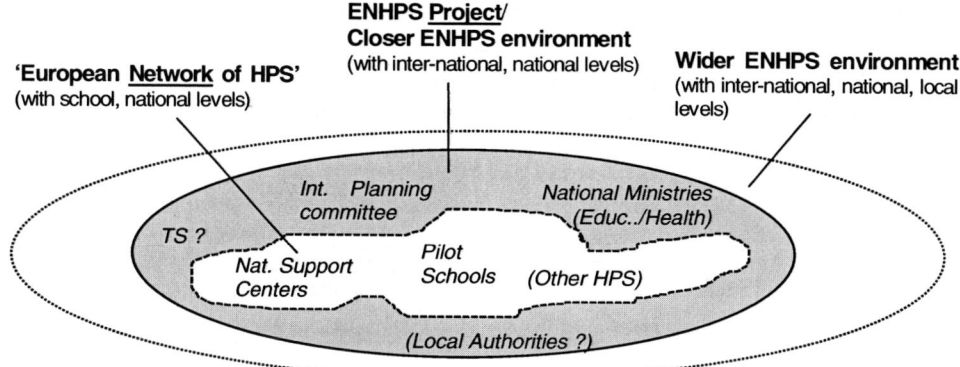

Figure 5.1.7: Re-conceptualizing the ENHPS initiative: a) in the European *Network* at least *two* types of organizational members (not one) cutting across at least *two* systems levels; b) in the 'ENHPS *project*' key actors at *several* levels (not only the international).

ENHPS:	"European Network (for the development) of Health Promoting Schools"	Int.:	International
		Nat.:	National
Educ.:	Education	TS:	ENHPS Technical Secretariat
HPS:	Health Promoting School(s)		

In light of the direct relations and interactions of the ENHPS Technical Secretariat with the National Support Centers the question arises whether this Secretariat is to be considered as ENHPS supporter or Network member. A common goal exists but are the relations based on mutuality and exchange? For now, this remains an open question.

After this elaboration of the interorganisational relations and interactions of National HPS Support Centers attention is drawn to those of the core ENHPS members, the 'pilot schools'.

II. Interactions and relations among health promoting 'pilot schools' and of those with other organizations

Similarly to the previous section, the relevant information has been derived by using a 'search scheme' as shown in table 5.1.3.

PILOT SCHOOLS' interactions/ relationships with:	organizations within the country ↓		organizations <u>outside</u> the country/ the European Dimension ↓
'local - local' →	1. other schools/ HPS: • other pilot HPS • schools 'linked'/ 'associated' to the ENHPS	2. local organizations in their community: • medical health care • others	3. schools outside the country • other (Health Promoting) Schools • other transnational school networks/ projects
'local - national' →	4. national ENHPS actors • NSC • NAB, MoH, MoE	5. other networks/ projects	
'local- international'→			6. Int. ENHPS actors • Secretariat (TS) • IPC
'the part & the whole' →	7. The European Network of HPS as a whole		

Table 5.1.3: Schema of potential interorganisational relationships of the ENHPS pilot schools with other key organizations within and around the ENHPS

ENHPS:	European Network of Health Promoting Schools	NSC:	National HPS Support Center
HPS:	Health Promoting Schools	MoEs:	Ministries of Education
IPC:	International Planning Committee	MoHs:	Ministries of Health
Int.:	International	TS:	Technical Secretariat

At *international* level there is only one information source with information systematically collected across countries: the "ENHPS Schools Data Base 1998", a publicly accessible online data bank created by the Technical Secretariat jointly with the National Coordinators and ENHPS pilot schools (see WHO/EURO 1998). This is the main reference for this section; additional others were used as indicated in the text. This ENHPS Schools Data Base, in the following briefly referred to as 'the Data Base', currently contains 219 portrays of mainly pilot schools from 22 national networks, i.e. about 40% of all pilot schools from roughly 60% of all 'ENHPS countries' are covered. Although not randomly selected, the portrays provide a better understanding and valuable insights into the realities, diversity and also commonalties that can be found among both pilot *schools* and their *national networks*. When reading across all portrays from an *interorganisational* research perspective much exciting information on the health promoting work of pupils, school staff and others *within* their schools had to be left aside; but it should be said that in spite of their variety the long list of activities at the local, regional, national and international levels points to some unifying themes and about five projects categories: the school's physical environment, health-related topics (AIDS, nutrition,...), building democracy in schools, policy development, and development of teacher training materials (Burgher et al 1999 p7). While school's worked in some or all of these action areas they engaged in relations and interactions with local, national and international organizations as follows.

The 'local - local' dimension - from neighborhood to neighbor countries

1. ENHPS pilot schools among each other, and with other schools in their countries

One of the aims of the ENHPS is for health promoting 'pilot schools' not only to *develop* but to *exchange* and *disseminate* information about *good practice* within the country and beyond. The ENHPS Data Base shows that almost all of the over 200 pilot schools from 22 countries undertake activities not only at school but also national level, with two of three activity categories clearly indicating interactions *among* pilot schools and often mentioned in combination: About three quarters participate in national 'meetings'; and about half are involved in 'cooperation between schools'.

It should be noted that national meetings and conferences have their limits as means for inter-school networking for experience exchange and mutual learning, for reasons such as the limited number of staff per school that may be able to attend, and depending on opportunities for participants to share their knowledge with their school community at home (Parsons et al 1997). In addition, national meetings tend to be less frequent per year because of travel costs and geographical distance in many cases. However, they have also been an effective means of network building in countries (e.g. Slovenia). From the organizational sciences it is known that face-to-face meetings are important to establish sustainable and productive interorganisational relations or networks; but the supportive function and potential of e-mail (or 'hard' networking to use Hastings terms) is known, too. It may well be that the vision of a *European* network *of schools* may only come true once a good balance is reached between inter-school collaboration at local and regional level, twinning across borders, national and trans-national meetings, and computer links. The German case study presented later draws particular attention to this issue. However, the main issue remains the *common purpose* around which schools may network and over time, this may need further specification beyond the general notion of 'developing Health Promoting Schools' - as experienced and successfully done in Healthy Cities Networks by means of Multi City Action Plans (see chap. 2.2.6).

Relations and interactions of *pilot schools and 'other' schools* in the same country vary as much as approaches to disseminate the HPS concept vary between countries. Therefore, this issue needs to be taken up in individual country case studies as done later on. As said before the originators of the European Network have laid out high expectations towards the ENHPS pilot schools: they should act as key players when their national HPS project moves from pilot to dissemination phase; they should give their experiences and knowledge to other schools, and also to their local communities and all levels of the health and education sectors. School health promotion in 'ENHPS countries' has been found to often spread from school to school, and also through local networks; and key people in national HPS networks frequently identified the increased school-to-school relations and exchange as 'success' of the European Network in their country (Piette et al 1999).

2. 'Pilot schools' and other organizations in their local community

As explained before, the schools' commitment to the Health Promoting Schools (HPS) concept includes the improvement of links with other organizations in their local communities, to promote the health of the school community but also that of the local community as a whole. Strengthened school-community links have been identified as one of the remaining challenges for the 'second phase' of the European Network. In accordance with their mission, all 'Health Promoting Schools' (HPS) covered in the ENHPS Data Base have planned to impact on the health of members of their school community (usually pupils, and teachers, but also parents) which usually leads schools to focus first on co-determinants of health *within* or directly related to the school. But in addition, some of these pilot schools have already planned to impact also on the wider 'local community', and some of them report first success. This indicates that 'HPS in the making' may first tend to establishing networking 'within' their school, before turning towards networking 'with others' locally. However, for about two thirds of the 219 schools covered in the Data Base *medical health services* are part of their 'HPS project'. This does not necessarily mean that these schools practice interorganisational collaboration with local medical or school health services, as school nurses or other health professionals may be part of the school staff, or just visit for the routine services to be provided to all schools by law (screening, dental care,...).

With regard to partners locally, parents are perhaps the most frequent and important groups but pilot schools also have inter*organisational* relations (Burgher et al 1999). Asked for 'support' received from others, most pilot schools mention their National Coordinator and many 'medical staff'; a variety of 'others' is less often mentioned, but if, then this refers to local *organizations* and often to a whole range of them. The number of active local agents available for support varies between countries and between schools in the same country, and also their power and access to resources varies (see e.g. Parsons et al 1997). The opening up of pilot schools towards their local communities has been frequently identified as 'success' by key people in ENHPS countries in the EU (Piette et al 1999).

The findings suggest that in general, within the European Network interorganisational links between Health Promoting Schools and local communities need strengthening. However, individual success stories are encouraging signs of development, particularly when considering the big organizational development challenges most schools are facing when starting to implement the HPS concept, and also in light of the traditionally high degree of insulation between schools and local communities pointed out by Parsons et al (1997). *Diversity in interorganisational school-community links* or -

from the European Network perspective in networking 'with local others' - will remain the 'common characteristic', because HPS development as other development effort in countries need to build on the specific local circumstances and needs.

3. Pilot schools and schools outside their country

As to this aspect of networking 'within' the European Network the ENHPS Data Base shows that (about four, five years after the launch of the ENHPS) many pilot schools were undertaking activities with an international or European dimension. Cross-border inter-school relations ranged from the *exchange* of information or materials to that of teachers and/or pupils to mid or long term *'twinning'* arrangements with another school. In almost 40 cases twinning had been established or was being prepared. Whether the schools linked up with are also ENHPS network schools is not known but within the European Network members are actively encouraged to twin (and specific channels towards funding are provided). Several network schools are also members of other transnational initiatives, for example, by UNESCO or the EU, including those on cultural exchange, peace, and 'Europe against cancer'.

When looking at these findings, it can be said that the involvement of 40 pilot schools out of overall roughly 500 in often cross-border 'twinning' arrangements represents a significant extent of formally established bi-lateral inter-school- relations within the European Network. That with view to the European Network as a whole the majority of pilot schools do obviously not (yet) engage in such cross-border school-to-school twinning in support of Health Promoting School (HPS) development is not surprising: On the one hand, the implementation of the HPS concept in each pilot school alone - the main aim of the European Network during its first years - is an organizational, school development innovation that takes time and binds attention and energy of all those involved. On the other hand, the innovation taken up by all ENHPS pilot schools to do the above in *mutual learning with other* pilot schools in a European Network context is for various reasons usually approached within *national* 'HPS networks' or '-projects'; and this *second* innovation likely binds already a pilot school's time and energy for interorganisational relations or networking. In the light of this, the existing 'twinning' among ENHPS pilot schools definitely reflects a remarkable degree of realization of networking 'within' the European Network, the so called 'European dimension'. But it is questionable whether it also represents a first step towards realizing the overall vision of a "European *Network of* Health Promoting Schools" - at least if 'interorganisational networks' as discussed in chapter 2.4 are in mind.

However, as of now *interactions and relations of pilot schools* with other organizations at *local* level have been addressed, with all respect to the limitations of the data available. As the assessment of the European Network as a *whole* remains the goal (to test the network assessment framework developed) this examination has yet to be extended to the national level.

The 'local - national' dimension

4. Pilot schools and ENHPS actors at national level

Pilot schools can only enter the ENHPS when selected by the national level. Their relations with national actors will be influenced by the way this selection process was shaped. The limited information available indicates that an open invitation approach with a competitive selection process is fairly common, that some countries 'hand pick' schools at regional level, and also random selection can be found. From the interorganisational research perspective important is whether schools joined the European Network *voluntarily* or were obliged to do so. The former can be assumed in light of the kind of guidance provided by the International Planning Committee and Technical Secretariat to countries (see above). That drop out at school level is no issue confirms this assumption (see Piette et al 1999).

Relations and interactions of pilot schools with the *National Support Centers* have been addressed already in section A above and will be further exemplified through the two country case studies later on. With regard to the *National Advisory Board, Ministries* of Health and of Education it is usually the *National Support Center* that serves as a kind of *'spokes person' for the pilot schools* and other health promoting schools in the country. Of course, all schools have their more or less indirect links to their Ministry of Education through the country specific channels within the education sector. But the National Support Centers (through the national HPS project teams) are the core partners of European Network schools at national level. And as an increasing number of countries has moved beyond pilot phase into a dissemination stage often *Regional* Support Centers have become the main HPS network partner of schools at levels above the local.

5. Pilot schools and 'other' national networks or projects

Pilot schools' relations with projects or networks outside the European Network represent interactions between the ENHPS and its environment. Remarkable is a link repeatedly found between Health Promoting Pilot Schools and Healthy Cities Networks in Europe. The ENHPS Data Base shows such links in about 15% of the cases covered, spread over 13 countries. In two countries, half or even more of all pilot schools identified themselves as Healthy City Network members. Also in light of 'EVA 2' study results it can be assumed that in Europe the two health promoting Settings networks (Healthy Cities and Health Promoting Schools) are linked in *individual* cases at local level rather than at national or European network level, - although both networks benefit from leadership and administrative support of the same international agency, WHO/EURO. In this sense, the *European Network* (for the development) of Health Promoting Schools (ENHPS) seems yet to be much *inward oriented*, but the same applies to other Settings networks, too. In several ENHPS countries a lack of links between national or regional HPS networks and other school health promotion projects or networks has been found (Piette et al 1999). The 'Canterbury' study (Parsons et al 1997) indicates that the involvement of network schools in other national projects helps to strengthen the work in their own HPS projects.

The 'local - international' dimension

6. Pilot schools and the international actors of the European Network or 'ENHPS project'

As shown in chapter 5.1.3 the contacts of national HPS networks or projects with the ENHPS Technical Secretariat are usually exercised by the National Support Centers, not by network schools themselves. *As at the national level, also at international level the National Support Center (via the Coordinator) is the voice* of the health promoting network schools; and the Coordinators' contact or networking partner at European level is the Technical Secretariat who is the bridge to the International Planning Committee (EC, CE, WHO/EURO).

"The parts and the whole"

7. Pilot schools and the "European Network of Health Promoting Schools" (ENHPS) as a whole

As elaborated before, the vision set out by the ENHPS initiators is the creation of a *network of 'Health Promoting Schools' (HPS) throughout Europe*, but starting off with a limited number of 'ENHPS pilot schools'. First, these were to develop - *in mutual learning* - good practice of Health Promotion in the school setting (*demonstrations site function*) and then - in a second step - to become *active disseminators* of the HPS concept as to both *other* schools (support of good practice development) and even in the education sector as a whole. Obviously, the combination of *both* the health promoting Settings approach and some kind of 'network for mutual learning' approach genuinely means very high expectations of *all* those involved towards a) the ENHPS 'pilot schools', but also b) those that encouraged them to go down this route. Without saying, European Commission, Council of Europe and WHO/EURO have invited pilot schools together with national level actors, first and foremost the National Support Centers, to create *interorganisational* networks, i.e. to try out an *innovative organizational form* to reach the common goal of creating Health Promoting Schools (HPS) throughout Europe. Thus, *all* those involved in the **ENHPS initiative**, pilot schools included, face **two significant innovations at the same time**:

1. the 'health promoting Settings' approach at *school* level, an innovation meaning organizational/school development and touching the core of education systems in countries;
2. the *inter*organisational *network* (ION) approach, to implement the first innovation in mutual learning and on a larger scale throughout Europe.

And obviously from all organizations involved the **pilot schools are those most concerned** by both because as the first innovation directly applies to themselves (*their* transformation into a 'Health Promoting School'). The Health Promoting Settings approach includes challenges of organizational development in most if not all school cases, and inevitably will feed back into the education sector as a whole the more schools transform themselves into 'Health Promoting Schools'. Thus, within the European Network over the long term the (pilot) network schools could indeed play a key role in influencing the network's closer institutional environment: the education systems in countries. But the national level actors or network members have a crucial role, too.

However, as to **the 'network dimension' of the European Network** the data available indicate that *interorganisational collaboration is not (yet) a main focus of ENHPS 'pilot schools'*, at least during their first years of development (before HPS related dissemination becomes an issue). The several 'snapshots' taken of smaller or bigger Network parts at different points in time, mainly at the end of the European Network's 'first phase' and during the transition years that followed, indicate (see ENHPS Data Base/WHO-EURO 1998; 'Canterbury' study/ Parsons et al 1997; and 'EVA 2' study/

Piette et al 1999): **Pilot schools** show a 'pattern of diversity' with regard to their ***self-identification as members*** of the *European* Network and/or their *national* HPS 'project' or 'network'. While the European level actors define all 'pilot schools' as *core members of the ENHPS*, several years after the Network's launch a significant number of pilot schools did *not* identify themselves as such: While most pilot schools from 23 countries covered in the Data Base did identify themselves as *either* national *or* European HPS Network member, many did *not* (with a ratio of roughly 3:2). But *among those who did state membership* in a HPS network or project, the vast *majority* identified themselves as *European* Network member (solely or combined with national membership). Double membership (European/ national) was expressed as often as sole European membership. - A look by ENHPS countries did show that several years after the launch of the ENHPS in several cases **a mixed pattern of network related identification** of pilot schools existed: with some stating membership in the *national* HPS project, some in the *European* Network, and some *both*. In other ENHPS countries, pilot schools did not identify with *any* HPS network or project yet; in one country the *Healthy Cities* network was the main reference network; in the host country of the first ENHPS Conference the *sole* identification with the European Network was remarkable. - Recognizing this insufficient level of identification as European Network member among 'ENHPS pilot schools' of the time the European level planned for a public relations campaign (ENHPS 1996, 1997).

Further insight into the extent to which ENHPS 'pilot schools' fulfill their role as *members* of the overall "European *Network* of Health Promoting Schools" provides a look at their activities undertaken in interorganisational collaboration: All of the over 200 pilot schools covered in the ENHPS Data Base reported on HPS activities directed at their school community (i.e. *inward oriented* action) but at the same time almost all engaged in what Hastings (1993) has called *'soft' networking* among each other and with their National Support Center within country borders (national meetings etc.). In light of the general tendency of schools towards insulation (Parsons et al 1997) this can be interpreted as a *remarkable extent of realization of the network approach* of the ENHPS initiative at its school level by member country. And such interorganisational linking or networking has even been found *across* country borders: Several pilot schools (particularly those that in several ways are nationally involved) have also cross-border exchanges or twinning arrangements which indicates that within the European Network there is indeed some potential for realizing not only a national but *European* network dimension at school level.

The Health Promoting (pilot) Schools and the European Network - intermediate synthesis and discussion

As of now it can be summarized that the limited information available at international level on the *'pilot school' level of the European Network* indicates an encouraging extent of interorganisational collaboration among pilot schools *and* with National Support Centers - in Hastings' terms this refers to the *networking 'within'* the European Network as to its local and national levels. The findings support the earlier assumption that - from an interorganisational network research perspective - not only the (pilot) schools but also the National HPS Support Centers have to be considered as *members* of the so called "European Network 'of' Health Promoting Schools" (ENHPS). The ENHPS is an *interorganisational* European network not 'of' but *'for the development of'* Health Promoting Schools (HPS). This clarification of the European Network's borders from an interorganisational research perspective is the base needed for addressing other network assessment issues, for example, the extent of networking 'within' this European Network: As of now it remains unclear whether ENHPS pilot schools indeed form an interorganisational *network* within and across country borders as implied in the idea of the "European Network *of* Health Promoting Schools" and in the sense of "interorganisational networks" elaborated in chapter 2.4. Also the *quality* of the various interorganisational interactions and relations remains a question, particularly as to actors at national and sub-national levels. Also Health Promotion related issues such as the extent to which interorganisational *school-community-links* are realized (a genuine part of the HPS concept) remain unanswered. As 'diversity' has been generally found to be a 'common characteristic' as to various ENHPS dimensions, only ENHPS *country* case studies promise to provide some answers.

To shed some light on the open issue of the role of the international ENHPS Technical Secretariat within or around the European Network its interactions and relations with key actors remains to be examined, before the planned 'synthesizing analysis I' on network *structure and processes* can meaningfully begin. As documents often do not distinguish between Technical Secretariat and International Planning Committee (IPC) to various others, both will be addressed in the following and last section of this *overall* 'basic case study' on the European Network as a whole.

III. The international level actors of the ENHPS initiative and other organizations within and around the European Network

Documents on the European Network initiative as a whole are usually written by the two main European level actors, the International Planning Committee (IPC) and ENHPS Technical Secretariat, and a distinction between positions of the one or the other have not been found. The relations and interactions of the IPC (with WHO/EURO, European Commission and Council of Europe) and the ENHPS Technical Secretariat with the (assumed) European Network members at national and local level have been already addressed: as to the 'National Support Centers' in section A above, as to the 'pilot schools' in section B - but from the perspectives of the national and local actors, not the European. That of the latter is taken now.

IPC and Technical Secretariat have often been the *originators and 'transmitters'* of a package of innovations that representatives of countries - as Parsons phrased it - are *'invited* to contract in' (Parsons et al 1997). From the start, **with view to the overall**

ENHPS initiative the three European agencies as **IPC members** saw themselves as the *'leading organizations'* (that set the broad course, raise funds, etc.) with view to both National Support Centers and network schools, i.e. the organizational ENHPS *members* identified so far. The IPC never intended to engage in direct *continuous* interactions or networking with the latter. This was left to and done by the Technical Secretariat at least regarding the National Centers. From an interorganisational network research perspective this suggests that the **Technical Secretariat**, too, may reasonably be interpreted as organizational ENHPS *member* - in contrast to the IPC which remains an external partners and supporter in the network's closest environment.

With view to important **organizations in the European Network's environment**, *two* systems levels have to be considered. First, as to the **national level**, the IPC members (rather than the Technical Secretariat as such) have their formal relations to the *Ministries* of Health and of Education in 'ENHPS countries' and, thus, direct links to key organizations shaping the closest environment of the ENHPS *within countries* (see chap. 5.1.1). But the information available gives rise to the thought that during the European Network's first developmental phase, once that various Ministers had signed the initial 3-year-agreement on their countries' formal ENHPS membership, neither IPC nor Technical Secretariat pursued regular ENHPS-related interactions with the ensemble of Ministries concerned. Only during the European Network's 'transition phase' identified above attention was shifted back to these important actors (see chap. 5.1.4). Second, as to the **international level**, relations and interactions of the European actors with 'others' in the European Network's environment have hardly been an issue. Only at the very beginning of the ENHPS initiative, the three initiating agencies invited 'others' to join their 'ENHPS project' but it remained a tripartite endeavor. Overt time the Technical Secretariat started to actively encourage 'ENHPS countries' to join the WHO led HBSC-initiative (Health Behavior in School-aged Children surveys). Already earlier ENHPS specific evaluation projects such as the 'Canterbury study' and 'EVA 2' resulted in recommendations including *more* interorganisational relations of the ENHPS project with other *international* organizations, projects or programs (such as UNESCO, other 'Health Promoting Settings'- networks and school health related projects). (Piette et al 1998, 1999, w.y.; Parsons et al 1997; Barnekow-Rasmussen 1997; Wold 1996) - The latter is yet to be realized.

In recent years, International Planning Committee and ENHPS Technical Secretariat started to strive for some changes that also relate to their relation with the National Support Centers (see Burgher et al 1999): The **Technical Secretariat** wishes to shift some tasks in support of the 'networking within' the European Network to the **National Support Centers** (organizing business meetings/ editing the Newsletter). While keeping up its *support* function towards the National Centers it would shift its focus towards new challenges identified during the transition years such as the renewal or strengthening of the commitment to the ENHPS initiatives goals at governmental level. For the Technical Secretariat this means an *intended shift from 'networking within'* the European Network *to 'networking with external others'* at governmental level where needed; for the National Support Centers this means an expected expansion of responsibilities as to the 'networking within' the European Network as a *whole* (i.e. beyond their countries). Information on how far this has been realized has not been found. However, IPC and Technical Secretariat via 'twinning programs' continue their support of 'networking within' the ENHPS at the level of both network schools *and* National Support Centers. - Overall, interactions between ENHPS Technical Secretariat and **(other) network members** represent *'international-national'* rather than *'international-local'* links: Established is a certain degree of networking with the ensemble of National Support Centers; direct links or visits to individual network schools are sporadic only. The latter may nevertheless be crucial to avoid that the European level looses touch with the *core* network members, the schools, i.e. the only places where the Network goal of creating 'Health Promoting Schools' can be achieved.

As to the **quality of interactions and relations within and around the European Network** (for the development) of Health Promoting Schools (HPS), the International Planning Committee (IPC) and Technical Secretariat have formulated expectations. Less has been said on quantitative aspects such as frequency and types or numbers of interacting parties. The **motto "partnerships as method and goal"** is emphasized. It should *enable schools* to determine their needs and work to meet them in their own ways.

"To prevent duplication of efforts and to provide a framework within which to foster and sustain innovation, disseminate models of good practice and make opportunities for Health Promotion in schools more equitably available throughout Europe, the ENHPS requires *cooperation at and between every level* of European society (international, national, regional and local) and *within and between several sectors* (particularly education and health)" (Burgher et al 1999 p5 italics not in original). The tripartite **International Planning Committee**, the *key* external partner, sponsor and supporter of the ENHPS, presents itself as a *role model* in 'interagency collaboration' for HPS development that should be mirrored in countries. However, during the ENHPS transition years Scicluna (1997) from the European Council rightly pointed out that the *intersectoral* collaboration expected and practiced between *national* health and education ministries in ENHPS member countries needs yet to be matched at *international* level. There, it is still the *health* sector that carries out the 'ENHPS project' - although EC and CE also encompass education and other relevant sectors. The **partnership attitude** of the IPC is nevertheless put into practice as reflected, for instance, in the *joint planning and decision making* with National Coordinators and Technical Secretariat (business meetings) and *demonstrated flexibility* with regard to changes by network members of cornerstones or rules of the game set our by the IPC at the beginning of 'their project'. Examples of the latter include letting go of the criticized "12 criteria of a Health Promoting School" as guiding 'standard', and accepting more than one independent HPS network per ENHPS country.

Already now, from an *international* and interorganisational *network* perspective and on the basis of the above analysis of interactions and relations among the various organizational actors within and around the European Network (ENHPS), the following can be summarized: For long, the European Network (for the development) of Health Promoting Schools has been quite *inward oriented*, i.e. focused on two types of organizational network *members*: National HPS Support Centers and ENHPS pilot schools. This applies clearly to the European level of the European Network or ENHPS initiative, and *in general* also to national and local levels. However, in light of the limited data available at international level (on [groups of] ENHPS countries and their 'national HPS projects' or '-networks') the latter needs surely further examination country by country. The only remarkable '*outward* oriented' activities identified so far are those of the three ENHPS initiators and Technical Secretariat to recruit new ENHPS 'country' members, and may be the 1st ENHPS Conference held and evaluation studies that interviewed external others. Latest plans express intentions to pay more attention to the Network's closer environment *in countries*, particularly the education sector.

Another remarkable finding refers to the European Network's closest environment at *international* level: the far reaching *stability* of the so called tripartite "ENHPS project". Its core actors, structural set-up and operational processes have been hardly changed, i.e. a) the troika of the WHO Regional Office for Europe (WHO/EURO), European Council (CE) and Commission of the European Union (CE) as long term partners in the International Planning Committee (IPC) and key network sponsors, supported by the ENHPS Technical Secretariat; as well as b) the strong and sustained emphasis on partnership approaches and use of joint planning and decision making mechanisms (business meetings) with view to the representatives of the European Network's sub-systems in 'ENHPS countries' (the 'national HPS projects' or '-networks'). Only the emphasis on the *network* approach seems to have faded since the ENHPS initiative left its first three (pilot) years behind and entered into a transition phase to identify the way forward towards the desired large scale dissemination of the HPS concept to all European schools; at least some uncertainty arose in this regard.

There are other issues worth discussing but these will be addressed in the synthesizing analyses that follow. This applies also to open questions such as the that of the nature of ENHPS 'country members', the network membership or not of the ENHPS Technical Secretariat, and whether the distinction found at European level between the network supportive 'ENHPS *project*' and European *Network itself* holds also at national level or below.

Now, that the overall 'basic case study' of the "European Network (for the development) of Health Promoting Schools" has been finalized, i.e. the first major step in the 3-step-case study approach chosen for this research project, the way is paved for the second step, the 'synthesizing analysis I': As said in chapter 4, a **more specific pilot application of the ION assessment framework** will examine distinct features of network structure and processes.

5.2 Synthesizing analysis I - Structural and process features of the ENHPS

The previous chapter on interactions and relations of key actors has laid the final ground for a synthesizing analysis of the European Network's core features in terms of those identified in the ION assessment framework developed in chapter 3. As explained earlier (in chap. 4), in this 'synthesizing analysis I' the focus is on *selected elements* of the network assessment framework proposed: **The emphasis is on distinct basic, structural and process features of the network from an interorganizational network research perspective** (not on the network's functioning as a *whole*). As such, this part of the ENHPS case study concentrates on the declared foci of this network research project whose goal is to develop a practical instrument that helps to assess networks 'in terms of both structures and processes' (chap. 1).

A look back to overview figure 3.1.1 on the ION assessment framework and its partial presentation in figure 4.2.2 helps to keep the 'overall picture' in mind and at the same time quickly grasp the selection of foci made for this step of framework application: a) membership/ network borders; b) network structure (size/ complexity/ differentiation/ connectivity/ centrality); c) operational processes (methods of coordination); d) purpose of interactions within the network e) perceived effectiveness/ levels of conflict; f) the network's networking 'with others' and the relation of networking 'within'/'with others'; g) the network's 'hard' networking, means of 'soft' networking, and the relation of 'hard'/'soft'-networking; h) geographical distance among network members; i) (self-)reflection/ observation/ evaluation processes and feed back loops within the network; and j) "organizational networking" of network *schools*. Thus, that part of the network assessment framework will be tested that contains most of the base line indicators on networks. But 'satisfaction' of network actors (as an outcome) will be already addressed, too. - Thus, this 'synthesizing analysis I' of the European Network will reflect a combination of the Alter/Hage network theory and Hastings' model of organizations capable of networking (see chap. 2.4). The first crucial step to do is taking the *final decision on the unit of analysis* of this research project, i.e. on the European Network *borders*.

5.2.1 Membership or borders of the European Network (for the development) of Health Promoting Schools (ENHPS)

In chapter 3 interorganizational networks have been defined as based on *trustful* relationships, as bounded clusters of organizations that, by definition, are non- or less central collectives of legally separate, laterally linked units. It has been pointed out that network boundaries are co-defined defined by the *quality* of the interorganizational *relationships* and not just formal institutional status. Qualities such as the extent of reliance on mutuality, feed back, and joint decision making, and factors known to create far reaching and sustainable change in complex social systems (consensus orientation, accountability, participation, etc.) have been underlined. If one not only takes formal 'membership status' or position as the criteria for defining who is member of the "European Network (for the development) of Health Promoting Schools" and who is not but also the quality of interactions and relations among various actors and their commitment and action on the network's vision and goal then the following interpretative summary can be given:

As assumed before, the "ENHPS" has never been a pure "Network *'of'* Health Promoting Schools" but a network 'for the *development* of' Health Promoting Schools (HPS): This is already indicated by the term 'ENHPS *country* member' used (in addition to ENHPS pilot schools) and for which formal ENHPS specific membership criteria are applied. Whether the term 'ENHPS *country*' refers to a) the whole *sub-system* of the European Network created *within a country* due to ENHPS membership or b) the *national* level such as the Ministries of Education and of Health that signed an agreement on joint action for national infrastructures in support of ENHPS pilot schools - a precondition of 'their' country's ENHPS membership - remains unclear. And even as to the ENHPS *sub-systems in countries* (point a) there is the question of distinction between so called 'national HPS *projects*' and 'HPS *networks*'. The overall case study of the ENHPS initiative from the international and interorganizational network research perspective in chapter 5.1 has shown:

In practice (as to concrete activities, interactions and relations of core actors) the so-called "European Network of Health Promoting Schools" (ENHPS) is a unique inter-*organizational* network rather than a 'country network' as typically known in intergovernmental development work. And not only the ENHPS (pilot) schools are European *Network members* (as formal documents announce) but also the National HPS *Support Centers* that are required of all participating 'countries'. Among all important ENHPS related actors identified these *Centers* are the key inter-actors or exchange agents with almost *all* other groups of actors in the pursuit of the Network's goal: the creation of 'a group of' model- Health Promoting Schools across Europe that later on disseminate their experiences and good practice developed to more and more schools. In comparison the National Support Centers, national *Ministries* of Health and of Education are generally spoken in the role of key sponsors and political supporters as to ENHPS activities *within* their countries (at least they formally committed themselves to do so for at least the first three years of ENHPS membership). Thus, the Ministries play at *national* level a role complementary to the financial and political supporters at *international* level, i.e. to the members of the *International Planning Committee* (IPC) WHO/EURO, European Commission and Council of Europe. The examination of roles and responsibilities, actions and interactions of the latter confirmed their self-stated position as ENHPS supporters outside the European Network, i.e. in the closer *network environment*. Unfortunately, the position of the ENHPS *Technical Secretariat* as to European Network membership or not remains a border line case: It regularly interacts with one of the two groups of ENHPS members identified: the National Support Centers. It does so, too, with the Network's closest *international environment*, the IPC, but *not* with the second group of ENHPS members, the (pilot) schools. Since the launch of the European Network it not only organized the two major mechanisms for *networking 'within'* the European Network at large (business meetings/ Newsletter) but also *engaged* in networking as network members did. Most recently it reconfirmed its 'supportive' role towards the National Coordinators but clearly expressed the intention to shift its focus - in Hastings' terms - *from networking 'within'* the ENHPS (which should be taken over by the group of National Support Centers) *to linking up 'with external others'* (those that shape the Network's policy *environment* within countries). (Burgher et al 1999) It may well be that the ENHPS *country* case studies that follow later and the perspectives from within countries shed light on the position of the Technical Secretariat as ENHPS member or external supporter. For now it will be considered as a unique network *member* with special tasks and capacities, which may intend to 'retreat' into the network's closest supportive *environment* in the future. - Overall and in sum, the border of the **European Network for the development of (not 'of') Health Promoting Schools** that draws the line between its **members and important actors in its closer environment** can be illustrated as in figures 5.2.1 and 5.2.2.

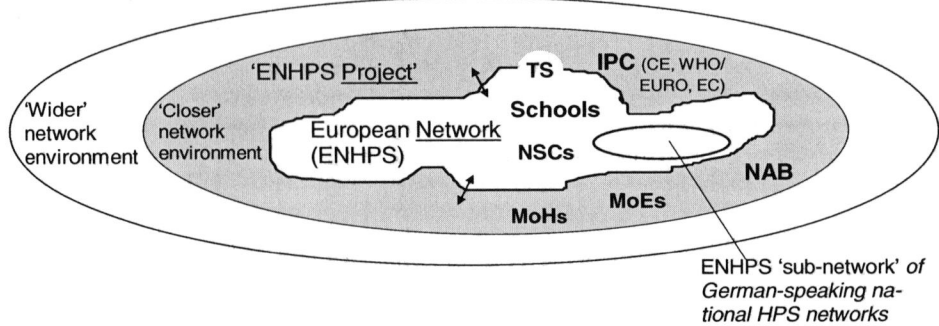

Figure 5.2.1: Members of the European Network for the development of Health Promoting Schools (ENHPS), its sub-structure, and actors or supporters in its closer environment. (The latter refers to the participants in the 'ENHPS project with both international *and* national actors.)

CE:	Council of Europe	MoHs:	Ministries of Health
EC:	European Commission (EU)	Nat.:	National
ENHPS:	"European Network of Health Promoting Schools"	NABs:	National Advisory Boards
		NSCs:	National HPS Support Centers
HPS:	Health Promoting Schools	TS:	ENHPS Technical Secretariat
IPC:	International Planning Committee	WHO/EURO:	World Health Organization/
MoEs:	Ministries of Education		Regional Office for Europe)

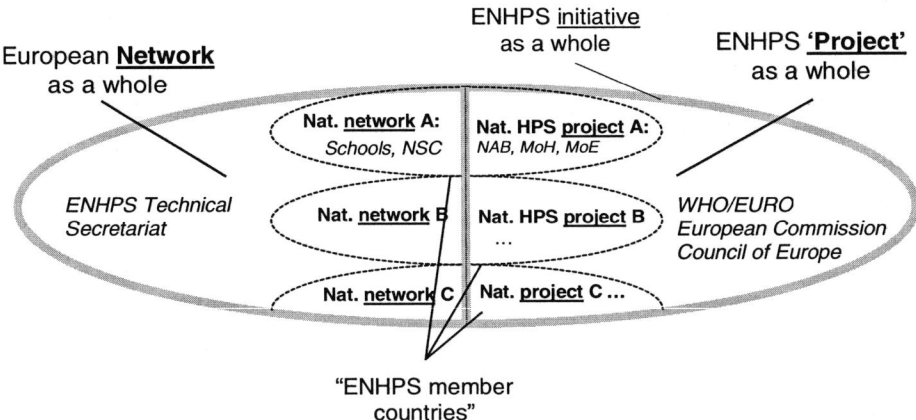

Figure 5.2.2: The international ENHPS initiative unraveled: A multi-system, multi-layer entity. - Interorganizational networks (left side) are distinguished from supportive ENHPS projects (right side). Each has at least two layers: the European (outer ellipse) and the country level (inner ellipses). National networks for the development of Health Promoting Schools make up the European network. Each network is a *distinct* social system on its own and thriving within or through the support project.

An assumption made earlier still holds: The distinction found at European level between *two* distinct ENHPS related systems (European *Network vs.* supportive 'ENHPS *project'* in the network's closer *environment*) applies at the national level of the ENHPS initiative, too. But to be confirmed it needs further examination through *country* case studies as exemplified with the Slovenian and German cases later on. This approach to *clearly distinguish* between the European 'Network' for the development of Health Promoting Schools (ENHPS) and a ENHPS 'project' or supportive closer environment - and this in *both* cases *explicitly* at *two* systems levels, European *and* national – is beneficial not only for the network assessment effort at stake in this pilot research but the European Network itself: On the one hand, it helps to develop and sustain a *network identity* among long term committed organizations that engaged or wish to engage in mutual exchange and even concerted action to achieve a common goal; and it creates a certain degree of *network stability*. At the same time, it offers and maintains *flexibility to all those 'others'* that wish or are obliged to support the network's goal or specific objectives over a limited time span and/or with limited involvement and/or foci only. The differentiation between European 'Network' and its *'closer supportive environment'* labeled as ENHPS or HPS *'project'* allows to offer also the latter group of actors a positive *network related identity* (as e.g. 'HPS project participant' or 'ENHPS partner'). Most importantly, this makes them positively distinguishable from the many other, more passive or less supportive actors in the network's wider environment.

Finally, the member organizations of the European *Network* for the development of Health Promoting Schools (HPS) have been identified and clearly positioned in relation to a range of 'other' important actors, actors that share (or have shared at least for three years) the network's overall goal and play a key role related to the network's development or functioning. Therefore, now the *specific,* structural and process characteristics of the European Network can be examined one by one in the pursuit of this research project's goal.

5.2.2 The structure of the European Network for the development of Health Promoting Schools

According to Alter and Hage (1993) an interorganizational network's 'structure' has five features (size, complexity, differentiation, connectivity, and centrality). Now, that the borders of the European Network and, thus, the unit of analysis within the overall ENHPS initiative has been clarified, these can be addressed.

Network size and its development over time

As to 'the size' of the European Network (ENHPS) two points are important: a) to distinguish between 'country' members and *organizational* ENHPS members, as well as *several types* of organizational members; and b) to note that developments of network size over time *differ* by types of members. From the international and interorganizational network research perspective *network size in terms of organizational members* are of main interest, i.e. National Support Centers (one per 'country' member), the initial "ENHPS pilot schools", the European level members (suggested is the one Technical Secretariat), and - from a certain point in time - also 'other' (non-pilot) schools, i.e. schools that joined the European Network in one way or the other *after* the 'pilot schools'. Table 5.2.1 summarizes the figures available and visualizes the change in network size by member types. The growth in number significantly differs not only by member type but also by network development phase.

	'First phase' (first 3 years)		Transition years (about 3 years)	
A) Changes in total network size:	roughly from 80	to 440	to	490 "plus thousands"
B) Changes in size by member type:				
"country" members	++	times 5 (from 7 to 37)	+	little increase (plus 4)
National HPS Support Centers	++	times 5 (from 7 to 37)	+	little increase (plus 4)
'pilot' schools*	++	times 5 (from about 70/80 to 400/450)	+	little increase (plus about 40/50)
'other'/ 'new' schools	(++ ?)	(at int. level no formal recognition yet)	++++++	(scale of thousands; in 2/3 of ENHPS countries as of 1998)
ENHPS Technical Secretariat	*no change* (one only)		*no change*	

Table 5.2.1: The size of the European Network for the development of Health Promoting Schools (ENHPS) from the inter-organizational network research perspective: Illustration of changes over time by types of network members.

* = figures estimated on the base of ENHPS recommendations of 10-15 pilot schools per ENHPS 'country'

The **'first phase' of ENHPS development** was characterized by a *rapid network expansion*: The number of National Support Centers increased *times five* (from 7 to 37) and so did that of 'ENHPS pilot schools' (from roughly 70 to 400). Whether the Technical Secretariat is one additional member as assumed before or not does not matter as to size. Overall, during the first three years the European Network grew *from roughly 80 organizational members to over 400*. This increase shows that overall, the so called 'first phase' of the European Network needs to be understood as a 'mixed stage' of network development: with an information *exchange network* in place whose rapid expansion indicates that the network as a whole is still being *built up*. - During the **transition years** that followed (about 3 years), *total* network size increased much slower with a hand full of new national level members (National Support Centers) and an estimate of 40 additional 'pilot school' members in new ENHPS countries. - If one does *not* count the many 'new' (non-pilot) schools that joined the European Network sooner or later (and which - at least during the 'first phase' - were understood as 'associated' but not full 'ENHPS schools'), then it can be concluded: The *size of the European Network after five to six network years reached more or less stability on a scale of 500* organizational network members. However,

when analyzing the European Network's growth over time and in light of its main goal (large scale dissemination of the HPS concept...) it has to be noted: Already during the first three network years and even more during the transition years that followed, the number of 'other' (non-pilot) or *'new' network schools* within the ENHPS sub-systems in countries increased significantly: *either* through *planned* dissemination efforts of national HPS networks or projects, *or* informal *spontaneous* dissemination around the ENHPS 'pilot' schools. In the sixth year of ENHPS development (1998), in at least two thirds of ENHPS countries a higher number of 'new' health-promoting schools (beyond the limited number of 'pilot' schools) were found (Piette et al 1998, w.y.). It remains to be examined whether these 'new' schools truly interact and network across the *European* Network or rather their *national* HPS networks. In case of the former the size of the European 'Network' in the true sense of the word would have increased dramatically to a scale of 'thousands' rather than 'hundreds'.

An interesting fact regarding the European Network's *size* concerns the ENHPS *sub-network* of the five German-speaking *national* HPS initiatives established early on: It accounts for roughly *one fifths* of all organizational *ENHPS members* (and this while considering only National Support Centers and pilot schools, not the 'other'/ 'new' schools). I.e. 20% of all ENHPS members (from both national *and* school level) are engaged in special efforts of networking across country borders, i.e. in Hastings terms in true *networking 'within'* the European Network as a *whole* (rather than mainly at its national and international level).

Network complexity

This structural feature of the European Network (ENHPS) refers - in Alter/Hage-terms - to the number of different services, products, sectors etc. present within the group of network members. As of now, two to three types of organizational members of the European Network for the development of Health Promoting Schools have been identified: National Support Centers; 'pilot schools'; and eventually the ENHPS Technical Secretariat and/or the 'new' schools that joined national HPS networks after the 'pilot' schools. However, these do *not* necessarily represent a fairly low complexity of the European Network. For example, the National HPS Support Centers are *not* a homogenous group and, thus, likely offer *different* resources and services to the European Network as a whole: the EVA 2 study by Piette et al (1998, 1999) indicated that half of the National Centers may be located in the *education* sector (mainly national Ministry), half in the *health* sector (Ministry or other); most in (national) *governmental* institutions, some *elsewhere* (e.g. universities). Also, even the resources or services potentially offered by National Support Centers located in the *same* type of organization will differ as, for example, their host organizations' capacities, responsibilities and/or priorities differ from country to country, from Eastern to Western Europe, - and as the professional qualifications of National Coordinators differ, too (e.g. the EVA 2 study found roughly 50% teachers, 25% social scientists, one medical doctor). - Similarly, the group of 'network schools' is *not* homogenous: Not only have 'pilot' schools more years of practical experiences in networking for and/or implementing the Health Promoting Schools (HPS) concept than 'other'/ 'new' schools. Even within these groups, secondary and primary schools will offer different resources, experiences or services to the network; and some schools will have more experiences and knowledge than others regarding HPS relevant methods or action areas such as school-to-school networking, parent involvement, and/or curriculum issues.

Thus, it has to be noted that the European Network's *complexity is much higher than the fairly low number of types of members suggests*. This can be stated although exact data on network members are lacking and the *extent* of network complexity cannot be accurately identified. However, the country case studies will provide further insight.

Network differentiation

As to the European Network's differentiation, i.e. according to Alter and Hage (1993) the extent of the *division of labor or function* within a network, data at international level are hardly available. However, the *tasks, roles and responsibilities of different groups or types of network members* defined provide valuable information in this regard:

Those of the **first type of network member**, the ENHPS *'pilot' schools,* did change over time: **A first set of tasks** relates the European Network's 'first phase': pilot schools were expected to engage in a) health supportive *intra-organizational development* (transforming themselves as schools into Health Promoting Schools and demonstrating the impact of this approach); b) inter-organizational *networking 'within'* the European Network (exchanging HPS related knowledge and experiences on the way); and c) shaping the *network-environment-link locally,* a limited outward orientation (building the school/community-link). Early on **a second set of task** was outlined for the time *after* the 'first phase' of the ENHPS (here called transition years). From this time, 'pilot' schools were expected to somehow expand their *network-environment-links* or *'outward'* orientation beyond their local communities to the health and education sectors at large (by disseminating experiences and practice models to these sectors 'to influence policy and practice nationally and internationally').

In comparison to the 'pilot' schools the **second type** of ENHPS members, the National HPS Support Centers, had complementary tasks and as of now these remained fairly stable over time: **A first set of tasks** relates, thus, not to the first phase of ENHPS development but to the European Network's *sub-systems within countries* as a *whole*. From the start and in network research terms National Centers were expected to engage in: a) *networking 'within'* the European Network's national sub-systems (enable, coordinate, manage and support the national 'HPS projects' or '-networks'); b) technical *guidance and support* functions (develop strategies, organize evaluations, and provide political support and credibility); and c) the shaping of the *network/environment-link*, a general 'outward' orientation (importing information from abroad and providing access to 'external others'). **A second set of tasks** relates to the European Network's *international* dimension. From the start National Centers were expected to: a) engage in *networking 'within'* the European Network as to national and international level members (direct exchange across national borders; contact point for the ENHPS Technical Secretariat); and b) serve as network *contact point for* interested actors in the network's *environment.*

It was suggested before that the *ENHPS Technical Secretariat* represents a **third type** of network member whose tasks, roles and responsibilities indicate the extent of "network differentiation" of the European Network for the development of Health Promoting schools (HPS). Its **first set of tasks** relates to the *'first phase'* of the ENHPS during which the Technical Secretariat was expected to: a) serve as the European Network's technical and managerial *support entity* (support of National Support Centers/ National Coordinators as a group or individually; initiation, production and dissemination of training courses/ information/ materials); b) strengthen and engage in *networking 'within'* the European Network particularly internationally (ENHPS business meetings, but also newsletter and documentation of developments); and c) shaping the *network/environment-link* with focus on the network's *international* level and closest environment (serving and taking part in the International Planning Committee; recruiting new 'country' members). **A shift in emphasis rather a second set of tasks** was initiated *during the transition years* that followed the 'first phase' of the ENHPS: The Technical Secretariat now planned to a) *decrease* its responsibilities in the area of *networking 'within'* the European Network (National Support Centers are called upon to take over) and b) *increase* its efforts to shape and reinforce the *network/environment-link* with focus on the network's *national* level and closest environment (more contacts towards national Health and Education *Ministries* to reinforce their commitment and collaboration as to the ENHPS initiative).

At *international* level and with view to the **fourth type** of ENHPS members, the 'other' *(non-pilot) schools* that joined the ENHPS sub-systems in countries more or less **after the network's first phase,** specific roles and responsibilities have not been defined. Their being part of the European Network's sub-networks or –projects *within* countries inherently requires them to at least tackle *some* of the tasks that 'pilot schools' took up at the beginning: a) health supportive *intra-organizational development* (becoming a HPS) and b) shaping the *network-environment-link locally* (building school/community-links). The information available gives the impression that for the European Network as a *whole* further requirements are not formulated but consciously left to the actors responsible within the ENHPS sub-systems in countries. Thus, whether and where the 'new' network schools have not only Settings-focused tasks but *networking* tasks, too, is an issue for the country case studies below.

Overall it can be concluded that the European Network's 'network differentiation' (or division of labor or function among members) follows, on the one hand, the line between organizational networking *by systems levels,* with two of the overall four organizational networking processes identified by Hastings (1993) in the foreground. As of now and from the *international* perspective, the following general picture emerged: The **division of labor as to the 'networking within' the European Network** was and is organized as follows: as to the local and national network levels, it is always the network members of the level *concerned plus* those at the next higher network level who are responsible for organizational networking 'within' (i.e. at the network's *local/school* level the 'pilot schools' and National Centers, at its *national* level National Centers and international Technical Secretariat). Here hardly any change occurred over time. This is in contrast to the **division of labor as to the European Network's linking up or networking 'with external others'** where important changes occurred over time: During the *first years* of ENHPS development, each group of network member focused on approaching 'external others' at its *own* systems level and mainly as to the network's closer environment. For the time *afterwards*, the *original* idea put forward by the ENHPS initiators was that the main *local* level network members, the pilot schools, should start to somehow influence policy and practice not only at school level but within the health and education sectors as a whole (*'nationally and internationally'*). However, years later the European actors stressed that it is the *European level* network member, the ENHPS Technical Secretariat, that will focus on linking up with the health and education sectors, but particularly the *national* level actors therein (national Ministries). This is visualized in table 5.2.2.

	ENHPS members:	'pilot' schools		National Support Centers		ENHPS Technical Secretariat		'other' schools (non-pilot)	
	Phases:	I	II	I	II	I	II	I	II
Networking 'within' ENHPS as to:	network schools	x	x ?	(x)	(x)				(x)
	national level actors	(x)		x	X +	x	X -		(x)
	internat. Level actor			x	x				
Linking up 'with' external others'	other local actors	(x)	(x)						
	national level actors		(x)	x	x		X +		
	internat. level actor		(x)			x	x		

Table 5.2.2: The European Network's 'network complexity' form the organizational networking perspective: overview by both a) two major networking processes ('within' the net and with 'external others') and b) systems levels.

(x): networking limited to the own school, community, country,...
+ / - : intended increase/ decrease

In addition to the above, information available suggests that there is also a **division of labor as to technical support functions** directed at the European Network's overall goal of creating Health Promoting Schools (HPS) and follows the lines of the level of knowledge at a given period in time in terms of the HPS concept and its implementation. During the first network years, technical guidance and support functions were particularly ascribed to the international and the national network levels (ENHPS Technical Secretariat, and National Support Centers) and both were focusing on the *local* network level (the pilot schools); but for a while the international level directed its technical support also to the national network level. As country case studies show, over time the picture became more diverse as *all* groups of network members gained knowledge and experiences, even if this did not necessarily occur equally across the network and/or all relevant knowledge areas.

Network connectivity / a network's 'networking within'

As explained in chapter 4, this synthesizing analysis of 'connectivity' (Alter, Hage 1993) is merged with that of the network's 'networking within'-dimension (Hastings 1993), as the latter encompasses the former. **Reciprocal contacts** and interactions **among groups of network members** rather than individual members are the focus. 'Networking within' is used as the overriding term and to shed light on the network's *structure* is still the goal. Further issues of *quality* of interactions are addressed separately below (see network 'processes' and 'purpose of interactions'). Each *network organization's networking with other member organizations* taken together reflects the *'networking within' the European Network 'as a whole'*. As this network case study is undertaken in order to *pilot test* the comprehensive network assessment framework developed in chapter 3, the aim is providing an **overall** picture of the European Network's 'networking within' (including connectivity).

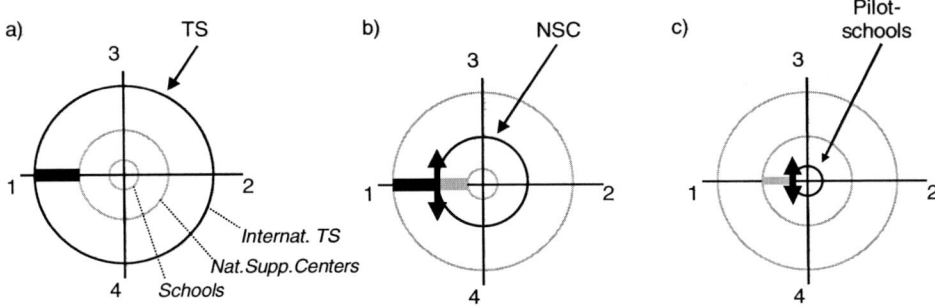

1 = Hastings' organizational networking-dimension 'networking with others'
2,3,4 = the other three 'Hastings-dimensions' (not yet of relevance here)

━ = 'networking' between network levels/ groups of members
▬ = 'interorganizational relations of some kind' between network levels/ groups of members (i.e. not necessarily 'networking')

↕ = networking at that network level/ within that group of members

Figure 5.2.3: Networking within the European Network. Who is networking with whom? - Illustration of interorganizational relations or networking *between* and *within* member groups, group by group:

a) TS = ENHPS Technical Secretariat;   b) NSC = National HPS Support Center;   c) Pilot-schools.

Guiding questions were which of the first three, later four groups of European Network members had the mandate and/or did regularly interact (in pursuit of the common goals) and which not? And which changes occurred over time in this regard?

The tasks, roles and responsibilities of network members related to the European Network's networking 'within' have already been synthesized above because the division of labor by groups of members follows this line (see 'network differentiation' and table 5.2.2). Figure 5.2.3 illustrates the *picture that emerged.*

Hastings' *model of the 'new' organization* has been taken as the *orienting framework*, particularly the axes of the "organizational networking" processes, - with the poles of the x-axis representing the two dimensions of networking 'within'/'with others', those of the y-axis 'soft'/'hard' networking, and the concentric circles geographical distance between network members (see chap. 2.4.2). The latter element of the graphic on this model has been slightly modified and translated into the three *systems levels* of the European Network identified so far. These represent the three major *groups* of network members (the network's local level: schools; national level: National Support Centers; international level: ENHPS Technical Secretariat). At least during the first years of European Network development this matches well with Hastings' issue of 'geographic distance' among network members with: pilot schools mainly interacting *within their country* (inner circle/ lowest distance); National Centers across Europe (middle circle/ bigger distance); and the Technical Secretariat eventually with other Regional centers of this kind across the world (outer circle/ maximal distance).

Summarizing and illustrating in this way the **networking 'within' the European Network** and in Alter/Hage-terms **the network's 'connectivity'** is of advantage: During the further course of this synthesizing analysis of the European Network's various 'network features' identified in the proposed network assessment framework (chap. 3), the European Network's "organizational networking" as a whole can be unraveled and illustrated step by step. The first step, the analysis of the **networking '*within*' the European Network by *groups* of network members** unravels a simple pattern visualized in figure 5.2.3. However, it should be noted that this refers mainly to **'soft networking'** among the groups of members (i.e. direct person-to-person links) rather than 'hard' networking (via e-mail etc.) The latter is not documented. Also there is a lack of data regarding those 'new' (2nd generation) network schools that joined the European Network and/or its sub-systems in countries *after* the 'pilot schools' (i.e. the "1st generation" of network schools).

Within the European Network for the development of Health Promoting

Schools (ENHPS) during its **first network years,** all **pilot schools** were *expected* to 'network' with each other (however defined) *across Europe.* The data available indicate that after a few years a scale of *three quarters* of them engaged in inter-school relations or networking *across their country*; and a scale of *5-10%* had *'twinning'* relations with another school (*within or across national borders* and likely but not necessarily with other ENHPS member schools). In spite of variations across the European Network, from the international perspective this is an encouraging extent, particularly if one considers the immense organizational development challenge inherent in the HPS concept and taken up by these 'pilot schools' at the same time. (see figure 5.2.3 c) - **Over time**, and there where the ENHPS *sub*-systems in *countries* were expanding, the expectations towards the pilot schools regarding their networking 'within' (parts of) the European Network did increase the more 'new' schools were able to enter the European Network or sub-networks therein. Overall, due to the lack of data at international level a judgment about how far the vision of creating a *Network 'of'* Health Promoting Schools has been realized is not possible - whether across Europe or the individual ENHPS countries in *general*. The *qualities* of the inter-school relations in terms of interorganizational 'networking' as elaborated in chapter 2.4 are not known at international level. Again, the country case studies later on will provide some insight.

Similarly to the pilot schools, from the start the ENHPS members at national level, i.e. the **National Support Centers,** were *expected* to engage in *networking amongst each other across Europe* and they do so on a regular basis: annually face-to-face, plus to *various* degrees via e-mail and other means. There is not much information on the networking 'within' the European Network in ENHPS documents, although a few ENHPS assessments called for attention in this regard (e.g. Parsons et al 1997; Sub-regional network... 1997). However, a yet unpublished effort on 'ENHPS indicator' development by a small group within the ENHPS considered all network levels (see chap. 3). The minimal frequency of *reciprocal contacts among* National Centers is once per year, but several Centers engage in additional networking relations such as bilateral twinning arrangements, defined ENHPS sub-networks (e.g. the German-speaking one), and/or for a limited time span around joint productions of manuals or other ENHPS products. - As to the interorganizational *relations* of National Support Centers to the *next higher and next lower network levels* there is a mixed picture: Regarding the *international* level (Technical Secretariat) *reciprocal 'networking'* takes place but with low frequency (annual business meetings); the National Centers' pre-defined role of 'contact point' for the international level indicates *mono-*directional contacts. Regarding the network *schools* relations *may vary* from country to country; pre-defined *expectations* towards National Centers (enable, coordinate, manage, support national HPS projects) indicate *mono*-directional and/or *reciprocal* contacts with network schools. The two country case studies that follow (Germany and Slovenia) will exemplify the situation in this regard. (see also figure 5.4.3 b)

The European Network's assumed *international* member, the **ENHPS Technical Secretariat**, was *expected* to have and realized mono-directional support relations towards the national network level (National Centers) plus had reciprocal *networking* relations as mentioned above. It does not network directly with the school level. (see figure 5.4.3 a)

Now, that the European Network's 'size', 'complexity', 'differentiation', 'connectivity' and 'networking within' the network has been analyzed a last *structural* network feature remains:

Network centrality

According to Alter and Hage (1993) 'network centrality' addresses how much in the European Network for the development of Health Promoting Schools (ENHPS) the overall 'work' flows through one or a few network members which is a question of dominance of these members. From the international perspective on the European Network as a *whole*, in general it is the group of **National Support Centers** who are involved in most information flows and experience exchanges within the network and also in joint actions, - as to international or cross border activities as a 'group', as to those at sub-national level 'one by one' in most cases. The overall image that emerged is captured in figure 5.2.4: an image of **a multi-centered system** framed as a combination of two types of circles: *One first type of circle* encompasses those *groups* of network members who (are to) network *across Europe* (National Centers and ENHPS Technical Secretariat); within this circle additional bilateral or even multi-lateral 'work' flows can be found. This is complemented by a whole *set* of a *second type of circle* which encompasses network members by ENHPS country, i.e. one National Center plus the 'pilot' schools of the same country each. - At least during the first (pilot) years of ENHPS development National Support Centers often had additional bilateral relations with individual pilot schools (see fig. 5.2.4 a). From the international perspective, during the transition years of the ENHPS as a whole (and with more and more ENHPS countries moving from the 'pilot' phase to one of 'dissemination' of the HPS concept to a second generation of 'new' network schools) the relations of National Support Centers and network schools in their countries cannot be judged anymore (the picture is fuzzy and variety has generally been stressed). However, as illustrated in figure 5.2.4 (a and b) over time the National Centers remain in their central role as to the European Network as a *whole*.

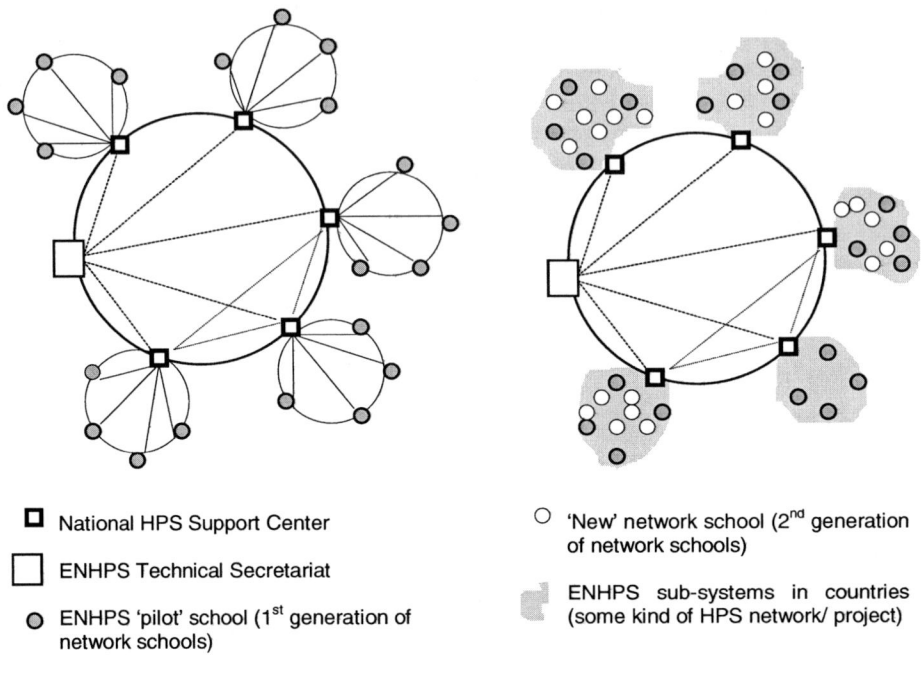

□ National HPS Support Center

☐ ENHPS Technical Secretariat

○ ENHPS 'pilot' school (1st generation of network schools)

○ 'New' network school (2nd generation of network schools)

ENHPS sub-systems in countries (some kind of HPS network/ project)

Figure 5.2.4: The 'centrality' issue - The European Network for the development of Health Promoting Schools as a multi-centered system, with National Support Centers in central roles. (This figure should not be misinterpreted as illustrating size or connectivity.)

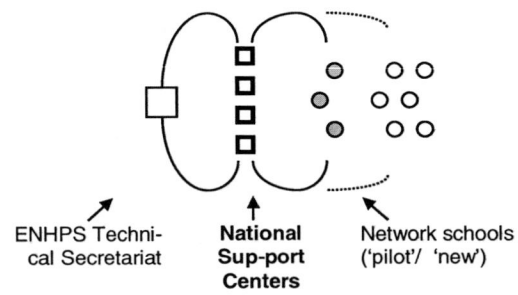

ENHPS Techni-　　National　　Network schools
cal Secretariat　　Sup-port　　('pilot'/ 'new')
　　　　　　　　　Centers

Figure 5.2.5: 'Centrality' in the European Network: Simplified illustration of the National Support Centers' central position.

The European Network is a multi-centered network but at the same time, when looking by *groups* of network members, exhibits high centrality (with the group of National Support Centers in the most central role) (see fig. 5.2.5). However, due to the guiding motto 'partnership as a method and goal' as well as high commitment to basic principles and values of Health Promotion such as participation it can be assumed that their potential dominance over other network members will have been buffered. But only country case studies can examine this issue.

5.2.3 The European Network's 'operational processes' and 'organizational networking'

Operational processes: Methods of coordination used

In contrast to the network structure, the synthesizing analysis of *this* important feature of interorganizational networks does not need many words. Alter and Hage (1993) point to the extent of *joint decision making* and *reliance on mutual adjustment and feed back* as well as of staff *working together interdependently across* organizational boundaries. Categories of related methods of coordination are with increasing utilization of feed back: a) *impersonal* methods (e.g. contracts/ rules and regulations); b) *personal* methods (e.g. designation of coordinators/ direct contact among staff); and c) *group* methods (e.g. face-to-face communication of *several* people planning and taking decisions by *consensus*) (see chap. 2.4.3). From the start the European Network for the development of Health Promoting Schools and its initiators focused on the latter two: At both the European Network's national and school level, the **designation of a coordinator** (capable of team work etc.) was *the* personal method of coordination used and even a condition for network membership. **'Group' or team methods of coordination** were **most emphasized and implemented** and this with view to both the network itself and its closer environment. Within the network, such methods were a) applied to *individual member organizations:* obligatory for network schools (as HPS project teams), desired around National Coordinators (as national HPS teams). They were b) applied to interorganizational work *across the network*: in the form of 'ENHPS business meetings' for information exchange, joint planning and decision-making. Also with view to the European Network's *closest environment* (or 'ENHPS project') group methods of coordination were applied: in the form of the International Planning Committee of the three ENHPS initiators and sponsors (that stress participation, consensus orientation, and democratic approaches to coordination, management and governance of the ENHPS initiative). Even as to the *network/environment-interface* at *national* level group methods of coordination are recommended (in the form of 'National Advisory Boards' as decision making bodies).

Besides this clear preference within and around the European Network for a combination of 'group' and 'personal' methods of coordination, **'impersonal' methods** have been used mainly in the network's *environment:* as written cooperative agreements between a) Ministries of Education and Health for at least three years, b) among the international ENHPS initiators (WHO, EC, CE). How far within the European Network these group or team methods of coordination have been realized is at *international* level not much documented. The ethos of partnership highlighted in most documents, the principles laid out in the 1st ENHPS Resolution (1997) and selected evaluation findings indicate that group methods of coordination are not only called for but also indeed implemented. The regular international business meetings are perceived as important. The situation at national and sub-national network levels across Europe is hardly known but the country case studies below provide some insight.

The general purpose of interactions within the European Network

This point refers to the interorganizational network typology by Alter and Hage (obligational/ exchange networks, promotional/ joint action networks, systemic/ joint production networks) that reflects stages of network *development* (see chap. 2.4 and table 2.4.4). On the one hand, the European Network for the development of Health Promoting Schools from the start was an information and experience **exchange network**, even if different groups of members were not equally involved into such exchange. Pilot schools were expected to *exchange* experiences and information among each other and many did - some (an estimate of 5-10%) even beyond national borders (school twinning). National Support Centers had the responsibility to not only share experience among each other but also be a main mediator for rather indirect *cross-border* experience *exchange* among network schools (as disseminators of 'international experiences' within the ENHPS in their countries). On the other hand, after a few years the European Network also engaged in some *joint actions* that no single (group of) members could have done alone such as creating an ENHPS Data Base and the 1997 Resolution with 10 guiding principles for the ENHPS initiative. In Alter/Hage-terms these products addressed supra-ordinate member issues, accomplished a functional purpose, and needed 'moderate' cooperation as well as peripheral and segmented (rather essential and enduring) interorganizational activities. Thus, in addition to being an exchange network the European Network evolved to **a 'promotional' (joint action) network**. – Similarly the German-speaking ENHPS *sub-*network exchanges information and experience but also shows joint actions (e.g. publication of a position paper).

After this synthesizing analysis of a range of specific, more or less *internal* features of the European Network now the analysis will be continued with view to Hastings model of the "new" organization capable of networking (see also figure 2.4.1). This brings the network's interactions with its (organizational) *environment* back into the picture.

Synthesizing analysis of the European Network's "organizational networking" ('within'/'with others' and 'hard'/'soft')

The European Network's networking 'with external others' and relative emphasis given to networking 'within' versus 'with others'

Already the examination of 'network differentiation' in chapter 5.2.2 above did show: For the first network years, regarding the European Network's networking with 'external others' there was a clear division of labor, which began to be changed during the transition years. *First*, each group of network member (schools, National Centers, ENHPS Technical Secretariat) was **responsible to** link up or network with 'external others' at the *same* systems level (schools with local authorities and NGOs; National Centers with national level actors; etc.). And a look at the information available about links **realized** indicates that during **the first network years** this was indeed the main direction, and mainly limited to the European Network's *closest environment*. Both national and international level members had from the start interorganizational (likely dependency) relations with public education and/or health agencies (National Support Centers with the national Ministries, the ENHPS Secretariat with WHO/EURO, Council of Europe (CE) and European Commission (EC)). Many National Centers also linked up with *additional* 'others' but constellations and extent are reported to *vary* widely among cases. Only the third group of network members, the network schools, did generally *not yet* realize the European Network's intended links to its *closer, local* level environment: After several years, the 'school/ community-links' still needed strengthening in most cases. However, an estimate of 5 to 15% had links with *additional* 'others' such as other national (network) projects or individual members thereof. (see also chap. 5.1.5)

From 1996, during the European Network's transition years (chap. 5.1.4) documents increasingly express **a shift** regarding the European Network's 'networking with others': To strengthen the commitment to the ENHPS initiative of *national* actors in the European Network's *closest environment* is presented as an issue for the 'ENHPS' rather than for individual network members (the National Centers) as before. With the intent to strengthen and sustain the ENHPS in countries particular *plans* or calls for action mirror an **expanded view and awareness of 'external others' in the networks closer environment particularly** within countries and beyond each network school's local community. Directly addressed or targeted are: all 'national governments'; policy and decision makers; stronger interministerial collaboration between Health and Education and even other Ministries; the national education (and health) *sectors as a whole* rather than individual schools; and collaboration *between systems levels*. With view to this, published information reflects overall a *new division of labor proposed* among Network members: The *international* level member moves into the foreground as major actor. *National* level network members are considered *individually* and as in need of support - rather than as the major member *group* within the European Network that could act jointly. – Meanwhile, the task of network *schools* to link up with *local* community organizations and authorities in support of HPS development remained unchanged.

Hastings pointed out that organizational systems must take decisions on whether they need for a particular task to focus on networking 'with others', or networking 'within', or in one way or the other on both. As to the European Network all in all it can be summarized: This network - challenged by the self-set goal of large-scale sustainable development of 'Health Promoting Schools' throughout Europe - during the *first years focused mainly on networking 'within'* the network in support of two organizational innovations taken up at the same time: the network schools' organizational development towards "Health Promoting Schools" (HPS) plus with view to this a systematic experience exchange and mutual learning process across Europe via an interorganizational network. *A few years later*, while the ENHPS projects or networks in many but not all participating countries indeed expanded to include more or less increasing numbers of (health promoting) schools, the *focus shifted towards the Network's closest institutional environment:* newly to the national education and also health sectors, and as intended before to local community organizations and agencies. But, the overall impression is that this did happen less by 'the European Network' as a whole and more by its *international* level *member* with view to individual ENHPS countries and in support of *individual* national network members concerned (National Support Centers). In comparison to this, continued networking 'within' the network (such as among network schools and National Centers) receives less attention in important documents and national education policy development is highlighted instead (see Piette et al 1998, 1999; Burgher et al 1999). Only the innovation of 'Health Promoting Schools' development is reconfirmed as a focus. Figure 5.2.6 illustrates these developments, i.e. the European Network's shift over time **from an inward oriented towards an outward oriented network, with a shift - in Hastings terms - from mainly 'networking within' the European Network to mainly 'networking with others'** in its closer environment.

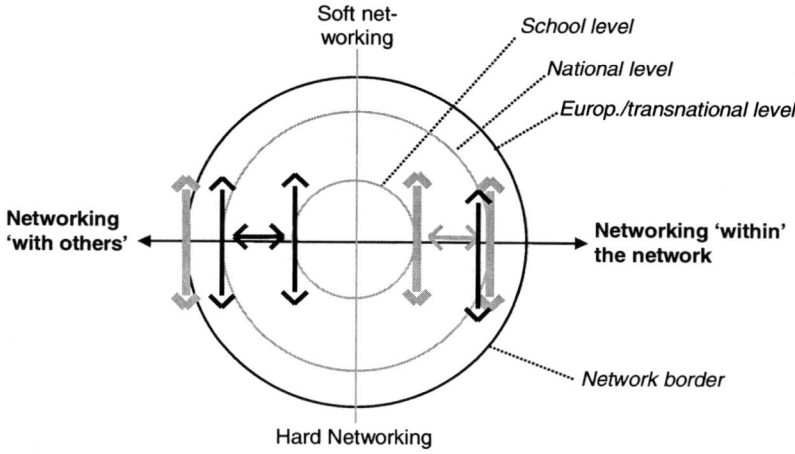

▬▬ Gray: 'first phase' of network development
▬▬ Black: transition years that followed the 'first phase'

Thinner arrow: less emphasis/ thicker arrow: more emphasis/ no arrow: hardly any emphasis

x-axis/ left side: The European Network's networking with *external* organizations at local, national and European level [mainly from the education and health sector]

x-axis/ right side: the networking within and among groups of Network *members* (school, national, international)

Figure 5.2.6: The European Network's *emphasis* on networking 'within' and 'with others', differentiated by partners at various systems levels, and as to developmental phases (Gray: 'first phase' 1992-1995/ Black: transition years from 1996 to 1998/99).

The first Network years are characterized by a higher emphasis and also realization of networking *within* the European Network (x-axis, right side) both within and among the major member groups, i.e. network schools and National Support Centers (gray arrows). Then, the European Network starts to turn to its *closer environment* at national or lower levels (x-axis, left side), i.e. the education and health sectors in individual ENHPS countries. This was accompanied by a significant decline in emphasis on school-to-school networking (dark arrow, right side), i.e. of the original innovative idea of large scale 'Health Promoting Schools' development throughout Europe by means of creating a network *of* health promoting schools for mutual learning and exchange.

The European Network and 'hard' networking, means of 'soft' networking, and the relative emphasis on 'hard' and 'soft' networking

'Hard' networking within the European Network for the development of Health Promoting Schools (HPS) such as the creation of links via e-mail and Internet is **hardly documented**. But from the start, at *inter-country and international* level hard networking in the form of e-mail access of National HPS Support Centers. - With view to a) *national and international* level network members and *international* level supporters, regular face-to-face meetings (i.e. **'soft' networking** opportunities) were emphasized (and implemented with low frequency (once per year) as common internationally). With view to b) the *school* members, the (more limited) information available suggests that in many countries these, too, engage(d) in soft networking but mainly confined to their countries. But this needs further clarification as exemplified in the country cases studies below.

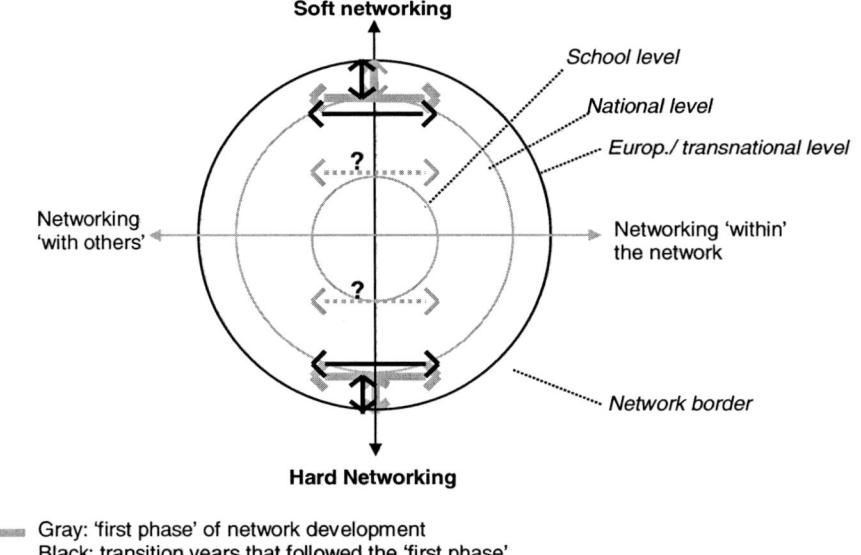

▬ Gray: 'first phase' of network development
▬ Black: transition years that followed the 'first phase'

Thinner arrow: less emphasis/ thicker arrow: more emphasis/ no arrow: hardly any emphasis;
?: insufficient information (hard and/or soft networking among network schools?)

Figure 5.2.7: The European Network's *emphasis* on 'soft' and 'hard' networking, differentiated by partners at various systems levels, and as to developmental phases (Gray: 'first phase' 1992-1995/ Black: transition years from 1996 to 1998/99).

x-axis/ left side: The European Network's networking with *external* organizations at local, national and European level [mainly from the education and health sector]

x-axis/ right side: the networking within and among groups of Network *members* (school, national, international)

The overall picture of the relative emphasis on 'hard' and 'soft' networking <u>within</u> the European Network (ENHPS) is illustrated in figure 5.2.7.

That in figure 5.2.7 the black and gray arrows are much alike shows that from the international perspective, the European Network from its *first* to its *transition* phase *maintained* the levels of emphasis on soft and hard networking - at least as far as *national and international* actors are concerned: Networking *within* the European Network at its **inter-country or international level** rested on the systematic use of **both 'hard'** *and* **'soft' technologies.** The *extent* of the use of the former is not known but e-mail access was *required* for all ENHPS National Coordinators. The frequency of face-to-face meetings (a 'soft' technology) decreased after the first few years from a few to once per year, but due to the reduction of training seminars. Thus, not the emphasis on soft networking was decreased but on training provision internationally. This is supported by the fact that over time soft networking across the whole of the European Network was complemented by a 'twinning strategy' at national network level. As to the **level of network** *schools,* international level actors have *repeatedly* pointed to the desired "European dimension" of the European Network initiative but (as indicated by the dotted arrows in fig. 5.2.7) the *means* of such networking have not been spelled out.

Regarding the realization of the over time increased emphasis on **networking <u>with others</u>** the information available does not allow a judgment as to the European Network's preferences of soft and/or hard networking. But with view to 'external others' at *national* level 'visits' (i.e. soft technologies) have been proposed.

The European Network's 'organizational networking' -intermediate synthesis and discussion

Now that all four networking processes have been analyzed (within/ with others; soft/ hard) the overall picture of - in Hastings terms - the **"organizational networking" of the European Network as a whole** can be outlined. This is visualized in figure 5.2.8 in terms of the *relative emphasis on each* of the four networking processes - and changes over time (see a and b). At least for Network members at national and international level, the relative emphasis of *soft and hard* networking remained fairly the same over time - but this applies to the European Network's *internal* networking (right side) rather than that with external others (left side).

From the international perspective, the European Network's relative emphasis on *networking within and with external others* has clearly shifted towards the latter. After the first years of network development with special attention to *internal links among and between network members* at national and school level (i.e. pilot schools and National Support Centers) the focus of attention shifted towards actors in the closer environment of those (the local 'community' and national education ministries) - to improve or renew the environmental support and involvement into the overall efforts of creating 'Health Promoting Schools' (HPS). This relies likely on soft networking processes (rather than hard networking).

The reminder of this chapter will round up the 'synthesizing analysis I' of structure and processes of the European Network for the development of Health Promoting Schools (ENHPS) by addressing remaining network features: geographical distance; culture of self-reflection/ evaluation/ feed back; 'reasonable' network outcomes (perceived effectiveness/ levels of conflict); - and briefly the network schools' "organizational networking", too (as an inherent demand of the 'Health Promoting Schools' concept).

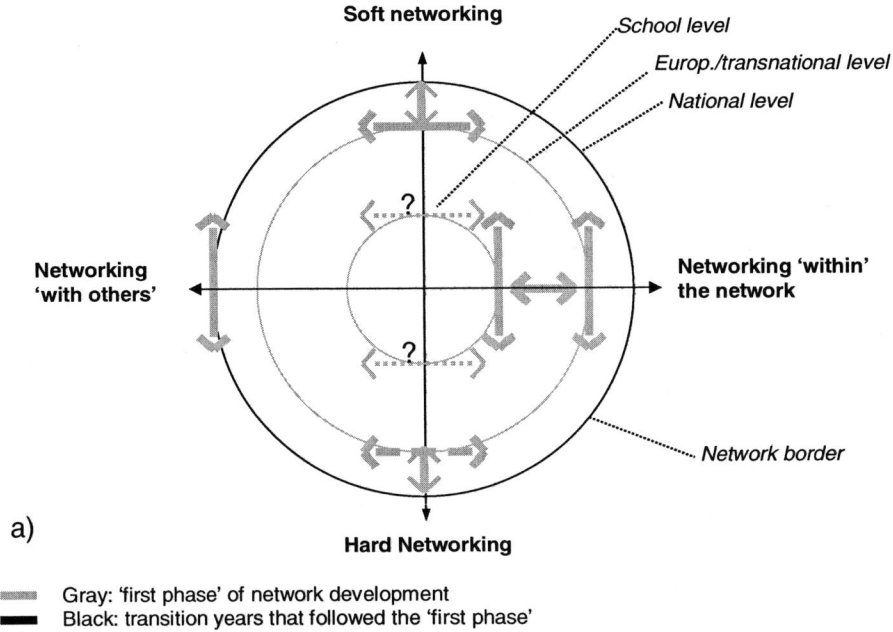

Gray: 'first phase' of network development
Black: transition years that followed the 'first phase'

Thinner arrow: less emphasis/ thicker arrow: more emphasis/ no arrow: hardly any emphasis; ?: insufficient or no information (hard and/or soft networking among network schools?)

Figure 5.2.8a: "Organizational networking" of the European Network for the development of Health Promoting Schools (ENHPS) - Emphasis on networking 'within' the net, 'with others' (x-axis) and 'hard' and 'soft' networking (y-axis) during a) the first phase and b) the transition years that followed.

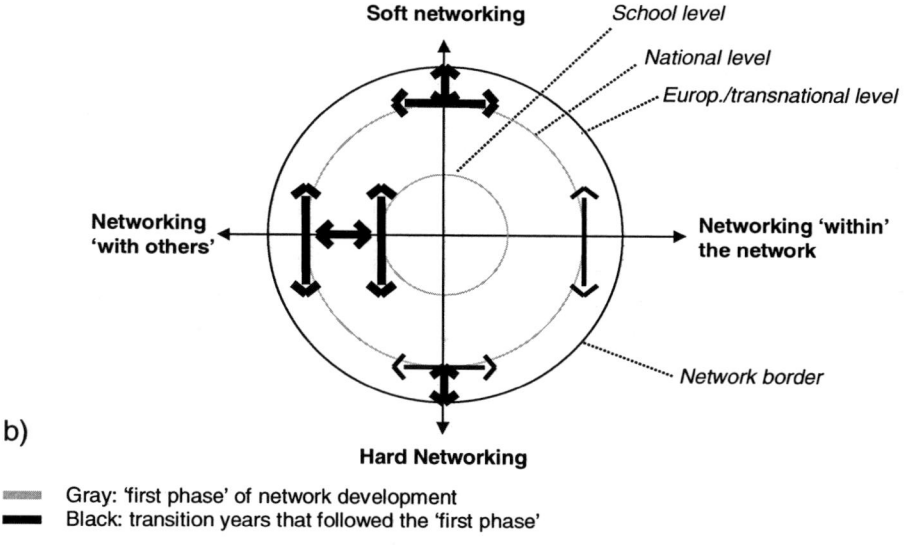

b)

■■■ Gray: 'first phase' of network development
■■■ Black: transition years that followed the 'first phase'

Thinner arrow: less emphasis/ thicker arrow: more emphasis/ no arrow: hardly any emphasis; ?: insufficient or no information (hard and/or soft networking among network schools?)

Figure 5.2.8b: "Organizational networking" of the European Network for the development of Health Promoting Schools (ENHPS) - Emphasis on networking 'within' the net, 'with others' (x-axis) and 'hard' and 'soft' networking (y-axis) during a) the first phase and b) the transition years that followed.

5.2.4 Distance, assessment culture, and satisfaction within the European Network

Geographical distance among network members

Hastings has pointed out that even with full use of new information technologies (i.e. 'hard' networking) psychological barriers for collaboration generally increase with geographical distance. Obviously, interorganizational networks with geographically dispersed members that lack 'hard' networking have, in addition, to overcome *physical* barriers of geographical distance to engage in 'soft' networking and meet face to face. The members of the *European* Network for the development of Health Promoting Schools (ENHPS) generally face both of these barriers. This applies to the National HPS Support Centers that due to travel costs meet only once per year. This will apply also to the pilot schools, which were consciously selected from all over a particular country - to facilitate the spread of their experiences in implementing the Health Promoting Schools (HPS) concept to other schools evenly across countries. Thus, it can be expected that over time networking within the European Network with view to both network members at national and school level, will intensify by geographic regions (and shared culture). An example is the German speaking 'Sub-regional network' of national ENHPS networks; and it would be no surprise if the country case studies would unravel processes of sub-national/ regional sub-differentiation of such national networks.

The culture of (self-)reflection, observation, evaluation processes and feed back loops within the network

Both Alter and Hage, and Hastings refer to this issue: the former as part of the network feature 'operational processes' (discussed above), the latter as a central element of his 'radar beam model' of the 'new' organization (see fig. 2.4.1). The radar beam symbolizes the *needed culture* of ongoing or repeated *self-reflection, self-observation, evaluation and feed back loops* within organizational systems capable of networking. **From the start**, the initiators of the European Network for the development of Health Promoting Schools (ENHPS) implemented **some mechanisms for self-reflection and feed back:** *regular reports* required of National Support Centers to the international Secretariat; *annual business meetings* for joint reflection and planning; the recommendation of a 'National Advisory Board' for all national ENHPS initiatives; and *membership criteria* for both ENHPS 'countries' and (pilot) schools such as 3-year-'project'-plans and *commitment to facilitate evaluation* and dissemination of results. Thus, with regard to self-reflection and evaluation the ENHPS initiative *inherently called upon* the Network members *within* countries (National Support Centers and network schools).

After the first three network years (at the end of the 'first phase'), a small range of **single events** of self-assessment and/or evaluation occurred. **Systematic self-reflection** was demonstrated by the 1995 'strategic review' (ENHPS 1996, 1997) involving *all* National Support Centers or HPS networks. This was complemented by a voluntary 'first provisional appraisal' of the ENHPS by the German-speaking sub-network (Sub-regional Network... 1995) - the first (published) effort within the ENHPS of a systematic analysis of *all* European Network levels (schools to national/ international levels). - **A survey** to create a first 'ENHPS Schools Data Base' required self-reflection particularly of network schools (by addressing also needs assessment/ progress made/ evaluation activities) (WHO/EURO 1998). - During the European Network's transition phase, several **international evaluation projects** were undertaken; but these did *not* cover *all* ENHPS countries but larger or smaller parts of the European Network only. The first focused narrowly on school health (education) interventions ('EVA'/ CE et al 1996); a study on six

ENHPS countries and 'EVA 2' then addressed a wide array of different issues each (Parsons et al 1997; Piette et al 1998, 1999). One finding was that, after six years of existence of the ENHSP initiative, at least two thirds of all national networks had evaluators in place that indicates a widespread recognition of the need of (some kind of) evaluation in ENHPS countries. After all these activities, the first and only attempt of the European Network (or its international Secretariat) to move from increased awareness **towards more appropriate evaluations** was a ENHPS indicator development initiative end of the 1990s (ENHPS w.y.): It systematically addressed *all* ENHPS systems levels or types of members (schools to international Secretariat; see chap. 3) but the lack of referral in documents indicates that results did neither receive wider recognition nor were they implemented yet.

Overall, the series of *international* **evaluation projects** and important ENHPS documents produced during the transition years (ENHPS 1996, 1997; ENHPS conference report 1997) show: On the one hand, within the European Network initiative the *awareness of the need to expand the evaluation focus* (beyond school program effectiveness to include aspects of the European Network as a whole) *increased over time* - at least among those involved at international level - and concrete evaluation activities demonstrate this. On the other hand, *more appropriate evaluations* of the European Network as a whole have not been undertaken (or documented) yet. While one may speak of a *general culture of self-reflection* within the European Network since its inception, a *culture of systematic, comprehensive and repeated evaluation is still lacking.*

The 'organizational networking' of network *schools*

As explained in chapter 5.1.2, the implementation of the concept of the Health Promoting School (HPS) is expected of all network schools and inherently requires schools to both start networking 'within' their organization and develop interorganizational relations with 'others locally'. As members of the European *Network* for the development of Health Promoting Schools they are also expected to engage in interorganizational networking with 'others across and outside their country'. The over 200 school portrays in the ENHPS Data Base show that many pilot schools *did* or do engage in *interorganizational networking,* but mainly within the network and less with other organizations locally. (WHO/EURO 1998; see chap. 5.1.4) The country case studies below will allow a closer look at these issues.

Satisfaction of network members - perceived effectiveness and levels of conflict

The principle of a 'reasonable outcome approach' was consciously integrated into the proposed network assessment framework (see chap. 3). From the organization science perspective and following Alter and Hage (1993) two outcome indicators were chosen: effectiveness and levels of conflict *as perceived by* key actors in the network. The limited information available in this regard stems from critical reviews of network members, written statements by key actors, and an evaluation study EVA 2. (see also chap. 5.1.4) Unfortunately, there is some bias towards EU or Western European countries and supra-local actors.

Reviews of the European Network as a whole **after the first three network years** (or 'first phase') by **network members** in countries as well as at international level led to several conclusions on successes, remaining challenges, and weaknesses (see chap. 5.1.4). Written statements fall into three groups (general, organizational, health related). a) A range of *general statements* expressed general satisfaction such as the 'good reputation' gained by the ENHPS as a 'sound investment' in the health of young people and first successes in 'agenda setting' for education and Health Promotion. But an important weakness remaining was the lack of appropriate approaches to measure the European Network's quality and effectiveness. b) With view to *organizational change and interorganizational collaboration,* positive statements referred on the one hand, to schools (e.g. more democratic management/ teaching styles; links between schools, even beyond national borders), on the other hand, to the European level (e.g. contributions to building consensus, cooperation and a 'sense of unity' among the three key network supporters WHO/EURO, European Commission and Council of Europe). Stated weaknesses included insufficient commitment of health and education sectors to collaborate, and lacking resources to allow effective national HPS networks to occur. Some pointed specifically to remaining training needs of teachers and heads of schools (in organization and HPS development), and needs of further investments into school-to-school networking ('soft' and 'hard'). During the first 3 years, statements of satisfaction referred less often to c) *health related* effects of the European Network initiative. But some particularly confirmed the Health Promoting Schools (HPS) concept as the 'right framework' and a 'workable guide' that indeed contributes to solving problems related to health risks at schools for pupils and teachers. Negatively seen were too narrow approaches in many (health education) curriculum projects.

With view to the European Network's **external supporters at international level** it is remarkable that, **throughout the first phase**, the three

ENHPS initiators (WHO/EURO, EC, CE) jointly or individually underlined their *satisfaction* with the ENHPS initiative. On the one hand, they referred to various *Network features* (such as essential mission, growth, complexity (however defined), and European dimension), and on the other hand, to *environmental features at European level* (such as successful inter-agency collaboration and management arrangements that 'minimize bureaucracy while maximizing results', and the Network's positive perception by health and education sectors). But challenges in the form of developmental variations between countries were stated, too.

After five years and more, i.e. during the European Network's **transition years,** *general satisfaction remained* or at least its dominance over dissatisfaction: The first 'ENHPS Conference' 1997 (i.e. network members *and* external others) concluded that 'successes so far' warrant the European Network's further implementation while not denying persisting basis weaknesses (such as in the area of evaluation). Over the years, network schools and national ENHPS initiatives as a whole did show remarkably *low drop out* rates. The EVA 2 study interviewed the **National Coordinators and a spread of other 'key' people** in ENHPS countries, mainly officials and staff from the health and education sectors and some evaluators. It did seek spontaneous answers as to *perceived successes of the 'ENHPS in countries'*: The majority referred to successes of *individual* pilot schools (e.g. health concepts or approaches to problems used). Also repeatedly mentioned were features of pilot schools in *general*, a) aspects of *interorganizational* relations (increased relations or exchange among schools/ opening up towards the local community) and b) improvements of teachers' capacities (e.g. knowledge/ empowerment). Successes related to sub-national, i.e. *regional networks* were brought up seldom. Overall, the study confirmed that in the vast majority of (EU) countries the European Network had a positive image among those involved - tendency increasing (Piette et al 1999). - The **external supporters at *international* level** continued to be satisfied (also with European level management structures and the Technical Secretariat). (see also chap. 5.1.4)

The second 'reasonable' outcome suggested, **perceived levels of conflict** within the European Network, have not been addressed in (evaluation) reports on the European Network. A **source of tension** between European Network *schools* and 'external supporters' for the time after the pilot phase has been documented: While in a European survey pilot schools often reported financial problems when looking at 'activities carried out with difficulties', the EVA 2 study reported on national actors favoring non-monetary rather than monetary support to health promoting schools (WHO/EURO 1998; Piette et al 1998, 1999). EVA 2 and also the

Slovenian case study (below) show that public donors may not be willing or able to finance the support provided to the limited number of 'pilot schools' during a limited period of time to all those other schools that (wish to) join the ENHPS.

5.3 ENHPS country case 1: The "European Network of Health Promoting Schools" in Germany

5.3.1 The German network initiative - context at the outset, concepts, goals

In the Federal Republic of Germany, the fairly sovereign States (Laender) rather than the federal level are responsible for most of the education and health matters. Nation wide developments are coordinated in the standing Conference of the Ministers of Health (GMK) and of Education (KMK). The 'Federal-State-Commission' (BLK) is an important bridge between 'Laender' and Federal level and through its financing of three so called 'model experiments', has been a core actor in the large scale development of Health Promoting Schools in Germany. A first one on health promotion in school's daily life (1990-1993) took place in only one of the German Laender, Schleswig-Holstein. Its Ministry of Education documented strong leadership with regard to a nationwide effort to create Health Promoting Schools in Germany within the European Network of Health promoting Schools (ENHPS) initiative. The latter was organized, financed in parts and anchored in the public education sector in the form of a second Federal/State- 'model experiment', i.e. as a four year *project with an applied research component* (1993-1997): the German "Network Health Promoting Schools" project. Developments were to be sustained beyond the project phase and found again public support in form of a preceding three year long Federal/State-'model experiment' called "OPUS - Open Participatory Network and School Health" (1997-2000). Then, this type of support was ended, the supporting and coordinating office at *national* level was closed and documentation of processes stalled. Therefore, this case study covers the developments from 1993-2000. However, by now, i.e. within about two years, the former evaluator and core actor of the two network projects succeeded to achieve a private foundation's mid term commitment in support of further developments.

As will be shown below, in Germany between 1993 and 2000 a trans-State network for the development of Health Promoting Schools has been developed, and this in two formal steps: from 1993 to 1997 as a project entitled German "Network Health Promoting Schools", from 1997 to 2000 as a follow-up project called "OPUS/ open participatory network and school health". In the following, the former will be also referred to as "the Network", the latter the "OPUS-network".

The German context

The German 'Network Health Promoting Schools' was created time wise parallel with some legislative and regulative developments in the **health sector** that were of particular importance also for the field of Health Promotion: These include the *"paragraph 20"* of the Social Law, Book V (SGB V) which in its versions from 1988 and

1992 formulated the sickness funds' role or task to act on health promotion. In addition, in 1991 the *64. Conference of Health Ministers* of the German States (GMK) recognized Health Promotion as task of the State and local level authorities. For the EU member Germany also of relevance is article 129 of the *'Maastricht Treaty'* from 1992 that supports Health Promotion (see chap. 5.1.1). Within this climate and on the basis of the 'paragraph 20' one German sickness fund became a key 'cooperating partner' of the network initiatives on Health Promoting Schools in Germany. In 1996, however, its legal basis changed when the "paragraph 20" was modified to forbid sickness funds Health Promotion activities from 1997 (Lehmann 1997). But in 1999 it was altered again; from 2000 prevention, self-help and also health promotion at the work site were included again (Meierjuergen 2001b). A related position paper of the German statutory sickness funds explicitly includes the Settings approach and not only as to work sites but also schools.

Of course, school health promotion programs in Germany are legitimized on other grounds such as through various State level regulations within the **education sector**. Germany's joining in the European Network of Health Promoting Schools (ENHPS) happened against the background of an increased level of technical debate around school health education and promotion in the early 1990s. The 'Soest theses and guidelines for health education and health promotion in schools' by experts and practitioners called for a comprehensive, school-related prevention and health promotion concept (Soester Thesen 1991). Also highest political levels took stock: At State level, the Conference of the Ministers of Education (KMK) published a report on 'the situation of health education in schools' which in the outlook refers to the option of the 'healthy schools' approach (KMK 1992). The then 'Federal Ministry of Education and Research' (BMBW) initiated intersectoral cooperation with the Ministry of Health and the German umbrella NGO for health (the 'BfGe') and conducted a 'health and school' project. This took a Health Promotion and co-determinants of health perspective and developed federal recommendations for a health-promoting school reform (Broesskamp 1994; Broesskamp-Stone 2000). Not all of these efforts were already linked when, in 1993, the German 'Network Health Promoting Schools' started as a *multi-State project* of the Ministries of Education of 13 out of 16 German States and the Federal Education Ministry. It was this project that allowed Germany to become a **member country of the European Network** of Health Promoting Schools (ENHPS). This step was perceived as a possibility to *exchange* experiences and *disseminate* successful models, an important *'precondition' to learn about* how to: put aspects of 'health literacy' higher on the agenda at all levels of the educational system; develop methods for information dissemination applicable across subjects or areas; overcome organizational barriers; clarify incentive and training issues regarding teachers in support of HPS development; and increase parents' and (head) teachers' awareness of their role as health promoters. ('Health literacy' refers to the cognitive and social skills that determine an individual's motivation and ability to gain access to, understand and use information in health promoting and maintaining ways (WHO 1998a).

Vision and key concepts at the outset and changes over time

There is not the vision or goal statement of the German "Network Health Promoting Schools" at its outset to be quoted but various network or project descriptions show: The German Network had a **vision of schools** as 'places in which people feel well', which provide 'healthier living and learning conditions' - as a precondition for productive learning and good interpersonal relationships (NGS w.y.).

As to **key concepts** it is interesting to note that with regard to the **'Health Promoting Schools'** (HPS) concept, key actors of the German Network initiative refer to its root concept *'Health Promotion'* rather than to the 'Health Promoting *Schools*' concept as expressed by the European Network. The Settings approach is being applied without much use of the term. The 'five Health Promotion action areas' and levels as identified in the Ottawa Charter are broken down for the education system and school. Already early network leaflets show emancipation *from the ENHPS criteria* for a Health Promoting School. A different but compatible set of 'goals' is presented, on: the school as *a good place* for living, learning and working; supporting healthy lifestyles; and opening up towards the community and *interorganizational relations locally*. (BLK-Modellversuch Netzwerk… 1993; NGS 1994, w.y.; GNHPS 1994)

In Germany, the HPS network projects had strong concept and knowledge development components. At the beginning, much effort went into further developing the 'Health Promoting School' concept: From early on, a 'Health Promoting School' has been described as *transferring Health Promotion principles and action areas into political discussions of education and school reform*. For schools, building 'healthy public policies' implies bringing Health Promotion into the political horizon; creating 'supportive environments for health' implies the schools' opening, networking, and use of public resources; 're-orienting health (relevant) services' implies organizational development, a focus on school culture and a 'healthy' school profile; strengthening 'community action for health' implies team building and the creation of co-operative working modes; and finally, 'developing personal skills' implies strengthening personality, and trying out and enabling healthy lifestyles. The *whole* school (i.e. class room teaching, school life *and* school environment) is to profit from these developments that are understood as **'health promoting school development' from 'within'** rather than externally imposable. The concept's great potential to link up with and *integrate* other school development initiatives and concepts (such as the 'good', 'just', 'open' school) are stressed, as are *'everyday life'* conditions and the specific situations and interests of individual schools as starting points. (Barkholz, Paulus 1998) **Eight interrelated 'dimensions'** of a Health Promoting School are being distinguished and guide evaluation activities: the conceptual, curricular, social, further education/training, ecological, 'communal'/neighborhood, organizational, and acceptance dimension. To avoid that health promoting school development looses its unique **health specificity**, the German Network developed a list of *school related 'health factors'*. Each school is invited to develop its *own* profile of a 'Health Promoting School'. (Paulus 2000; Barkholz, Paulus 1998)

As the European Network, also the German Network at its outset did not present the Network's definition of **'health'**. However, one of the 'goals' of the Health Promoting School is the development of a *'holistic understanding of health'* which recognizes the interrelationships of physical, mental and social *'health factors'* (NGS w.y.). This shows that in general, the German "Network" initiative rested on a perspective on health and 'co-determinants of health' that underlies the Health Promotion concept (see chap. 2.2).

Contrary to the Slovenian case, early documents on and by the German "Network Health Promoting Schools" contain frequently the terms **'network' and 'networking'** (the latter in the sense of "Vernetzung"). Various descriptions and ideas of the project's network dimension can be found. *Building and maintaining* the network in Germany and its being part of the European Network are the foci of a whole set of *'ques-*

tions to be examined' by the model project (BLK-Modellversuch Netzwerk... 1993; GNHPS 1994 - see below). The German Network has been described as a **"multi-Laender support system** which is to enable" participating schools to develop their own, situation specific 'health promoting profiles' and to exchange experiences (GNHPS 1994 p3). A year or two later, a brochure states that networking as the **working mode** of the German HPS Network project means: *'thinking interrelations'* and understanding the multiplicity of options; *joint action and interest in external stimuli*; overcoming professional narrowness; developing contacts and exchanging experiences; and *helping oneself and thereby supporting others*. 'Networking' is also **an 'area' that influences a school's development** towards a Health Promoting School: here, reference is made to a *school's exchange and cooperation with other organizations* in its closer environment. Elsewhere it is stressed that 'the whole is more than the sum of its parts'; the interrelations of individual parts are increasingly important; and this applies also to schools. (BARMER w.y.) - This shows that German "Network" initiators or actors were very aware of and actively reflected upon the *network* dimension of their (and the European) Health Promoting Schools- development project. But a clear conceptual basis and understanding of networking had yet to be developed. How far, nevertheless, an interorganizational network has been established is being examined throughout this case study.

The first four-year-project on large-scale development of HPS via the German "Network Health Promoting Schools" represents the ENHPS pilot phase in Germany. At its end, the (national level) actors had clarified their understanding of the 'network(ing)' dimension – an important basis of the next project **"OPUS/ open participatory network and school health** - health promotion through networked learning" (1997-2000). Networking (in the sense of "Vernetzung") was understood as a *'new mile stone' of school health promotion* to be achieved and a principle within the 'guiding idea' (or "Leitbild") newly formulated for the OPUS-network. From 1997, the **'network'** was understood as **a multi-centered and multi-level organizational system** with one or more *"network nods"* at each level (local, regional/State, supraregional/trans-State, international). These nods are *organizations* with one *appointed coordinator* each who are embedded into a *team* (see below). An important developmental step from the "Network Health Promoting Schools" to the "OPUS" project was the shift in focus from supporting individual schools to *creating links among schools, to 'networking schools'*. The network strived for has the following **network features**: It is a *multi-centered* network, a 'self-active field', in which network actors participate actively in a *joint, self-organized process*. It lives from *'give and take'* (i.e. reciprocity). (Barkholz et al 1998) The **local network level** received particular attention: Key national actors stress that an OPUS network is a **network of 'learning schools'** which indicates an orientation towards the concept of the 'learning organization' introduced in chapter 2.4. But it is stressed that this learning happens in new ways, as **mutual, self-organized, 'networked learning',** starting with the needs of individual schools and 'leading via empowerment' to their strengthening. *Differences* (e.g. in knowledge and 'know how') are declared *positive assets and potentials* of the network. (Barkholz, Gabriel, Hahn, Paulus 1998, 2001) - Thus, after the first four years the network (for the development) of Health Promoting Schools in Germany had reached a significant increase in understanding of *interorganizational networks and its members*, the 'learning' organizations, which guided the next three years of further development under the heading 'OPUS'. Structural features and roles and responsibilities of core actors are further addressed below.

With regard to the **Health Promoting schools** (HPS) concept, also under the heading 'OPUS' the German network for HPS development continued to apply the HPS concept developed and already implemented by the pre-succeeding "Network Health Promoting Schools" project. The newly formulated 'guiding idea' ("Leitbild") of the OPUS network made the understanding of **'health' and 'health development'** more explicit: by highlighting "the *systemic*-holistic understanding of health", referring to health as dependant of complex *'living conditions'*, and explicitly pinpointing to the *'salutogenic approach* of Health Promotion' (Barkholz et al 1998 p18). Particularly the network's scientific advisor Paulus strengthened the 'resources for health' perspective within the OPUS network and brought Antonovsky's concept 'sense of coherence' (chap. 2.1.2) into the project. The **'Health Promotion'** concept (Ottawa Charter) remained the reference concept.

Core concepts and approaches - intermediate synthesis and discussion

As to the understanding, clarity and use of core concepts and approaches of Health Promotion as elaborated in chapter 2.2 (i.e. as to health, determinants of health, Health Promotion, and *both* the *Settings* approach and a *network* approach), it can be summarized: The large scale efforts to develop Health Promoting Schools (HPS) in the 1990s in Germany led first to a deeper understanding and operationalizing of the Settings approach in schools, in the form of an eight dimensional HPS concept. Soon, 'factors that influence health' in the school context were carved out which made the co-determinants or resources for health perspective more visible. Over time, a better understanding of the network dimension emerged and an explicit conceptual framework was developed. And from 1997, *combining* the Settings approach and modern organizational models such as the 'learning organization' with an *interorganizational network approach* was an explicit goal. The developments at conceptual level show that with view to the *individual* network schools from early ideas of modern organizational development guided the efforts. With view to a *network of* schools and/or other organizations they show that only over time an understanding of such interorganizational systems emerged but then significantly and matching with some core features of interorganizational networks as identified in modern organization sciences (see chap. 2.4).

Network rational and goals and objectives

For the first seven years, the large scale development of Health Promoting Schools in Germany was organized in form of *two* successive 'model experiments' or projects and one distinct set of questions was 'to be examined' each time. This raises the question whether these '*questions* to be examined' by the network *projects* should be understood as implicit statements of the goals or objectives *of* the *network* being developed *through* these projects. As network assessment needs to consider the tasks of or goals set by a network this issue is important.

At the start of the 'pilot phase' of the ENHPS in Germany, i.e. of the German **"Network Health Promoting Schools"** in 1994, a clear **rational for the network approach** was lacking, but the *'international collaboration'* through the ENHPS membership was seen as important as health-harming factors do not stop at national borders. And a 'multi-State system' should *enable* the *'project schools'* to a) *develop their own,* situation specific 'health promoting profile' and b) *exchange* experiences among each other (Barkholz, Paulus 1998 p25). For two "Network" related entities **goals** were more clearly formulated: a) **'Project schools'** (for the project years 1994 to 1997) 'set themselves the task' to *comprehensively promote the health* of pupils, teachers and other school staff. *Collaboration with other schools* in their region was 'strived for'. b) The 'Federal-State-Commission model experiment' or **"Network" project as a whole** set out to examine three detailed sets of questions which reflect a wide range of objectives with different foci: Set A of questions focused on the *individual school* (its main groupings and organization), set B on the *school/community link*, and set C on *'network' issues* (GNHPS 1994; Barkholz, Paulus 1998; BLK-Modellversuch Netzwerk... 1993).

Set A asked *how teachers, pupils and parents can be enabled to act* in a health-promoting fashion at school and at home, and *which organizational aspects of schools and school development need attention* for schools to become 'healthy organizations'. Sub-questions reflected a range of objectives related to school and class-room teaching and issues of further education of teachers and headmasters. Question set B asked *how local resources can be made accessible* for Health Promoting Schools (HPS) and *in what ways schools can be opened* towards their social surroundings. Related sub-questions reflected objectives related to local policy makers' awareness of the features of Health Promoting Schools, the consideration and use of relevant technical competencies, and school/community cooperation that supports the schools' development into health promoting work-sites. **Questions on network dimensions** were the focus of set C: *How could the German HPS Network be set up and maintained across all types of schools, and how could it be linked with the European Network and this in a sustainable way.* Here, sub-questions implied a *range of objectives* of particular interest from the network research perspective:

- a *communications network* that facilitates the information flow between German schools within and across the States; (which hints at an information exchange network)
- the 'right' amount and forms of *seminars, conferences or workshops* for the right participants and on the right subjects; (an issue also of soft networking opportunities)
- the interlink and complementary function of the German Network's *new impetus* and of *goals and plans of other* national and European (non-governmental) organizations; (an issue of network-environment-interaction)
- understanding *how* German project *schools link up with those in other countries*; (a difficult issue of realizing interorganizational networks over larger geographic distances)
- identification of European *pupil exchange programs and seminars* that are suitable to test and support Health Promotion measures in everyday school life, and

- achieving national or European *sponsorships* for development projects. (the latter two points are issues of mobilizing external resources and hint at resource dependency)

For the full sets of questions see NGS 1994, GNHPS 1994 or Barkholz and Paulus 1998.

After this look at the various statements on goals or 'questions to be answered' on, by or related to the German "Network" (1993-1997), two interrelated questions remain: that of the genuine goals *of* that Network, and that of its boundaries or members. The distinct bundle of 'questions to be examined' was developed by those that applied for the funding as FSC-model project, i.e. the later staff members of the network's national Project Support Center. Thus, they can be understood as reflecting goals and objectives of this national center and external expectations towards the network. Should it turn out that the Project Support Center is a *member* of the "Network Health Promoting Schools" (1993-1997) and that *all* Network members subscribed to the tasks formulated by the Center, the set of questions would be part of self stated goals of the Network and thus, reference point to assess its outcomes. The membership question is further addressed below, but first the network rational and goals formulated for the second phase of network development as 'OPUS network' will be addressed.

Rational and goal of the 'OPUS' network (i.e. of the ENHPS in Germany from 1997/ its second phase of development) are not clearly separable. As reflected in its title 'open participatory network and school health - health promotion through networked learning', the OPUS network was to **create opportunities for** schools to communicate with each other about health themes, exchange experiences and information, and learn with and from each other. *Networking* as de-central, active and self-organized participation and learning was to represent **a context within which** "health promoting school development through *empowerment* in a salutogenic perspective" could take place and "the social and *social-ecological* as well as *pedagogical* dimension of Health Promotion" be realized (Barkholz et al 1998 p16). The assumption was: In a network as described above *'courage and power for self-activity'* is growing; a health promoting culture of learning and living will be *exchanged* not only within but among schools as well as their surroundings. The **goal 'of OPUS'** (the network and/or the project) was to achieve *sustainable* networking ("Vernetzung") of Health Promoting Schools that is oriented towards *'open participation'*. In contrast to the first phase of the ENHPS in Germany, a 'central' aim of OPUS was to clarify, *whether, how and to what extent, through the networking among schools and/or of schools and other organizations, the development of individual schools towards Health Promoting Schools can be actively and appropriately 'driven forward'*. From the start, a 'multi-centered' network was strived for (see conceptual base above). (Barkholz et al 1998)

As for the pre-succeeding model experiment "Network Health Promoting Schools" also for the 'OPUS' network **a whole set of questions** to be examined was formulated which raises the same question as before: whether these reflect goals and objectives or expected outcomes of the OPUS *network* or the OPUS *model experiment*.

The first interim report on OPUS refers to them as work priorities 'of OPUS' and as thematic foci 'of the experiment', the final report as 'questions of the *model experiment* OPUS' (Barkholz et al 1998 p26, 2001 p13). **Three areas** are covered: a) *forms and levels of networking among schools* (knowledge exchange, use of data networks, 'networking', transfer within the European Network); b) *regional support* ("rationalization" concept, sub-regional and local forms of network building/ networking ("Vernetzung"), conditions and possibilities of schools' entering the network, cross-regional transfer); and c) *creation of health promoting school profiles* (school program, guiding vision, organization development, 'Health Promotion/networking' as school profile). These were translated into a set of '*objectives*' of the OPUS-*model experiment*' at five 'levels':

1. and 2. level: through networking or network building ("Vernetzung"),

- changes in 'school related health status' of *persons* in schools involved;
- a qualitative and quantitative improvement of the 'health promoting *school development* processes';

3. level: a functioning network ("Vernetzung")

- *among* schools,
- *of* the schools *with external* 'cooperating partners',
- which in both cases are perceived a) by the *schools* as helpful for planning and implementation processes in the context of health promoting school development, and b) by the cooperating *partners* as meaningful as to their contribution;

4. level: Regional Coordinators establish functioning, self-sustainable regional network(ing) structures;

5. level: 'efficient cooperation' between the individual Regional Coordinators with view to their coping with their (everyday) tasks.

Formulated by staff of the OPUS-National Coordinating Office (the former 'Project Support Center') and the scientific evaluator for funding application and evaluation purposes, the above sets of 'work foci', 'questions to be examined' and 'objectives' can be reasonably understood as reflecting goals and objectives in the area of *knowledge development* of a) the National Coordinating Office and b) the external donor, the Federal-State-Commission and, thus, the State Ministries of Education involved. Whether these goals and objectives became indeed also those of *all* OPUS network members and, thus, those of the OPUS network as a *whole*, needs further examination. Should membership include commitment to these goals and objectives the answer would be 'yes'. In this case, the *set of issues or questions* would be an important reference point for assessing the OPUS network's outcomes.

The German network's task or goals -intermediate synthesis and discussion

According to the Alter/Hage network theory a wider *scope* of an interorganizational network's *tasks or goals* calls for different network structures and operational processes than a more narrow scope. Also, the network outcome *'perceived effectiveness'* will related to the goals set. Thus, the German *network's* tasks or goals should be well understood. With regard to the two German network development 'projects' ("Network Health Promoting Schools" and "OPUS") a **range of expected outcomes have been more or less explicitly expressed**: The range of questions to be answered put forward each time need systemization to improve the understanding of the German network's tasks or goals at the outset and after the first four years of development. When using the Health Promotion outcome model adapted from Nutbeam as shown in figure 3.1.3 above the following picture emerges:

For the years 1993-1997, the sets of questions 'to be examined' by the 'model experiment' entitled 'Network Health Promoting Schools' (which again, may or may *not* be the same as the network itself) reflect the following: With regard to the *'project schools'*, i.e. network members, goals were expressed in terms of *ultimate or long term outcomes* (improved **health** of members of the school community). As to both *'project schools' and the German "Network"* goals were expressed in terms of *direct or short term outcomes*, particularly in the form of changes in **organizational practices,** both within individual schools and in their interorganizational relationships. (The Network initiative expected that *schools are enabled to* develop health promoting school profiles and exchange experiences; project schools strive for *collaboration with* other schools.) - Overall, goals, objectives and/or expected outcomes related to the first phase of the ENHPS in Germany, addressed almost solely *direct or short term* outcomes and, in addition, included many 'how to'- questions that can be understood as referring to - in Nutbeam's terms - *'Health Promotion actions'* to achieve Health Promotion outcomes. Only once a intermediate outcome (in terms of 'healthy lifestyles') was explicitly addressed (…pupils, teachers, parents act in a health promoting fashion…):

a) With regard to the level of direct or short term Health Promotion outcomes:

- *a few* objectives address issues of the outcome category *'health literacy'* (motivation for healthy lifestyles) or *'social action and influence'* (participation in Health Promotion actions, health conscious consumers, peoples' influence on environmental changes);

- *none* address issues in the outcome category *'healthy public policies'*; and
- the vast majority of objectives address issues in the outcome category 'health promoting organizational practices'.

From an interorganizational research perspective, the latter can be grouped as follows: objectives related to

inwards oriented organizational development of individual schools (aspects to be addressed remain unspecified; participation of organizational members is an issue);

interorganizational relations of individual schools, with (a) organizations in their local surroundings or (b) other schools;

interorganizational networks as regards (a) *German schools* (addressing geographical dimension/ 'across Germany', communication/ information exchange function, sustainability) or (b) the link between the *German and European Network* (ways of linking, sustainability);

and - cross-cutting to these three groupings - objectives related to

means of 'soft networking', here seminars, conferences, and workshops (the forms, foci and target groups of which are to be identified).

b) With regard to **'Health promotion actions' or inputs to achieve desired outcomes,** the set of questions to be examined implies objectives related to:

- *training or further education* of teachers and headmasters, as well as *advocacy and capacity building* for their joint actions in developing Health Promoting Schools (HPS);
- *awareness raising* and sustaining regarding the HPS among local politicians; and
- *learning about* several issues: ways of *network development and maintenance* among schools (in Germany; in the European context); potential links of impulses by *the Network and existing goals or plans of other* organizations; as well as options for resource mobilization (at national or European level).

This analysis of the explicit or implicit objectives of the German "Network" or network project shows: German "Network" initiators have taken seriously the health promoting Settings approach with its emphasis on contextual and organizational co-determinants of health and everyday life. The interpretation of the Health Promoting School concept as a 'school development approach' is fully reflected in Network related goals and questions to be examined. It remains the question whether all of these are indeed goals and objectives of the German '*Network* Health Promoting Schools' or in parts external expectations towards it. The answer lies in the identification of the Network's boundaries, of who is member and who is not. It may well be that, as in the case of the European Network initiative, also in Germany key actors fall into two categories: network members, and network supporters or actors that are part of the network's closer environment. This will be examined below.

Also for the from 1997 reshaped and renamed German network, the OPUS network, the set of questions to be examined and objectives of the 'model experiment' put forward reflects on the *scope* of the tasks, or goals and objectives of, the network or at least the National Coordinating Center. When again applying the *adapted Nutbeam-Health Promotion outcome model*, the following picture of expected outcomes of the second phase of the ENHPS initiative in Germany emerges: In comparison to the first phase, now **organizational and inter-organizational issues are clearly in the foreground**:

a) With regard to the level of **ultimate or long term outcomes:**

- there is only *one* objective: changes in *'school related health status'* of those persons in schools involved, but this "only" as to the *influence of* the inter-organizational *networking* on this issue;

b) All other expected outcomes fall into the category of Nutbeam's **direct or short term Health Promotion outcomes** and two broad groups can be distinguished:

- first, *organizational development* of the schools (*one* objective: improvement of the 'health promoting school development processes')
- second, *interorganizational networking or network building* (*all other* objectives as explained above: school to school, school/external co-operating partners, among Regional Coordinating Centers, and 'within regions')

The latter aspect refers to 'functioning, sustainable' network structures within *regions* that may or may not refer to inter-organizational networks, although this is likely if sustainability is the goal.

Overall, it is obvious that the second phase of network development for developing Health Promoting Schools shifted its focus almost entirely on the network dimension of the initiative. That there is less emphasis on the *health* promoting developments in individual schools is not surprising if one considers the following: a) the German network as part of the ENHPS initiative, which overall only during the *first* phase focused on creating 'models of good practice' of individual Health Promoting (pilot) Schools, and then encouraged its 'member countries' to shift the focus towards *disseminating* the 'good practice' developed; b) the 3-year-project period, i.e. the relatively short time for achieving measurable changes in health status in school community members; and c) the fairly limited resources for evaluation of the overall very complex network initiative - as will be further unraveled now.

5.3.2 Structural set-up and key actors of the 'model experiments' and network in Germany

Particularly during the first four years, written presentations on the German large scale effort to develop Health Promoting Schools in the context of the European Network (ENHPS) do not clearly distinguish between the 'Federal-State-Commission-model experiment' or 'project' *entitled* "Network Health Promoting Schools" and the German *network* itself. This raises the question whether these are the same or separate or overlapping interorganizational systems. This needs clarification to understand the unit of analysis of the intended 'network' assessment. From the project or network reports the following picture emerges:

The two **'Federal-State-Commission model experiments'** 1993-1997 and 1997-2000 are understood as the 'contributions' of the German *government* to the joint WHO/Council of Europe/EU- initiative 'European Network of Health Promoting Schools' which is recognized as the 'right strategy at the right time'. German *States* (the "Laender") are the *participants* of the experiments, first 13, later 15 of the overall 16 German States. Statements such as the 'model experiment started working' in August 1993, the identification of a *formal leadership* agency, here the *Ministry of Education* of the State 'Schleswig-Holstein', and the experiments' being 'attached' to the University of Flensburg indicate that it is an own entity. As regards content, the model experiments were *'oriented towards'* the guidelines put forward at the European level (ENHPS vision, rational, HPS concept, and pre-conditions to join as explained in chapter 5.3). Through these two projects, a network for the development of Health Promoting Schools in Germany was created. Although name and logo were changed over time one may reasonably speak of *one* network continued to exist and mature between 1993 to 2000, because the overall vision and long term goal (i.e. that German schools become Health Promoting Schools) as well as key actors remained the same while the network approach was strengthened and additional members joined. Key actors or members were the following:

For **the first four years**, from 1993 to 1997 the network was called "**Network Health Promoting Schools**" (and not, as the European Network, network *of* Health Promoting Schools): As required of ENHPS member countries, a national level **support structure** was established: the *'Project Support Center'* at the University of Flensburg with the required 'National Coordinator' (full time) and desired further staff (here a full time 'educational advisor', two part-time secretaries, and two professors as part time 'scientific advisors'). Overall, **key organizational actors** within or close to the German "Network" included 15 State level *Ministries of Education*, 29 network or 'project' *schools* (usually 2 per State), the network or Project *Support Center* and *its formal host*, the University of Flensburg, as well as three so called 'national *cooperating partners*' (one sickness fund, the public accident insurance association, and a further education academy). In addition, and as part of the so-called "rationalization" (or decentralization by States), a limited number of so-called 'associated schools' entered the system. Also, about three 'advisors' per State played important roles but often in their personal capacity as experts rather than as organizational representatives (Paulus 2001).

Germany became ENHPS member country although the requirement of cooperation between Health and Education Ministries was not fulfilled; up to date, neither the Federal Ministry of Health nor most of the State Ministries got involved in the large-scale development of Health Promoting Schools. This may explain the wording in official documents of Germany's 'contribution to' the European Network rather than its membership. The roles and responsibilities of the various actors are addressed later when *interactions and relationships* of and among members of the German network are being examined.

With the beginning of the new funding period, from 1997 the network approach was changed as explained above. During **the following three years** the network was called **"OPUS - open participatory network and school health"**. The former Project Support *Center* changed its approach, reflected also in its new name 'National *Coordinating* Office'. Staff members and human resources remained more or less the same (with one new team member and a change in the area of scientific advice). Overall, several **key organizational actors** within *or* close to the former German "Network" *continued* to be involved with regard to the "OPUS network", i.e. the 15 State level Ministries of Education, the *reoriented* national network office (still hosted by the same university), the three 'national cooperating partners', as well as those schools that were already part of the former "Network Health Promoting Schools". But **some new** organizational actors came 'on board': Fifteen *"OPUS-Regional Centers"* (one per State) and sometimes even 'sub-centers' were established and *organizationally anchored* in network schools, State level NGOs for health, and also teacher training institutes; some had been involved already in the previous "Network". The 'regional coordinators' did not necessarily work in the same organization. Most importantly, a *large number of new schools* decided to join the OPUS network, reaching a scale of about 500 over time. The often **modified roles and responsibilities** of all these actors are addressed below in the context of the examination of *interactions and relationships* of and among OPUS-network members.

Table 5.3 1 illustrates and summarizes the basic structural frame in which various actors were located and which early on was laid out by key actors at national and State level for the OPUS-network. The *'team' structure* chosen shows that the network systematically and *actively* shaped its **network/environment-interactions** by system levels: The National Coordinating Center recommended that Coordinators involve the following *members in the teams*: 'locally' (i.e. at *school level*), the members of the school community; at *'regional'/State level,* the School Coordinators, regional cooperating partners, State Ministry of Education and other 'supporters'; at *'supra-regional' level*, in the national work group, the 'project leading team' (leading State Ministry of Education/ National Coordinator/ pedagogical coordinator), all Regional Centers and all 'national cooperating partners'.

Societal level	Network nod	Contact person	mechanism for shaping the network/environment -link ← Team	→ Environment Coop. Partners
local	Network-School	School Coordinator	School Steering Group	local cooperators
regional (State)	Regional Center	Regional Coordinator (RC) ↘	State Steering Group; subregional arrangements	regional cooperators
supra-State (National)	National Coordinating Office	National Coordinator (NC) ↘	Project leader; RC-Work group; Scientific advisor;	nationwide cooperators
international	ENHPS Technical Secretariat (TS)	ENHPS Consultant →	ENHPS business mtgs.(of National Coordinators)	European cooperators

Table 5.3.1: Structural frame of the German network for the development of Health Promoting Schools in its second phase, as 'OPUS-network' 1997-2000 (adapted from Barkholz et al 1998, 2001)

As shown with table 5.3.1, from 1997 network 'knots' are organizational entities only and, thus, the reshaped German network is clearly an *interorganizational network*. As *national* networks are sub-systems of the *European* Network (see chap. 5.1) this supports the thesis put forward in chapter 1 of international networks for the development of Health Promoting Schools being interorganizational networks. Cooperating partners may or may not be organizations, and may provide infrastructures, resources or know/how supportive of the networking. Already the table shows that in the reshaped (OPUS-) network a higher awareness and clarity of **network borders** exists ('nods' are clearly identified and distinguished from cooperating 'partners'). In the early phase of network creation a whole range of organizations had been presented as the "structural components *of* the (German) *Network*" (Arnold et al 1994 p29; italics not in original) but later these were (more rightly) referred to as 'structural components' in the closer *'environment of the project support center'* rather than 'of the network' (Barkholz, Paulus 1998 p30). Organizations listed included further education institutes and universities; NGOs and sickness funds; the leading State Ministry of Education (MoE), ministerial health education focal points as well as the Federal Education Ministry; the 'project schools' and even 'cooperatives in the European context' and WHO/EURO; and the national 'Project Support Center' in a central position. Not only as to the network borders but also the *mechanisms for* **network-environment-interactions** a better awareness and understanding was reached, with different 'teams' systematically offering opportunities. The emphasis on a 'team' structure also shows that from 1997 the German network (as OPUS-network) actively and visibly promoted a **team approach** (or group methods of coordination) for its operations, according to the Alter/Hage-network theory desirable if goals or tasks have a wider scope. All this indicates that over time the understanding of the *network* dimension of the large scale 'Health Promoting Schools'-development in Germany as distinct from its *environment* clearly improved and with this an *interorganizational network* took shape. (Barkholz et al 1998; Gabriel 1999)

External resources

As to the apparently external (financial and other) resources the two successive multi-State *'model experiments'* (on the "Network Health Promoting Schools" and "OPUS") were financially supported by the **public education sector**: the *Ministries of Education* of the participating States and the Federal Ministry. While during the first four years, via the State Ministries, it were the project *schools* who received about 8 hours teaching reduction for their health promoting work, during the following three years, within the "OPUS"- project, it were *Regional* Coordinators and Centers. The Commission of the *European* Community (or EU) provided support for specific activities (e.g. translations and adaptations of ENHPS materials and transnational activities). Attempts to achieve additional funding from the German government's initiative to 'link schools to the Internet' failed. In addition to the public sector's involvement, support was provided also by three organizations of the **non-governmental** or half-autonomous sector from both the **education and health** system. One sickness fund and the public accident-insurer association provided resources for particular projects. After four years, *legislative changes* improved the options of the latter to support the network's 'prevention' activities. But from 1997, German sickness funds lost their legal basis to undertake health promotion courses, project days or teacher training which lessened the as of then intense cooperation between the one sickness fund and the German network; however, the cooperation was continued as far as possible (i.e. in the area of health information (events, materials) and counseling). A 'further education academy' provided access to *knowledge* and advice on *European* links and funding sources. Other support for network members varied from region to region. From its inception it was an integral part of the German Network for developing Health Promoting Schools to encourage schools and also regional level actors to seek additional resources in their closer environments. In light of gaps and inherent challenges particularly for the schools, from 1997 the reshaped network approach included more systematically and explicitly (team) mechanisms to facilitate the involvement of the range of stakeholders in school health promotion. (BLK-Modellversuch Netzwerk... 1993; Arnold et al 1994, 1995; GNHPS 1994; NGS 1994; Barkholz, Paulus 1998; Barkholz et al 1998, 2001) At the level of individual network schools, during the first four years of network development in Germany (via the 'Health Promoting Schools'- project), only 3 of 19 'project' schools questionnaired (i.e. at least 10% of *all* network schools) had a budget on its own (WHO/EURO 1998). But network schools received 8 hours teaching reduction and had access to project specific financial resources, which sine 1997, via the OPUS-network project, was not any more the case (Meierjuergen 2001).

'Soft' and 'hard' networking

Implementing soft technologies increases the likelihood that exchange networks develop. From the start, the national Project Support Center of the German "Network Health Promoting Schools" (1993-1997) used soft technologies to create links among selected organizational representatives or individuals within or around the "Network" (**soft networking**). These included consciously designed network meetings, a network newsletter, an own logo for the German network (the European Network had none at the time), and providing access to and active and wide distribution of up-to-date address lists of various actors. Work conferences helped to link up also with external partners within and beyond the national borders. For example, within the first year one international conference was held as well as three 'working conferences' for school coordinators and then also for other members of the project schools and regional level actors (Arnold et al 1994). The latter aimed not only at information exchange and technical work but also at *personal motivation and experience exchange* (such as on special roles within the network). Nevertheless, evaluations did show that network actors such as school coordinators and national Support Center staff perceived the networking among schools as not yet sufficient. After four years, the national Project Support Center went so far to describe the then "Network Health Promoting Schools" as an (information) 'distribution network' with one-sided information flow from the Center *to* schools rather than extensive information exchange directly *among* schools (Barkholz/Paulus 1998, Barkholz et al 1998, 2000). This led to the **reshaping of the network approach** of the German network for the development of Health Promoting Schools towards what has been labeled an 'open participatory network', the 'OPUS'-network. This was pre-succeeded by a process in which the *network* dimensions moved more and more into the foreground, so that from 1997 and in support of *mutual learning* and *participation of schools*, the reshaped and renamed German network focused in modified and expanded ways on both 'soft' and 'hard' networking.

The **OPUS-network** continued to initiate, support and strengthen 'soft' networking but the focus shifted towards other actors. *National* work meetings (2-3 per year) now brought together staff of the national Coordinating Office and cooperating partners and the *Regional* Coordinators rather than network *school* representatives as before. The latter were now meant to meet at regional or sub-regional level. Within the reshaped network approach the **'team approach'** (in support of the evolving of ideas, *joint* planning, decision making and practical implementation) was even more stressed - and this at *all* network levels: as before within schools and the national Coordinating Office, but now newly or with more emphasis at community, regional and also sub-regional levels (e.g. as 'round tables' on health) and with one Coordinator as contact point each (see table 5.3.1). While team building in one way or the other was defined as a *'must'*, types and ways of their creation were decided at the level concerned and by those involved. Recommendations by the national Network Coordinating Office provided some guidance (see Barkholz et al 1998 p22).

The potential of **'hard' networking**, i.e. linking computers for effective information exchange was already acknowledged during **the first four years** of HPS network development in Germany, at least by the national Project Support Center. First efforts resulted in the use of existing 'school networks' to offer an electronic 'news forum' on school health promotion (EP.HEALTHY.SCHOOLS), conceptualized as a permanent conference with opportunities to provide information, pose questions, exchange experiences, and follow and/or participate in discussions; a special training module; the data bank 'index health and schools' (IGUS) with commentated publications (mainly in German) and also practice models; and the Network's bilingual website. The use of these means was repeatedly promoted at national network conferences and meetings, i.e. particularly among network *school* representatives. Although the capacities including 'hard ware realities' of the potential or intended users, particularly network schools, did not match up to the offers made, the national actors continued to emphasize 'hard networking' during further network developments. They were convinced that both 'health promoting school development' and school-to-school networking via the Internet were *two complementary innovative approaches* that match overall societal developments and school development needs, and help to enhance *direct* information exchange among *schools* and training and information flow in general. **After four years**, the national level of the now **'OPUS'**-network expected particularly the *Regional Centers* to step into electronic information exchange among themselves and with the national Network Coordinating Office, and the network newsletter was sent in electronic format. Governmental funding was sought to create the hard networks at regional level but failed. How far 'hard' and 'soft' *networking* (and not only electronic information *provision*) within the German network and beyond was realized will be addressed in chapter 5.3.1 below, when examining relations and interactions.

5.3.3 Developments over time: the evolution of the German network for the development of Health Promoting Schools

Systematic efforts to improve knowledge and practice of school related Health Promotion on a larger scale (i.e. involving 25 to 30 German schools or more at the same time) started with the *one*-State project "Health Promotion in a school's everyday life" (1990-1993). It turned out to be a valuable step towards a *multi*-State, almost *nationwide* network initiative on Health Promoting Schools. The one-State project worked at the interface of concept development and practical implementation. Mutual learning among schools was part of the project philosophy (but realized mainly among the nominated 'school coordinators'). Conceptual work included the translation of the five Health Promotion action areas for use in the school context, and the integration of health promoting and school development work. Project results shed light on and underlined the importance of 'school profiles', daily life conditions, school culture or climate in support of health, school/community-links, schools' self-organizing and innovation capacities and active role in shaping education policies. The term networking (in the sense of "Vernetzung") was already used, with view to school/community-links. Overall, the project provided *a conceptual basis* upon which the initiators of the German "Network Health Promoting Schools" could, and did built on. (Homfeldt, Barkholz 1993, 1994; Arnold et al 1994) The affinity of the German "Network" project with the pre-succeeding one-State project goes even further: The key actors at State level of this one-State project initiated and took the lead in the first almost *nationwide* project "*Network* Health Promoting Schools", namely the State Ministry of Education involved (at the time also chair of the committee of health education focal points of the sixteen State Ministries of Education in Germany), as well as academics and educational staff of the project office. Even the main donor, the German 'Federal-State-Commission for Educational Planning and Research Promotion ("BLK"), was the same. And the final conference of the first project was the 'start up' of the next (Barkholz, Gabriel 1994).

Towards a country wide "Network Health Promoting Schools" in Germany

Preparations for the German "Network" started already before the formal launch of the 'Network project' in 1997. In **preparatory meetings** of the health education focal points of the **State Ministries of Education** *'selection criteria' for schools* were defined and contacting of schools began. The formal launch of the project marked Germany's joining the European Network of Health Promoting Schools (ENHPS). The first six months served to prepare the successful start of a German "Network": with clarification of roles, responsibilities and relations among actors and issues of content and, most importantly, the creation of a *national* **'Project Support Center'** (PSC) and nomination of 'project schools'. The **school selection and nomination process** can be summarized as follows:

- identification of potential network schools (various types, two per State) by *State Ministries* of Education according to jointly defined **selection criteria**, i.e.: (a) a certain degree of understanding or experience with a 'pedagogical approach' to health promotion; and (b) preferably also experience with bigger projects or other model experiments;

- information of pre-selected *schools* about project goals and content by the same *Ministries*;

- phase of reflection on the project idea within *schools* and internal decision making on the school's participation in the German and, thus, European Network 'Health Promoting Schools'; this includes decisions by each of the school committees (teachers, pupils, parents) *and* by the 'school conference' (i.e. the whole school community);

- if *all* school committees decided positively, schools were designated as 'project schools' by their *State Ministry* of Education and, thus, were members of the "Network".

(Barkholz, Paulus 1998)

Hence, there was no open invitation to German schools to apply for "Network" participation in the early years and only those contacted by their Ministry could decide for or against their participation. In one case indeed a school decided against and another one was identified and nominated instead. From an international and interorganizational research perspective, the German *"Network Health Promoting Schools"* (rather than the Federal/State-project *on* a network) started to exist in February 1994, - when core network *members*, the 29 'project schools' started their practical work towards reaching the overall network aim: the creation of Health Promoting Schools. In 'project' terms, this was the beginning of the three-year 'main' project phase that ended in January 1997 and was followed by a four months 'analysis or final' phase. Table 5.3.2 provides an overview of "project development" and network initiation in Germany as presented by key national actors: the three 'phases' of the model experiment are complemented by six specific 'project steps' (from installation to securing results) which are not meant to be read in formal-chronological order. (Arnold et al 1994; Barkholz, Paulus 1998) Interestingly, for each step reference is made to different actors: First *'the network'* sets up the above explained pre-conditions for a successful start (installation step), a process with an *interorganizational* dimension. Then, the *schools* start working on their tasks: they step (jointly or individually?) into a process of health promoting *organizational development*: from needs assessment and team building across school staff, pupils and parents (initiation step) to planning, implementing and revising of activities including aspects of organizational development (implementation step) to critical reflection and selection of those activities and processes that should and could be part of the school's educational profile and 'daily life' as an organization (institutionalization step). When it comes to 'transfer' as one of 'the *Network's'* tasks, i.e. to report on experiences and results, other actors move back into the foreground of descriptions: the *'project support center'* (by deriving, synthesizing and disseminating new knowledge and the *'regional advisory structure'* (which supports 'project' schools in transferring experiences and are in contact with the other so called 'associate' schools). The final stock taking ('securing results') is linked to the development of perspectives for a continuation and expansion of the network project with the *'Project Support Center'* in the leading role.

Project Phases and Project Steps:

Pre-phase (8/93-1/94)		Main phase (2/94-1/97)			Analysis/ Final phase (2/97-5/97)
Installation	**Initiation**	**Implementation**	**Institutionalization**	**Transfer**	**Securing results**
Actors referred to:				'schools' - supported by **regional advisory** structure	
'the Network'	'schools'	'schools'	'schools'	'project support center'	'project support center'
				'the **network's** task' to reach visibility/ impact externally	
The German 'BLK'- *model experiment* "Network Health Promoting Schools"					
German *Network* (for the development of) 'Health Promoting Schools' ... → ... → ... →					

Table 5.3.2: Project steps of the German model experiment "Network Health Promoting Schools" and their foci (Project phases and steps from Arnold et al 1994 p23; Barkholz, Paulus 1998 p25)

What has been labeled German "Network Health Promoting School" did not cease to exist when the network initiating 'model project' ended. But from the formal reports by national Support Center and project leader on this first phase of large scale HPS development the Network's true nature remains vague. However, the education ministries prolonged their support for the creation of a network related to Health Promoting Schools in Germany and within the European context for another three years - in the form of another but reshaped network 'model project', "OPUS". (see Arnold et al 1994; Barkholz, Paulus 1998)

As illustrated in table 5.3 2, reports on 'network *project*' development much refer to the schools as main actors but also the Project Support Center. When '*the network*' is referred to there is no mention of who is exactly meant by that. The overall impression is that of a **strong 'school' focus within a vague and less stressed 'network'**

context. From an interorganizational research perspective the national 'Project Support Center' emerges as a likely network *member* - in addition to the 29 network schools. All other national or State level actors identified earlier as key actors 'within or around' the German Network appear to be rather external (supporters) to the network. This assumption needs further examination, though.

Expansion of the "German Network" or sprouting of 'regional' networks ?

From its inception, the German 'Network Health Promoting Schools' was meant to be both sustained beyond the length of the respective 'model experiment' 1993-1997 and expanded beyond the limited number of project schools to many more schools in each State. The latter has been conceptualized as **'rationalization'** with the creation of 'regional sub-networks' *within* the German Network over the long term (BARMER w.y.; GNHPS 1994; Arnold et al 1994). The technical support of the 'project schools' and in-service teacher training according to State and locally specific situations was central and much needed. Already for the only 29 pilot schools this would not have been possible by one central, national 'project support center', and definitively not for even more 'health promoting schools' to come. However, it took half a year before actors recognized the need for additional support structures in the regions. The action that followed aimed at establishing sustainable advisory structures at local and State level that would support 'project' schools and any others interested in Health Promotion. (Barkholz, Paulus 1998)

As important **actors in the regions** identified were 'health education focal points' of the **Ministries of Education** of the participating States, and **a special two-level advisory structure** for participating schools (a recommendation by the Ministries' health education focal points) (PUZ 1994). In May 1994, a) one 'advisor at *regional* level' per State and b) so called 'advisors at *school* level' (about one per project school) were nominated. The 'regional level' advisors came mainly from the public *education* sector (State institutes of further education/ ministries/ authorities), the 'school' advisors from a *wider range* of organizations (mainly public but also non-governmental) among them about 50% *health* (care) oriented NGOs or universities. (Arnold et al 1994) This indicates high network complexity. Quickly after nomination, the national Support Center brought the advisors together; training and work sessions followed, their roles within the network were clarified, consensus achieved on important project issues - i.e. *group methods of coordination* rather than impersonal methods were used. - State Ministries acted as financial *supporters* of advisors (travel costs/per diem). The network's national Support Center and the State health education focal points, with input from the regional advisors, **recommended the set up of 'regional work groups'** of pilot schools, regional advisors, and regional focal points of the national cooperating partners - which i**deally would** establish a *formal* **regional work committee** as *'central regional* information agency' for (project) schools. (PUZ 1994)

However, the German Network project unfolded its own dynamics and the Federal and State level initiators felt the need of **opening up for additional schools earlier than planned**. A year after the 29 Pilot schools had started their work, the national Support Center and later also the participating States explored and/or prepared the States' *nomination* of about 2 to 5 new *'associated schools'* per State. These were selected by the 'advisors' in close cooperation with the State concerned and the national Support Center. The developments that followed vary widely from State to State (also depending on the human and financial resources locally). The new 'associated schools' received materials and advice from 'advisors' as well as the German *Network's* 'cooperating partners'. Regional conferences were held in some regions. At the end of the 'model project', in six of the 15 participating States regional substructures were in place ('regional working groups' and/or HPS-'practice offices').

The first four years (or first phase) of network development in Germany - intermediate synthesis and discussion

During the first year of existence of the German 'Network Health Promoting Schools', the 29 'project' schools, Project Support Center and a few cooperating or supporting actors most involved in its practical work, were joined already by a new group of actors: special 'advisors' for project schools from a range of organizations. This supports the assumption that the title of the 1993-1997 'model experiment' - "Network Health Promoting Schools", *not* network *of* Health Promoting Schools - was consciously chosen, - a wording deviating from the European Network "of" Health Promoting Schools. (Only English translations of German documents show the term 'German Network *of* HPS' likely to harmonize with language used at international level rather than making a technical statement.) The name given to the German network together with the pursued sub-differentiation by region indicate that the large scale development of HPS in Germany was not meant to be undertaken in a pure network of *schools* but also of other actors. The lack of a clear 'network' concept at the beginning and the developments summarized above support the assumption that during the first phase of creation of a German network for the development of Health Promoting Schools (1993-1997) the network first *started to take shape around two types of actors* (and may be network members): core *organizations*, i.e. the 'pilot schools' and the national 'Project Support Center', and a group of core *individuals* related to them, the so called (school or regional level) 'advisors'. This is an important point as it relates to the theses of this research project that international networks for the development of Health Promoting Schools are inter*organizational* networks. As the *group* of advisors started to meet at national level the question arises whether it represented a new organizational entity, i.e. an *expansion* of the *German* network as a whole. Another interpretation is that the German network earlier than planned did branch out State by State: in this view, per State, the about three 'advisors' together with the two initial 'project schools', the regional outlets of national cooperating partners (sickness fund and accident insurers) plus eventually two to five newly nominated 'associated schools', formed the yet young *sprouts of regional networks* (for the development of) Health Promoting Schools. Some regional cases of the time demonstrate that these had the capacity, with some 'nurturing', to mature to *sustainable* regional networks (see Barkholz, Paulus 1998; Barkholz et al 2001).

Particularly in highly federalist and geographically big countries such as Germany sustainable '*regional* networks' would be a positive outcome, as sub-units of a nationwide initiative on a 'Network for the development of Health Promoting Schools'. However, the focus of this pilot research on assessing interorganizational networks for Health Promotion is on the *European* Network of Health Promoting Schools and two of its *member countries* to *exemplify* its structure. The *European* Network was conceptualized at national and school level and an examination of the variety of network spin offs or sprouts that occurred and still are occurring within and around it is not the focus of and cannot be covered by this research project. Rather, from an **international perspective**, it aims at developing and in a first round piloting the proposed assessment framework and indicators for interorganizational networks in Health Promotion, here international networks for the development of Health Promoting Schools. Therefore, the *nationwide* network dimensions of the ENHPS in Germany (and later in Slovenia) will remain the focus of research (rather than particularities of sub-national/ regional developments). Thus, the **examination of *Germany-wide* developments** will be continued:

At the end of the first four years of network development in Germany - from now on also referred to as the 'first phase' - documents still reflect an **ambivalence** with regard to the creation of a network *'of'* Health Promoting Schools and one *for the development* of such schools. On the one hand, **network membership** is clearly defined as to *school* members which is likely the influence of the guidelines of the European Network (ENHPS): On the one hand, members are the 29 *'project' schools* initially selected and several so called 'associated' schools that joined the network's regional branches. As the 'project' schools, also the latter needed to fulfill criteria and be formally nominated. Therefore, and as the "rationalization" was understood as a process *within* the overall German network, it can be assumed that 'associated' schools became members not only of a regional but also the German network as a whole and, thus, of the European Network. On the other hand, the status of *other important but 'non-school' actors* such as the national Support Center was not clearly declared: it remains to be examined whether these are 'participants' of the time limited Federal/State 'network project', 'members' of the longer living *'network'* (intended to be sustainable beyond project financing), and/or *external* supporters of both. This was the situation when from 1997 the network development in Germany was reshaped towards an "open participatory network and school health/OPUS".

'Open participation' - a door to network evolution and growth

As regard **content** (i.e. health promoting school development) the 'OPUS'-network represented a *continuation* of the existing German network for the development of Health Promoting Schools (see above). With view to the **network approach**, it represented *a new developmental step*. This was one of the outcomes of the conceptual work and knowledge development during the first phase of the ENHPS in Germany. Already during the final phase of that 'old' "Network Health Promoting Schools" a reshaped network was being prepared. The Federal Education Ministry's approval of another 'model project' on "OPUS" (1997-2000) provided the political, legal and financial framework to actively continue the development of a German network for developing Health Promoting Schools. The yet national 'Project Support Center' and the focal points of the *State Ministries* of Education discussed OPUS-structures, desired project development, and guiding questions (an issue of network project/environment-interactions less emphasized during the first phase of network development). Regular work meetings to continue discussions were agreed upon, as was a continuous information flow from OPUS to the State Ministries and 'OPUS-Regional Coordinators'. The latter were identified by the Ministries in *close coordination* with the national Center, 'rewarded' with about eight hours teaching reduction for their work, and supported in setting up one "OPUS-*Regional Center*" per State. This way, in contrast to the previous network phase, formally established *organizational entities* rather than individual advisors became regional cornerstones of the German network. This supports the thesis that inter-national networks for the development of Health Promoting Schools are interorganizational networks. - The national coordinating center and the three 'national cooperating partners' of the first network project soon agreed to continue their cooperation for another three years.

With the second phase of development the German network for the development of Health Promoting Schools (as 'OPUS'-network) reached another level of network development: Now, a network philosophy and not only network related questions did exist. The network's **guiding idea** ("Leitbild") was clearly formulated and *consensus reached with the Regional Coordinators* of the OPUS-network. Other members such as schools had to "buy in". This 'guiding idea' is in line with but goes beyond the guidelines of the European Network concerning the Settings approach. Six conceptual items and underlying values are made explicit: the understanding of health, the salutogenic approach in Health Promotion, the Settings approach as to schools, the participatory principle, the network principle, and the European dimension of the network. The new level of sophistication of the German network is reflected particularly in two points: The **'participation principle'** refers to the enabling of 'those concerned' to become 'participants' in a '*democratic* process of internal school development'. The **'networking principle'** ("Vernetzungsgedanke") is referred to as "we are going *our own* way, but we are going it *together*", and as making *agreements* and creating *suitable* structures to **exchange and share** knowledge, information, resources and experiences. Importantly, the **openness for new members** is explicitly stated: 'New comers *will be advised and supported*'. The European *Network* dimension is not mentioned but actors 'understand themselves as part of a European *initiative*'.

For this second phase of network development for Health Promoting Schools in Germany, i.e. the 'open participatory network'/ OPUS phase, the **school selection and nomination process and membership criteria were modified**: Now, the '*Re-

gional Centers' rather than the State Ministries of Education *decided* on which and how many schools became network member, but a) in coordination with the responsible Ministry and the National Coordinating Office and b) dependent on its own resources. The following selection or *membership criteria*, a mix of old and new ones, were to be fulfilled by network/ member schools:

- commitment and work according to the newly formulated OPUS-*guiding idea* (above);
- work on 'health promoting school development' according to the *step wise approach* developed during the first four years of network development in Germany;
- commitment to remain an active network member from the self-chosen point in time of joining the net until the formal end of the OPUS- project in May 2000;

Besides these new criteria some of the former continued to apply:

- the nomination of a school coordinator; creation of a school team to steer the project; and a positive decision on the network membership by the *'whole' school community*, i.e. by a clear majority of the so called 'school conference'.

The reshaped German network for developing Health Promoting Schools overcame the exclusive character of the first years or 'ENHPS pilot phase'. The OPUS-network aimed at offering **two possibilities to schools**: a) to apply for and eventually become full OPUS-member or *'network school'*, or b) to enter sooner or later into an information *exchange on selected topics via the Internet*. However, the latter was not realized as expected as many schools or teachers lacked capacities to access or use such opportunities (Barkholz et al 2001).

As shown more clearly below, the reshaped German (OPUS-) network did *not* pursue the original vague idea of a *nationwide* network of health promoting *schools*. Now 'network schools' were meant to network in *regional or sub-regional* arrangements; at the *national* level the new 'Regional Centers' were to meet. Criteria put forward for the **selection** of the **Regional Centers** were: a) technical competencies and experiences in health promoting *school development* that enables them to effectively support schools, and b) orientation towards the guiding principles and ideas of the *European* Network of Health Promoting Schools (Barkholz et al 1998).

From an international and network research perspective, the **'Regional Centers'** rather than network schools appear as new core members of the reshaped *nationwide* (i.e. multi-State) or 'German' network. Regional Centers met regularly with the National Coordinating Office; and their tasks included the networking among network schools within their regions. The new network picture emerging is clearly that of an almost *nationwide* 'German' Network *for the development of* (not 'of') Health Promoting Schools - with regional *sub*-networks for the development of Health Promoting Schools (HPS). The following examination of the relations and interactions of the key actors or network members of the German network in both developmental phases (first under the heading "Network Health Promoting Schools", then as "OPUS") aims to clarify these and other issues raised before.

5.3.4 Interactions and relations of network members

Organizational systems → Key actors ↓	German 'network project' participants	German network members "Network HPS"	from 1997 "OPUS"	Regional HPS- projects*/ networks participants*/members
national level	Federal MoE/ 'Laender-beirat' (advisory board with State level MoEs) Core cooperating partners (BARMER, BAGUV/BUK, Th.-Morus-Academy)	Project Support Center	National Coordinating Office the *leading* State MoE (Schleswig-Holstein) ?	
regional level	State MoEs (participating States only)	'advisors' in the regions ?	Regional Centers	*'Advisors' ? * a regional work group/ formal 'work circle' in some States
local level		ENHPS pilot schools/'project' schools (HPS) Associated schools?	OPUS- or 'network' schools (HPS)	'pilot' and 'associated' /network schools (HPS) *'other' schools ? *local organizations ?

Advisors': 1 at regional level; 1 per project school (per State)
BARMER: a German statutory sickness fund
BAGUV: Association of the German public accidence insurers
ENHPS: European Network of Health Promoting Schools
HPS: Health Promoting School(s)
NHPS: here: 'Network Health Promoting Schools'
MoE: Ministry of Education
MoEs: Ministries of Education
*: assumed participants of regional HPS project
?: actor positioned with less certainty

Table 5.3.3: The ENHPS in Germany or the German network for the development of Health Promoting Schools 1993-2000: key actors and assumed membership status as well as related social systems (projects).

To examine interactions and relations of network 'members' the **question of membership** or network borders needs to be answered. There is no easy response because the German network was initiated and over the first years implemented without a clear network concept. As at European level, also for the first (pilot) phase of network development in Germany it seems useful to distinguish between a) the network '*project* (here Federal/State-'model experiment') and b) the *'Network'* itself. Another yet open question is whether during the first four years the German network, the then "Network Health Promoting Schools", was an inter*organizational* system or a mixed one with *individual* members, too. Much reference was made to 'advisors' many of which did this job in their personal capacity rather than with an organizational mandate; and it remained unclear whether these advisors were *'network'* members or parts of the network *'project'* or supportive and enabling *environment* of the network. Table 5.3.3 on the *ENHPS in Germany* provides a summary of both key (organizational) actors during **the first four years or phase one,** and their assumed membership or participant status as to the German "Network" and 'network project'. It also provides a simple framework for the examination of the inherent assumptions about the German network's boundaries.

It needs to be recalled from chapter 4.2, that the following exploration of interorganizational *relations and interactions* within and around the German network for the development of Health Promoting Schools during the years 1993 to 2000 attempts to capture **an *overall* picture.** It aims at improving the understanding of Network *membership and environment* - as - as the crucial base for applying the proposed network assessment framework (chap.3) as to a) basic structural network features (i.e. size, complexity, differentiation, connectivity, and centrality) - and b) the extent of organizational networking processes. *Other basic features* of interorganizational *networks* need to be kept in mind, too (non-/less hierarchical, lateral links, self-regulation; informal or formal relations; direct person-to-person-connections, trust, mutual benefit/reciprocity, information/resource sharing, long term perspective, etc.). (see chap. 4.2) The Alter/Hage network typology is an issue of reference, too (exchange, promotional, systemic networks). As before, the examination of interactions and relations is organized around one selected key actor per system level whose relationships with all others is being examined (see figure 4.2.1 above). **For the first (four year) phase** of network development in Germany **(1993-1997)** these are the *national* 'Project Support Center' and the *'project schools'* which (as shown in chap. 5.2.1 before) are both ENHPS members. For the next three years or the **second phase** of network development **(1997-2000)** chosen are the then so called *'National* Coordinating Office', the *'Regional* Centers', and the *'network schools'*. For both phases, also the relations of the German network *as a whole* (the "Network Health Promoting Schools" and later "OPUS"-network) will be reflected upon: 'inwards' looking (as to the German regions) and 'outwards' (as to the European Network).

I.	Interactions and relations of the national support/coordinating centre with other organizations

To derive the relevant information the following 'search scheme' presented has been used:

THE NATIONAL SUPPORT/ COORDINATING CENTER'S **interactions and relations with:**	*organizations within their countries* ↓		*organizations outside their countries/ the European Dimension* ↓
'national - local' →	**1. the network schools/ HPS:** A: Pilot HPS; 'other'; B: OPUS/network schools;other		
'national - regional' →	**2. key actors in regions:** A: advisors* (at regional or school level) B: Regional Centers		
'national - national' →	**3. key national actors:** A, B: Federal-State-Commission; MoEs; 3 'Cooperating Partners';	**4. other national organizations or networks** (A,B)	**5. other ENHPS 'countries'** (A, B)
'national-internat.' →			**6. IPC & TS** (A, B)
the part & the whole →	**7. The German network as a whole / the "ENHPS" as a whole** (A , B)		

ENHPS: European Network of Health Promoting Schools
HPS: Health Promoting Schools
IPC: International Planning Committee of the ENHPS
MoEs: Ministries of Education (Federal / State level)
TS: Technical Secretariat of the ENHPS

Table 5.3.4: The ENHPS in Germany: Schema of potential interorganizational relationships of the national support or coordinating center with others within and around the ENHPS or the national network for the development of Health Promoting Schools.(A: 1st phase of network development 1993-1997; B: 2nd (OPUS) phase 1997-2000).

The 'national - local' dimension

1. National support/coordinating center and the (health promoting) network schools

A) Among other tasks the Project Support Center of the then **'Network Health Promoting Schools'** was responsible for coordination, information and advice *'within* the network', creation of links *with and among* the 29 pilot schools, *evaluation and feed back* on developments to the schools (as well as to external partners and the general public), plus for *concept and knowledge development* (the 'concept of the network' included). This shows its role as intellectual leader and overall 'motor' of network development. Preparing the *opening up of the "Network" beyond the 29 'project schools'* towards other schools was the future oriented task. To support *experience exchange and networking among 'project' schools* (in support of their effective work locally) the Center focused on regular national face-to-face meetings with school coordinators and head teachers of pilot schools (i.e. 'soft' networking) realized about three times per year, and electronic information and experience exchange (i.e. 'hard' networking) which was less realized. In its final report the Center critically stated that overall the German "Network" had turned out to be a centralized 'distribution network' as the Center had remained the main information *provider,* schools mainly information *receiver,* and direct information or experience *exchange among* schools was hardly realized (Barkholz/Paulus 1998). However, as to German project schools' 'activities at national level' the ENHPS Schools Data Base (WHO/EURO 1998) shows: Towards the end of the first four network years in Germany, 17 of the 19 pilot schools covered (i.e. at least a good half of all network schools) mention their national level 'meetings'; and 11 (i.e. at least a third of all) network schools report of 'cooperation between schools'. At least a third of all pilot schools reported 'support received' from the National Coordinator (the same amount referred to the national network partner 'sickness fund').

From an interorganizational research perspective the labeling of the German Network as 'distribution' network appears too harsh of a statement that indicates a degree of disappointment of the national Center's staff. Documents show that schools did not only receive but also *provide* much information to the Center; and that 'soft networking' among schools *took* place and successfully (during national meetings), even if schools would have loved to do even more. But surely the Center's increasing expectations towards *'hard'* networking directly among schools were not fulfilled. But these appear to have been just too high when looking at the still quite limited Information Technology related capacities of German schools in *general* of the time. However, after the ENHPS 'pilot phase' the German network's network approach was reoriented and the national Project Support *Center* became the National *Coordinating Office:*

B) This renaming as well as that of the German network as a whole - from 'Network Health Promoting Schools' to **'OPUS- network'** or an *'open'* and *'participatory'* network on school health - matches with the reformulation of the national network body's roles and responsibilities. The **National Coordinating Office** set out to fulfill a kind of 'bridge' function, in coordination with those participating in the "school net": With view to **actors external** to the network the national Office was to serve as motivator or contact point for *'non-network schools'* (to raise or respond to their interest in the network), but also liaise with *supra-regional 'partners'* (e.g. Federal Ministries/ NGOs/ and model projects working on similar issues). With view to the **network itself** it was to publish an electronic newsletter, identify experts where needed, and advise and support *network schools* as to issues of planning, implementation and evaluation and this *in cooperation with the 'Regional Centers'.* (Barkholz et al 1998) The National Coordinating Office kept track of OPUS- school members and *formally confirmed network membership* at school level (certificate). Overall, an **interesting change** in approach is that since the reshaping of the German network as 'OPUS', the *national coordinating center* was not anymore in systematic or regular contact with the network *schools*; the newly established 'Regional Centers' took over this task.

From an interorganizational research perspective this is an essential change: as opposed to the first four years of network development in Germany - where the national center was positioned as rather *within* the German network for the development of Health Promoting Schools (of which both schools *and* the National Support Center were a part) now another picture emerged: a) a separation of the *national* coordinating body from the network that is encompassing the network (or OPUS) *schools*, and related to this b) a rise of a second network encompassing the *National* Coordinating Office and the *Regional* Centers. While it remains to be further examined whether the former is conceptualized and/or developing itself as a network *of* (health promoting) schools, the latter clearly points to the development of a national/regional-level network 'for the development of' Health Promoting Schools and not 'of' schools. With the transformation of the former "Network Health Promoting Schools" into the "OPUS" network, the ENHPS in Germany seems to have split into *two types* of sub-networks: on the one hand, a network *for the development of* Health Promoting Schools spanning national and regional level only; on the other hand, a type of network that links participating *schools* (and may be other actors). As shown below the two are linked through the participation of the Regional Centers in both.

The 'national - regional' dimension

2. National support or coordinating center and 'non-school' actors in the regions

A) During the **first four years** of network development, the national Center's relations or interactions with two groups of actors are of relevance here: those within the 'advisory system' created in each State, and the State Ministries of Education. As to the latter the Project Support Center's tasks included informing and liaising with them; it kept them informed. As to the **'advisors' in the regions**, the Center *identified and mobilized* them and jointly with the project leading State Ministry *qualified and financially supported* them. It *organized* face-to-face-meetings for advisors ('soft' networking) and *jointly with* them created a list of 'school-related health factors' and national workshops.

B) **From 1997**, with the OPUS-network the national-regional dimension was significantly modified: the National Coordinating Office - now having *organizational* counter parts at regional level (the **'Regional Centers')** - was to *closely cooperate* with these Regional Centers and take part in their selection processes of network schools. The 'guiding idea' for the whole network (originally outlined by the National Office) was jointly discussed and launched before its acceptance became the precondition for network participation (also of, Regional Centers). Towards Regional Centers the national coordinating office played a key role in *information provision and further qualification,* as it was responsible for all *supra*-regional information and advisory services within or by the German network. Regional Centers perceived experience exchange, developmental work as to network structures, key concepts and (network) competencies of members, as well as the links to the European Network as important and helpful. With view to the National Office **regional coordinators** felt predominantly or fully 'acknowledged and accepted', 'benefiting' from the national meetings organized, and in most cases also effectively 'supported'; all three items ranked among the first 5 (out of 25) that were most positively assessed (Barkholz et al 2001 p342-373).

The 'national - national' dimension (within and across borders)

3. National support/coordinating center and the Federal and State level

The mechanism of a 'Federal-State-Commission/FSC- model experiment' by which Federal and State level can jointly fund projects of nationwide interest was the one used by the Education Ministries in Germany to set up the two successive model projects on network development for Health Promoting Schools in Germany (1993-2000). In this context, the national 'Project Support Center' and 'National Coordinating Office' *were set up* by the project leading State Ministry of Education, which provided crucial (teaching) staff. Throughout the network development projects, the national center was not only *accountable to but also clearly financially dependent on* the Federal-State-Commission and the leading Ministry. From 1997, the reshaped network concept put forward by the national center did *not* consider Education Ministries as 'network knots', in spite of their increased involvement in the overall developmental work. - These points confirm an assumption made earlier on the German network's boundaries that places the Education Ministries *external* to the German network from its inception: the Ministries are participants of the Federal/State- network '*projects*' or closer network environment, important donors and supporters rather than network members.

4. National support/ coordinating center and other (national) organizations or networks in Germany

Here, throughout the years the national center's interactions and cooperation focused on the three formal "*national cooperating partners*" (sickness fund, accident insurers, education academy) and on implementing respective cooperative agreements. All parties continued their cooperation beyond the first four years of agreement (in one case even in spite of legal constraints) which indicates what has been repeatedly stressed: that this in Hastings' terms 'networking with external others' of the German network via its national center has been perceived as meaningful and successful and mutually beneficial. There was also regular contact and some joint activity (e.g. a network conference) with the 'Institute for Health Education' at the University of Flensburg, the host of the national coordinating center. Ideas to permanently establish the national center within this Institute after project financing have not been realized. - The national center was also a driving force towards the creation of (Internet based) services and materials that would stimulate those *'other'* *schools* that did not (yet) become network members but searched for information on school health promotion.

5. National support/coordinating center and actors in other ENHPS member countries

The national center and the leading State Ministry of Education played a key role in strengthening and expanding the ENHPS related cooperation of *German speaking countries* towards the transnational 'sub-network' of the European Network (see chap. 5.1.4). In the midst of the first phase of network development (in 1995) Germany hosted the first transnational conference of about 50 health-promoting *schools,* the national coordinating centers, and also advisors, cooperating partners, Ministries of Education in charge, and the European Council. And the national center continued to play an active role as to the transnational conferences that followed and where not only materials were *exchanged* but also *joint applications* for EU funding delivered. The latter indicates that - in Alter/Hage terms - the German coordinating center not only engaged in a transnational *exchange* but also *promotional (joint action)* network. ('Subregional' Network... 1997; Barkholz, Paulus 1998)

The 'national-international' dimension

6. The national support/coordinating center and the 'European Network of Health Promoting Schools'

Throughout the German 'network projects' (1993-2000) the national center *kept in touch* with the European Network (or ENHPS) initiators and Technical Secretariat as well as the National Coordinators of other ENHPS member countries (see also chap. 5.1). From the national perspective this is an 'outward orientation', from the European Network perspective an orientation towards 'lateral links' as expected of all ENHPS member countries. To secure experience exchange and knowledge transfer, the German center *actively participated and contributed* at European level in several ways (e.g. manual adaptation/ Conference contributions). Notably in the area of evaluation the German network through its scientific advisor moved into a *leading role* (e.g. with the first international HPS evaluation conferences 1999/2001). Also, the national center *provided the first bilingual website* of all ENHPS country members and, thus, made itself (potentially but actively) *accessible* throughout Europe and beyond. It also *used opportunities for direct support* from WHO and the EU to realize the German network's 'European dimension' (such as in national events).

'The whole and its parts'

7. The national support/coordinating center and the German "Network" as a whole

A) During **the first four years,** the Project Support Center played a key role in cooperatives with *external* others at national level (see above) and also as to linking up with regional level actors. Its role in 'networking *within*' the network and even within other network members, the schools, is addressed below. Overall, the Project Support Center was crucial in the various country wide '*soft*' networking processes and tried to provide as far as possible opportunities for 'hard' networking, too. Particularly with regard to the network 'project' schools and the 'advisors' in the regions the Center provided essential *technical guidance* and support and organized the crucial face-to-face network meetings and related financial support. With regard to '*hard*' networking the national Support Center over the first three years created the network's website with electronic newsletter, key documents, contact lists, etc. - a means for both information dissemination supportive of 'soft' networking *within* the network as well as to the network's *environment*.

B) **From 1997,** within the OPUS-network the national Coordinating Office's *role changed* twofold: On the one hand, it limited its direct networking mainly to the Regional Centers and supra-regional actors, 'giving up' the direct networking with network schools of former times. Here the Regional Centers took over. As to its role as evaluator the focus shifted from 'school development' evaluation (of individual schools) to *'network' evaluation*. Besides various aspects related to the Regional Centers, network dimensions evaluated included the extent of contacts among actors *within regions*, the purpose of these contacts, and the role and extent of *'hard'* networking.

The national support/ coordinating center and the German network as a whole - intermediate synthesis and discussion

In light of the findings above and with view to **(A)** the first phase of network development in Germany, it is reasonable to define not only the 29 pilot schools but also the national 'Project Support Center' as organizational *member* of the ENHPS sub-system in Germany, the then German "Network Health Promoting Schools". It shared and acted on the common goal of creating Health Promoting Schools (HPS); took part in regular, national level experience and information exchange among and with pilot schools; and it seems to have had trustful and supportive relationships with them. Also, it fulfilled its role as national support center as required for a country's *European* Network membership. With view to **(B)** the second phase of the ENHPS in Germany, i.e. with the reshaping of the German network as OPUS and the national 'Support Center' as 'Coordinating Office', the role of this national body changed. Nevertheless, it is reasonable to define it as network *member* also of the *reshaped* German network: While the 'old' national network was sub-differentiated into *regional* networks with one Regional Center each, a modified but *national* network system *remained*. The national office not only continued to share and work towards the network's overall goal (large scale HPS creation) but was systematically placed within the reshaped and specified, multi-level network and team structure. It continued to take part in regular, national level experience and information exchange - but now with the new Regional Centers rather than the increased number of network schools. Also these relationships seem to have been mutually beneficial. In comparison to the national support or coordinating center, the Ministries of Education were key participants in the national 'model *projects*' (as co-funders and supporters).

Thus, the results of the general German case study support the perspective derived from the European case study (in chapter 5.1): that the European Network for the development of Health Promoting Schools (ENHPS) has at least *two* types of members: *national support centers* and Health Promoting (network) *Schools*. The overall ENHPS *'project'* can then be understood on the one hand, as being in a supportive and guiding role towards that European *Network* and, on the other hand, - so the suggestion from this country case study - as encompassing *not* only the *international* level actors (WHO, EC, CE) but *national* level actors, too: a) the *national Ministries* of Education and of Health and (particularly in the case of federalist member countries) in the future potentially also b) committees or associations of State Ministries or even local level authorities. (see also fig. 5.2.2)

Now, the attention will be shifted from the interorganizational relations of the German *national* support or coordinating center to those of the network (or 'project') *schools* in Germany.

II. Interactions and relationships among the health promoting network or 'project' schools and of those with other organizations

The 'search scheme' shown in table 5.3.5 has been used to derive and present the interrelations of the German 'pilot' or 'network' schools with other organizations. The *main* information sources are intermediate project reports and final reports/book publications (Arnold, Barkholz, Gabriel, Heindl, Paulus 1994, 1995; Barkholz and Paulus 1998, Barkholz, Gabriel, Jahn, Paulus 1998 and 2001). A range of other sources was used as mentioned in the text.

THE NETWORK SCHOOLS' interactions and relations with:	*organizations within the country* ↓		*organizations outside the country / the European Dimension* ↓
'local - local' →	1. **other HPS:** • other Project/ Network Schools • 'associated' schools • other schools	2. **local organizations in their community** • health care; others	3. **schools outside the country**
'local – regional' →	4. **regional actors** • Advisors • Regional Centers • MoEs		
'local - national' →	5. **national actors** • national support and coordinating center • 'National Cooperating Partners'		
'the part & the whole' →	6. **The German network as a whole** 7. **The 'European Network of HPS' as a whole**		

ENHPS: European Network of Health Promoting Schools   MoEs: Ministries of Education
HPS: Health Promoting Schools

Table 5.3.5: Schema of potential interorganizational relationships of the 'project' or 'network' schools in Germany with other key organizations within and around the German network for the development of Health Promoting Schools (or the ENHPS in Germany)

As explained in chapter 4.2 the 'local - *international*' dimension is irrelevant as schools have *cross-border* contacts with *schools* or may be *national* actors of other countries but hardly ever with actors at European level such as the ENHPS Secretariat.

The 'local - local' dimension (from neighborhood to neighbor countries)

1. German 'project schools' among each other, and with other schools

A) **During the first four years** of HPS network development in Germany, the task of project or network schools in Germany was to develop 'health promoting school profiles' that would be an *example for other* schools in their region. School-to-school networking as a goal was expressed more indirectly: as the school's *involvement in the planned sub-differentiation by region* of the German Network. The focus was on three areas one of which includes networking and interorganizational relations: a) overall school development; b) development of successful examples for practical implementation; and c) internal 'opening up' of the school (i.e. beyond the classroom) and towards outside, 'its networking', and its involvement in 'rationalization' structures and processes. Measures of organizational development, and in-service teacher training within *and* across schools should support this.

The halfway evaluation of the then "Network Health Promoting Schools" asked the 29 project schools and some 'associated' schools what in their **cooperation with other network schools** is *good or can stay* as is. Over a third did not respond but the others highlighted the *experience exchange* at the Network's *national* conferences that facilitated getting in touch with others. As to *difficulties* for cooperation, more than half of the network schools did *not* mention anything, others pointed particularly to geographical distances and differences in school types. Regarding *missing aspects* in their cooperation a fifth did not respond, others pointed to the *exchange* of information and practical materials *outside* national meetings, because of *geographical distance and lack of time*. Finally, two thirds of schools expressed that they wish **more experience exchange, a more continuous communication and more contacts among schools**. The national work conferences were perceived as not sufficient enough for experience exchange among network schools, and *regional* meetings and training as meaningful and desired. (Barkholz/Paulus 1998 p118)

Overall, during the first phase of large scale development of Health Promoting Schools in Germany (1993-1997) eleven national and two transnational conferences - described as 'important information and communication points' - brought together all network schools, the national Project Support Center, and also other actors of the German 'Network project'. As to the network schools' **links with other schools** such as 'associated schools' in their regions no overview has been published. However, *examples* of network school activities such as neighborhood conferences with other schools and links with schools abroad have been found.

These findings indicate that after the first phase of network development in Germany, the *network* dimension *among* schools at the level of an interorganizational exchange network still needed strengthening. But it is also apparent that many network schools already realized stronger school-to-school- exchanges within the German Network. However, limitations to realize this equally across a big country like Germany and the need and potential of stronger networking within *regions* are apparent, too.

B) Matching with the above, **from 1997**, within the reshaped German network OPUS the increasing number of network schools was not anymore to meet at national but at *regional* level. The team structure to be developed in all regions, the 'regional steering group' was to encompass among others the coordinators of all network schools in the region; but as said before by the year 2000 these did exist in less than half of the States only - leaving many schools without this mechanism for regular 'soft' networking among each other and with other cooperators. However, Regional Centers had the task to organize regular work meetings for schools. Therefore, and also because schools had to sign the 'OPUS-guiding idea' including the 'networking principle' (resources exchange/sharing) and the European dimension therein, one can assume: During the second phase of German network development network schools were more conscious about and committed to networking with external others (be it schools or not). In the 'old' network (before OPUS) network schools had to sign "only" the 'Health Promoting Schools'-concept which inherently calls for (in Hastings' terms) 'networking within' schools but lacks a clear school-to-school-networking dimension; it stresses school-community links, though. Unfortunately, the up to day published results of the German network's evaluation part called "network analysis" (undertaken by region) does not provide information on the degree of school-to-school networking and other links of network schools to specified partners (e.g. their Regional Center) (see Barkholz et al 2001 pp373-398). However, the evaluation of **Regional Coordinators' perspectives** on networking issues after two and a half years of existence of the OPUS-network provides two specific insights on **networking among schools**: As to the effect of the networking ("Vernetzung") in their region, a) roughly 55% are fully convinced and 30% agree in general that it '*enables schools to exchange experiences* among each other informally' (with positive trend). But b) only good 5% are fully convinced and good 20% agree in general that the networking in the region 'serves the cooperation between schools' in the sense of '*developing joint plans'*. However, over 70% agreed that this is realized at least to a *low* degree, a point that was only a year before yet fully denied by over 30% and agreed on by only good 50%.

With view to the interorganizational network typology by Alter and Hage (1993) these findings indicate: Within the German 'open participatory network' on health promoting schools - after 2 to 3 years and with view to the *regional* level - in the vast majority of States 'exchange relations' (and may be even 'exchange networks') among network schools had emerged. They also indicate that many of these regional sub-network's developed the potential to 'mature' beyond 'exchange' relations or networks towards 'promotional' joint action relations or networks - according to Alter and Hage a logic evolutionary step.

2. Project/network schools (HPS) and other organizations in their local community

A) During the course of the "Network Health Promoting Schools" project (**1993-1997**) project schools began to increasingly use local resources and cooperate with external others but overall, they mainly focused on *networking 'within'* their school. Yet, most schools reported on and acknowledged support received by the local outlets of

the sickness fund in formal cooperation with the national network project, in spite of initial skepticism. This support was continued within the reshaped (OPUS-) network.
B) **From 1997,** network schools were explicitly asked to commit themselves not only to 'networking within' their school but motivate, cooperate and keep in touch with *local* cooperating partners or supporters, be it organizations or individuals, and plan *joint activities* with them. And indeed close cooperation between school teams and local others has been found. This was always a dimension of the 'Health Promoting Schools'-concept but in the reshaped OPUS-network more emphasized. From an interorganizational research perspective this represents high expectations as, according to Alter and Hage, interorganizational 'joint action' relations pre-suppose 'exchange' relations. In any case and initiated by the *national* network level, schools were offered and/or received support by the local offices of the public accident insurer and sickness fund in formal cooperation with the network. It has been reported that schools closely cooperated with external partners (Barkholz et al 2001).

The 'local - regional' dimension

3. 'Project'/network schools (HPS) and actors in their region

A) During **the first four years** of network development in Germany, as to the **regional advisors**, identified to provide technical support to schools in their region in implementing and evaluating health promoting activities, the interrelations vary among schools and regions. Many network schools report *good contact* and the *development of continuity* in cooperation over time (covering mainly aspects of capacity building and networking *within* schools but also links with *external* experts). About a third of project schools do *not* report negative, insufficient or lacking aspects of school/advisor- cooperation. Others miss one issue or another (e.g. continuity, initiative, sufficient time) and/or wish *more* cooperation and support of school activities, training, and *regional networking*. Obviously, for the various project schools the advisory system has functioned more or less well. And with view to individual project schools cooperation seems to have been more inward oriented than toward networking with external others. 'Advisors' spent over 50% of their advisory hours with school actors. Little is reported on the **State Ministries of Education** (MoE) in relation to Network activities, which indicates that project schools, once nominated by their Ministries did not have much to do with them beyond the usual school/ school authority-link. For about three years each Ministry sponsored its two 'project schools' with seven hours teaching reduction. This confirms the earlier assumption that these Ministries were *external supporters* rather than member organizations of the German "Network Health Promoting Schools".

B) **From 1997**, with the establishment of the OPUS-Regional Centers the situation significantly changed. A main responsibility of these *Regional* Centers was to create and maintain a 'regional net of health-promoting schools' for mutual support. For schools these Centers were the gates to network membership. In case of successful membership application they received direct impulses and support for their health promoting work but at the same time were encouraged to take this work jointly with other schools in their own hands. School coordinators were (to be) invited by 'their' Regional Center to regular work meetings of all network schools in the region. Where "regional level team structures" were established as planned (table 5.3.1), network schools met and worked with the Regional Center and regional cooperating partners on various issues.

The 'local - national' dimension

4. 'Project'/network schools (HPS), the national center and other national level actors

A) The interactions and relation between network schools and the *national* Project Support *Center* have been already addressed above (part I). After one and a half years and as to the cooperation with regional entities of the network's 'national cooperating partners' (sickness fund BARMER and public accident insurer association/BAGUV) the network schools judged quite differently: Cooperation with the former was perceived as *very satisfactory*, that with the latter *rather insufficient*. In the cooperation with the sickness fund schools appreciate the technical support, training, information/ materials, and financial support received as well as the openness for the schools' individual needs. As to *aspects missing* in the cooperation, two thirds of schools responded pointing mainly to the public accident insurers and their *lack of activity and effectiveness*. B) It has been said before that **from 1997**, within the OPUS-framework network *schools did not anymore meet regularly at national level*, i.e. with the national network office. And as during the years before their cooperation related to the official 'national cooperating partners' of the German network was if, then realized at the level of the local or regional organizational entities of these partners.

"The parts and the whole"

5. 'Project'/network schools (HPS) and the German network as a whole

A) The evaluation of the German **"Network Health Promoting Schools"** did show that project schools perceived much *support by* a range of partner organizations, particularly by the cooperating sickness fund and also the national Project Support Center. The 'school advisors' ranked high, too. Also regarding their *'networking with others'* project schools point strongly to the sickness fund but also to other schools and public administrations, i.e. organizations structurally involved through the Project Support Center's initiative. Organizations the cooperation with which depended on the school's *own* initiative, ranked clearly more low (e.g. health services, non governmental organizations, teacher training institutes). However, among the 'forms of networking' developed through their project work, the *networking within project schools was clearly outweighing their interorganizational networking*. These points of analysis of *national* level actors are confirmed by statements of project *schools* themselves: After one as after two years of network membership in all but two network schools more than 75% of school community members did know about their school's membership in the German network. However, in another questionnaire after about three years of membership only five out of 19 project schools identified themselves as 'national HPS project'-member. All but two did, however, report to be involved in *national level activities* (in national 'meetings', and half of them also in 'cooperation between schools') (see also point 6 below).

B) This pattern may or may not still apply during the reshaped German network as **OPUS-network**; the information available does not allow a judgment. The focus of evaluation had shifted away from internal developments within *individual* network schools to the situation of *Regional Centers* and *network* related issues. But as said before, the new network approach expected and directed network schools to be active part of their *regional* OPUS-network rather than the *German* network as a whole. How far network schools nevertheless developed an identity also as part of a 'German' network (i.e. beyond their regional sub-network) remains an open question.

6. 'Project'/network schools (HPS) and the "European Network of Health Promoting Schools" (ENHPS) as a whole

Obviously, within this case study on the European Network and its taking shape in selected countries this point addresses a core question: Did or does the plan of the European Network's initiators to create a *European* network *of* Health Promoting Schools (ENHPS) work out? For the ENHPS in Germany the following has been found:

A) **During the first four years** of network development, there were only first signs that German 'project' schools integrated a European dimension into their health promoting work, not only as to school-to-school links across borders but also their *identification* as 'network members'. The ENHPS Schools Data Base (WHO/EURO 1998) shows that of the 19 (of overall 29) German pilot schools covered, only four joined the network project with **motives** related to exchange, networking, or relations with *external* others (school *internal* issues dominated in 9 cases and several did not express any motive at all). As to the **membership** question, only five reported membership in the 'ENHPS', another five in the 'national HPS project', and nine neither one (with two reporting even 'Healthy Cities'- or 'self effective school'- network membership instead). I.e., statements by German "network" schools themselves confirm reports of national level actors: After about three years of membership in the 'ENHPS' and German "Network Health Promoting Schools", and in a *European* questionnaire, at least a third of all German pilot schools did identify themselves neither as member of the European nor German network initiative. As to (local, national, 'European') *activities* undertaken the picture is more positive: 8 of the 19 German 'project' schools (i.e. at least 25% of all project schools) report activities with an international or 'European' dimension, and six of those (or 20% of all) even in relation to longer-term *"twinning" plus pupils/teachers exchange* rather than one-off activities only. The occasional 'transnational conferences' of the German speaking ENHPS-sub-network have been mentioned before. According to national actors, German project schools did not get involved in *"electronic" (or 'hard') networking* neither across nor within national borders (see below).

It should be noted that the information derived from the ENHPS Data Base has to be interpreted carefully because of the low response rate of German schools (about 55%) and as it documents only one point in time. Nevertheless it is valuable to see that the analyses of the *national* Network actors concerning network schools and the schols' embeddedness in the German and the European Network match with statements by schools themselves.

B) **From 1997**, in the reshaped German network (OPUS) the 'European dimension' and networking were essential and visible parts of the 'guiding idea' that all network members did formally commit themselves to when joining the network. However, how far the network schools realized this European dimension is not documented. Overall, the network became stronger 'network oriented' but by regions (i.e. more inwards oriented). The occasional opportunities for cross-border meetings of network members through the conferences of the transnational ENHPS-sub-network of German speaking networks continued.

III. Interactions and relations of the 'OPUS- Regional Centres' with others

As shown above the creation and emphasis on Regional Centers within the reshaped German network for the development of Health Promoting Schools as **'OPUS'** moved the *regional level much into the foreground of overall network development* and evaluation activities. Interactions or relations between Regional Centers and *national* coordinating office as well as network *schools* have been addressed in sections I and II. Regular meetings of the national work group of National Office, Regional Centers and the network's 'cooperating partners' (about three per year) served experience exchange and qualification purposes, and were the ground on which feelings of close **cohesion and high levels of trust** among Regional Center staff emerged. Foci were issues of networking and also organizational/school development and the link of both. - Regional Centers were to *facilitate participation processes* in the *regions*, supported by the national office through newsletter, technical meetings and the scientific advisory work. One challenge was to find the right balance between providing ideas and guidance to schools and stimulating schools and their partners to develop their own perspectives. Regarding the *European Network*, Regional Centers as all other actors of the German network were 'oriented by' the guidelines set at European level but usually had no direct relations to European level actors. Within **the German network as a whole** (and the regional sub-networks therein) the **role of Regional Centers** can be summarized as follows:

Each Regional Center committed itself to the OPUS-'guiding idea' including the 'European dimension' but their **tasks were directed towards their region** only: From the perspective on the *German network* a) an *inwards* oriented task, the creation and maintenance of a *'regional net of Health Promoting Schools'* (including school selection in cooperation with State Ministry of Education and National Coordinating Office); b) an *outwards* oriented task, the clarification of the *division of labor among State/regional level actors* and supporters; and c) tasks in further education and public relations. Regional Centers were the **translators of the overall network framework into practice**. Depending on their own resources they were potential *'exclusion* factors' as they were expected to accept only as many new school members as they could effectively support (Barkholz et al 2001 p157/8). They were to identify, **mobilize, reach out, mediate between, and support** network *schools* and 'regional cooperating *partners*' alike; **keep up contacts and information flow;** and support the establishment of mechanisms such as 'round tables' *close* to network schools where these jointly with partners would stir developments and ensure quality work. These cooperatives were expected to over time evolve as *self-organized* entities for *exchange and planning of joint activities* that would have access to a 'regional network for Health Promotion' as needed - which hints at the striving for new smaller network structures linking geographically close 'OPUS-network schools' and 'external others' to *locally focused, independent, self-sustainable* "exchange" and/or "promotional" networks (to use the Alter/Hage-network typology).

Thus, with view to the regional sub-networks of the reshaped German network (and potential sub-regional or local spin-off cooperatives) the Regional 'Centers' were truly in a 'central' role both towards network members and supporters. Within the system of 'team structures' (table 5.3.1) - or the network/environment-link - the Regional Centers played the key role as to the (sub-)regional level (e.g. 'regional steering groups'). An inherent, yet unanswered question was how a 'networking' between schools and their partners (i.e. the German network's network/environment-interactions at (sub-)regional levels) could be shaped to achieve a win/win situation for all.

Against this background, part of the German network's evaluation addressed the goals of Regional Coordinators as to the networking process in their region, the extent of **realization of goals**, and their work situation. In the third year of the reshaped German network Regional Coordinators assessed 15 (of 22) suggested 'networking goals' as important; on the first three ranks were informal *experience exchange* among schools; support of health promoting organizational/ *'school development';* and central *information provision* for all. This matches with the **work focus** set by all Regional Coordinators' on 'general coordination and maintaining contact with *schools*'; only a few mentioned as foci also 'maintaining contact' with the National Coordinating Office and/or cooperating partners or 'creating round tables on health'.

As to **support received** from other network members or network supporters most Regional Coordinators felt 'effectively supported' by their host organization, National Coordinating Office and State Ministry of Education, but some did less or not agree. From the second to the third network year the perceived support by State Ministries sank. With regard to other actors (e.g. regional steering groups) satisfaction was expressed, too, particularly as to the German network's formal "cooperating partners". Regarding the support by other network *members* there was a positive trend towards full satisfaction with the *National Office*. That there is a benefit of *cooperation with other Regional Centers* and as to the *national work meetings* finds agreement (predominantly or fully) by 70 and 80% in the second network year, and 80 and 90% in the third. As to their coordinating functions 80-90% of Regional Coordinators agree predominantly or fully that they feel **recognition and acceptance** by the National Coordinating Office; the same applies to 'schools and cooperating partners' (but here with a negative trend from the second to third network year). This all points to good *quality relations and interactions within* the German Network as a whole, and as to its regional sub-networks also with some core actors in these networks' closer environments.

Overall, with view to the *German and the European Network as a whole* two further points are of interest: a) According to the German network's own analysis **supra-regional network structures need further improvement** (also in the area of 'hard' networking). b) In the second network year only 40%, but in the third about 70% of Regional Coordinators agreed (mainly or fully) that 'the **networking created transparency** between local, regional, nationwide, Europe- and worldwide impulses and initiatives for health promotion'. (Barkholz et al 2001 pp364-368)

IV. The German network for the development of Health Promoting Schools and the "European Network of Health Promoting Schools/ ENHPS"

'The part and the whole'

From the start the initiators of the German **"Network Health Promoting School"** were very conscious about the 'European dimension' of their ENHPS membership. The sets of 'questions to be examined' included distinct questions on how this could be realized. Already the start-up conference of the network (1993) had a European dimension, and the participation of EU and WHO representatives as well as National Coordinators of the ENHPS in other countries allowed German actors to get a first impression of the 'European dimension' inherent in the German Network project.

It has been stated repeatedly that being part of the "European Network" has stimulated significantly and sustainably motivation and contributions of all actors involved within and around the German network. Although both successive network projects in Germany did not succeed to fulfill one core ENHPS membership criteria, i.e. the cooperation between education *and* health sector at ministerial level, the German network has been recognized and its national center has acted as true ENHPS member. The ongoing dissemination and *widespread use of ENHPS manuals* in Germany indicates that Germany's education sector is politically in accordance with the principles of the Health Promoting School as accepted across Europe. Since its inception the German network, through its national support or coordinating center actively participated in ENHPS business meetings, conferences, and evaluation projects; over time, its scientific advisor became a key actor in European HPS *evaluation* efforts in general. The *regular experience exchange* at European level formed the basis for increasingly intense cooperation in areas such as *pupils and teacher exchange, joint development* of educational material, and finally the development of the before mentioned **ENHPS sub-network of *German* speaking networks** in which Germany was a **driving force** (Barkholz et al 1998). The German network hosted the first of by now four or five transnational conferences that followed and which proved to be good means of cross-border information transfer, *experience exchange*, comparison of developments, cross-border *school-to-school relations*, and *development of joint strategies* to successful work in networks with Health Promoting Schools (Barkholz et al 2001).

From the perspective of the European Network, the reshaping of the German network as **OPUS-network** did not change much: Germany continued to be ENHPS member and participation in ENHPS meetings and activities remained the same. Nevertheless, documents reflect some important changes. As said before, the 'European *dimension*' became an explicit part of the German network's 'guiding idea': as members' commitment to 'understand themselves as part of a European *initiative*', not the European *Network*. With regard to the German network as part of the European one an ambivalent picture emerges: On the one hand, a brief presentation of the European Network is repeatedly reprinted within network reports, and the OPUS-network structure (table 5.3.1) shows the ENHPS Technical Secretariat as a network knot as the national center, Regional Centers, and network schools. On the other hand, the term 'European Network' does hardly appear in documentation or examinations of issues of Regional Centers and network schools. However, in their review of seven years of large scale HPS development through a network approach the national center staff concludes: "through the integration of the networking in Germany in the European Network of Health Promoting Schools (HPS) a significant increase in motivation and a higher degree of identification of the participants can be reached"; they further state that *the German network needs to be part of the European Network* as the *related exchange is 'essential'* for the development of 'concepts, models of good practice, evaluation and quality assurance' in school health promotion (Barkholz et al 2001 p161 and 25). - Even a *global perspective* emerged over time: Network reports refer to the outcomes of *all* WHO global conferences of Health Promotion (not only to 'Ottawa') (see chap. 2.2); the network's scientific advisor participated in some of these events and disseminates contents; and since 1997 the German network's new 'guiding ideas' explicitly mention the global dimension of Health Promotion.

However, it should be recognized that several points indicate that, since the German Network was reshaped and strongly "regionalized", its ENHPS membership as perceived by German network members may be changing: a) In contrast to the first four years of network development the network schools have no direct contact to the national Office anymore, the only German network 'knot' with direct link to the European Network for the development of Health Promoting Schools (ENHPS); the Regional Centers are a new layer between schools and European Network level. b) The Regional Centers, who now meet with the National Office, appear to be very focused on sub-national or intra-regional network development. c) The OPUS-guiding idea that all members 'sign' leaves the European dimension 'network in-specific' and without any call for network links across national borders. In addition, d) within the German network use and access to the Internet, a facilitator of cross-border networking, is not far developed; and finally e) in contrast to the first phase of network development, the new network label 'OPUS' and the new logo do not remind at all of the ENHPS initiative nor of the Health Promotion movement since Ottawa. Therefore, it would be no surprise if the majority of network members in Germany (network schools and eventually some Regional Centers) have sooner or later a low if any awareness of their fairly indirect ENHPS membership. The German network's strong "rationalization" suggests that network schools may not even have a strong identity as members of a nation-wide/ German network, only as regional network members. Meanwhile, European level actors continue to perceive and label the about 500 German network schools as schools of the 'European Network in Germany'. From the international perspective there is a risk that the vision and goal of a European Network 'of' Health Promoting Schools will less and less match with the realities in Germany. Regional Centers are in a key position in this regard: Depending on whether they make sense and effectively communicate both that 'their' regional network is part of a nationwide network initiative and Germany's ENHPS membership, the European Network dimension may fade - leaving several smaller, inward looking 'regional OPUS-networks' for health-promoting school development in Germany with a weak if any identity of being part of a bigger 'whole'. However, the transnational conferences of the German speaking sub-network of the European Network may help to prevent such developments.

5.4 Synthesizing analysis I - structural and process features of the German Network

The ENHPS in Germany received increasing recognition for its evaluation. For this research project only those results of evaluations and analyses have been selected that relate to the network's *interorganisational network* dimension (which leaves out most of the evaluation results from the first four years). The previous chapter (on interactions and relations as well as roles and responsibilities of key actors) has laid the ground for a synthesizing analysis of the German network's core features in terms of those identified in the proposed assessment framework for interorganisational networks (IONs) (chap. 3). As in the other two case studies (and explained in chap. 4) for now the focus is on *selected elements* of the ION assessment framework: **Yet, the emphasis is on distinct basic features of the network rather than the network as a whole and its Health Promotion dimension** (the foci of the *final* chapter 6). A look back to overview figure 3.1.1 on the assessment framework and its partial presentation in figure 4.2.2 helps to keep the 'overall picture' in mind while recalling the selected foci: a) membership/ network borders; b) network structure (size/ complexity/ differentiation/ connectivity/ centrality); c) operational processes (methods of coordination); d) purpose of interactions within the network e) perceived effectiveness/ levels of conflict; f) the network's networking 'with others' and the relative emphasis on networking 'within'/'with others'; g) the network's 'hard' networking, means of 'soft' networking, and the relative emphasis on 'hard'/'soft'-networking; h) geographical distance among network members; i) (self-) reflection/ observation/ evaluation processes and feed back loops within the network; and j) "organizational networking" of network *schools*. Finally, 'satisfaction' will be addressed, too.

5.4.1 Membership or borders of the German network for the development of Health Promoting Schools

The German network's membership will be addressed as explained before (chap. 4) and done for the "European Network of Health Promoting Schools" (ENHSP) (see chap. 5.2.1). Matching with defining criteria of interorganisational systems such as being collectives based on trustful relationships, non-or less central, laterally linked, etc. the synthesizing analysis of the German network's borders and membership needs to take into account the *quality* of interorganisational *relationships* and not just formal 'membership status' or position. (see also chap. 3) This leads to the following interpretative summary:

A) During **the first four (ENHPS 'pilot') years** of network development in Germany, i.e. as to the then "Network Health Promoting Schools" the assumption put forward earlier can be confirmed: From an interorganisational research perspective not only the formal ENHPS and German network members, the 'project schools', have to be considered as network members but also the national 'Project Support Center' of the time. The latter also represents the 'ENHPS country membership' of Germany (see chap. 5.2.1). With view to the *nationwide* German network (rather than regional sub-networks!) the status of the individual 'advisors' remains in a 'gray zone' between the network and its closer environment. What has been made explicit later (under 'OPUS') applies already during the pilot years: It is useful to distinguish between the core network *members* (or network 'nods') and 'partners or supporters' (i.e. a network 'project' or closer network environment). The latter includes actors at all levels of society such as the formal 'national cooperating partners, the Ministries of Education involved, and potentially others in individual regions or local communities of network schools.

B) During the next three years of network development (**from 1997**) this picture slightly changed: Besides the above mentioned members (now identified as network 'nods') the newly established OPUS-Regional Centers emerged as *a new group of network members* (replacing the individual advisors system). *This marked a sub-differentiation of the German network* in one *supra*-regional network part (with National Coordinating Office and Regional Centers) and 15 *regional* sub-networks (with from a national perspective at least the Regional Center and a varying number of network schools each). Documents pay hardly attention to the former and much focus on the Regional Centers. Overall, from a national perspective these are in the main and crucial position to link both *among regional* sub-networks as well as *between regional and national* level. However, as before, the National Office formally *remained* responsible for all supra-regional affairs, including the direct links between the German and the European Network or its components (a division of labor sometimes overcome during the conferences of the transnational German-speaking ENHPS sub-network with its *direct* cross-border networking by not only national but regional and school level actors. - Network membership from the perspective of *individual regions* has been not always presented like this (and actors that, from the national perspective are network supporters, may be perceived as network members).

Overall, it can be firmly concluded that from the beginning (and as the network names indicate) the ENHPS in Germany has never been a pure Network *'of'* Health Promoting Schools but a network 'for the *development of'* Health Promoting Schools, but nevertheless and increasingly with special attention to the creation of an *inherent*, self-sustainable network 'of' Health Promoting Schools for mutual learning (for now by regional or sub-regional units). The German network evolved and increasingly was presented as an inter-*organizational* network which supports the thesis put forward by this research project: that international networks for the development of Health Promoting Schools such as the European Network and its sub-systems are *inter-organizational* networks (chap.1). The borders of the ENHPS in Germany or the German network for the development of Health Promoting Schools, its membership, closer environment and sub-structure, can now be illustrated as follows:

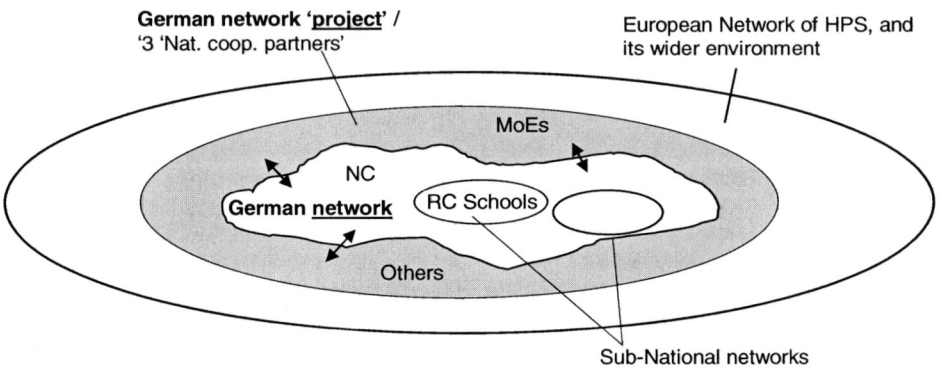

BARMER:	the sickness fund with formal status as "national cooperating partner"	MoEs:	Ministries of Education
		NC:	national support/ coordinating center
HPS:	Health Promoting Schools / network schools	RC:	Regional Center

Figure 5.4.1: The German Network for the development of Health Promoting Schools: its borders, members, sub-structure, and closer environment. (The latter consists of 'network model projects' and three formal 'national cooperating partners'.)

The findings suggest that the ENHPS and its sub-networks in countries are well conceptualized as *a network systems with a kind of double-border*: a first border around the *core* called the "network" with clearly identified and nominated network members (at least including the health-promoting network schools and a national coordinating body) and a more permeable second border around the network's "closer supportive environment" (with e.g. formally or informally bound 'network partners' or 'supporters', or the key actors in so called 'network projects', or otherwise defined). As said before (chap. 5.2) this conceptual approach benefits not only network assessment efforts but the networks itself: It helps to develop and sustain a network identity among long term committed core actors and a certain degree of network stability, while at the same time offering and maintaining flexibility to all those that wish or have to support the network's goal or specific objectives over a limited time span only, or with limited involvement and/or foci only. The differentiation of the 'network' and its 'closer supportive environment' (e.g. labeled as 'network project' or '- cooperative') allows to offer also the latter group of actors a network related identity (as e.g. 'network partner' or 'network project participants') and be distinguishable from the many others, more passive actors in the network's wider environment. - One particularity of **the reshaped German network** should be mentioned: as to its *borders at the level of 'school' members* (not at that of others) *the network was made more flexible*: Now, schools could enter the network *any time,* but they had to *stay at least until a defined point in time* (here the formal end of the Federal/State Commission "OPUS-project" in 2000). School membership has been conceptualized in 'three phases': 'entry' into, 'work within' and 'leaving' the net (with no information available on the latter which suggests that by the time of final report writing on the second phase of network development in Germany (as 'OPUS') 'school drop out' was not an issue.)

5.4.2 The structure of the German network for the development of Health Promoting Schools

Alter and Hage (1993) identified five features of a networks 'structure' (size, complexity, differentiation, connectivity, and centrality) which now, that the membership question regarding the German network has been answered, can be addressed:

Network size

As to the German network's 'size', after the first four years of network development (or the ENHPS 'pilot' phase) *significant changes occurred* both as to the German network as a whole and as to two systems levels. With regard to *school members*, the network did grow within three years or less, from nationwide 29 'project' or pilot schools and some 'associated' schools to 500 (OPUS-)network schools. However, in light of the strong decentralization of the network the latter should not be over-interpreted and rather expressed as average number of schools per German sub- or regional network: with 15 regions this means an *average* of about 33 network schools per region (but with big variations among regions: e.g. two out of 15 regional networks did hardly unfold) (Barkholz et al 2001 pp373f./391-398). With regard to network members at *regional level* the number raised from zero to 15 (if one neglects the number of *individual* advisors in the 'gray zone' of membership during the first four pilot years). Only the *national level* remained the same: with the one network member, the national support or coordinating office.

As in the reshaped German network as OPUS net a) schools usually did not network beyond regional borders and b) the Regional Centers were focused on intra-regional networking, too, the *development of the 'size' of the German network over the first seven years* may best be looked at as follows: A) The first four years it was <u>one</u> geographically spread network of *30 members* (all but one schools plus the national coordinating center); after that B) the German network dispersed into at least <u>*15*</u> *subnational networks* 'under development' which over time reached an average size of about *34 geographically more concentrated members* (all but one schools plus one regional center each). Thus, **in terms of "size", the enlargement of the European Network in Germany represents a multiplication (times 15) of the type of network that existed before but with geographic concentration of network members, <u>plus</u> the creation of an additional sub-network of another type** (no schools) which with *16* members (National Coordinating Office and 15 Regional Centers) is of half the size of the others. In light of this, the question arises whether it will be meaningful to assess the German network *as a whole* in terms of 'size' defined as total number of members, here about 516 (500 schools, 15 Regional Centers, 1 national office).

Network complexity

This structural feature refers to in Alter/Hage-terms the number of different services, products, sectors etc. presented within the group of network members. The three groups of the German network's members (schools, Regional Centers, national center) do *not* represent a fairly low complexity. Not only will a national network coordinating office at a university likely have different competencies and access to other partners, resources, perspectives than a Regional Center or a locally oriented network school; the same applies to a Regional Center within a Ministry of Education in comparison to one located in a health related NGO. The German network's complexity is fairly high because, first, Regional Centers do <u>not</u> have all the same services, products, resources to offer. On the contrary, they are part of at least *six* types of host organizations from different sectors and systems levels (five schools, five State teacher training institutes, four 'Regional Associations for Health', two State education authorities, one university, and one further education agency/ - with 14 organizations of the public *education sector,* four of the *health* sector/ 11 at *State* level and 7 in individual education organizations). Second, also the network 'schools' are not a homogenous group but represent primary, secondary and other schools each potentially providing different resources or services to the German network. With this the network complexity is already quite high. In addition, from 1997 on, those (network) experienced 'health promoting schools' (the former 29 'pilot' schools) have to be distinguished from those newly entering the network. Obviously, an analysis of network complexity should be guided by the common goal of network members, here the creation of Health Promoting Schools, which calls for consideration of 'complexity' in terms of the prevalence of members with resources and experiences of particular relevance to achieve this goal (e.g. re. organizational/school development, fund raising, school/community- or school-to-school-cooperation, and particular health related themes identified as priorities and/or inherent in Settings work such as school climate and health, healthy canteen, school related 'health factors', etc. etc.). However, a nation-wide overview of relevant data was not available but it has to be assumed that the German network's complexity is quite high.

Network differentiation

As to the German network's differentiation, in Alter/Hage-terms the extent of division of labor or function within the network, from chapter 5.3 at least the roles and responsibilities of the three groups of network members are known (i.e. of national center, network schools, and since 1997 Regional Centers). In summary, within the German network throughout the years there was a clear division of function and labor between these groups: During the first four network years *pilot schools* were to both start and follow through a 'health promoting school development'-process (including opening towards the local community), develop models of 'good practice' transferable to other schools, and share and report back on experiences and progress made; they also were to get involved in the network's 'regionalization' planned. During this time, the national support center was responsible for various coordination and information processes at *supra-school* level (within the net and towards others), overall development of the network project (including school-to-school networking, expansion at school level, and preparations for decentralization), and evaluation.

After the reshaping of the network as OPUS, the national network office and the new Regional Centers shared labor: the former remained the only one responsible for *supra*-regional issues, and main contact point for actors outside the net; the latter took over responsibilities for various *issues within 'their' region* and with a focus on "networking"-tasks which were by now conceptually clarified (e.g. 'school network' building, network/environment-links and related information and coordination). Similar "networking" tasks but now at *supra*-regional level only were in the hands of the national center who remained responsible also for evaluation. Network schools were still responsible for *their own* 'health promoting school development' but had to build on lesson learned from the pilot years; and as *all* network members they became explicitly responsible for actively participating and engaging in the 'give and take' of networking within their regional context (as orchestrated by the Regional Center). To find the right balance between the provision of ideas and technical leadership of non-school members *towards* schools and stimulation of the schools' self-organized and self-responsible action has been pointed out as a 'challenge'. Network schools remained 'in charge' of *their* health-promoting 'school development'-process, but had more actively to seek and provide mutual support rather than just receiving it from the non-school network members:

While the 'network differentiation' of the 'young' German network followed more the line between tasks regarding *organizational development within* schools on the one side (task of schools), and all supportive *network related tasks* on the other (task of national center), within the 'maturing' reshaped German network (under the heading OPUS) this changed: Now, *all* members were explicitly responsible for "networking" within the network and network/environment-links - with a division of function or labor by system levels and by orchestration versus participation functions: at supra-regional level the national center orchestrated, regional centers participated; at (sub-)regional level the regional center orchestrated, schools participated; and all members at 'their' systems level and/or below were to reach out to actors external to the network (schools mainly at local level and surroundings, regional centers at regional and also sub-regional levels, and the national center from supra-regional level up - with members at 'higher' system levels being oriented towards support of those at lower levels in support of their *joint* goal: effective health-promoting *school* development in an increasing number of schools across Germany.

Network connectivity / a network's 'networking within'

As explained in chapter 4.2, this synthesizing analysis of 'connectivity' (as used by Alter and Hage) as a *structural* network feature is merged with that of the network's 'networking within'-dimension (Hastings), because the latter encompasses the former. The focus is on **'*reciprocal*' contacts (i.e. interactions) and these among '*groups*' of network members** (rather than *all individual* members). 'Networking within' is again used as the overriding term to present quantitative and basic qualitative information in an integrated and meaningful way to shed light on the network's *structure*. (As before, further issues of quality of interactions are addressed separately: under the headings network 'processes' and 'purpose of interactions' below). Also the evaluation of the decentralized **German network (OPUS)** addressed network connectivity as the extent to which every channel is used, complemented by data on frequency, reciprocity, and other aspects of contact quality. But, unfortunately, published results address only the *mix* of both network *members* and *external others* by region (Barkholz et al 2001 pp373f./391-398); thus, these data do not allow a statement on the regional sub-network's extent and quality of connectivity or networking *'within'*.

Each *network member's networking 'with other' members* taken together reflects the *'networking within' the German network 'as a whole'*. In light of the goal of this research project to undertake the network case studies only as a first *pilot test* of the comprehensive ION assessment framework developed for Health Promotion, with country cases undertaken only to enlighten the *European* network in focus, and also because of the general lack of specific data, here **an <u>overall</u> picture of the German network's 'networking within'** (including connectivity) is provided. Similar to the other case studies the guiding questions followed were *which of the three groups of network members (national center, regional centers, schools) had the mandate and/or did regularly interact (in pursuit of the common goal) and which not? And which changes occurred over time in this regard?* - without ignoring any additional information of relevance. Looking at the roles and responsibilities or tasks of network members and reported observations of practice (chap. 5.3.4) the following summary can be given:

Throughout, the only national level network member, the *national support or coordinating office* had the task and did network with other members in the country, but with a significant change: The first four years it networked directly with *all* other network members (i.e. network 'project' schools plus the 'advisors' in the 'gray zone' of membership); then, after the decentralization of the network (as OPUS) it mainly networked directly with the new network members, the Regional Centers and the national/school level networking stalled in favor of strong intra-regional links (fig. 5.4.2 a). Related to this the *network schools'* 'networking within' the German network changed significantly: The first four years they networked directly with not only the national center but among each other across Germany; the network's decentralization brought about that each network school was mainly to network directly with a) the Regional (instead of national) Center, and b) other network schools in its region or sub-regional unit (rather than across Germany) (fig. 5.4.2 b). Both issues vary by region. Each *Regional Center's* task as to 'networking within' the German network was geographically bound to its own region and directed at networking with and among the network schools in that region; however, they also networked at supra-regional level, directly with the National Office and each other (mainly via a national work group) (fig. 5.4.2 c). Supra-regional networking 'within' the German network has been identified as needing improvement.

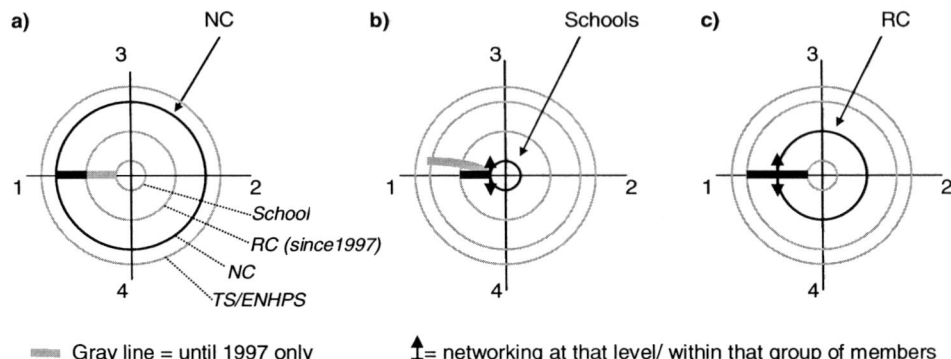

Gray line = until 1997 only   ↕ = networking at that level/ within that group of members

1 = Hastings' organizational networking-dimension 'networking with others'
2,3,4 = the other three dimensions of organizational networking (not of relevance here)
TS/ENHPS = Technical Secretariat of the European Network of Health Promoting Schools
a) NC = national support/coordinating office;   b) Schools = network schools;   c) RC = regional centers

Figure 5.4.2 : 'Networking within' the ENHPS in Germany: who is networking with whom? - Illustration of interorganisational relations or networking *between* and *within member groups*, group by group:

Obviously, *quantity and quality* of contacts within the German network need further specification. As to the *frequency* of contacts among national center and (until network decentralization) the *ensemble* of all network schools, afterwards all Regional Centers, information available refers mainly to 'soft' networking opportunities (here national level meetings) because 'hard' networking among network schools and/or Regional Centers hardly developed. National meetings were held three to four times per year. The national center, however, had additional bi-lateral contacts: until 1997, with all network schools, and after the network's decentralization mainly with the Regional Centers. The little further information found sheds some light on the 'networking within' the German network's **sub-national level:**

As to networking among network schools, it is interesting that after their first as well as their second year of network membership all but two of the original 29 pilot schools report that over 75% of the school community members did know of 'their' school's membership in the German network (Barkholz, Paulus 1998 p113) - i.e. *wide spread awareness of the net within almost all network member organizations*, a basis for active interorganisational networking, did exist. For the time **after the German network's decentralization** as OPUS, the published findings of the network's "network analysis" by region *indicate:* In half of the German sub-networks (those with a response rate of 75-100%) - and as to connectivity (reciprocal or not) among a *mix* of *members and external* others (here called 'network related actors'): a) **connectivity varies widely** between the 12 to 21 network related actors (once 40) identified per region; (in the lowest cases connectivity is 10-20/25%, in the highest case about 70%, in other cases somewhere between 35 and 60%); but importantly, b) **the degree of reciprocity is fairly high** (i.e. the number of reciprocal contacts in relation to the total number of contacts whether reciprocal or not) (of a scale of 65-85%), i.e. the *majority of contacts is reciprocal* rather than one-way. - For the other half of German sub-networks the data do not allow a meaningful interpretation. (Barkholz et al 2001 pp373f./391-398)

After size, complexity, differentiation and connectivity or 'networking within' the network, the last structural network feature of interorganisational networks to be looked at is:

Network centrality

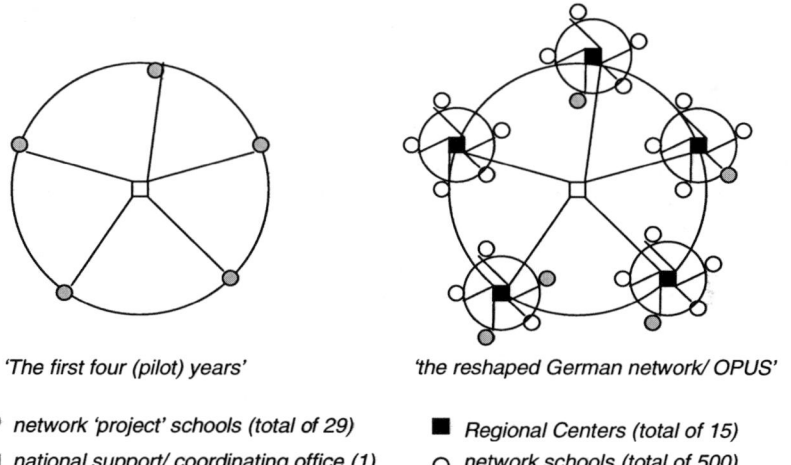

'The first four (pilot) years'   'the reshaped German network/ OPUS'

○ network 'project' schools (total of 29)   ■ Regional Centers (total of 15)
□ national support/ coordinating office (1)   ○ network schools (total of 500)

Figure 5.4.3: The German network for the development of Health Promoting Schools: Illustration of its 'centrality' during the first four (ENHPS pilot) years (1993-1997) and after its reshaping as OPUS-network (1997-2000). (This figure should not be misinterpreted as illustrating size or connectivity).

In Alter/Hage-terms centrality refers to how much in the German network the overall 'work' flows through one or a few members which is a question of dominance of one or a few members. In this regard, a significant change occurred. As shown in figure 5.4.3, during its first four 'pilot' years the issue of centrality of the 'young' German network may be best illustrated by a wheel with the national support center as the hub and the network schools on the rim. After the reshaping and decentralizing of the network as 'open participatory network' OPUS the image emerging is one of a wheel (of national and regional coordinating centers only) surrounded by several other wheels (one per (sub)regional network) firmly linked to the first.

The German network clearly achieved one of its goals set after four years of experience: to transform itself into a multi-centered network. However, in spite of the national center's, and later also the regional centers' central position their potential dominance has been buffered in self-regulation: by strong commitment to basic principles and values of Health Promotion and interorganisational networking alike such as participation, working in partnership, and also continuous self-reflection and learning and - matching with this - increasing emphasis on a 'team approach' within the overall network framework.

5.4.3 The German network's 'operational processes' and 'organizational networking'

Operational processes: methods of coordination used

As mentioned before (chap. 5.2.3), this feature of interorganisational networks is crucial but its synthesizing analysis does not need as many words as that of the network's structure: Alter and Hage (1993) point to the extent of joint decision making and reliance on mutual adjustment and feed back as well as of staff working together interdependently across organizational boundaries. It should be recalled that categories of related methods of coordination are with increasing utilization of feed back: a) impersonal methods (e.g. contracts/rules and regulations), b) personal methods (e.g. designation of coordinators/ direct contact among staff) and c) group methods (e.g. face-to-face communication of *several* people planning and taking decisions by consensus) (see chap. 2.4.3). From the start, the German network for the development of Health Promoting Schools clearly and increasingly focused on the latter two: As in the European Network, *the* personal method of coordination was the **designation of a coordinator**, a must for any organizations' network membership. In several ways **'group' or team methods of coordination** were required or recommended, too: a) *internal* to *member* organizations (in form of school internal 'HPS project teams' or OPUS-school teams, or the (voluntary) national project team); b) as to interorganisational work *across the network or sub-networks* (in form of national or (sub-)regional network meetings); and - most visible after the network's decentralization - c) as to the *network/environment-interactions* (in form of the OPUS-network's declared multi-level "team structure" - see table 5.3.1). Not only general reports but also specific evaluations indicate that "team" methods of coordination were indeed realized, also across 'systems hierarchies': For example, after the first two years of network development, all schools perceived the 'psychosocial climate' and the 'organization' of the 'cooperation' between schools and national center as very positive (reference is made to: feelings of acceptance, being taken seriously, dealing with each other very positive; and: information flow, non-bureaucratic administration, the national conferences) (Barkholz, Paulus 1998 p116). And as said before, Regional Centers did show high levels of satisfaction in this regard, too.

The German network underpinned the personal and group methods of coordination used also by *'impersonal methods of coordination'*: Latest since the network's decentralization as OPUS the principles of participation and networking as well as of the health promoting Settings approach became the explicit 'rules of the game': in the form of *the network's published 'guiding idea'* to which *all* organizations entering the network had to commit themselves. Overall, the principle of participation led to a high level of identification of network members with the common goal, i.e. the goals of the Health Promoting School (Barkholz et al 2001 p22).

The general purpose of interactions within the German network

This point refers to the interorganisational network typology by Alter and Hage (obligational/exchange-, promotional/joint action-, systemic/joint production-networks) which also reflects stages of network development (see chap. 2.4; fig. 2.4.6; table 2.4.4). Throughout the documents on the German network for the development of Health Promoting Schools or the ENHPS in Germany *exchange* has been repeatedly and consistently referred to as a major purpose of choosing a 'network approach' (however defined if defined at all). Most often stated are information exchange and experience exchange but also exchange of practical materials, of 'models of good practice' and 'mutual or joint learning' on the way. All observations and particular evaluation results such as the OPUS-network's "network analysis" confirm that and individual groups of network members and the German network as a whole intended and achieved to be (part of) **an exchange network**: along the lines of the *patterns of connectivity* identified above and with - in Alter/Hage-terms - 'limited cooperation' and a focus on the needs of individual members (rather than supra-ordinate member goals). The latter refers particularly to the needs of individual network schools and their process of self-transformation to 'Health Promoting Schools' (HPS), but also to the interests and needs of e.g. the national coordinating center which strived (and was accountable) for knowledge development and dissemination in a variety of HPS and network related areas. Barkholz et al (2001 p17f.) point to intensity of experience exchange as a factor positively related to sustainability of network structures.

There are indications that the German network as a whole or in parts is not only an exchange network but develops **towards a promotional network**, i.e. a network where joint or concerted action to achieve functional objectives and/or solve supra-ordinate member problems takes place. Not only the in Alter/Hage-terms 'rather quasi-formal' membership approach (as opposed to informal loosely linked 'obligational' networks) hints at this. German network members did jointly developed things of functional purpose such as practical materials for everybody's use (e.g. a list of 'health factors in schools', the 'steps towards a health promoting school', and a data bank on good practice models). Particularly striking is one result of the German network's "network analysis" undertaken after its decentralization as OPUS, although it refers to a *mix* of network members *and* external others (Barkholz et al 2001): The results of a questionnaire among 350 of this mixed group of network related actors identified region by region (total response rate 57%) shows: Throughout Germany, when asking **regional network related actors** for the purpose of network contacts **'information and experience exchange' ranked first** - which is no surprise as by then such exchange was an explicit part of the German network's 'guiding idea'; but, in *several* sub-networks (and on *average across Germany*, too) **'joint projects' ranked clearly second** (before mutual support, qualification purposes and other issues). In one selected case presented in more detail a degree of connectivity as to 'contacts for implementing joint projects' of almost 20% was found. These findings match with the Alter/Hage-network evolution theory that postulates that 'exchange' networks are a precondition for 'promotional' or joint action networks to occur (and the latter for systemic networks) but which may occur simultaneously.

After this synthesizing analysis of a range of specific, more or less *internal* features of the German network now the network will be analyzed (again in a synthesizing way) against Hastings model of the "new" organization capable of networking (see also fig. 2.4.1). This brings the network's interactions with its (organizational) environment back into the picture.

The German network's networking 'with external others' and emphasis given to networking 'within'/ 'with others'

In relation to the 'German network for the development of Health Promoting Schools' as a whole, the issue of organizational 'networking with others' has **two dimensions**: a) networking with other *members of the European Network* (in its role as 'ENHPS member' actively contributing to the 'networking within' the European Network); b) networking with *external others outside this realm*, particularly within the own country. First, as to the German network's **networking with other 'European Network/ ENHPS' members**, all tasks *beyond* the realm of *individual* (school) members (such as the twinning of school x with school y) have been *mainly undertaken by one network member*, the *national* support or coordinating office. This is required by the ENHPS Technical Secretariat and International Planning Committee. Only *from time to time the whole network or a bigger part of it* has been actively involved in cross-border 'networking within' the European Network (e.g. related to the transnational conferences of the German-speaking ENHPS sub-network). As to the *quantity* of contacts with other ENHPS country networks and the European level, the German Network may have been above the average of ENHPS country networks as it participated not only in the routine or widespread activities (e.g. business meetings, EVA projects) but via its national center was increasingly active and recognized at international level (e.g. in the initiation of the German-speaking ENHPS sub-network and in the area of evaluation). Little has been said about the *quality* of these contacts but the latter point and acknowledgments of the benefit of ENHPS membership from the German side indicate mutual recognition, acceptance and 'win/win'.

Second, the German Network's **networking 'with others' within the own country** has partially changed over time. As to *'others' at national level* its networking remained consistent, focused on the public funding agencies as well as three formal "national cooperating partners", and was repeatedly pointed out as successful and effective. The network member formally responsible for supra-regional issues within the net, the national coordinating center, took care of such networking. Regarding networking with *'others' at local or community level* the German network as a whole had no specified tasks (besides those inherent in supporting the 'Health Promoting Schools'-concept). In the form as school-community-links network schools were always responsible for such networking. However, in the early years of network development only four of 19 'pilot' schools expressed motives to join the German network related to exchange or external others (WHO/EURO 1998; Barkholz, Paulus 1998). As said before, after four years this motive became explicit part of the 'guiding idea' that all network schools had to buy in and was explicitly extended beyond the local towards the (sub)regional realm. As to the network's networking with *'others' at regional level* first the national center, after the network's decentralization the Regional Centers acted on behalf of the network. It has been reported that cooperation with and among key regional actors, the State level Ministries of Education, 'developed positively' and that 'State specific interests and supra-State perspectives' were successfully 'linked' (Barkholz, Paulus 1998 p130).

Overall, with view to Hastings' point that organizational systems must take decisions on whether they need for a particular task to focus on networking 'with others', or networking 'within', or in one way or the other on both the following can be summarized:

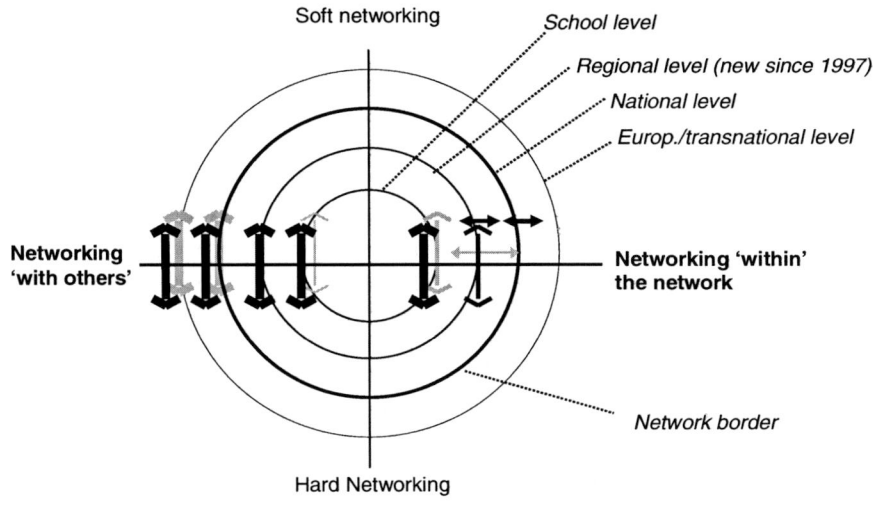

Gray: first phase of network development
Black: second phase of network development

Thinner arrow: less emphasis/ thicker arrow: more emphasis/ no arrow: hardly any emphasis

x-axis/ left: The Slovenian Network's networking with external organizations at local, regional, national and European level
x-axis/ right: The networking within and among groups of network members (school, regional, national, European)

Figure 5.4.4: The German network's *emphasis* on networking 'within' and 'with others', differentiated by partners at various systems levels, and as to developmental phases (Gray: first phase/"Network Health Promoting Schools" 1993-1997; Black: second phase/"OPUS"-network 1997-2000).

Figure 5.4.4 illustrates that the German network, challenged by the self-set goal of large scale development of 'Health Promoting Schools' throughout Germany (or - in the network's own terms – of initiation and support of 'health-promoting school development'), focused on both networking 'within' and 'with others' – in far reaching division of labor. It not only networked with 'others' in the European Network but built alliances with other German (national and State level) organizations that in one way or the other are structurally responsible for (school related) health promotion (one sickness fund; public accident insurers) and/or school development (Education Ministries). However, it did not link with the public health sector as such. with view to the *national* level the emphasis on the German network's networking 'with others' remained constant over the years (with a few but high quality links). But with view to actors at both *regional and local* level, after four years the reshaped German network brought about a significant shift towards more, and more consciously constructed networking with 'others' while at the same time intensifying its internal networking between these levels.

The German network and 'hard' networking, means of 'soft' networking, and the relative emphasis on 'hard' and 'soft' networking

As to the **'hard' networking within the German Network** the picture is clear: Throughout the years of network development, the *national* support center created Internet based services and intensely propagated 'hard' networking (linking computers) and its active use in support of soft networking purposes. But inherent potential to significantly increase the frequency of contacts across the network was not at all realized as expected: neither with and among network schools (in focus the first four years) nor Regional Centers (in focus after the network's decentralization in 1997). Many network members lacked financial resources, some also other capacities. After one to two years in the network, Regional Centers assessed 'hard' networking via Internet or e-mail as clearly less beneficial than 'soft' networking technologies. *Within the regions* electronic networking remained *marginal*, and even *among national and regional* centers it was realized only slowly and *partially* (e.g. in 2000 still two Regional Centers were outside the electronic info-exchange). Overall, from the start 'hard' networking *effectively served* the network's (supra-regional) networking with *external others* and, since 1997, increasingly also supra-regional networking 'within' the net as here the national center was in charge. The network's various electronic services, particularly used by external others, led to widespread public recognition. (Barkholz, Paulus 1998; Barkholz et al 2001)

Thus, **networking *within* the German network remained depended**

on the systematic use of 'soft' technologies, printed newsletters (stalled in 1997) and face-to-face-meetings (from national conferences to regional 'steering groups'/'work groups'/'round tables' implemented in many regions). With the new (OPUS-) "team structure" of the network (table 5.3.1) the **emphasis on 'soft' networking increased;** and while at national level the *frequency* of meetings remained the same (about 3 per year) it did significantly increase within regions (with often monthly encounters). - For the German network as a whole, the *national work conferences* were the *crucial means for networking 'within' and with external* key partners. As long as they were the main means for 'soft' networking among network schools (i.e. during the first four network years) they have been assessed as too seldom which may be explained by the lack of 'hard' networking in between these events and otherwise mainly bi-lateral national center/school-contacts. The quality of these conferences as means of 'soft' networking has been continuously improved and much valued by network members. (Barkholz, Paulus 1998 p130)

The German network's "organizational networking" - intermediate synthesis and discussion

Following Hastings' organizational model, now the overall picture of the "organizational networking" of the German network as a whole can be summarized - on the base of the synthesizing analysis of the German network as to each of the four networking processes that together constitute an organizational systems' "organizational networking". Figure 5.4.5 visualizes not only the network's 'organizational networking' in general but provides insight into the **relative emphasis on each of the four networking processes** as well as **developments over time.** In sum, from the start (figure a) within the 'German network for the development of Health Promoting Schools' as a *whole* (which refers to the *ensemble* of its members): a) 'soft' networking overall was much emphasized, 'hard' networking very little. [The national center could not pull its 'hard' networking-goals through.] b) Inter-member networking (the networking 'within' the net) was moderately realized but not much spoken of (or not much emphasized). [The network's attention was bound to *intra*-school development in the pursuit of health.] As to the networking with 'external others' the network's main emphasis was on national, supra-national or trans-national level.

With regard to **changes over time**, a look from the first through the second phase of network development (fig. 5.4.5 a, b) shows: In general, there was neither a reduction in emphasis in any one of the four networking processes nor a shift in the *relative* emphasis on **networking 'within' versus ' with others'** (x-axis). The *emphasis on both of these network-*

ing dimension was increased in the form of further differentiation: The existing focus on networking 'with others' (such as network 'partners' or 'supporters') was broadened to include strong regional and sub-regional foci. The overall emphasis on networking 'within' increased by: a) the creation of Regional Centers (as new network layer) and regional sub-networks (with reduction of geographic distance among an increasing number of members); and b) the integration of clear networking-related expectations into the network's 'guiding idea' (complementary to the already existing focus on health-promoting school development of individual network schools).

As to the **'hard' versus 'soft' networking** -dimension (y-axis) the *relative* emphasis *did* change, with a shift even more towards 'soft' networking (through implementation of a sophisticated system of '[interorganisational] teams' at regional and sub-regional levels while 'hard' networking hardly changed).

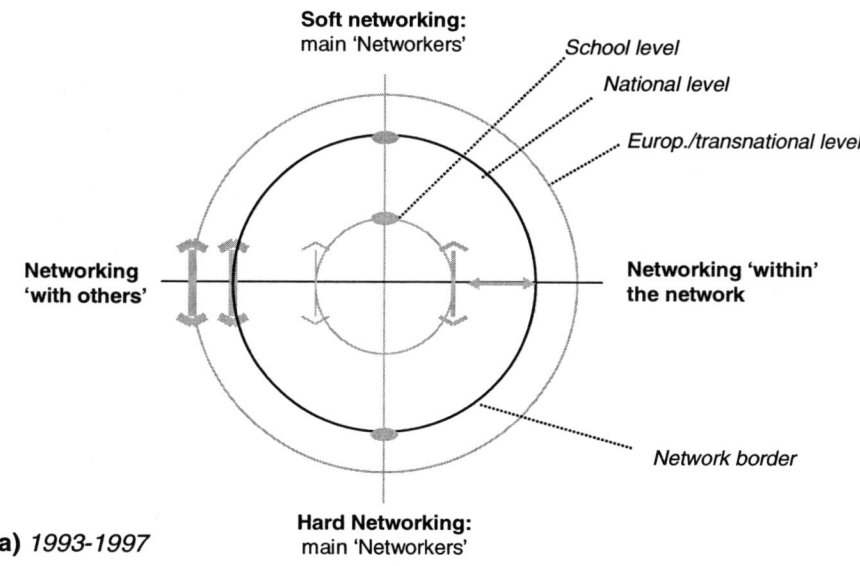

a) *1993-1997*

Figure 5.4.5a: "Organizational networking" of the ENHPS in Germany – Illustration of the German network's emphasis on networking 'within' the net, 'with others' and 'hard' and 'soft' networking by developmental phases: a) first phase 1993-1997/ "Network Health Promoting Schools"; b) second phase 1997-2000/ "OPUS").

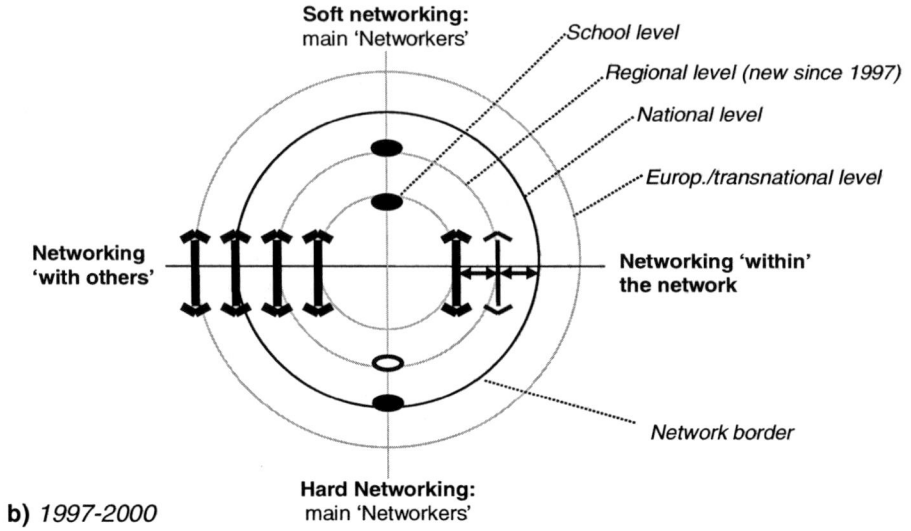

x-axis/ left:	The Network's networking with external organizations at local, regional, national and European level
x-axis/ right:	The networking within and among groups of members of the German network (school, regional, national, European)
y-axis/ upper half:	The Network's emphasis on soft networking by member groups (i.e. by user groups of 'soft' technologies)
y-axis/ lower half:	The Network's emphasis on hard networking by member groups (i.e. by user groups of 'hard' technologies)
Thinner arrows:	less emphasis/ thicker arrows: more emphasis/ no arrow: hardly any emphasis

Figure 5.4.5b: "Organizational networking" of the ENHPS in Germany – Illustration of the German network's emphasis on networking 'within' the net, 'with others' and 'hard' and 'soft' networking by developmental phases: a) first phase 1993-1997/ "Network Health Promoting Schools"; b) second phase 1997-2000/ "OPUS").

The reminder of this chapter will round up the synthesizing analysis of the German network as a whole, by addressing the yet outstanding features of interorganisational networks as identified by Hastings or Alter and Hage: geographical distance; the culture of self-reflection/ evaluation/ feed back; and network outcomes in terms of perceived effectiveness and levels of conflict - with a short look at the network schools' "organizational networking", an inherent demand of the creation of 'Health Promoting Schools' within a network context.

5.4.4 Distance, assessment culture, and satisfaction within the German network

Geographical distance among network members

Hastings has pointed out that even with full use of new information technologies (i.e. 'hard' networks) psychological barriers for collaboration increase with geographical distance. Obviously, interorganisational networks with geographically dispersed members that lack 'hard' networking have to overcome in addition the *physical* barriers of geographical distance to engage in 'soft' networking and meet. German network actors have reported that **geographical distance** between organizations was an important factor in the overall networking process or work of the German network for the development of Health Promoting Schools (with a general notion of 'closer is better'). They found *schools* to need understanding, flexible 'support systems' in their *closer* geographic environment *to ease daily-life-compatible and successful cooperation with other schools and external partners* in support of their Health Promoting Schools activities. The network's "network analysis" of the mixed 'schools and others'-networks in regions did find indications of more *'successful' networking* where organizations were *geographically close* to each other (Barkholz et al 2001). However, it should be recalled that these results stem from (the parts of) a network with very low levels of 'hard' networking in support of 'soft' networking. The contrary could change the results as to the impact of geographical distance.

The culture of (self-)reflection, observation, evaluation processes and feed back loops within the network

Both Alter and Hage, and Hastings refer to this issue, the former as part of the network feature 'operational processes' (discussed above), the latter as a central element of his *'radar beam' model* of the "new" organization (fig. 2.4.1). The radar beam symbolizes the needed culture of *ongoing or repeated* self-reflection, self-observation, evaluation and feed back loops within organizational systems capable of and involved in networking. The reports on the German network contain various hints that such a culture has emerged. For example, (as in Slovenia) at least the first 29 network (pilot) schools systematically documented their work in a 3-months-rhythm for both self-reflection and evaluation purposes (Barkholz, Paulus 1998). The national coordinating center, in charge of evaluation, regularly fed back results to network members and published yearly overall progress reports. The emphasis on soft networking, mutual learning, participation, regular face-to-face-discussions among network members and meetings for joint planning, external and self-evaluation, etc. supports the assumption that the in general the German network did work towards and implemented various 'radar beams' into its daily network work. How far this remained equally spread throughout the network after the network's decentralization remains an open question.

The 'organizational networking' of network *schools*

As explained in chapter 4.2 before, the implementation of the HPS concept - the goal of the German network as a whole - explicitly expects network schools to develop school-community-links, i.e. the school's networking 'with others'. Calls for *joint* planning, decision making, and action to achieve locally relevant and sustainable Health Promoting Schools programs reflect an emphasis and need of *'soft'* networking. During **the first four years** of network development in Germany, the overall picture is that network schools clearly focused on networking *'within'* their organization (using *'soft'* networking technologies such as 'school teams'). As to the their networking *'with others'* they all networked with other network members (particularly the national center); but 'school-community-links' (and, thus, interorganisational relations of schools with local others *'external'* to the network) were less developed. **After the reshaping of the German network (as OPUS)** the emphasis on the schools' networking *'within'* may not have changed much as the guiding concept (HPS) and practical tools remained the same. However, networking was now explicitly stressed as a 'principle' for all actors. And as shown in chapter 5.3.4, network schools were now not only more conscious about and committed to networking *'with others'* in their region but also realized such networking indeed (mainly for school-to-school exchange and external support).

In sum, overall and over time German network schools remained or even strengthened their focus on *internal* networking to transform themselves into Health Promoting Schools but did - through the reshaping of the German network as a whole - started to significantly strengthen their networking with external others - according to Hastings the right step as schools did not have all the needed resources to achieve their goal internally available. And matching with a more regional (rather national focus) soft networking was the means of choice (in parts due to lacking capacities regarding 'hard' information technologies).

Satisfaction of network members - perceived effectiveness and levels of conflict

Now, that the various structural and process features of the German network for the development of Health Promoting Schools have been analyzed another step towards the network's final analysis will be taken: the analysis of 'reasonable' network outcomes. Satisfaction of network members in terms of perceived effectiveness and levels of conflict is a common indicator for 'reasonable' network outcome used also by Alter and Hage (see chap. 2.4 and 3). Although during the first four years the evaluation by and of the German network for the development of Health Promoting Schools did address this issue only as to the then (sub-)regional 'advisors' in place and also afterwards mainly as to the Regional Center staff, reports show the following:

Overall, the **national support or coordinating center**, in its regular progress reports expresses indirectly or directly and in various ways high levels of satisfaction (Arnold et al 1994, 1995; Barkholz et al 1998, 2001; Barkholz, Paulus 1998; BLK Modellversuch Netzwerk... 1993): *Statements* of intermediate and final stock taking or syntheses of results are **predominantly positive without denying areas of yet insufficient development**; a wide range of statements of specific 'successes' as part of the overall work within and by the network can be found. These reach far beyond the quoting of numbers of network schools or health-promoting school projects implemented. **A)** Regarding *the first four years* of network development, and as to the core goal of *Health Promoting School (HPS) development,* success messages refer to, for example, the network schools' progress made along the 'steps towards a HPS' and successful implementation of the HPS concept. In the area of *cooperation, exchange, and 'networking' (however defined)* success messages refer to, for example, the schools' 'networking' (within/ with others) that has 'developed successfully'; cooperation with and among Ministries of Education (i.e. actors in the network's closer environment); continuity of network development; meaningful and successful transnational information transfer; etc. Other success messages fall in the category of *impact on the network's closer or wider environment,* for example, higher acceptance of the HPS concept as 'school development model' in Germany; and successful links of supra-State and State level interests. **B)** Regarding the three years of work within the reshaped German network as *OPUS,* success messages as to *HPS development* point out that the Settings approach has proven to be an 'important basic innovation intervention' in school health promotion that complements well the problem based approaches, and that related, previously developed 'valuable support tools' are being used. The majority of success messages refer to *networking and the network approach* chosen: With its high flexibility, opportunities for wide participation and learning, involvement of a variety of partners, its refraining from quick expansion, its goal orientation and at the same time ability to address locally or State specific needs, etc. it is assessed as an 'appropriate instrument' for large scale 'school health promotion' (with about 500 schools involved, and high levels of trust within the network reached). Pointed out, too, is the German network's significant contribution to the European Network, 'one of the most successful approaches' of Health Promoting Schools and a 'high innovation potential'.

The national office is satisfied with the **continuous progress made** over, overall, ten years of large scale development towards Health Promoting Schools in Germany, with reference to: concepts and testing of models that make health the theme of the school; sustainable cooperation with non-school partners; valuable experiences as part of the European Network; the extent of successful mid-term oriented fund raising; significant know-how development and of practical 'tools'; recognition of the OPUS-approach in 'technical discussions' beyond national borders; effective and sustainable use of (OPUS) network structures developed (including the 500 network schools and 15 regional coordinating centers); the important perspectives derived for educational and related political reorientation and reform; and the extent of progress as to school development and network development within a relatively short time of three years.

When asking for the **satisfaction at regional network level,** for **(A)** the first four years of network development the **'advisors in the regions'** come to mind. After almost two years of involvement, *'advisors'* when questionnaired (response rate 10 out of 18) express: as to 'their job' in general at least half of *all* advisors were satisfied; as to support received from the national level (financial, information, meetings) at least 25-30% of all were very satisfied, another 25-30% somewhat (e.g. further experience *exchange* among each other was yet desired); advisors felt positive about the materials received from the European Network; but they did have conflicts (which may or may not be related to interorganisational relations). **B)** As to the OPUS-**Regional Centers** the evaluation has shown that *all* Regional Coordinators, after two years of work, are fully (60%) or predominantly (40%) 'satisfied with what they achieved as regional coordinator as of then' (a year before 30% were still little satisfied and only a few fully). The many other indicators of satisfaction in various facets of (net)work include that *most* coordinators after two years: perceived their cooperation among each other as beneficial (with positive trend), succeeded in their main self-set networking goal (effective transfer of useful information within the net), were satisfied with the support received by national center and cooperating partners, felt acceptance and acknowledgment of work by school and national network members; 70% had overall enough financial resources for coordination tasks (positive trend), and 80% felt positive that in their State the OPUS-concept could be implemented successfully (but with negative trend). Regional Coordinators found it more difficult to mobilize new network schools than new cooperating partners, felt over time less accepted and recognized by these actors, and as said before felt a need for improvement as to supra-regional networking.

At least at national level, only little or partial information is available on the **satisfaction of network schools** in Germany. During the first four years, a few evaluation results provide a glance at school satisfaction: The 29 *pilot schools perceived much support* by a range of organizations, particularly one external 'partner' and the national support center. As to school-to-school-*cooperation within the net,* limited data point into the direction that overall, more, and more *regional* opportunities were needed (although national ones are valuable). The reshaped German network took up this point and after good two years the vast majority of Regional HPS Coordinators judged 'networking among schools' positively: as enabling experience exchange among schools. - *Inequalities of access* to various resources among the 29 formal 'project' schools and 'associated' schools during the first four network years left caused dissatisfaction of the latter (Meierjuergen 2001). Also this issue was taken up when after four years the German network was reshaped (as OPUS), in the form of an '*open* participation' approach; this gives reason to assume that schools' satisfaction did increase over time also in this regard. - With view to *school coordinators' 'work satisfaction'* in the reshaped German network, a small group of OPUS-school coordinators provides a *mixed picture*: with some factors indicating low levels of satisfaction (e.g. financial resources/ teaching reduction) and others indicating high levels (e.g. self-responsible working/ room for creativity/ subjective perceptions of 'good success', positive feed-back from the side of the school, support by (head) teachers) (Michaelis 2001).

Key donors or **actors in the German network's closer environment,** after seven years of network development projects, highly acknowledged the results achieved and expressed **much satisfaction** (e.g. the Federal and the project leading State level Ministry of Education and the cooperating sickness fund; see Boppel 2001; Brackhahn 2001; Meierjuergen 2001b).

Reports on the German network for the development of Health Promoting Schools do not specify **'levels of conflict' within the network** (the second general network outcome indicator used in the network assessment framework). But there are statements that the work has not always been easy.

5.5 ENHPS country case 2: The "European Network of Health Promoting Schools" in Slovenia

This case study rests on the fairly rich, mostly unpublished material in *English* language on the European Network (ENHPS) in Slovenia (i.e. NSC 1998a, 2000a; SLNHPS 1995; Stergar: from 1993a to 2000; Stergar, bevc Stankovic 1998; Turnsek 1995a; Turnsek, Stergar 1994, 1995a). The language barrier between researcher and country did not allow to use additional information potentially available in Slovene. Therefore, it is not claimed that this network analysis rests on a *complete* review of existing written material of the times and here or there information may have been missed and interpretations affected. However, the researcher is confident that a) the *overall picture* of the Slovenian network as a sub-network of the European Network derived, provides a very good ground to fulfill the primary purpose of this research project, i.e. the first pilot testing of the ION assessment framework developed in chapter 3. She also feels confident that b) overall, the analysis provided does justice to the Slovene 'Network of Health Promoting Schools'. In May 2001, the National Coordinator of the Slovenian network project, Eva Stergar, kindly checked the detailed summary of the Slovene material produced, i.e. the data basis for the analysis undertaken in this chapter. And she found it to be very comprehensive and complete, had hardly any corrections to make, and only filled in some valuable specific information on particular issues in question. (The latter is referred to as 'Stergar 2001')

In Slovenia, the *initiative* to enter the 'European Network of Health Promoting Schools' (ENHPS) and create such a network in the country came from the *health sector,* while it is being *implemented* within the *education sector.* The Ministry of Health appointed the required ENHPS National Coordinator at the national Institute of Public Health even before a first intersectoral meeting with the Education Ministry took place and the National Support Center was established. According to the National Coordinator, from the start there were 'no problems with the idea of intersectoral cooperation' (Stergar 1997). The Slovenian 'Network of Health Promoting Schools' has been developed in as of now two main phases with a short transition phase in between, and a new phase seems to emerge (NSC 2000a; Stergar 1993a): Matching with the terminology used at European level and with some similarities as to developments in Germany (chap. 5.3), *the first four years* of Slovenian network development or the 'ENHPS in Slovenia' (1993-1997) represent **the first main phase, the 'pilot' phase** in which 12 selected 'ENHPS pilot schools' started joint work. After a **short transition phase** in 1997 followed **a second main phases, the so called 'dissemination phase'** (from 1998) the beginning of which was marked by the **formal launch of the "Slovenian Network of Health Promoting Schools"**, an *expanded Network* with now 130 network schools (including the 12 former 'pilot' schools). After two years of work of this expanded Slovenian Network (in 2000) considerations of yet another phase emerged towards a 'nationally adopted program for Health Promoting Schools (HPS) in Slovenia'. However, the focus of this research project remains the Slovenian '*Network* of Health Promoting Schools', and it covers the years since the network's inception (in March 1993) until the year 2000.

5.5.1 The ENHPS in Slovenia - context, concepts, goals

The Slovenian context

Since Slovenia declared its independence in 1991 (and since it prepared itself to became a member of the European Network in 1993), several major reform initiatives included those on the health care and education system. Over a decade, the health care sector - a key actor in the Slovenian Health Promoting Schools (HPS) initiative - has been changed significantly, oriented by the new 'Health 21' policy of the WHO European Region (chap. 5.1): A considerable amount of 'health'/disease care legislation was passed including a few of relevance to the field of Health Promotion and the HPS initiative in Slovenia: on investment in health (1994), use of tobacco products (1996), and a *Mental Health* Act (still under review in 2001). The latter addresses a key topic of the Slovenian Health Promoting Schools initiative ("mental and emotional health") and matches with two of the major public health concerns identified for Slovenia: 'high suicide rates' (twice of EU average) and 'high consumption of alcohol and tobacco' (ECHP 2000). The new Slovenian 'National Health Care Programme - Health for All 2004' - under development throughout the years of Slovenian HPS network development covered in this study, and accepted by the Parliament in May 2000 - has no specific Health Promotion program component; but it includes a *proposal on strengthening the role of 'health promotion and disease prevention' and assuring conditions* so that individuals can take care and responsibility for their own health. The incorporation of *health education in the school curriculum* became one of the government's interventions to promote '*equity* in health'. The **Ministry of Health finances health education** programs of governmental and non-governmental organizations (also to increase public participation) and **over time** developed *intersectoral collaboration* with other Ministries (such as *Education*, Labor, and Social Affairs) which in 1996, while overall still assessed as 'just in the beginning', was already positively acknowledged in the areas of 'Healthy Schools' (or the Slovenian HPS project) and 'Healthy Cities'. Intersectoral initiatives include life-style and young people oriented research and programs - the latter also on 'the *development of* programs to prepare *young people* for' living a life free of tobacco and drugs and to promote healthy food and physical activity; and the 'use of different **settings to promote health** among certain groups' ('**healthy schools**', child care institutions, hospitals). '*Educational bodies*' and the Ministries of Finance and of Agriculture were consulted as to tax and subsidy policies; taxes e.g. on *tobacco, alcohol and 'unhealthy foods'* have been levied as a punitive measure and part of that **tax is used for health promotion.** This and other information (below) indicate that the Slovenian (network) project on Health Promoting Schools and health promotion related parts of the public health sector reform did reinforce each other. The WHO 'investment in health appraisal' 1996 in Slovenia, undertaken on *request* of the country and involving high level discussion on Health Promotion, will have had an influence, too (see also chap. 2.2.5). It strongly recommended Slovenia a 'comprehensive development of Health Promotion approaches for children and young people' (Rivett 2000). (ECHP 2000; HEA, WHO/EURO 1998, 1996) Over time, the *Ministry of Health* developed the stand point that *Health Promotion should be coordinated by the National and Regional Institutes of Public Health* (i.e. key actors in the Slovenian network project on Health Promoting Schools as shown below); thus, the Health Ministry claimed the leading role in the field. However, the Slovenian HPS network development did not take place only in a positive 'pro-Health Promotion' political climate: After high emphasis on health promotion in the first halve of the 1990s, 'Health Promotion' started to 'struggle with little political support' (Krech 1999). But in late 2000, there were plans to establish a 'national center for health promotion' in the National Institute for Public Health (Stergar 2001).

With view to the **education system,** the overall reform since Slovenia's independence (1991) includes the reform of the whole school curriculum. The introduction and implementation of the Health Promoting Schools (HPS) concept happened time wise parallel (from 1992). The idea of developing an 'education for health curriculum' as part of the overall curriculum (or "education for health" as a cross-curricular theme) arose during this time and has been acted upon since 1998. It is guided by the *vision* that all subjects contribute to 'education for health'. In Slovenia, **general education reform, Health Promoting Schools development, plus later the "education for health" curriculum development, have gone hand in hand - the latter two in high-level intersectoral cooperation of the education *and* health sector.** By 2002/2003 all schools have to start implementing the new school curricula. How *both* sectors are involved in *each others* domains shows the following: The national 'Institute of Public Health of the Republic of Slovenia', through its *Health Education* Department links both 'Health Promoting Schools' (HPS) and 'education for health' development at national level (with the Director serving as both National HPS Coordinator and also in the national expert group for the latter). (Stergar 2000; see also chap. 5.5.3 below) The Ministry of Education plays a key role in HPS development, too, and for example, has a program on *'healthy physical activity';* complementary a law on sport from 1996 focuses on availability of facilities and youth (ECHP 2000).

Vision and key concepts at the outset and changes over time

There is not the vision or goal statement of the Slovenian network to be cited. The vision of the European Network is shared, embedded in the network's 'Health Promoting Schools'- concept.

From the beginning, the following **Health Promoting School (HPS) concept** has guided the work in Slovenia: It comprises three basic elements situated in a kind of nested structure: the *'education for health curriculum'*, the *'hidden curriculum'*, and the *'community'*. This HPS model, known as "the kite", stems from one of the earlier business meetings of the European Network (see fig. 5.5.1). The model emphasizes the value of the different *cultures* within countries which for Slovenia has been underlined as 'grown over centuries' and a 'positive resource for every school'. (Stergar 2000)

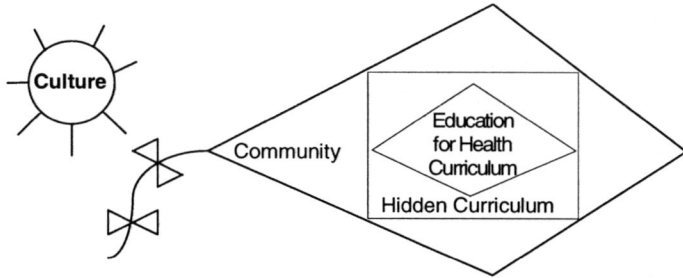

Figure 5.5.1: The 'Health Promoting School' -concept used in Slovenia: "the kite" (NSC 2000a)

The first element, **the "Education for Health Curriculum"** aims that all subjects taught during primary and secondary school contribute to health development and guidelines and practical materials developed build on the experiences gained by those involved in the HPS project (new teaching methods included). While the importance of what pupils learn is acknowledged, the second element of the HPS concept, **the 'hidden curriculum'** is stressed as even more important. The perspective *of schools as health supportive environments* encompasses many aspects: some focusing on the schools core business *'teaching'* (such as appropriate teaching and learning methods ('with children not for them'), or teachers awareness of their 'role model' functions); many relate to *intra*-organizational development in schools and health supportive environments (e.g. a 'positive climate', 'good' interpersonal relationships, food services, environmental protection/ promotion within and outside the school, sensitive and/or joint decision making, consideration of needs/ wishes of children, organisation/ management issues such as timetable, project days, etc.). Also *inter*-organisational relationships of schools are addressed: in the aspect of the school's *openness* to parents' involvement and the community. As to the third element of this HPS model, the *reciprocity* **of close school/community-links** is emphasised: with on the one hand, schools to be places where everyone feels welcomed and teachers continuously keeping in touch with and involving all parents, and on the other, efforts from the side of the community (including decision makers' awareness and support of Health Promoting Schools (HPS) in their community); stressed are interorganisational relations between Health Promoting Schools and all services that could support or take part in its work (such as 'school doctor's teams'/health care services, counselling centres, and centres for social work) (Stergar 2000) The *'12 criteria of a Health Promoting School'* put forward by the *European* Network (and introduced in chap. 5.1.2 above) serves as an additional complementary conceptual framework. (Stergar 1997; Stergar, Stankovic 1998). Network schools are invited to translate this HPS concept into 'their' positive vision of their future school and published self portrays of ENHPS pilot schools in the first network newsletter show some results (SLNHPS 1995).

While **Health Education** is an accepted inherent element of the Health Promotion concept in general and Health Promoting Schools (HPS) concept in particular, in Slovenia it is particularly stressed. Health Education in Slovenian HPS development is understood as 'a combination of different learning processes planned for predisposing, enabling and reinforcing voluntary adaptation of individual or group behaviour conducive to health'; it is distinguished from 'traditional health education' and always addressed as embedded in the Health Promotion concept. (Stergar 2001). This emphasis is likely reinforced by the interrelations of the overall educational reform and HPS development in Slovenia mentioned above and matches with research findings on reforming 'expert organisations' (such as schools) suggesting first to strengthen their 'core business areas' (here class room teaching) (see chap. 2.4.2).

As the European Network, also the Slovenian network did not present the Network's definition of **'health'**. In general, as in overall Slovenian health care policy, the WHO definition of health is referred to (see chap. 2.1). The specific aims of network school projects include the 'promotion of *mental, physical and emotional* health' (Stergar 1996). In the ENHPS Data Base 1998 the Slovenian network answers the question of 'which are the *determinants used to describe the concept of health* in the *country*' by referring to behavioral changes, action possibilities, well-being, lifestyle, and living conditions (WHO/EURO 1998). This indicates that the Slovenian network supports and is guided by a holistic comprehensive understanding of health that matches with that elaborated in chapter 2.1.

As to the key concept of **Health Promotion** (national) representatives of the Slovenian network usually refer to the Ottawa Charter (1986) and declarations of succeeding global Health Promotion conferences such as the 'Jakarta Declaration' (1997) and the 'Mexico Ministerial Statement for the Promotion of Health' (2000) (Stergar 2001; see chap. 2.2). As the National HPS Coordinator put it, schools that participate in the European Network (the 12 'pilot' schools in Slovenia included) "*adopt an integrated, holistic approach to Health Promotion, prioritizing it within* the curriculum, school management practice, and the school's physical and social environment" (Stergar 1997 p2). As to *principles* guiding the Slovenian network reference is made to the First ENHPS Resolution (1997) which highlights principles such as democracy, equity, and empowerment (see chap. 5.1.4; Annex IV).

Documents do not provide much information on conceptual reflections as to the terms **'network' and 'networking'**. However, there are indications that the network approach chosen by the initiators of the European Network (ENHPS) is reflected upon and appreciated, for example: From the start of Slovenia's ENHPS membership, the National Support Centre always presents the 'national HPS *project*' as part of the European *Network* and when triggering applications for network membership all schools received material including pro's and con's of network membership (unfortunately unavailable in English). And although during the first years of network development national actors speak mainly of the 'national Health Promoting Schools *project*' its network focus is made explicit latest from the second year on - in form of the newsletter entitled the "Bulletin of the Slovenian *Network* of Health Promoting Schools" (SLNHP 1995).

In summary, the development and work of the Slovenian "Network of Health Promoting Schools" and the national HPS project build on the conceptual basis as put forward and supported by WHO and the international field of Health Promotion in general (see chap. 2.2) and the European Network of Health Promoting Schools in particular. As to the set of concepts identified as 'core' for the case studies (i.e. health, co-determinants of health, Health Promotion, the 'Settings' approach and the 'network' approach) Slovenian documents elaborate mainly the terms

'Health Promoting Schools' and 'education for health' therein. While it can be reasonably assumed that the *general* understanding of 'health' and 'co-determinants of health' is matching with that in the field of Health Promotion internationally, that of the 'network approach' remains an open question; the range of regular reports and the presentations analysed lack a systematic reflection but its value is clearly expressed.

Network rational and goals and objectives

There are not the statements on network rational, goal and objectives of the Slovenian network to be quoted. And similar to the European level and Germany, a *range* of goals exist. Via the first network newsletter, which was disseminated throughout Europe, Slovenian key actors express the following rational for and goal of the network: "Fostering *interaction* between all those involved in the project is an important aim set out by the network of health promoting schools" (SLNHPS 1995 p4) - a goal **related to nation-wide developments**. Documents reflect the strong identification of the Slovenian network initiators as *'European Network'*- members; and the concepts and HPS related goals defined at *European* level are used and repeatedly referred to. After three years of network development, the National Coordinator presents the '*specific aims*' of the *projects* in Slovenian Health Promoting *Schools*' in a way that remind of the 12 HPS criteria internationally defined. These can be interpreted as not only the objectives of the *individual* network schools but the national HPS project or network as a whole. The focus is on *intra*-school development without neglecting the 'school/community-link'; on the contrary, the latter is specified as inter*organisational relations* between schools and community *organizations* rather than left unspecified as often done in the field (see Stergar 1996). Similar to European Network, the objectives **related to HPS development** are a mix of both specific and general, school development and health education related goals; aspects showing the organization development dimension are highlighted:

- education and enhancement of personal and *professional growth* of teachers;
- *systematic integration of health-promoting issues into the daily life* of the school;
- promotion of mental, physical and emotional health (a nation wide priority theme);
- qualification of pupils and teachers (better knowledge and promotion of their responsibility for health);
- reduction of stressful events in the school setting;
- promotion of healthy dietary habits and developing physical skills of the pupils;
- stimulation of parents to take an active role in the life of the school;
- developing *communication skills* among pupils, teachers, parents;
- providing *health-promoting work conditions and environment* (ecological projects);
- fostering *better links with community institutions*;
- providing preventive programs and activities (on general health education, nutrition, drug abuse, stress, smoking, family planning/sex education, pupil-to-pupil

communication, self-esteem, oral health, accidents, cancer, AIDS, ...)

As one of the pilot school teams phrased it the "*global aim* pursued by all those participating in the project is 'to do their utmost for the health of school children, the family and the community at large'." (Marija Broz Primary School in SLNHPS 1995 p4)

As said before, the Alter/Hage network theory suggests that a wider *scope* of an interorganisational network's *tasks or goals* calls for different network structures and operational processes than a more narrow scope. Also, network outcomes such as *'perceived effectiveness'* will depend on the goals set. Therefore, network goals should be well understood if network assessment is a goal. When using again the Health Promotion outcome model adapted from Nutbeam 1999 to systematise the Slovenian network's or network projects goals (see fig. 3.1.3) the following picture emerges: As the name implies, the "Slovenian Network of Health Promoting Schools" formulated and communicated its overall goal mainly in terms of what 'Health Promoting Schools' (HPS) are about. The range of objectives cover *all* levels of the outcome model, and a few focus on selected groups of the school community only:

a) With regard to the level of **ultimate or long term outcomes**, i.e. health and quality of life outcomes:

- the Slovenian network's HPS related objectives include *one:* the promotion of 'mental, physical, and emotional health'.

b) With regard to the level of **intermediate outcomes**, i.e. changes of the *co-determinants of health*, both of the two broad categories of factors are addressed:

- health promoting lifestyles (dietary habits and physical skills; and more or less directly drug/tobacco use, sexual and accident related behaviours);

- health promoting environments (reducing stress full events in schools; healthy ecological environment; health promoting 'work conditions'; - the latter also relates to the next level);

c) With regard to the level of **direct or short term outcomes** *all three* categories are addressed:

- 'healthy public policies and organisational practices'

Interesting from an interorganisational research perspective, objectives relate to **organisational practices** rather policy and can be grouped as follows:

objectives related to

inwards oriented *organisational development* of individual schools (teachers' professional growth/ integrating health-promoting issues into daily school life/work);

interorganisational relations of individual schools with a) organisations in their local surroundings and/or b) other schools.

Matching with the HPS related goals formulated at European level, also the Slovenian network does not specify objectives in terms of 'Health Promoting Schools' as interorganisational 'network members' or their 'organisational networking'-capacities (in spite of the overall emphasis given to the 'European Network'-membership). However, *one* general objective was widely communicated by national actors that relates to

interorganisational network building (fostering interactions between all those involved in the project).

Other objectives fall into the other two categories of direct or short term outcomes:

- **'health literacy'** (aspects addressed include knowledge, responsibility for health, communication skills, stress coping ability, self esteem); and
- **'social action and influence'** (stimulation of parents to play an active role in school life).
- d) With regard to the fourth dimension of the 'Nutbeam-Health Promotion outcome model', **'Health promotion actions' or inputs to achieve desired outcomes'**
- *one* HPS related objective of the Slovenian network falls into this category (provision of *'prevention programs'* including *'general health education'*).

Other objectives address education or qualification measures as to pupils and teachers, too.

This analysis guided by the adapted Health Promotion outcome model (elaborated in chap. 3.1.4) shows that **overall, at the level of objectives** put forward by the Slovenian network there is a) *equal emphasis on intermediate and direct or short term* Health Promotion outcomes; b) as to intermediate outcomes *equal emphasis on life-style and school-related environmental* co-determinants of health; c) re. ultimate or long term outcomes a *focus on health literacy* related aspects but also on *organizational or school development* issues (rather than on social action and influence, policy issues or interorganisational relations). The latter, however, *is* indirectly considered (as schools' outreach into their local communities).

5.5.2 Structural set-up and key actors of the Slovenian 'HPS project' and 'Network of Health Promoting Schools'

The development of the Slovenian '*Network* of Health Promoting Schools' (SLNHPS) or the ENHPS in Slovenia was started as a 'national Health Promoting Schools (HPS) *project*'. Its structure changed slightly over the three phases of development identified in this research project between 1993 and 2000: a four-year-'pilot phase' (1993 to 1997); a eight/nine months long transition phase (in 1997); and from 1998 a 'dissemination phase' with first network expansion. Over several years, particularly national actors have predominantly used the term national 'HPS *project*' rather than 'network'. During the pilot phase it was *organized at two systems levels*, national and local; later a third, regional level moved into the foreground, too. In light of the network definition derived in chapter 2.4 it is interesting, that the Slovenian '**HPS *project* organization**' has been described as a *'non-hierarchical'* structure that spans local and national level which during the first four years encompassed **four groups of 'key actors'**: a) a high level, intersectoral *'National Advisory Board'*; b) twelve selected *pilot or 'project' schools* (11 elementary, 1 secondary school); c) one *'National Support Center'*; and d) two so called *'peer teachers'* operating across the country. (Stergar 1996, 1997, 2001; SLNHPS 1995) This structure fully matches with the European Network's requirements (re. national support structure and interministerial collaboration) and recommendations (e.g. on a national advisory body).

The *intersectoral collaboration* between the national Ministries of Health and of Education and Sports (MoE) is up today anchored in the **National Advisory Board**, i.e. the national level **decision making body** newly established for the development of Health Promoting Schools in Slovenia. From early on the Advisory Board (with first 10, later 20 members) encompassed: the national *Ministry of Health and Ministry of Education and Sport* (each represented by several high level functionaries including the State Secretaries); the *'National Institute of Public Health'/ National HPS Support Center* (strongly represented, too); a *counseling center* for children, adolescents and parents; an increasing number of faculty members/ *academia;* and over time also the *'National Education Institute';* and a primary *school* representative. From its inception meeting regularly twice a year, the Advisory Board itself can be interpreted as an inter-*organizational*, national level network for the development of Health Promoting Schools in Slovenia. The participating individuals (faculty professors) are not just members in their personal capacity but expected to integrate the innovation of 'Health Promoting Schools'-development into their teaching to strengthen capacities in the field. - Presided by the Education Ministry, the Advisory Board *suggested and approved the selection criteria for schools* wishing to join the Slovenian and, thus, "European Network of Health Promoting Schools". Due to governmental changes and elections the Board has not been re-nominated since 1999 (Stergar 2001).

The reputable National 'Institute of Public Health' (IPH) serves as **National Support Center** for the Slovenian network of Health Promoting Schools (HPS); the Director of the Department of *Health Education* therein was nominated by the Health Ministry as 'National HPS Project Coordinator'. The official contact points in the Ministries of Education and of Health are the State Secretaries. During the first four 'pilot' years, there was a small 'national HPS project team' with 1,3 staff positions (National Coordinator position 33%; one professional/professor 100%). These were to support the Slovenian 'project' schools (see below). At the end of the first phase of network development and with view to the HPS 'dissemination phase' another full time professor joined the team. The disciplines covered (psychology, sociology/later pedagogy, and health education) match with the network's foci as regards content.

Following an initiative at the European level, during the first four years of network development **two "peer teachers"** played an important role. Nominated by the Ministry of Education, they a) had to 'teach the teachers' in the network's pilot schools, and b) advocate for Health Promoting Schools development in general by implementing the ENHPS manual on 'Promoting the health of young people in Europe' (EC, CE, WHO/EURO 1993; EC, CE, WHO/EURO, Health Education Board of Scotland 1994).

At school level, the Slovenian network of Health Promoting Schools (HPS) was and is organized in **multi-professional 'HPS project teams',** with one 'project leader' each (often the head master or school counselor) plus sometimes an assigned 'assistant'. These teams were to combine *school* staff, at least one local *health care* professional, and a high level *community* representative. After about a year of ENHPS membership, the vast majority of the 'HPS school teams' in the 12 Slovenian 'pilot schools' indeed reported to be well anchored within the school (staff, head master, school counselor involvement), two thirds also as to local *health care* services (nurse/ school doctor) as well as parents involvement, and half as to other *community* representatives. In a few cases special *pupils' teams* existed either complementary to the 'HPS project team' or as part of it. During the first four years of network development, school teams usually met monthly and invested 5 to 15 hours per month in the school's HPS project (SLNHPS 1995; Stergar 1996, 1997; Stergar, Bevc Stankovic 1998)

(External) resources

From the start, the development of the Slovenian network of Health Promoting Schools (HPS) was **co-financed by the national Ministries** of 'Health' and of 'Education and Sports'. As a national 'Health Promoting Schools (HPS) *project*' it was financed by systems levels and funds had *to be renewed on a yearly basis* - a burden for the National Coordinator. The *Health* Ministry covered costs at *'national level',* i.e. for the first four (pilot) years: 1,3 professional staff of the National Support Center, in-service training of teachers, and the production of manuals and network newsletter. This was complemented by some 'WHO donations'. Later, after the start of the 'dissemination' phase, a second National Support Center position was added. - Other than the Health Ministry the *Education* Ministry covered the costs at *'school level',* i.e. for the first four years: 7 hours teaching reduction per week for the HPS teams of each of the 12 'pilot' schools, plus the travel costs for in-service training. After six years, (in 2000) the support of the former 'pilot' schools was reduced to 4 hours teaching reduction per week, and fees and travel costs were to be covered by participants themselves. - The Education Ministry also supported the two 'peer teachers' operating during the network's 'pilot' years (by 1 day duty reduction per week); their training was supported by the *European* Network initiative.

The *in-service training* for participating teachers, a core activity in Slovenian Health Promoting Schools (HPS) development, benefited from the fact that in Slovenia, every school receives resources for five days training per year per teacher. During the network's pilot years, the Ministry of Health provided additional resources to pilot schools for special HPS courses. Overall, through *health* sector funds the National Support Center had a budget allowance of its own to implement the HPS project at national and international level. - However, over time (also due to financial crises in the country) the allocation of public funds has not always been timely. (Stergar 1996; 2001)

In summary, the development of the Slovenian 'Network of Health Promoting Schools' depended a) mainly on financial support (in cash or in kind) by two public Ministries (Education and Health) and b) on internal resources of the national Institute of Public Health i.e. the nominated 'National Support Center'.

'Soft' and 'hard' networking

Implementing 'soft' technologies to link people (as opposed to 'hard'/ new information technologies) increases the likelihood that exchange networks develop (see chap. 2.4). The National Support Center played a core role in **'soft' networking** processes to link people within the network: During the **pilot phase** central were the *3-monthly national meetings* of key actors (here National Center and 'pilot' schools) to *exchange* experiences and jointly *evaluate* developments on an ongoing basis. This shows that a) a Slovenian exchange network '*of*' health promoting schools did exist but that b) the *national* Support Center was part of the exchange network, too. The meetings also provided opportunities for network members to link up with *external* others because repeatedly potential partners were invited to present themselves and their services (Stergar 2001). During the first four network years, the 4 to 6 training courses per year provided frequent additional opportunities for soft networking *within* the network. Soft networking was also supported by occasional site visits of the national Center to schools and soon by an annual newsletter, too. The latter made the name "Slovenian *Network of* Health Promoting Schools" widely visible, introduced an own 'Healthy Schools' network logo, and thereby facilitated the identification of members with the network. (At the time the *European* Network had no logo yet and many member countries created their own.) From an interorganisational research perspective, the teacher training program, a strong, remarkable and *integral* component of the Slovenian HPS network initiative, provided throughout valuable opportunities for 'soft networking' *within* the network. this applies particularly the pilot years when teachers of all of the yet limited number of network schools frequently met in the same course. In times phases when schools newly *entered* the network, some training courses were organized for both school and *non*-school actors (i.e. staff of local school health services).

From the second larger phase of network development (or **'dissemination' phase**), national *meetings of a larger scale* emerged as new means of soft networking, starting with the 1st Meeting of the (now formally launched) "Slovenian Network of Health Promoting Schools" in 1998. Training courses likely played now a smaller role in soft networking *within* the Network: Documents indicate that the number of courses relative to the increased number of network members was reduced and with now 130 instead of 12 network schools it follows naturally that only some would repeatedly meet in training courses.

'Hard' networking, in the sense of linking computers (e-mail etc.) in support of soft networking and effective information exchange *within* the network, has not been an issue in documents on Slovenian network development. While it is known that the National Support Center from the start had and used e-mail as a means of networking across Europe, for the national network's *internal* networking this seems *not* to have played an important role if any. However, traditional 'hard' information technologies such as fax and phone have been crucial (WHO/EURO 1998).

5.5.3 Developments over time: the evolution of the Slovenian 'Network of Health Promoting Schools'

Network development during the 'pilot' years

The initiators and key actors at national level, as members of the National Advisory Board of the Slovenian 'HPS *project*', chose an **'open invitation approach' to select 'pilot schools'**: They invited *all* elementary and secondary schools (a total of about 650) to apply for participation in the national HPS *project* as part of the European *Network* in Slovenia. With the invitation, <u>all</u> *Slovenian schools received basic information* about Health Promotion, the European Network of Health Promoting Schools (HPS), and Slovenia's 'HPS project'. This means that the closer institutional environment of the 'HPS network in the making', the school system, was being influenced early on by information dissemination. To guide the selection of a limited number of ENHPS pilot schools out of all those schools that would show interest to join, the National Advisory Board developed the following **selection criteria** (Stergar 1993a, 1996, 1997; NSC 1998a) that may be grouped as follows:

a) *formal* criteria, here: schools with at least 8 classes, size of school (i.e. of school population), geographic location/ region, and urban or rural district;

b) *health (factor) related* criteria, here: health status of school children; material and social development of the school district; and integration of children with special needs;

c) *organizational innovation related* criteria, here: existing project work (presence of other projects at the school); connections with the local community; and - as a more general issue - the quality of the application/proposals made.

From an interorganisational *network* perspective interesting is the attention given to the schools' geographic location which as shown below guaranteed a geographically dispersed Slovenian 'pilot' network (with one 'pilot' school per region) as a crucial stepping stone towards network expansion later on. The criteria related to the schools' 'experience with project work' hints at organizational innovations outside the class room walls as does that on 'connections with their local community'. The latter also points to potential interorganisational relations locally. This reminds of two of Hastings' 'organizational networking' dimensions (1993): an organization's networking 'within' and 'with others'. - From a *Health Promotion* perspective interesting is the consideration of pupils' health status and of social factors influencing health such as the schools' socio-economic environment.

As shown in figure 5.5.2 the **'pilot school' selection process** did not only involve the *schools* as potential network members but also two *other* groups of organizations in the schools' *institutional environment* that potentially would have a key role to play in the development of Health Promoting Schools across Slovenia: the *local* health services (here 'school doctor's teams') and the *regional* Institutes of Public Health, i.e. the regional 'outlets' of the *national* Institute serving as National Support Center. Thus, local and regional *health sector* institutions were invited to support local *educational* institutions (the schools) near by - in their decisions for or against an application for ENHPS membership. The national actors supported this process, e.g. by spreading information on health and the HPS concept within the *wider environment* of the HPS network project (via mass media).

The small national *selection committee* spanned the health and education sector, here the National Institutes of Education and of Public Health/the 'National Support Center'. About 10% of all Slovenian schools applied for joining the ENHPS; 12 of these 60 schools (i.e. 20%) were selected: 11 elementary schools (age 7-15) and 1 secondary school. This matched with European level recommendations of the time for 'ENHPS member countries' to limit themselves to 10 pilot schools. From an international and interorganisational research perspective, the Slovenian network (for the development) of Health Promoting Schools started to exist in spring 1993, when the 12 'ENHPS pilot schools' and core network *members* first met with the National Support Center and started joint work towards the network's aim: the transformation of themselves (as pilot schools) into 'Health Promoting Schools' and - while doing so - helping to pave the way for more schools to follow this route.

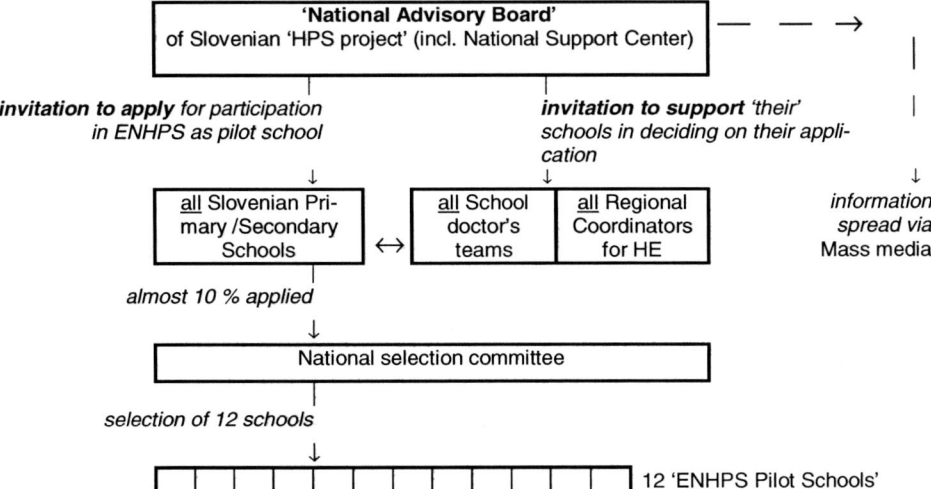

Figure 5.5.2: The 'open invitation approach' of the ENHPS initiative in Slovenia as applied to the selection of 'ENHPS *pilot* schools' for the first four network years. (on the base of Stergar 1993a, 1997)

A **range of activities** have characterized the first (pilot) phase of Slovenian network development (NSC 2000a; Stergar, Stankovic 1998; Stergar 1996). From an interorganisational research perspective these may be categorized as follows: a) *technical support and evaluation* activities (including provision of health promotion materials/ information/ advice); b) activities for *capacity development of organizational actors* at both local and national levels (team building *within* schools and National Center; intensive in-service training for national project staff and local actors both within *and* external to schools (e.g. school doctor's teams)); c) activities related to *organizational networking* (as elaborated in chap. 2.4.2) (network newsletter; involvement of an increasing number of people locally both *within* and *external to* schools;) and d) activities directed at the *network's wider organizational environment* (dissemination of information on HPS concept, Health Promotion and Education, and the European Network across the education and health sectors). In this regard - so the National Coordinator - these sectors were 'not up to date' and training was generally lacking (Stergar 1997). While in three of the four action areas (a,b,d) the *National* Support Center was the main actor (and in the first two the European Network, too), the key roles in the area of 'organizational networking' within the network and with local others (c) were played by both *National* Center and pilot *schools*.

The (teacher) **training** component of the Slovenian HPS network initiative, understood as "a must for quality and effectiveness" (Stergar 1996), has been shown to successfully *trigger desired actions* in pilot schools - while apparently not compromising the Health Promotion principle of self-controlled priority setting at local level. Addressed were both themes related to *health* (and the overall priority theme of 'mental and emotional health' that emerged during the pilot years) and issues supportive of *organizational innovations* in schools (such as Health Promotion program planning, project evaluation, interpersonal communication and 'managing change'). (Stergar 1995c, 1996, 1996a,b, 1997, 1997c)

The overall picture of the Slovenian network that emerged so far is one of a system that remained fairly constant over time as far as *types* and *numbers* of key actors and/or network members are concerned. The regular 'national meetings' of pilot schools and National Support Center plus school-to-school- encounters during training courses indicate that indeed a 'network *of* Health Promoting Schools (HPS)' was formed; however, consideration of the National Support Center's regular participation in these meetings as well as its roles and activities as compared to other key national actors suggests that the National Center, too, might be a 'network *member*' rather than 'external supporter'. The latter may be the role of, for example, the National Advisory Board. If this assumption holds, the ENHPS in Slovenia from early on was a 'network *for the development* of Health Promoting Schools' but with a strong 'school-to-school network'-component. Obviously, this issue needs further examination.

A 'planned' approach to network growth

From the very beginning of Slovenian network development the number of *additional* (non-pilot) schools interested to join grew and yet, the National Advisory Board insisted on a *'planned dissemination'* of the Slovenian 'Health Promoting Schools *project*' based on an *evaluation* of the pilot schools' activities. For this purpose and over a year before the end of the pilot phase, a **strategic 'dissemination (and evaluation) group'** was formally established. As the National Board, also this group reflected the principle of intersectoral collaboration between health and education sector and this even at *two* systems levels local and national (with pilot schools, a local health center and the 'peer teachers' being represented as well as the National Institutes of Education and of Public Health). The group was crucial in the development of the Slovenian HPS related 'evaluation-' and 'dissemination plans' (school selection included). These were approved by the National Advisory Board. The results of the process evaluation of the pilot phase were crucial for the Board's decision to 'disseminate' the national 'HPS *project*' which meant that the Education and Health Ministries prolonged their cooperation and support. Overall, pupils, parents, and teams of school doctors had favored the dissemination of the 'project', too (Stergar 1999). During 1997, a **short transition or preparatory phase** of about nine months resulted in *dissemination activities that were planned and timed with active participation of the school project teams* of the Slovenian pilot schools.

Network expansion and formal launch

With the beginning of the so called **'dissemination phase'** in early 1998, the Slovenian network (for the development) of Health Promoting Schools reached a new stage of development marked by *significant changes concerning* a) the total number of school members, b) number and type of regional level actors, and related to this c) the 'pilot' schools' roles and responsibilities. The network's expansion at school level and, thus, the move towards large scale development of Health Promoting Schools in Slovenia, rested on the idea to now build on *three* types of key organization actors: first, the group of the twelve by now experienced *pilot schools* who would start to serve *as new 'regional centers of excellence and training'* for the dissemination of the Health Promoting Schools (HPS) concept - with a shift in focus towards *regional* development; second, the group of the existing *Regional* Institutes of Public Health, who would become more visible and reinforced actors in HPS development; and third, and as before the *National* Institute of Public Health, i.e. the National Support Center.

Thus, **a regional level** of the Slovenian network initiative **clearly emerged** and the number of core *non*-school actors raised. Both regional and national Institutes were to jointly support the pilot schools in their new, regionally focused leadership role - a role foreseen for all 'HPS project teams' of pilot schools since the network's inception. (Stergar 1996b, 1997a-d, 1999, 2001; NSC 1998a) During the first four network years the pilot schools had focused on tasks defined for all 'ENHPS pilot schools' in Europe: the implementation of the Health Promoting Schools concept as outlined at European level and - on the base of a systematic planning, documentation and reflection process - exchange their experiences and develop transferable 'models of good practice'. The Slovenian pilot schools had also been actively involved in overall network development tasks such as the preparation of the Slovenian network's expansion. After four network years, in an expanded Slovenian network, they were willing and prepared to take on new responsibilities: to serve as regional *'centres of excellence and training'* for Health Promotion in the school setting or **'regional HPS centres'**. Due to the original pilot school selection process each region had such a regional centre. (NSC 1998a; Stergar 1999) Pilot schools as regional centres were expected to *actively exchange* ideas, information, and experiences as well as *exchange and develop* HPS and teacher training programs *with the new* network schools in their region. As to the latter they could build on some European materials, particularly the ENHPS manual on the promotion of mental and emotional health which addresses a key theme of Slovenian HPS development.

Not only the role of the pilot schools changed. Documents indicate expectations that ideally the *Regional* Institutes of Public Health would take over tasks that the *National* Institute had had before. However, in response to the pilot schools' request for continued support from the **National Support Centre** the latter - now strengthened through another full time position - continued to serve as national information point and provide technical support. It also took care of in-service training and materials for the new network schools to come, as well as to organise national meetings for the now *expanded* Slovenian network.

As to the **Regional Institutes of Public Health** little information has been found. Their 'health education focal points' had already been invited to play a role in selecting the very first Slovenian 'pilot' schools; via their routine meetings with the *national* Institute of Public Health they had been kept informed about Slovenian network developments throughout the years; and when the Slovenian 'HPS project' moved on into its 'dissemination phase', supporting the development of Health Promoting Schools (HPS) became part of their regular duties. The Regional Institutes attended at least one of the regular meetings of National Support Centre and pilot schools *before* the Network's expansion, an opportunity to early on step into *direct* interorganisational relations with *all* core network actors. As to the expanded Slovenian Network the Regional Institutes were to *actively support the 'pilot' schools* in their new role as 'regional HPS centers' in a way that would support the *new* network schools in their region. Since the network's expansion network related reports of the National Coordinator refer frequently to cooperation and quarterly meetings with the 'network of regional coordinators for health education' of all Regional Institutes of Public Health (Stergar 1998b,c,d) which indicates that their direct role in Slovenian network development did increase indeed.

When taking together the information available on a) the redefined roles of the pilot schools and b) the Regional Institutes of Public Health it becomes visible that, after four years of network (project) development in Slovenia, the network that spanned two systems levels evolved into one that spanned three. Its *regional* level (only latent and hardly visible during the pilot years) took now shape: on the one hand, by building as planned on the strengths and experiences of the 'pilot schools' and moving them clearly into the center stage of regional Health Promoting Schools and network development; on the other hand, by (re)activating and giving formal HPS related responsibilities to the existing regional Institutes of Public Health - and this in a way that made *the latter supporters of the former*.

After having identified *pilot schools, National Support Center and Regional Institutes of Public Health* as **key actors within or around the 'expanded' Slovenian network** for the development of Health Promoting Schools, one group of core actors remains to be addressed: the so called *'new' network schools*. A look at school selection criteria and process provides some valuable additional insight into the evolution of the Slovenian network as a whole:

It is interesting to note, that for the 'dissemination' phase (or the phase of network expansion) the **selection criteria for 'new' schools** interested in joining the "Slovenian Network of Health Promoting Schools" in 1998 are quite *different* from those for the 'pilot' phase (see Stergar, bevc Stankovic 1997); and they may be grouped as follows:

a) *'health promoting Settings' specific* criteria, here: the school's willingness 'to work towards meeting the 12 criteria of a Health Promoting School' (chapter 5.1.2); and 'more than half of school *staff has agreed* that the school should join the HPS network';

b) *organizational innovation related* criteria, here: the school's commitment to establish a 'multidisciplinary school project team' comprising representatives of the school community ('pupils, teachers, parents, management') as well as external others (the 'local community' and 'other organizations'); commitment to annual 'in-service training courses for *all* teachers (devoted to health, health promotion, health education or related topics'), and plans to undertake 'some extra-curricular activities for pupils' on health;

c) *interorganisational relations related* criteria, here: the 'school doctor's and dentist's teams' willingness to take part in the *project*; the school's commitment to 'cooperate with specialist institutions and professional organizations'; - and the already mentioned issue of staff's agreement "to join the HPS *network*" needs to be listed here, too.

Overall, in January 1998 **120 'new' network schools** were selected among all the elementary, secondary and/or boarding schools that followed the again open invitation to apply for network membership. The first year was a crucial one: All 'new' schools and the 12 'pilot' schools became '*official members*' of the Slovenian Network; soon, the National Support Center met a first time with all 'new' network schools; the "Slovenian **Network** of Health Promoting Schools" was **formally launched**; the provision of *in-service training* courses, already at the heart of network development during the four pilot years, was continued (particularly on 'planning and evaluation of Health Promotion programs' and the key thematic issue of 'mental and emotional health') (Stergar 1999); later on, the new schools started to create and implement the required 3-months-"Health Promoting Schools" plans; and towards the end of this first year of the <u>expanded</u> Slovenian Network, its *"first network meeting"* was held - on the occasion of receiving the "*WHO* 50th Anniversary *Award*". Yet before the 'new' schools started their planned Health Promoting Schools (HPS) activities, *base line data* were collected covering not only a) general school data but b) issues of *health promoting school development* (HPS project team/ in-service training/ school climate/ 'areas of change') and - interestingly and explicitly - c) *interorganizational relations and network* issues (involvement in other networks and cooperation with other Health Promoting Schools/ cooperation with school doctor's teams).

When comparing the selection criteria for network schools by both a) main phases of network development (pilot/ dissemination phase) and b) categories of criteria (as introduced above) an interesting *development over time within the Slovenian network as a whole* becomes visible. After four years of ENHPS membership and national network experience and at the point in time of opening up the ('pilot') network to many more network schools, the changes concerning the selection criteria for *school* members reflect *a more differentiated perspective on the organisational and inter-organisational aspects* of this work: the group of purely formal criteria disappeared; the group of health/ health factor related criteria was replaced by a *Settings specific* group (which nevertheless encompasses the former); the category of '*organisational innovation* related' criteria remained but is now complemented by a *new* separate group of criteria that is '*inter-*organisational relations' related. The overall impression emerging is one of *greater conceptual clarity* on the side of network actors although this remains somewhat hidden. - When looking at these findings against the background of the Health Promotion outcome model adapted from Nutbeam (see fig. 3.1.3) an additional thought comes to mind: the school selection criteria indicate an interesting shift in emphasis within and around the network as to 'base line' information required of schools interested to join the network: with view to the *selection* process, *less emphasis* is on information related to ultimate or long-term and intermediate Health Promotion outcomes, and *more emphasis* on information related to - in Nutbeam-terms - direct or short-term Health Promotion outcomes and here only as to the schools' (inter)*organisational* practice. It seems that the first network years have helped to see more clearly the importance of favourable organisational starting conditions for a school's fruitful membership in an interorganisational network for the development of Health Promoting Schools. The dealing with the still desired Health Promotion outcomes in terms of health and social outcomes as well as those related to co-determinants of health are now clearly and *solely* addressed as part of the commitment required of all network schools to implementing the European 'Health Promoting Schools' (HPS) concept (such as to the 12 'European' HPS criteria).

Unfortunately, the further evolution of the *'expanded'* Slovenian *Network* is not well documented. The new network schools stepped into the three-monthly planning and documentation process as did the pilot schools but in 2001 this material had not yet been analyzed. However, good two years after the Network's expansion key actors of the European Network's Technical Secretariat as well as the National Support Center perceived the developments as very positive: The European level called already for working towards the 'ultimate goal' of the European Network (ENHPS): 'nationally adopted *programs for* Health Promoting Schools' or the *'ENHPS as a national program'* in Slovenia; and pointing to the key role of the Education Ministry it also called for the support of other 'influential' educational organizations with whom first discussions had just begun (namely the national Institute of Education, Education Development Center, and education faculties) (Rivett 2000). Rivett goes so far to describe the goal of a next developmental phase in Slovenia as "the move *from a management* program for a *network of* schools *to a national program for* health promoting schools" (HPS) which would require both high level recognition and maintaining a 'strong experienced team' (Rivett 2000 p2/ italics not in original).

Also the *National* HPS Support Center after by then eight years of work with or within the Slovenian network, supported the above **direction suggested**; and as the European level, it called for an 'official agreement' for this type of national development beyond the dissemination phase at highest level. Reasons for this relate to the Slovenian *Network's closer and wider environment*: on the one hand, the ongoing educational reform, the new 'education for health curriculum', and the fact that still more and more schools wish to join the network; on the other hand, Slovenia's entering the European Union, and the identified need for the development of health promotion activities for young people. **'Strengths' to build on** included *the "Network* of Health Promoting Schools" itself; the systematic and partnership approach and existing cooperation *within and around the network*: among and across sectors, experts, organizations and countries; and *network capacities* such as manuals, in-service training and professional support in place. However, **threats** were identified, too, particularly as to the *network's environment:* a) re. the wider environment, such as the lack of a national Health Promoting strategy, of young people's issues on political agendas, and understanding of the Health Promotion approach among key actors; b) the network's closer environment such as the lack of integration of this approach into mainstream education and health policies, of professional training and research, and also of motivation among school or local community members and others. With view to the *network itself*, the lack of (human, material etc.) resources was pointed out.

The ENHPS Technical Secretariat suggested to create a Slovenian '*Association of Health Promoting Schools*' as an *additional infrastructure* that should help to maintain the level of support and networking activities provided to as of then 130 network schools even if the rest of Slovenian schools (i.e. 80% of all) would join the net, too.

The *Education Ministry did indeed* nominate its 'council for health' to develop a national strategy for Health Promotion within schools but - work did not progress due to government change, modification of the council, and loss of supportive State Secretaries on the way. The National Advisory Board for Slovenia's ENHPS initiative has not been re-nominated since. (NSC 2000a; Stergar 2001) The expanded Slovenian network did not cease to exist and work but its closest political environment changed dramatically and the National Board as the central basis for ongoing and systematic interorganisational collaboration at highest level got lost for the time being.

Network development over time - intermediate synopsis and discussion

From its inception and as the German network, the Slovenian network (for the development) of Health Promoting Schools was meant to be both sustained beyond the 'pilot phase' (1993-1997) and expanded beyond the limited number of pilot schools to many more schools across the country. As of now the following general picture of the network is emerging: The network took shape around *two main types of organizational actors* (and may be network members): a) *individual organizations*, i.e. the 'pilot schools' and the 'National Support Center' or Institute of Public Health, and b) a newly established intersectoral and *multi*-organizational body called 'National Advisory Board'. Thus, interorganisational relations and/or networks are at stake. With regard to **types and numbers of key actors and/or members** the network *remained constant* over time with during the first eight years *one exception,* the network's modification and expansion at the beginning of the 'dissemination phase'. This network behavior was caused by the National Advisory Board (and the major funding agencies, the national Ministries, therein); as the decision making body of the 'national HPS project' the Board exercised control over the timing and choice of processes for network school selection. That network 'membership' was only defined as to *school* members is likely the influence of the guidance of the *European* Network (ENHPS) which as explained before distinguishes between *country* members and *school* members only.

As to the Slovenian network initiative's relation to its **environment** the information available suggests: First, the Slovenian network (for the development) of Health Promoting Schools *started well anchored within the national level of the Public Health sector* and this was *strengthened over time* (reputable national Institute as National Support Center/ after the pilot years, support of 'Health Promoting Schools'- development as part of the formal work plans of the national *and* regional Institutes of Public Health). Second, the network's *structural anchors within the national level of the public education sector was reasonably strong*, at least as far as the use of the established teacher training system is concerned. However, there was *some decline over time* (decrease of teaching reduction per pilot school from 7 to 4 hours per week at a time when their tasks as regional key actors increased). - In general, the Slovenian network seems to have satisfied key actors within and around it but it remains an open question whether the *loss of its high level National Advisory Board due to political changes* after six years will have a weakening effect over time or not. The next wave of network expansion beyond the 20% of Slovenian schools already involved was in 2001 not yet in sight, - at least not in the way exercised before (i.e. with a joint decision and co-ordinated support by both Education and Health Ministry).

The Slovenian actors did not present an explicit or refined network concept; they followed the *general idea* of the 'European Network of Health Promoting Schools'. However, from the perspective of interorganisational network research it is interesting that *from the start at least one* **non-school actor** worked regularly and jointly with the schools towards a common goal, the 'National Support Center' or national Institute of Public Health. This shows that the latter may be reasonably understood as network *'member'* rather than external 'supporter'. If this assumption holds the Slovenian network is one 'for the development' of Health Promoting Schools and not a pure network 'of' schools as its name suggests - but with a strong 'school-to-school'- network component. In comparison to the National Support Center the National Advisory Board may have been a core actor more *external* to the network (as coordinator of decisions in the network's closest institutional environment (health/ education) such as on funding but without direct links to the main group of network members, the schools). It remains to be further examined whether National Support Center, National Advisory Board, and also the Regional Institutes of Public Health are participants of the time limited national 'HPS *project'* and/or 'members' of the longer living *'network'*. The examination of interactions and relations of and among various actors in the following chapter aims at clarifying this and other open issues identified above.

5.5.4 Interactions and relations of network members

To examine interactions and relations of network 'members' the **question of membership** or network borders needs to be answered. However, as the initiation and implementation of the Slovenian network was guided by the overall idea of 'the European Network of Health Promoting Schools (ENHPS) in Slovenia' and not an explicit interorganisational network concept there is no easy answer. What applies to the European level (see chap. 5.1) seems to be useful also for the network development in Slovenia: to distinguish between a) the 'network *project*' (here the 'national Health Promoting Schools (HPS) project') and b) the *'network'* itself.

Table 5.5.1 on the *'ENHPS in Slovenia'* provides a summary of both key (organizational) actors identified in Slovenia and their assumed membership or participant status as to the Slovenian 'Network' and 'network project'. The table provides a simple framework for the examination of the inherent assumptions about the Slovenian network's boundaries. A main question is whether the National Support Center and may be even the National Advisory Board could be reasonably understood as *members* of the Slovenian network for the development of Health Promoting Schools or not. A related question is whether the *regional* Institutes of Public Health formally in charge of supporting *HPS* development in their region since the first network expansion, are to be understood as network members or rather external supporters. The information below stems mainly from the analysis of the full set of regular reports of the National Support Center to the WHO representative in Slovenia (see Stergar 1993a to 1998d). Where information from the WHO Schools Data Base 1998 has been used this is noted (WHO/EURO 1998). Where ever possible the perspective of the national actors has been complemented by that of the pilot schools.

What has been explained in chapter 4 needs to be recalled: The following exploration of interorganisational *relations and interactions* within and around the Slovenian network for the development of Health Promoting Schools during the years 1993 to 2000 attempts to capture **an <u>overall</u> picture**. It aims at improving the understanding of Network *membership and environment* - as a base for clarifying basic structural network features (in Alter/Hage terms i.e. size, complexity, differentiation, connectivity, and centrality) - as well as the extent of *organizational networking processes* (i.e. Hastings' soft/ hard networking, networking within/ with others). *Other basic features* of interorganisational *networks* need to be kept in mind, too (non-/less hierarchical, lateral links, self-regulation; informal or formal relations; direct person-to-person-connections, trust, mutual benefit/reciprocity, information/resource sharing, long term perspective, etc.).

Organizational systems → key actors ↓	Slovenian 'network project' participants	Slovenian **network** members	
		'pilot' years	after network expansion in 1998
national level	National MoH National MoE 'National Advisory Board'(NAB) other organizations (e.g. Open Society Fund)	National Support Center = National Institute of Public Health (IPH) National Advisory Board [?] 2 'peer teachers'	
regional level	Regional 'Institutes of Public Health' (IPHs)		'pilot' schools* now as 'regional centers of excellence and training' Regional 'Institutes of Public Health' [?]
local level	local health care services (school doctor's teams) ? other local organizations other HPS outside the country;	ENHPS 'pilot' schools*	120 new network schools (HPS)

ENHPS: European Network of Health Promoting Schools
HPS: Health Promoting School(s)
IPH: Institute of Public Health
MoE: Ministry of Education
MoH: Ministry of Health
NAB: National Advisory Board

Table 5.5.1: The ENHPS in Slovenia 1993-2000: The Slovenian "Network of Health Promoting Schools" - key actors and assumed membership status as well as related social systems ('national project').

Also the Alter/Hage network typology is a reference issue (exchange, promotional, systemic networks). As before, the examination of interactions and relations is organized around one selected key actor per system level whose relationships with all others is being examined (see fig. 4.2.1 above). For Slovenia these are the *'National Support Center'* and the *'ENHPS pilot schools'* which as elaborated in chapter 5.2 both are ENHPS members. The network's *regional* level that emerged with the network's expansion in 1998 (dissemination phase) will be *examined as part of the examination of the pilot schools' relations and interactions* as these, in the second phase of network development, became nominated key actors at regional level. - In the following, where needed the interactions and relations will be presented *separately* for the first/ 'pilot' phase of network development (marked as A) and the years after network expansion/'dissemination' phase (B). The relations of the Slovenian network *as a whole* will be looked at both 'inwards' oriented (as to regional developments) and 'outwards' (as to the European Network/ ENHPS).

I.	Interactions and relations of the National Support Center with other organizations

To derive the relevant information the following 'search scheme' has been used:

THE NATIONAL SUPPORT CENTER'S **interactions and relations with:**	*organizations within their countries* ↓		*organizations outside their countries/ the European Dimension* ↓
'national - local' →	**1. the network schools/HPS:** A: 'pilot' schools (HPS); 'other'; B: 'pilot' and 'new' network schools;	**2. local others** health care services (school doctor's teams)	
'national - regional' →	**3. key actors in regions:** A/B: Regional Institutes of Public Health; B: pilot schools as 'regional centers of excellence and training' for HPS;		
'national - national' →	**4. key national actors:** A: 2 peer teachers A/B: National Advisory Board; MoE; MoH;	**5. other national organizations or networks**	**6. other ENHPS 'countries'**
'national-internat.' →			**7. ENHPS, IPC, TS**
'the part and the whole' →	**8. the Slovenian network as a whole / the "ENHPS" as a whole**		

Table 5.5.2: The ENHPS in Slovenia: Schema of potential interorganisational relationships of the National Support Center with other organizations within and around the ENHPS or national network for the development of Health Promoting Schools. "A" refers to the first or *'pilot'* phase of network development (1993-1997), "B" to the second phase or the *expanded* Slovenian network (1998-).

ENHPS: European Network of Health Promoting Schools
HPS: Health Promoting Schools
IPC: International Planning Committee of the ENHPS
MoE: Ministry of Education
MoH: Ministry of Health
TS: Technical Secretariat of the ENHPS

From the start, the **roles and responsibilities** of the National Support Center of the Slovenian ENHPS initiative have been *directed at the network schools.* A) For the first four years of network development the tasks can be summarized as follows (Stergar 1997): a) *'support'* of the Slovenian 'school project teams' and b) development/ provision of *print media*. From a network perspective, the latter focused on both the work of individual *members* and the network as a *whole* (teaching and teacher training manuals/ network newsletter). The former focused on human resource development and resource mobilization for network *members* (school staff) but to a limited degree also as to selected *others* (school doctor's teams) (development and provision of an accredited, financially supported training program/ motivation of teachers/ negotiating teaching reduction for HPS teams of network schools). While the National Center's tasks addressed mainly issues *internal* to the network, it also identified and distributed relevant information on the networks *environment* (on organizations, programs and events of '*external* others') (Stergar 2001). B) Documents on the expanded Slovenian network (or the 'dissemination' phase) do not present redefined roles and responsibilities of the National Support Center. However, as explained below some tasks were (planned to be) handed over to regional level actors, including the *direct* support of 'new' network schools. This brought about a shift in focus towards supra-regional issues.

In the following the interactions and relations of the National Support Center with key actors within and around the Slovenian Network will be examined.

The 'national - local' dimension

1. National Support Center and the health promoting network schools

A) Various information found reflects what has been stated by the National Coordinator towards WHO early on (Stergar 1997 p4, italics not in original): "*Nothing* that is going on in the Slovenian Network of HPS is *prescribed or imposed* or has to be done. From the very beginning **some premises were accepted**: Involvement in the project is not obligatory, but *after entering the network,* work towards the 12 [European HPS] criteria should begin. Every *school plans* its project on the basis of its own situation. Priorities are chosen according to the school/ local situation." But, planning models *should* be used and evaluation *should* be done. And *participatory* learning methods and close school-community-*collaboration* are *suggested*. National Support Center and pilot schools had a **voluntary relationship** to achieve a shared goal: the transformation of pilot schools into 'Health Promoting Schools' (HPS). In the before mentioned 'national meetings' with the schools' project *leaders* and/or school managers *joint* planning, review and evaluation took place - mainly with view to the 'evaluation and planning sheets' to be filled out by all pilot schools for 3-month-periods at a time. Beyond activities or concerns of the individual schools major ones concerning the *whole network* were jointly addressed, for example, the work around a country visit of European Network representatives and Slovenia's participation in a ENHPS related pilot project on 'mental and emotional health of school children' (Stergar 1996a).

Early on, when HPS program planning, evaluation and monitoring were on the agenda, the Slovenian 'ENHPS pilot schools' expressed their *desire to collaborate closely* with the National Support Center. And the latter not only confirmed the schools need of support and monitoring but also hoped that through continuous contacts their motivation would be sustained. The first full time professional joining the National Center was to enhance the 'vivid contact' with the pilot schools. The national project (or network) meetings, first always held at the National Center, were later hosted by *pilot schools*, too. Several *training courses* for staff of pilot schools were not only organized but held by the National Center and represented not only further meeting opportunities: in some courses, staff of National Center and pilot schools *jointly developed* health education programs for health promoting (pilot) schools. In addition, National Center and schools remained in frequent (likely bi-lateral) contact via *phone and fax*.

Apparently the interactions and relations between National Center and pilot schools were to a certain degree of **mutual benefit** rather than one-sided only: For example, the National HPS Support Center did benefit from the regular (network) meetings with pilot schools as these meetings were central to the process evaluation for which the Center was responsible; the schools did benefit from the technical and mutual support as to their HPS project planning and evaluation efforts and were able to provide input into national debate.

Nevertheless, within the Slovenian network the National Center was in a special and **supportive role**, too: For example, on behalf of the pilot schools it *negotiated* with the Education Ministry to achieve *financial support* for school activities on the base of the schools' proposals. It developed and/or organized the intense training program related to the schools' health promotion work and through this provided *technical leadership*. The individual pilot schools indeed did perceive the National Center as supportive as the results of a European questionnaire during the pilot phase show: of the two thirds of Slovenian pilot schools that responded all report on *technical support* received (via seminars or evaluation related activities), some also *organizational support*, and a few *moral support* and/or (facilitation of) *financial* support (WHO/EURO 1998).

Overall, the information above supports the assumption put forward earlier that both the Slovenian pilot schools *and* the National Support Center formed an *interorganisational network for the development of Health Promoting Schools* in Slovenia. There are close, *mutual, long term work relations* between National Center and pilot schools and this not only for information or experience *exchange* and (may be mutual) learning but also *joint action*. This means that, at least the Slovenian National Support Center and 'pilot schools' formed - in Alter/Hage-terms - an *exchange network* and to some degree even a *promotional network*.

B) **After the Slovenian network's expansion** (i.e. after the pilot and short transition phase) the national level meetings of National Support Center and pilot schools did continue (at least throughout 1998 - and likely beyond) (Stergar 1998a-d). Unfortunately, from 1999 the regular activity reports of the National Center to the WHO representative (i.e. the main source for *detailed* information for this research project) stopped. The remaining documents, however, indicate that the interactions and relations between National Support Center and pilot schools were continued. Although now the *regional* Institutes of Public Health were nominated partners of the pilot schools in their new role as regional HPS centers 'of excellence and training', pilot schools asked the *National* Support Center to continue its work in several areas (e.g. training).

These findings show that with the Slovenian Network's expansion the pilot schools in their new role as regional centers for 'Health Promotion within the school setting' were expected to cooperate and receive support by the *regional* Institutes of Public Health (by then formally responsible to support Health Promoting Schools). The information available gives the impression that the National Center expected that sooner or later pilot schools, supported by the regional Institutes of Public Health, would take over at least part of its tasks - but with a regional focus. How far this changed the interactions and relations between the National Support Center (i.e. the *national* Institute of Public Health) and the pilot schools remains an open question. At least during the first year of the expanded Slovenian network schools *continued* their regular national meetings and the National Center continued supportive actions.

2. National Support Center and local 'non-school' actors

With view to the Slovenian Network's goals indications of *regular* interactions between the National HPS Support Center and **local organizations** other than schools have not been found. However, the National Center did have contact to all *'school doctor's teams'* in the local health care services at particular points in time. At the network's inception, they received general information and were invited to support 'their' schools in their decision for or against network membership application (see fig 5.5.2). Then those in communities of the network schools were encouraged to become active members of these schools' 'HPS project teams'. And they were invited to participate in some of the HPS related training courses of the network. However, it were the pilot schools and not the National Center that had the direct links to the local (school) health care services.

The 'national - regional' dimension

3. National Support Center and actors at regional level

A) During the pilot years of the Slovenian Network (for the development) of Health Promoting Schools no network specific regional actors appeared. However, there was a link between the *regional* Institutes of Public Health and the *national* Institute (i.e. the National HPS Support Center): The health education focal points of the former met routinely with the Health Education Department of the latter; and the Director of the latter was the nominated National Coordinator of the Slovenian network project. From the start the National Center used this constellation to keep the regional Institutes of Public Health informed about developments related to the Health Promoting Schools and the Slovenian Network. Already for the pilot school selection process they were invited to play a role and advise schools as to their network membership application (fig. 5.5.2). And early on they were also invited to attend (some of the) national network meetings of National Center and pilot schools (Stergar 2001). But during the pilot phase regional Institutes had no explicit mandate to engage in the Slovenian network or overall Health Promoting Schools (HPS) development and did not get much involved. Their focus on health education (a core element of the HPS concept) was, of course, an indirect link.

B) By the time that the **Slovenian network** was **expanded** from 12 to 132 health promoting schools (HPS), the situation had changed. The support of HPS development was now formally integrated into the national public health goals and objectives and the work plans of both national *and* regional Institutes of Public Health (Stergar 2001) - a decision in which the National HPS Support Center or national Institute of Public Health will have played a role. The National Center and the network as a whole now expected *regional Institutes to support the pilot schools in their new roles* as regional HPS centers *'of excellence and training'* (e.g. in organizing meetings with the new network schools in their region, or - in Hastings' terms - in creating 'soft networking' opportunities at regional level).

Overall, the information available on the development of the Slovenian Network of Health Promoting Schools gives the impression that the National Support Center would have liked to see the regional Institutes of Public Health earlier and stronger involved into the large scale development of Health Promoting Schools in Slovenia than realized. It seems that the regional Institutes need(ed) more time, motivation (and may be even technical support) than desired to grow into this role. The (for traditional systems) somewhat radical decision taken early on to from the start build up the *pilot schools* (not e.g. the regional Public Health Institutes) as future key actors for regional HPS (network) development, may have had a restraining influence, too. In Slovenia, staff of pilot schools (after four, five years of HPS work in a national network context and intense training) were indeed ahead of the regional Institutes as to implementing the Health Promoting Schools concept. This, of course matched fully with the vision laid out by the European Network initiators of a Europe-wide network *'of'* Health Promoting Schools.

The 'national - national' dimension (within and across borders)

4. National Support Center and the State level

The mechanism of an intersectoral 'national HPS project' was used by the Slovenian **Ministries of 'Education and Sports' and of 'Health'** to initiate, guide and support the development of (the European) network of Health Promoting Schools in the country. In this context the 'National Support Center' *was set up* by the initiating Ministry of Health, in coordination with the Ministry of Education. Throughout, the National Support Center was *accountable to both Ministries* (and other Board members) but mainly *financially dependent on the Health Ministry* (and may be politically, too), because: a) the National Center was the national Institute of Public Health, the National HPS Coordinator a high level staff member therein, and additional staff was financed by the Health Ministry; and b) with the **National Advisory Board** an intersectoral decision making body was in place. With regard to the *Education Ministry*, the National Support Center on the one hand, had a *mediating role between network schools and their Ministry* (negotiation of financial support for schools). On the other hand, the National Center itself *depended* on it *as to one core task*, the provision of the training program (each course needed Ministerial approval and detailed documentation so that participating schools would receive financial support and credits). However, at the same time the National Center was a *member of the National Advisory Board* and, thus, had influence on the national level decisions made. And the National Support Center had *direct links to each Ministry* individually and this at highest (State Secretary) level.

5. National Support Center and other (national) organizations or networks in Slovenia

As discussed above, national or nationally relevant actors were brought together in the National Advisory Board. This was the main mechanism for the National Support Center's systematic cooperation with other key actors in the country. Other *regular* or outstanding interorganisational relations with national level organizations have not been found. However, the National Support Center actively *reached out and tried to influence the network's organizational environment beyond* National Board members: It frequently participated in national events of important national organizations (of preventive medicine, school principles, teachers etc.). At least at times it worked strategically with Slovenia's mass media (e.g. in times of network school selection). It also actively contributed to key developmental steps of the Slovenian field of Health promotion as a whole, notably the first Parliamentarian 'Health Day' (1998), and its activities did not stop at national or European Network borders. - Two years after the first expansion of the Slovenian Network the ENHPS proposed that the National Center should link up *further* and plan ahead with influential educational organizations, i.e. with organizations in the Network's *environment,* in order to speed up progress towards nationwide HPS development.

6. National Support Center and actors in other ENHPS member countries

Beyond the contacts within the European Network as a *whole* (see below) one specific bi-lateral link emerged: After the expansion (or pilot phase) of the Slovenian Network the National Coordinators of Slovenia and Wales, UK met and planned some kind of 'twinning arrangement' in the area of HPS development (NSC 2000a, Rivett 2000) but how far this has been realized remains an open question.

The 'national-international' dimension

7. National Support Center and the "European Network of Health Promoting Schools" (ENHPS)

As to the *European Network as a whole*, the National Center regularly participated in the *ENHPS business meetings* (the main 'soft networking' opportunity of the European Network), repeatedly contributed to ENHPS newsletters and publications and responded to questionnaires. In sum, it quite actively *shared and exchanged* information and experience with all ENHPS members and beyond. National Center staff participated in the series of ENHPS training seminars offered during the pilot years. From the national perspective this shows an 'outward orientation' of the National Center, from the European Network's perspective an orientation towards 'lateral links' (or in Hastings' terms 'networking within') as expected of all ENHPS members. In addition to these *exchange relations* and encounters for (mutual) learning, the National Center worked closely with the ENHPS Technical Secretariat and some other ENHPS members to *jointly produce* ENHPS products or services: It engaged in the pilot testing and refinement of the ENHPS training manual on mental and emotional health and the preparations of general program components of the First ENHPS Conference (chap. 5.1). Overall, the National Center was in regular contact and close collaboration with the ENHPS Secretariat and responsive to the technical guidance offered - which was likely supported by a stronger general presence of WHO in the country at the time (due to ongoing societal and health sector reforms).

8. The National Support Center and the Slovenian network as a whole

Particularly during the first four years and with regard to the 'pilot' schools, the National Support Center (or national Institute of Public Health) provided essential *technical guidance* and support. From early on, the National Center generally identified with the idea of the *European* 'Network'. With view to the developments within the country it took some time until the term *'national HPS project'* was complemented and almost replaced by the term *'Slovenian network* of Health Promoting Schools'. the Center's full identification with the latter is indicated by its publishing the network newsletter under the network's *and* its own name. Throughout the years the National Support Center was the main **orchestrator of networking *'within'*** the network: on the one hand, by organizing and taking part in the *national meetings* with *pilot* schools (although over time pilot schools started to host these meetings, too); on the other hand, by starting to prepare the *'National Conference(s)* of the Slovenian Network of Health Promoting Schools' once the network had been expanded beyond pilot schools (in 1998). However, **after the network's expansion** the situation as to the 'soft networking within' the network changed: In their new roles as regional HPS centers the **pilot schools stepped into a role similar to that of the National Support Center** but each with a regional rather national focus. From a network research perspective, this move planted the seed for a prospective sub-differentiation of the Slovenian network into *sub*-national networks *'of'* Health Promoting Schools. Unfortunately, by 2001 regional developments were not yet documented to allow a further analysis.

The National Support Center was the network's major **link to external others** but within some limits: First, *local* actors were generally to be involved by network schools directly. Second, after the network's expansion each pilot school as new regional HPS center stepped into direct interorganisational relations with 'their' regional Public Health Institute; but the National Center remained the main link between the Slovenian network as a *whole* and *all regional Institutes*. As said above it seems that at least for the first years of the expanded network the latter remained *external supporters* of the Slovenian Network rather than members, but nevertheless might become integral parts in the future.

National Support Center, other actors and network borders - intermediate discussion

In light of the above, some assumptions made as to the Slovenian network's borders can be followed up further. The two Ministries (Education and Health) individually can be clearly defined as *external* to the Slovenian Network (for the development) of Health Promoting Schools. From the start, they were key funding agencies for the network initiative. They directly influenced and were a powerful part of the network's closer institutional environment (the public health and education sectors) and as such they set the cornerstones of the framework in which the 'ENHPS in Slovenia' operated and thrived. They placed themselves as key actors within the *'national HPS project'*. As creators and part of the multi-organizational 'National Advisory Board' for this *project* they directly involved and communicated *with 'other'* nationally relevant actors in the network's environment as well as the *National Support Center* itself. But neither the Ministries nor the National Advisory Board as a whole did strive to engage in direct and reciprocal relations with the core group of the Slovenian Network, the network schools. This was left to the National Support Center.

The regularly meeting National Advisory Board might have been an interorganisational network in itself, for monitoring and guiding the overall HPS related development in Slovenia. But as the Ministries it is *external* to the Slovenian Network (for the development) of Health Promoting Schools (HPS) if one uses not only a common goal (HPS creation) but also direct, reciprocal and lateral links and relations among actors as indicators for network membership. A question emerging is whether there are *two separate but interlinked interorganisational networks* for large scale development of Health Promoting Schools in Slovenia: first, the so called *"Slovenian Network of Health Promoting Schools"*, an interorganisational network that as argued before is - through the involvement of the National Center - rather a network 'for the development' of Health Promoting Schools and not a pure network 'of' such schools. Second, the so called *'National Advisory Board'* of the 'national HPS project' is *potentially a network, too* - one of mainly national level actors that are financially, politically and/or strategically important, met twice a year, and apparently shared the goal of supporting and/or guiding the sustainable development of Health Promoting Schools in Slovenia within the framework of the European Network. No matter whether this assumption of the Board as an interorganisational 'network' holds or not: those involved can be reasonably seen as *participants* of the 'Slovenian HPS *project*' rather than members of the "Slovenian Network of Health Promoting Schools" that evolved out of their efforts. Both interorganisational systems spanned health and education sector as well as were *linked* with each other (via the membership of the National Support Center in both). And the second system, the National Advisory Board, formed and shaped the closer environment of the first.

In sum, it is reasonable to define not only the 'pilot schools' but also the *National HPS Support Center as organizational 'member'* of the Slovenian Network 'for the development' of Health Promoting Schools, and the *national Ministries as key participants in the national 'HPS project'* but not the network. **So far, the Slovenian case supports results of the European case study** (chap. 5.2): There are at least *two types of members of the so called "European Network* of Health Promoting Schools" (ENHPS), National Support Centers and Health Promoting Schools, - at least during the pilot years. The overall *ENHPS 'project'* can then be understood as being in a supportive and guiding role towards the European Network and as *encompassing not only international but also national level actors* (i.e. the intergovernmental organizations WHO, EU and CE and the national Ministries of Education and of Health). However, the examination of the various interorganisational relations of the National HPS Center needs yet to be complemented by that of the Slovenian *network schools*.

II. Interactions and relations among health promoting 'pilot' schools and between those and other organizations

The 'search scheme' shown in table 5.5.3 has been used to both derive information from the sources listed at the beginning of this chapter and present the interactions and relations of the ENHPS pilot schools in Slovenia with other organizations. As explained in chapter 4.2, within the

European Network the 'local - *international* dimension is not relevant as schools may have direct *cross-border* contacts with *schools* or may be *national* actors abroad but hardly ever with actors at European level such as the ENHPS Technical Secretariat.

THE 'PILOT' SCHOOLS' interactions and relations with:	organizations within the country ↓		organizations out-side the country/ the European Dimension ↓
'local – local' →	1a. other HPS: • other 'pilot' schools* • other 'network' schools • other schools	2. local organiza-tions in their com-munity • medical health care • others	1b. schools outside the country • other ENHPS schools/ HPS • others (via other int. networks/ programs)
'local - regional' →	3. regional actors • Regional Institutes of Public Health • 'regional centers of excellence and training' as to HPS*		
'local - national' →	4. national actors • National Support Center/ National Institute of Public Health • National Advisory Board • MoE and MoH		
'the part & the whole' →	5. the Slovenian network as a whole 6. the 'European Network/ ENHPS' as a whole		

ENHPS: European Network of Health Promoting Schools
HPS: Health Promoting Schools
MoE: Ministry of Education
MoH: Ministry of Health
* Note: after network expansion 'pilot' schools served as 'regional centers' for HPS development

Table 5.5.3: Schema of potential interorganisational relationships of the 'pilot' schools in Slovenia with other key organizations within and around the Slovenian network (for the development) of Health Promoting Schools (or the ENHPS in Slovenia)

Descriptions of the Slovenian **pilot schools' roles and responsibilities** became differentiated over time. When entering the 'European Network of Health Promoting Schools' (ENHPS) in Slovenia the ENHPS pilot schools committed themselves to *work towards the set of 12 criteria of a 'Health Promoting School'* (HPS) defined by the European Network which were somewhat adapted over time. From an interorganisational research perspective and as explained in chapter 5.5.1 above, the vast majority of these criteria are phrased in terms of school-*internal* development and 'soft' networking but also include one on *inter*-organizational relations (oriented towards a school's *local* community). However, reports also indicate that in addition, the Slovenian pilot schools *from early on* were expected and being prepared to serve as *example for other* schools and - after the pilot years - started to play an active role in disseminating the HPS concept in their *region*, i.e. in interorganisational or inter-school cooperation. Later on, this was captured in the pilot schools' role as *'regional centers of excellence and training'* in Health Promotion within the school setting - directed at supporting 'new' network schools in their region.

The 'local - local' dimension (from neighborhood to neighbor countries)

1. Slovenian 'pilot' schools among each other, and with other schools

The interorganisational relations of health promoting **pilot schools among each other** have in parts already been clarified in section I above on 'National Support Center/pilot school'-relations. - A) During **the network's pilot years** and beyond, the 12 pilot schools through their HPS project leaders met regularly over five years or more. From the start they *exchanged* experiences and worked jointly on HPS issues that concerned them all, particularly process evaluation and planning of 'HPS programs'. Also they *jointly acted on 'school overarching' issues* that addressed the network as a whole rather than particular interests of individual pilot schools (such as the Network's expansion). The pilot schools indeed perceived themselves as *cooperating* with each other as a European survey during the pilot phase has show (WHO/EURO 1998): Two thirds of Slovenian pilot schools responded and *all* of them reported to undertake activities at national level categorized as 'meetings', 'cooperation between schools' and 'teaching materials'. This shows an equally spread networking *'within'* the Slovenian network. While most activities identified as 'successful' and 'or carried out with difficulties' referred to school internal activities, at least three of the 12 pilot schools mentioned also issues related to interorganisational relations (e.g. as to their local community, or successful cooperation with other schools). - The schools also confirmed that in-service training was systematically received by all staff involved in the 'HPS project' of each school; this supports the assumption made earlier that besides national meetings also training courses were opportunities for 'soft' networking *'within'* the Slovenian network.

B) The information available shows that towards the end of the Slovenian Network's pilot phase and throughout the **transition phase** that led into the **Network's expansion** by 1998, the *networking among pilot schools* and with the National Center continued - with an increasing focus on common objectives beyond the interests of individual pilot schools such as the preparation of a planned approach to the Network's expansion. Although from the second year of the expanded Slovenian Network, documentation (in English) is rare it is assumed that the networking among pilot schools and with the National Center did continue as during the first year: because on the one hand, the former did ask the latter to continue its support and on the other, a lack of indications of any strategy or policy change in this regard.

Overall, the information above supports the presumption expressed before that the Slovenian pilot schools form an 'interorganisational *network*' as introduced in chapter 2.4. Over years they met regularly face to face, exchanged knowledge and undertook joint action related to a common goal, and early on perceived themselves as *'cooperating'*. This indicates that pilot schools engaged - in Alter/Hage-terms - not only in an *exchange* network but also a *'promotional' joint action* network. It also shows that their foci in organizational networking as defined by Hastings were both networking 'within' *and* 'with others', with a strong 'soft' networking component.

As to the pilot schools' **links with schools outside the Slovenian network** it is interesting that most pilot schools were not only members of the Slovenian network on Health Promoting Schools (HPS) but also *other* networks or programs (e.g. on peace or cancer); in three cases this referred to another health promoting Settings network (Healthy Cities). With view to HPS development, *all* ENHPS pilot schools in Europe were expected to become models of good practice to motivate other schools to implement the Health Promoting Schools (HPS) concept, too. The Slovenian pilot schools were *involved in defining new selection criteria for the expansion of the Slovenian network* (or the first wave of 'new' network schools to come) which shows their orientation towards networking *'with others'*. Within the expanded network they started to serve as *'regional* HPS centers' to support 'new' network schools (see below).

Within the National Center's activity reports **school-to-school relations beyond national borders** were hardly an issue but some hints have been found (e.g. participation of *several* pilot schools in an international 'life style campus' in another ENHPS country) (Stergar 1995a-d). The ENHPS survey *during the pilot phase* provides some insight from the pilot schools' perspective: Five of the eight Slovenian pilot schools that responded (i.e. at least 40% of *all* twelve pilot schools) undertook activities with an international or 'European dimension' which in all cases included interorganisational collaboration: *'twinning' with another school* in Europe was established or on its way in at least three cases, the *exchange of pupils and/or teachers* in at least four, and the *exchange of teaching materials* in at least three (WHO/EURO1998). Whether the 'other' schools abroad linked up with were also 'Health Promoting Schools' remains an open question.

From the international perspective it is interesting that about a third of the Slovenian pilot schools, i.e. schools that started their HPS activities *explicitly* as part of the *'European Network of Health Promoting Schools'* (ENHPS), soon did show activities *across* national borders: in the form of some kind of interorganisational *exchange* and/or in school *twinning*. Should the Slovenian pilot schools have linked up with other 'Health Promoting Schools', the seeds for the development of *exchange networks* at *school* level within the European Network would have been planted, i.e. in Alter/Hage-terms the first evolutionary step towards systemic interorganisational networks (chap. 2.4).

Unfortunately, in 2001 interactions and relations among the 120 **'new' network schools** in Slovenia's expanded "Network of Health Promoting Schools" and of those with the pilot schools and others were not yet documented. The information available indicates that school-to-school networking was foreseen to be more frequent or intense within each *region* but without giving up the idea of a *nationwide* network which presented itself visibly with its First Conference in 1998.

2. Pilot schools and other organizations in their local community

The activity reports of the National Center don't address this issue but results of the ENHPS survey during the pilot phase (response rate Slovenia: 66%) resulted in portrays of Slovenian Health Promoting Schools that provide the following picture (WHO/EURO 1998): The *motives* of most pilot schools to join the network were health and/or educational improvements *within* their schools rather than improvements within their local community or links with other schools. Accordingly, *activities at local level* usually concerned the groups of the school community (pupils, staff, parents) rather than other local organizations. Nevertheless, pilot schools had *interorganisational relations* with non-school organizations locally, with health care services and others. The composition of the network schools' 'HPS project teams' (in the ENHPS school data base addressed as 'supporting teams') usually reflect at least one case of interorganisational relations, the link to the **medical health service** which in Slovenia is understood as an *integral part* of the country's overall '*HPS project*'. This is supported in two ways: a) that health care services are obliged by law to collaborate with other institutions including schools and this is being monitored (SLNHPS 1995); b) that implementing the 'Health Promoting School' concept inherently expects all network schools to develop links to local institutions. Early on, local health care services had been *invited* to get actively involved into the Slovenian large scale effort to develop Health Promoting Schools: as advisors at the point of *pilot school selection* (fig. 5.5.2 above) and via participation in selected training courses for the HPS teams of network schools. Indeed, all of the eight pilot schools that responded to the survey (i.e. *at least two thirds of all* Slovenian pilot schools) indicated to have interorganisational relations to local medical health services to various degrees. However, in three cases this was limited to the sole provision of obligatory medical services (routine check ups etc.). But in five cases, i.e. for at least 40% of *all* pilot schools, involvement went beyond this routine (from providing lectures to participating in training seminars or even regular round tables on health). At least half of all pilot schools saw medical staff among those from whom '*support*' was received but the National Support Center and *non-medical local* actors were listed more often.

From **other local organizations** at least two thirds of Slovenian pilot schools said to receive 'support'. *At least six (or 50%) of all Slovenian pilot schools had interorganisational relationships of some kind*, particularly with public agencies (e.g. social work, firemen) but also with local NGOs or initiatives (e.g. sports, scouts, addiction prevention). Type and content of contacts varied (from participation in activities and lecturing to information dissemination and financing) which may or may not have been 'one off' events. - The ENHPS survey did show that most (if not all) of the Slovenian pilot schools did strive to 'impact' on their *school* community and internal processes rather than their *local* community or environment. Only one pilot school explicitly stated to a) strive for '*impact*' *on both* the whole school community and other organizations (schools, local shops, nursery schools), and b) to have made already 'great impact' on other schools in the town and region. At this school worked one of the two Slovenian "peer teachers" of the national HPS project.

With view to organizational networking (as explained in chapter 2.4) the above findings suggests: During the Slovenian network's pilot years the pilot schools were much oriented towards networking 'within' the school and school development rather than networking 'with *local* others'. They were, however, oriented towards networking 'with other *network members*' which were spread throughout the country. As to the Slovenian network's borders the earlier assumption seems to hold: that the pilot schools' *local partner organizations including medical health services can be reasonably defined as 'supporters' of and 'external' to the Slovenian network* (for the development) of Health Promoting Schools rather than network members for several reasons: a) No *type* of *local* organization has been reported to be in far reaching and frequent or ongoing cooperation with *several* or even all pilot schools in support of their joint goal of transforming themselves into 'Health Promoting Schools' (HPS); b) *overall* the contributions of the medical care services remained focused on medical prevention services and/or punctual other contributions (e.g. lectures) - without indications that they worked directly with and as part of the Slovenian network as a *whole*. But the evaluation at the end of the pilot years did show most school doctor's teams supported the further dissemination of the HPS concept to other schools in the country and, thus, the core network goal. - After this examination of the pilot schools' interactions and relations with other *local level* organizations those with *regional* level actors will be addressed.

The 'local - regional' dimension

3. Pilot schools, other network schools and actors at regional level

As to the relation of school and regional level actors the Slovenian Network shows an interesting development. After the pilot phase *some network schools* became also declared *regional* actors and this at a time when *another* group of regional actors, the regional Institutes of Public Health, entered the stage, too.

A) **During the network's pilot years** the 12 pilot schools were the only network schools and these networked with the *National* Support Center/ *national* Institute of Public Health rather than any regional level actor. The *regional* Institutes of Public Health and the pilot schools did know from each other as both met regularly but separately with the national Institute. While the latter worked with the *pilot schools* on the large scale implementation of the Health Promoting Schools (HPS) concept it worked with the *regional Institutes* on health education matters, i.e. on a *component* of the HPS concept. As such the regional Institutes were a more or less indirect actor of the Slovenian HPS initiative.

B) Direct relations or interactions of pilot schools and the *regional* Institutes of Public Health began **with the Slovenian network's expansion**, when the pilot *schools* took over their new functions as '*regional centers* of excellence and training' for Health Promotion in the school setting. Thus, pilot schools as *regional* actors started to cooperate with the *regional* Institutes - in support of the 'new' network schools in their region. By this time the support of HPS development had been newly incorporated into the regular tasks of these regional Institutes (i.e. their 'health education coordinators'). The latter were meant to support the pilot schools in their new function as regional HPS centers. However, as this was not equally realized in all regions some pilot schools/regional HPS centers continued to work mainly with the *National* Support Center (Stergar 2001).

These findings show that with the Slovenian network's expansion and the emergence of *two* regional level actors directly or indirectly focusing on the 'new' network schools *in their region* the Slovenian network did a first step towards its sub-differentiation by region. The ground was prepared for the emergence of *regional sub-networks* "of" Health Promoting Schools (HPS) consisting of one pilot school (and regional HPS center) and a number of new network schools, but eventually also of the regional Institute of Public Health. However, as to the *country-wide network* for the development of Health Promoting Schools (HPS) it remains an open question whether after its expansion also the regional Institutes of Public Health may need to be considered as network members (as done for the national Institute as National HPS Support Center). Judging from the first year of the expanded network it were the *pilot schools* or now *'regional centers of excellence and training'* that continued to regularly meet at national level; the regional Institutes did not join this circle. As now declared 'supporters' of the pilot school (or regional HPS center) in their region they are surely core actors in the Slovenian network's closer *environment* but clear indications of their *membership* therein have *not* been found. During the first years of the expanded Slovenian network not all of them were able to 'support' the pilot school in their region as expected and needed; and their meetings at national level remained separate of those of the National Support Center and pilot schools as core network members. Regional Institutes are, however, candidates for network membership of *regional* sub-networks should these evolve. Therefore, the earlier assumption that *regional* Institutes of Public Health are *'external supporters'* of the network rather than network members is kept up for now - while recognizing that this could well change over time.

The 'local - national' dimension

4. Network schools and national level actors

The interactions and relation between *pilot* schools and the **National Support Center** have been already addressed in section I above. Less addressed have been those of the *'new'* network schools with the National Center that joined the network at the point of its first expansion. Their main contact point became the pilot school in their region as well as the regional Institute of Public Health rather than the National Support Center. It can be assumed that most of them had hardly any contact with the National Center outside the (sporadic?) national Network Conferences organized by the latter.

Interactions and relations of pilot schools or other network schools with the **National Advisory Board and the Ministries of 'Health' and of 'Education** and Sports' have not been identified for the two former actors, and with regard to the Education Ministry only as far as financing proposals for particular HPS activities at school level were concerned. However, as said before the National Support Center acted here as negotiator and mediator. *Direct* interactions between network schools and the national Ministries and Advisory Board did not exist. However, there *were* interorganisational relations between schools and Education Ministry *beyond* those deriving from a school's being part of the education sector. From the start, *network schools were directly dependent on the Education Ministry* as far as their HPS-specific activities were concerned. This applied particularly to the 'pilot' schools which received some essential hours teaching reduction per team. But also the 'new' network schools were to a certain degree dependent on this Ministry - because *all* training courses of the network needed its approval as a key to financial support of participants.

As to schools' relations to **'other' national actors** it is known that a few pilot schools are a member of another national network, too, the Healthy Cities Network (WHO/EURO 1998).

"The parts and the whole"

5. Network schools and the Slovenian network as a whole

The evaluation of the Slovenian network's pilot phase hardly addressed this issue but focused on activities *within* the individual network schools. It did, however, show that **pilot schools** were receptive as to inputs or ideas transmitted via the network's core activity, 'in-service training': The number of health promoting activities was increasing particularly after training seminars; knowledge transfer was more visible where more members of the school team attended; and the priority theme 'mental and emotional health' ranked third among the 13 topic categories identified (Stergar, bevc Stankovic 1998). The ENHPS survey during the pilot phase provides additional insights (WHO/EURO 1998): Two thirds of the pilot schools if not all were involved in overall *network activities* (national meetings, school-to-school cooperation, etc.) and *felt supported* from *within* the network (National Center) and *also* by external others locally. Their *identification as members of a 'Slovenian network'* had first to emerge which is no surprise, because also the national actors first referred mainly to the 'national HPS project' or 'European Network'; but pilot schools did truly and increasingly act as key *members* of the *country-wide Slovenian network* (for the development of) Health Promoting Schools, most strongly expressed by their taking over the role as 'regional centers of excellence and training' for the 'new' schools that entered their network later.

Those **'new' schools** that joined the Slovenian network at the point of its first expansion, were from the start declared members of the then soon formally launched *"Slovenian Network"* (rather a 'national project'). In-spite of an emerging *regional* focus within this network the identity as *Slovenian* Network member was likely maintained: the organization of the '*First* Conference of the *Slovenian* Network of Health Promoting Schools' indicates that all network schools will be encouraged and supported by the National Support Center to engage in 'soft' networking across the country.

6. Network schools and the 'European Network of Health Promoting Schools' (ENHPS) as a whole

Obviously, within this case study on the European Network and its taking shape in selected countries this point addresses a core question: Did or does the plan of the European Network's initiators to create a *European* network *of* Health Promoting Schools work out? For the ENHPS in Slovenian the following picture has emerged:

Several indications have been found for a *high awareness* within the group of **pilot schools** as to being part of the *European* Network: a) at the time of pilot school recruitment schools were invited to apply for membership in the European (rather than a Slovenian) network; b) during the pilot years five out of eight Slovenian pilot schools explicitly identified themselves as ENHPS members, with two pointing to ENHPS membership *only* (all others to 'national HPS project' participation, too); c) all pilot schools received international HPS certificates and some even visits from ENHPS representatives; one was invited to present itself internationally; and the Slovenian Network as a whole publicly received a WHO award. As shown above (point 1) at least 40% of Slovenian pilot schools already during the pilot years did translate their 'European' awareness into *school-to-school (exchange) relations across national borders*. - However, this may or may not be the case for the many **'new' network schools** that entered explicitly the "*Slovenian* Network of Health promoting Schools". Although the Network's link to the European Network will have been communicated it would not be a surprise if the 'new' schools would have less of an awareness as *European Network* members: in contrast to the 'pilot' schools, the 'new' schools were from the start directed towards interorganisational links within their *region*, i.e. at *sub*-national and not national level.

III. Interactions and relations of the new 'regional centers of excellence and training' for Health Promotion within the school setting

As shown above, establishing the pilot schools as new 'regional centers of excellence and training' **within the expanded Slovenian Network** (for the development) of Health Promoting Schools, did move the *regional level more into the foreground of overall network development*. The interactions or relations between these new 'regional centers' and the National Support Center as well as the 'regional Institutes of Public Health' have been addressed in sections I and II above. The regular meetings of National Center and pilot schools - now in their new regional functions - continued (as documented until 1999); but for the 'new' network schools the pilot schools as 'regional HPS centers' rather than the National Center were the *direct* contact points and network partners. Each pilot school/'regional HPS center' was now to be supported by the *regional* Institute of Public Health in their region rather than the national Institute; but this was realized only to various degrees and the national Institute served as 'back up' where needed and possible. From an organizational networking perspective and with view to the Slovenian Network as a whole, pilot schools as 'regional HPS centers' remained oriented towards 'networking within' the net; but they started to be outwards oriented, too, by cooperating with the regional Institutes of Public Health as network supporters.

The overall documentation gives the impression that pilot schools as 'regional HPS centers' and established core network members - in combination with the regional Institutes - were meant to take over the direct work with network schools that before was undertaken by the National Support Center itself. This started to allow the latter to focus more on supra-regional issues such as 'soft' networking *'within'* the Slovenian Network as a *whole* (e.g. the 'First Conference' of the Slovenian Network). While the pilot schools as 'Health Promoting Schools' remained committed to the idea and goals of the *European* Network, and that of the Slovenian Network, in their function as 'regional HPS centers' their tasks were directed towards their *region* only. With view to the Slovenian *regions* they were truly in a *central* role; but with view to the Slovenian network as a *whole* they remained one of the network schools - which systematically and actively shared their special knowledge and experience with others. Thus, it depends mainly on the pilot schools and National Support Center whether the Slovenian Network - while starting to shape up in regional sub-clusters or even networks - remains nevertheless *one* country-wide interorganisational network rather than falling apart.

IV.	The Slovenian network for the development of Health Promoting Schools and the "European Network of Health Promoting Schools" (ENHPS)

'The part and the whole'

As the name suggests the "Slovenian Network of Health Promoting Schools" explicitly followed the idea and guidance of the "European Network of Health Promoting Schools" (ENHPS). Overall it has rightly been called the 'ENHPS in Slovenia' - with pilot schools explicitly invited to join the *European* Network, the European HPS criteria as well as intersectoral mechanisms proposed explicitly being implemented, and so forth. Also the (fairly unspecified) idea of a network approach put forward at European level was taken as the orienting framework for the Slovenian network; the challenging idea of creating a network '*of*' Health Promoting Schools was taken seriously when experienced (pilot) schools rather than other organizations were asked and prepared to move into regional leadership roles. The Slovenian Network (via its National Center but also pilot schools) played an active role within the European Network in various ways (from information *sharing* to joint training manual *production*). Unfortunately, during the first years it was among those ENHPS member countries that for political reasons (lack of EU membership) were excluded from the European Network's evaluation project called 'EVA'. However, the Slovenian Network did receive much recognition from the European level for its work and progress. At times it was used as international 'model' (such as in a high level meeting of strategic importance for the European Network as a whole).

As elaborated in chapter 4, now that the interactions and relations of the various actors within and around the Slovenian network for the development of Health Promoting Schools (HPS) have been analyzed the way is paved for the next step of this ENHPS country case study: for the 'synthesizing analysis I' of the network's *structures and processes* on the base of the clarification of network membership.

5.6 Synthesizing analysis I - structural and process features of the Slovenian Network

As of now the Slovenian Network (for the development) of Health Promoting Schools (HPS) has undertaken one major evaluation effort, towards the end of its first or *pilot phase*. Similar to those of the time at European level (e.g. EVA) and in other ENHPS countries (such as Germany) this focused on the implementation of the 'Health Promoting Schools' concept *within network schools* and thus, mainly on issues of *internal* developments of schools or school communities. *Interorganisational* relations or networking among and of network members were generally hardly an issue - with the exception of minimal approaches to explore the network schools' contacts with 'others' in their local communities. For this research project only those results of evaluations or analyses have been selected that relate to the network's *interorganisational network* dimension (which as in the European and German cases leaves out most of the evaluation results from its pilot years). However, as shown in the previous chapter on interactions, roles and responsibilities of key actors, the regular progress reports have laid the ground for a synthesizing analysis of the Slovenian network's core features in terms of those identified in the assessment framework for interorganisational networks (IONs) developed in chapter 3. As in the other two network case studies (and explained in chap. 4 above) for now, *selected elements* of the ION assessment framework are in focus: **Yet, the emphasis is on distinct basic features of the network rather than the network as a whole and its Health Promotion dimension** (which are the focus of the final chapter 6). As before, a look back to overview figure 3.1.1 on the ION assessment framework and its partial presentation in figure 4.2.2 helps to keep the 'overall picture' in mind while recalling the selection foci of this analysis: a) membership/ network borders; b) network structure (size/ complexity/ differentiation/ connectivity/ centrality); c) operational processes (methods of coordination); d) purpose of interactions within the network; e) perceived effectiveness/ levels of conflict; f) the network's networking 'with others' and the relation of networking 'within'/'with others'; g) the network's 'hard' networking, means of 'soft' networking, and the 'hard'/'soft'-networking- relation; h) geographical distance among network members; i) (self-)reflection/ observation/ evaluation processes and feed back loops within the network; and j) "organizational networking" of network *schools*. Also the 'satisfaction' of (groups of) network members will be addressed.

5.6.1 Membership or borders of the Slovenian network for the development of Health Promoting Schools

Similar to the European and German network cases, also the Slovenian network membership will be addressed as explained in chapter 4. Matching with defining criteria of interorganizational systems such as being collectives based on trustful relationships, non-or less central, laterally linked, etc. (see chap. 5.2.1) this synthesizing analysis I of the Slovenian network's borders and membership needs to take into account the *quality* of interorganisational *relationships* and not just formal 'membership status' or position (see also chap. 3). This leads to the following interpretative summary:

Not only the formal ENHPS and Slovenian network members, the 'pilot' schools and 'new' network schools, have to be considered as network members but also the 'National Support Center'. The latter also represents Slovenia's 'ENHPS country membership' (see chap. 5.1/ 5.2). With view to the *nationwide* Slovenian network (rather than regional sub-units that may emerge) the regional Institutes of Public Health are still external to the network but core parts of its closest environment. And their status is such that they have the potential to become sooner or later indeed members of the Slovenian *network* for the development of Health Promoting Schools (HPS). Overall, it is useful to distinguish between the core network *members* on the one hand, and network partners or supporters (or a ENHPS 'project' or *closer* network *environment*) on the other. The latter includes actors at all societal levels: from the start the members of the National Advisory Board (the Ministries of Education and of Health included), as well as the local health care services and/or others in local communities of individual network schools; later on, the regional Institutes of Public Health, too.

For about five years this *closer environment of the Slovenian network* did remain fairly stable - with a few less visible or sneaking changes only (such as the expansion of the National Advisory Board and the increasing but rather punctual or indirect involvement of the regional Institutes of Public Health via their work on health education reform. Then *two significant changes* occurred: At the time of the network's expansion the regional Institutes had become mandated supporters. And about two years later, the intersectoral high level decision making body, the National Advisory Board, was not reconfirmed anymore - which left the two Ministries of 'Education and Sports' and of 'Health' as separate individual actors in the network's closest environment. - The whole time, the *types of network members* remained *unchanged*: the selected schools that voluntarily and successfully applied for network membership, and the National Support Center or Institute of Public Health. But the former gained a second role on the way: the 12 pilot schools became 'regional centers of excellence and training' as to Health Promotion in the school setting. - All in all, it can be concluded that **the 'ENHPS in Slovenia' is a network 'for the *development* of' Health Promoting Schools** rather than a pure Network *'of'* Health Promoting Schools as the name suggests - but **with *inherent* strong clusters (and potentially sub-networks) *'of'* Health Promoting Schools**.

Now that the borders of the ENHPS in Slovenia or the 'Slovenian network for the development of Health Promoting Schools' have been clarified, **its membership, closer environment** (and emerging sub-structure) can be illustrated as shown in figure 5.6.1. Apparently, the 'European Network of Health Promoting Schools' and its sub-networks in countries are well conceptualized as *a network systems with a kind of double-border:* a) a first border around the *core,* an "interorganisational network" with clearly identifiable members (usually nominated to play a particular role) that *include* the health-promoting network *schools* and also a national coordinating body; b) a second, more or less permeable border around the network's 'closer supportive environment' (encompassing the National Advisory Board, and other formally or informally bound network 'supporters' such as the regional Institutes of Public Health and potential others).

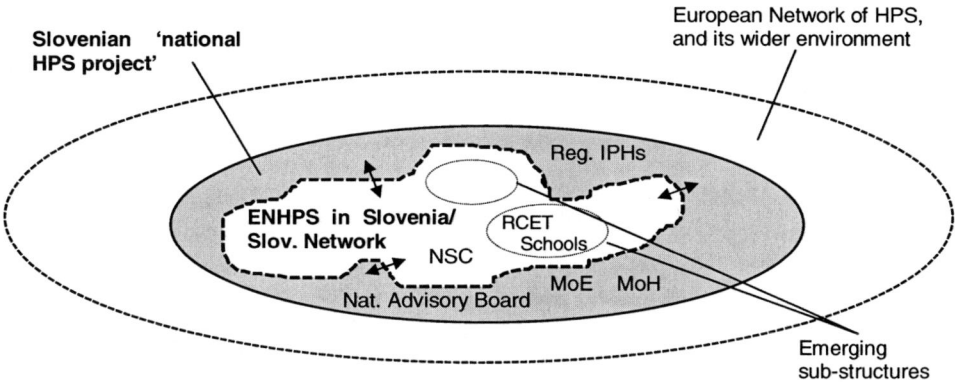

ENHPS: European Network of Health Promoting Schools
HPS: Health Promoting Schools/ network schools
MoE: Ministry of Education and Sports
MoH: Ministry of Health; Nat. National

NSC: National Support Center RCET: pilot schools as 'regional centers of excellence and training' for HPS;
Reg. IPHs: Regional Institutes of Public Health
Slov. Slovenian

Figure 5.6.1: The Slovenian network for the development of Health Promoting Schools: its borders, members, emerging sub-structure, and closer environment.

This conceptual approach benefits not only network assessment efforts but the network itself: It helps to develop and sustain a *network identity* among highly and long term committed core actors and a certain *degree of network stability*, while at the same time offering and *maintaining flexibility* towards all those that wish or are nominated to support the network's goal or specific objectives and this with limited interactions, time span, involvement and/or foci. The differentiation of the 'network' and its *'closer supportive environment'* (e.g. labeled as 'network project') allows to offer also the latter group of actors a network related identity (as e.g. 'network supporter' or participant in the national 'network project'); they become distinguishable from the many others that make up the network's overall wider environment.

5.6.2 The structure of the Slovenian network for the development of Health Promoting Schools

Alter and Hage (1993) identified five features of an interorganisational network's 'structure' (size, complexity, differentiation, connectivity, and centrality) which now, that the membership question regarding the Slovenian network has been answered, can be addressed:

Network size

As to the Slovenian network's 'size', *significant changes occurred* as of now only once - after the first five years of network development (or the ENHPS pilot phase) - and both as to the Slovenian network as a whole and two systems levels. With regard to *school members*, the network did grow at one distinct point in time from nationwide 12 'pilot' schools to 132 network schools. Yet, in light of the decentralizing effect of the pilot schools' new roles as regional HPS centers it remained that always a scale of 10 network schools had one network member as main contact point and direct support provider from within the net (during the pilot years the National Support Center, later the 'regional centers of excellence and training'). With regard to *regional level* network members the number raised from zero to 12 without affecting the total network size (because of the pilot schools' double role as network schools and regional centers). The *national level* remained the same: with the one network member, the National Support Center.

In light of this development the *development of the 'size' of the Slovenian network* may best be looked at as follows: It was first *one smaller, geographically spread network* of 12 members (all but one schools plus the National Center) and then *expanded to one bigger network but with emerging sub-national clustering around selected* (more experienced) *member schools* that are geographically equally spread. Thus, **in terms of "size", the enlargement of the European Network in Slovenia represents an expansion with view to one type of members only, the schools.**

Network complexity

This structural feature of interorganisational networks refers to in Alter/Hage-terms the number of different services, products, sectors etc. represented within the group of network members. The three groups of the Slovenian network's members (schools, regional HPS centers, and National Center) at a first glance do represent a fairly low complexity. Obviously, a *national* Institute of Public *Health* has different capacities and access to other partners, resources, and perspectives than a *school with five years experiences within a network on Health Promoting Schools (HPS)* and prepared to serve as regional HPS center, and the latter others than a school just joining a network on HPS. A closer look shows that the Slovenian network's complexity is yet a little bit higher: Even the 'new' network schools are not a homogenous group but represent primary, secondary and boarding schools, each potentially providing different resources or services to the Slovenian network as a whole. Thus, the network complexity is higher that it first seems to be.

An analysis of network complexity of course should be guided by the common goal of the network, here the creation of Health Promoting Schools on an increasingly large scale. 'Complexity' should be considered in terms of the prevalence of members with resources and experiences of particular relevance to achieve this goal (e.g. as to school development, school/community- or school-to-school-cooperation, in-service training, and particular health related issues prioritized or inherent in Settings work such as school climate, healthy school meals, etc.).

Network differentiation

As to the Slovenian network's differentiation, in Alter/Hage-terms the extent of division of labor or function within the network, the case study has shown that changes occurred over time: During the first years the division of labor followed the line between the two types of network members, National Support Center and pilot schools: The National Center identified and provided *(access to)* HPS related *technical* support and *national and European* resources and actors, engaged in *general* documentation and *evaluation,* and guided and supported the *network's* networking 'within' as well as links with external 'others' beyond the reach of individual schools. In comparison to this, all pilot schools were responsible for *implementing* the Health Promoting Schools (HPS) concept including the *school's* networking 'within' and its linking up with external others *locally, school specific* documentation, and developing and *sharing* of 'good practice' and experiences. Change occurred towards the network's expansion: some (e.g. information and training related) tasks were shifted from the National Center towards the pilot schools as now regional HPS centers, and in parts also towards the regional Institutes of Public Health. *Within* the group of network schools the new schools focused on tasks that the pilot schools had in earlier years. In sum, with the network's expansion the division of labor or *'differentiation' within the Slovenian network increased and changed*, also among organizational members of the same type (here schools).

While the 'network differentiation' of the 'young' Slovenian network followed roughly the line between tasks regarding *organizational development within* schools and *school/community*-links on the one hand (task of schools), and coordination, supportive or other *network related and supra-local tasks* on the other (task of national center), within the expanded (and may be 'maturing') Slovenian network this changed: Pilot schools became regional centers and increasingly responsible for tasks formerly covered by the national center. Overall, particularly as to national and regional HPS centers it appears that the lines were not rigidly or harshly drawn but somewhat flexibly, allowing consideration of particular circumstances in regions.

Network connectivity / a network's 'networking within'

As explained in chapter 4.2, this synthesizing analysis of 'connectivity' as a *structural* network feature is merged with that of the network's dimension of 'networking within' (Hastings), because the latter encompasses the former. The focus is on **'*reciprocal*' contacts (i.e. interactions) and these among '*groups*' of network members** (rather than *all individual* members). As before, 'networking within' is used as the overriding term to present the information available in an integrated and meaningful way to shed light on the network's *structure*. And further issues of quality of the interactions are addressed separately below: under the headings network 'processes' and 'purpose of interactions'.

The *networking 'with other' members of each individual network member* taken together creates the *'networking within' the Slovenian network 'as a whole'*. Similarly to the European and German case studies the aim is to provide **an <u>overall</u> picture of the Slovenian network's 'networking within'** (including connectivity): because the purpose of this case study is the network assessment framework developed in chapter 3 and the structural and process indicators therein (with the Slovenian country case to enlighten the *European* network in focus); and also because of the general lack of specific data in this domain. The *guiding questions* were *a) which of the first two, then three groups of network members (National Center, regional HPS centers, schools) had the mandate to and/or did regularly interact (in pursuit of the common goal) and which not? And b) which changes occurred over time in this regard?* Additional information of relevance was considered, too. When taking into account the roles and responsibilities of network members and reported observations of practice (chap. 5.5.4) the following summary can be given:

Throughout, the one *national*-level network member, the Slovenian **National Support Center** had the task and did network with the other members in the country, but with a significant change: As long as the network was small it networked *directly* with *all* other network members, i.e. the pilot schools. After the network's expansion it continued the networking established but did *not* start to directly network also with all the 'new' network schools. This means from a national perspective and generally spoken that: a) the direct national/school level networking was given up (in favor of regional/school level networking); b) national/*regional* level networking moved into the foreground instead (as pilot schools were now regional HPS centers); but c) without the national level stopping to be in direct touch with the school level (via the pilot schools) (see figure 5.6.2 a). Accordingly, the **network schools'** 'networking within' the Slovenian network changed, too: The first years they networked directly with not only the National Center but among each other across the country; the network's expansion brought about that each network school was mainly to directly link up with a) the regional (instead of national) HPS center and b) other network schools in its region (rather than across the whole country) (fig. 5.6.2 b).

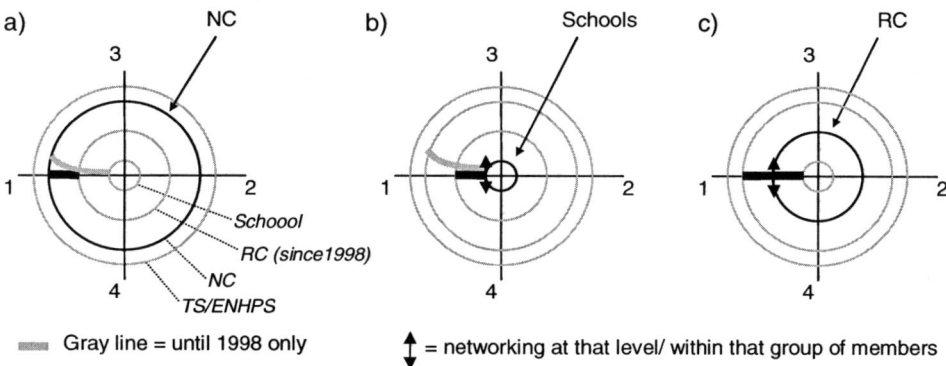

Gray line = until 1998 only   ↕ = networking at that level/ within that group of members

1   = Hastings' organizational networking-dimension 'networking with others'
2,3,4 = the other three dimensions of organizational networking (not of relevance here)
HPS: Health Promoting Schools/ network schools
TS/ENHPS: Technical Secretariat of the "European Network of Health Promoting Schools"
a) NC = National Support Center;
b) Schools = network schools;
c) RC = regional HPS 'centers of excellence and training (i.e. the pilot schools' new role)

Figure 5.6.2:   'Networking within' the ENHPS in Slovenia: who is networking with whom? - Illustration of interorganisational relations or networking *between* and *within* members groups, group by group:

The tasks of each **'regional center of excellence and training'** for

Health Promotion in the school setting (or the regional HPS centers) as to 'networking *within*' the Slovenian network were from their start in 1998: a) geographically bound to its own region; and b) directed at networking with and among the 'new' network schools in that region. The latter refers also to the regional Institutes of Public Health that for now have been defined as network supporters rather than members. However, c) the regional HPS centers also networked at supra-regional level, directly with the National Center and amongst each other (fig. 5.6.2 c).

Obviously, *quantity and quality* of contacts within the Slovenian network for developing Health Promoting Schools (HPS) need further specification. As the term 'networking' - consciously used above - implies, the connectivity within the small Slovenian (pilot) network was clearly meant to be and was **reciprocal**. This applies also to the time after the network's expansion, at least as far as the connectivity among National Center and pilot schools is concerned. The information available does not allow a judgment on connectivity among network members at subnational level, i.e. among pilot and 'new' schools within regions. However, fostering *interaction* among all actors within the network and its closer environment was an aim pointed out as important and acted upon from the start - as indicated by the overall emphasis given to face-to-face meetings and the intermediate valuation of the network's cooperation 'within' and with others as a main strength to build on in the future.

As to the **frequency** of contacts *among National Center and the ensemble of network schools* the two groups of schools need to be distinguished: pilot schools and 'other' or 'new' network schools. The information available refers only to *'soft' networking opportunities* (as opposed to 'hard' networking): As to the pilot schools/regional HPS centers, from the start there were three-monthly national meetings, the annual newsletter, and (during the pilot years) a few training courses per year. As to the other 'new' schools, national level networking was much less frequent: with a start up meeting at the very beginning and the "First Meeting of the Slovenian Network" soon after, but during the next year no networking opportunity of this kind. Meanwhile, National Center and *pilot* schools had quite frequent (e.g. weekly) bi-lateral contacts (at least during the pilot years).

Now, that four out of five the structural network features of interorganisational networks have been addressed (i.e. size, complexity, differentiation and 'networking within' the network or connectivity) the look at network centrality remains.

Network centrality

According to Alter and Hage (1993) this structural feature captures how much in a network the overall 'work' flows through one or a few members which is a question of dominance of one or a few members. The images emerging of the Slovenian network by its two developmental stages are presented in figure 5.6.3.

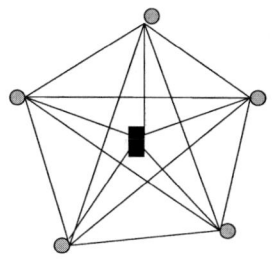
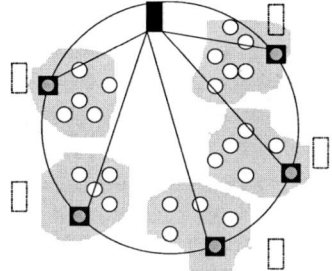

a) The young/ yet small Slovenian network

b) The 'expanded' Slovenian Network

○ network pilot/ 'project' schools (total of 12

■ National Support Center (1) = National Institute of Public Health

▨ Sub-clusters within national network

▣ pilot schools as regional centers of excellence and training (total of 12)

○ 'new' network schools (total of 120)

□ Regional Institutes of Public Health

Figure 5.6.3: The Slovenian network for the development of Health Promoting Schools: Illustration of its 'centrality' during the first (ENHPS pilot) years (from 1993) and after its expansion (from 1998). (This figure should not be misinterpreted as illustrating size or connectivity).

During the first years the network may be well illustrated as a polygon with the National Support Center in a central position but nevertheless links among *all* corners. Towards the network's expansion, with pilot schools getting more involved into a) general networking issues (holding national meetings, member selection, etc.), b) cooperation with regional others (Institutes of Public Health), and c) preparations to serve as 'regional centers', the 'National Support Center' moved somewhat out of the center of the Slovenian Network (fig. 5.6.3 b). However, while the pilot schools become centers of sub-national network units (symbolized with the gray fields) the National Center remains clearly in a central position as to the supra-regional (and in parts also regional) network *environments*. Overall, its inherent dominance has been buffered in self-regulation: by strong commitment to the basic principles and values of Health Promotion and interorganisational networking alike such as working in partnership, participation and continuos self-reflection. This can be reasonably expected at regional network level, too, i.e. as to the pilot schools as 'regional centers'. These had, of course, within the sub-clusters of the expanded Slovenian Network a central position (fig. 5.6.3 b).

This elaboration of the set of structural features of the Slovenian network for the development of Health Promoting Schools indicates that the *structural* network indicators identified in chapter 3 are applicable to this type of network. Before looking at the network as a whole this 'synthesizing analysis I' turns towards network related *process* indicators.

5.6.3 The Slovenian network's 'operational processes' and 'organizational networking'

Operational processes: methods of coordination used

As shown in the two case studies before (chap. 5.2.3 and 5.4.3), the synthesizing analysis of this process feature of interorganisational networks takes much less words than that of the network's structure. Nevertheless, it is equally important. Following Alter and Hage (1993) in focus are the extent of joint decision making and reliance on mutual adjustment and feed back, as well as staff working together interdependently across organizational boundaries. Related methods of coordination - with increasing utilization of feed back - are: a) impersonal methods (e.g. contracts/rules and regulations), b) personal methods (e.g. designation of coordinators/ direct contact among staff) and c) group methods (e.g. face-to-face communication of *several* people planning and taking decisions by consensus) (see chap. 2.4.3). The Slovenian network for the development of Health Promoting Schools (HPS) clearly focused on the latter two: As required of European Network members, within the Slovenian network on Health Promoting Schools *the* personal method of coordination was the **designation of coordinators:** one 'National Coordinator' within the National Support Center, and one 'HPS project manager' or 'leader' as to each network school. In addition, **'group' or team methods of coordination** were applied in various ways: first, *internal* to *member* organizations in the form of a) 'HPS project teams' within schools (an ENHPS requirement), and b) the 'national project team' of the National Support Center; second, as to interorganisational work *across the network* in the form of the regular meetings of National Center and pilot schools, and after network expansion also the intended regional meetings of network members; third, as to the *network/environment-interactions* in form of the National Advisory Board, the 'strategic dissemination and evaluation group' and 'selection committees'. Reports underline that particularly among network members 'team' methods of coordination were indeed realized. National coordinating groups increasingly encompassed also local level network members.

From the start, the Slovenian network did *not* focus on '**impersonal methods of coordination**' but the how and when of entering the network was clearly regulated. Voluntary membership and actions were a ground rule but active work towards implementing the Health Promoting Schools (HPS) concept, too. The principles of participation and orientation towards school specific needs were unwritten 'rules of the game'.

The general purpose of interactions within the Slovenian network

Following the interorganisational network theory by Alter and Hage (obligational/exchange-, promotional/joint action-, and systemic/joint production- networks) this indicator is one of network type and at the same time network evolution or development (see chap. 2.4; fig. 2.4.6; table 2.4.4). Throughout, documentation and activity reports on and by the Slovenian network for the development of Health Promoting Schools (or ENHPS in Slovenia), **exchange** has been repeatedly and consistently referred to as *purpose* of interactions and of choosing a 'network approach' (whether identified as such or not). Up today, *exchange 'within'* the network (but also with others) concerns *ideas, information and experiences* - whether among National Center and pilot schools or among pilot and new schools since network expansion. Particularly as to the latter the exchange of HPS knowledge, materials and training programs have been mentioned, too. (Mutual) learning has been brought up as well. The roles and responsibilities defined and observations reported confirm that the Slovenian network as a whole and the core group of member schools therein were and increasingly explicitly intended to be (part of) an **interorganisational exchange or 'obligational' network,** and this along the lines of the *patterns of connectivity* identified above.

But, the Slovenian network did not remain long at this level of (in Alter/Hage-terms) 'limited cooperation' and limited focus on the needs of *individual* members. In some training courses members developed jointly health education programs for Health Promoting Schools (HPS). The roles and responsibilities of pilot schools reworked towards the network's expansion explicitly stated not only exchange but *development* of HPS and teacher training programs *with* new network schools to come. Already during the first few network years cooperation was increasingly extended to *supra-ordinate* member goals which moved into the foreground for *all* members. Clear examples are the development of a planned approach and common strategy to the network's expansion (jointly with national actors external to the net) and the preparation of pilot schools to become 'regional centers of excellence and training'. Thus, network members undertook **joint action** to achieve functional objectives and soon formed - in Alter/Hage terms - **not only an exchange but 'promo-**

tional' interorganisational network. This conclusion is supported by the - in Alter/Hage-terms - 'rather quasi-formal' membership approach (as opposed to informal loosely linked obligational networks). - These findings match with the Alter/Hage-network evolution theory that postulates that 'exchange' networks are a precondition for 'promotional' or joint action networks to occur (and the latter for systemic networks) but which may occur simultaneously.

After this synthesizing analysis of a range of specific, more or less *internal* features of the Slovenian network for the development of Health Promoting Schools, now this network will be analyzed (again in a synthesizing way) against Hastings model of the "new" organization capable of networking (see fig. 2.4.1). This brings the network's interactions with its (organizational) *environment* back into the picture.

The Slovenian network's networking 'with external others' and emphasis given to networking 'within'/ 'with others'

With view to the Slovenian network as a whole, 'organizational networking with others' has **two dimensions**: a) networking with other *members of the European Network/* ENHPS (in its role as 'ENHPS member' actively contributing to the 'networking within' this European Network); and b) networking with *external others outside this realm*, particularly within the own country. First, as to the Slovenian network's **networking with other European Network members** there was both: on the one hand, active sharing and exchange of information with *national and European* level actors and even joint material development with some - with *one* network member (the National Support Center) coordinating and mainly acting on behalf of the network as expected of ENHPS country members. On the other hand, at least 40% of the pilot schools developed during the first network years direct cross-border exchange or 'twinning' relations with individual other *schools*. - No indications have been found that this changed after the network's expansion. How far also the 'new' network schools that joined the Slovenian net with its first expansion realized a 'European dimension' remains an open question.

As to the *quantity* of contacts with ENHPS networks in *other countries* and the *European level*, the Slovenian Network (via its National Center) may have been above the ENHPS average. It participated not only in the routine or widespread activities (business meetings, newsletter...) but over time engaged also in cross-border manual development and other special activities. - Little has been written about the *quality* of these contacts but active participation and acknowledgments of the value of ENHPS membership from the Slovenian side as well as the network's

WHO award and involvement in special occasions from the ENHPS Secretariat's side indicate mutual recognition, acceptance and 'win/win', particularly as to the relations between European and Slovenian national level.

Second, the Slovenian network's interorganisational **networking 'with others' within the own country** has mainly concerned *two groups of actors*, national and local (with one regional level exception). From the start networking with *national* actors was mainly realized through the National Center's being part of the intersectoral 'National Advisory Board' and related groups, and its bilateral links to the key Ministries of Health and of Education (i.e. the core resource providers of the network). In addition to these *ongoing* efforts, external others were irregularly invited to the national network meetings to expand members' links. - The dimension of (interorganisational) 'networking with *local* others' was developed from the start, too, but overall *weaker* and with local variations. It was mainly in the hands of the individual network schools, but with view to the local health care services there was also a systematic approach from the network as a whole (selective involvement in member selection, training, etc.). As said before, after a few network years at least half but not all pilot schools had interorganisational relations with the medical services somewhat beyond traditional service provision; and a similar proportion had contacts with other local actors. While such involvement of local others in network activities did increase over time, a 'lack of participation of the local community' remained a 'barrier' to the network's dissemination phase (Stergar 1999). - After the network's expansion its networking with one external supporter at *regional* level began, but as at local level (and in spite of a formal mandate for support of HPS development) the support capacities desired or needed were not equally or right away available across regions.

As to the *quantity* of contacts of the Slovenian *network with external others* little has been documented. The National Advisory Board met regularly twice a year, related special committees more often; bilateral contacts with the key Ministries apparently were more frequent. As to the local 'school doctor's teams' the pilot phase evaluation did show that 29% of those team members participated 'constantly' and 47% 'from time to time' (proportions similar to those concerning teachers which are *not* members of their school's HPS project team) (Stergar, bevc Stankovic 1998). National Center and regional Public Health Institutes met regularly but on their general Public Health functions rather than specifically on the network's issues. - As to the *quality* of contacts between the *network and 'external others'* a more general assessment by the National Coordinator in the network's seventh year applies: The 'existing cooperation' between 'sectors, experts, organizations and countries' is a 'strength' to build on in the future (Stergar 1999). This positive judgment is supported by statements of pilot schools of which already during the first network years at least half perceived 'support' by local health care services, and two thirds by non-medical others. The latter indicates one-way (rather than reciprocal) relations between network schools and local others in many cases (which supports the decision made to treat them as 'external' to the network). As to the regional Institutes the basis for interactions with the network changed over time: before the network's expansion they were invited by the network to participate in selected network building events (selection process, national meetings); by the time of expansion, these regional actors had received a formal mandate to support HPS development in their regions but realized this to varying degrees.

As Hastings (1993) pointed out organizational systems must take decisions on whether they for a particular task need to focus on networking 'with others', networking 'within', or in one way or the other on both. With view to the relative **emphasis on networking 'within' and 'with others'** of the Slovenian network for the development of Health Promoting Schools as a *whole* and the two developmental phases examined it can be synthesized: With view to *national* level actors, networking 'with others' was much emphasized from the start and remained more or less the same over that time (National Advisory Board). - Networking 'with *local* others' was the whole time less emphasized (with a slight increase around the network's expansion): There was some accentuation on network schools' collaboration with school medical services, and the school/community-link inherent in the 'Health Promoting Schools'- concept was fully supported, too. However, in comparison to the networking 'within' the network as a whole, 'within' local member organizations (schools), and 'with others' at national level it was less weighted (and overall less realized, too). - Finally, with view to actors at *regional* level both the Slovenian network's networking 'within' and 'with others' became an issue only later, with the network's second developmental phase (or first expansion): Since, the network much accentuated both (but it realized more the dimension of networking 'within' than 'with others').

Overall, networking 'within' the network among *all* network members (national/ school) was much emphasized *before* the network's expansion. With the expansion it became networking among national and regional level network members (pilot schools as regional centers) while networking among regional and local level members emerged. But soon the "first" national Network meeting was formally held showing the intention to keep up networking 'within' an even significantly *expanded* network among *all* members. - These developments are illustrated in figure 5.6.4.

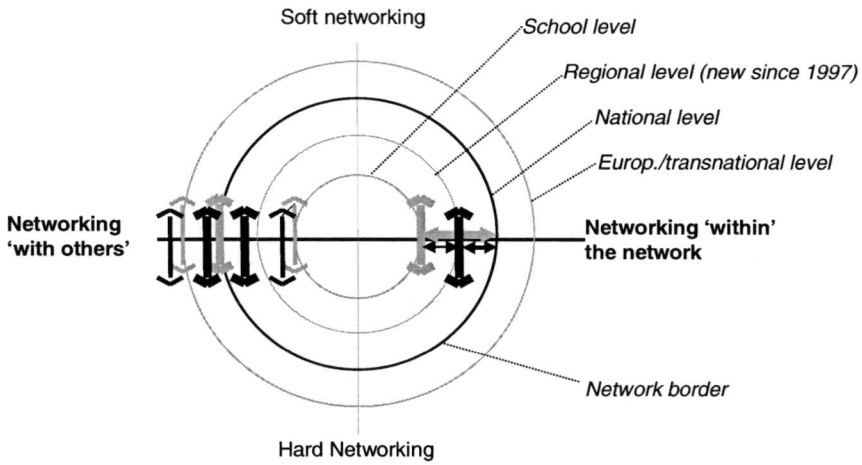

Gray: first phase of network development
Black: second main phase of network development/ sine network expansion

Thinner arrow: less emphasis/ thicker arrow: more emphasis/ no arrow: hardly any emphasis

x-axis/ left: The Slovenian Network's networking with external organizations at local, regional, national and European level
x-axis/ right: The networking within and among groups of network members (school, regional, national, European)

Figure 5.6.4: The Slovenian Network's *emphasis* on networking 'within' and 'with others', differentiated by partners at various systems levels, and as to the two larger developmental phases. (Gray: before network expansion/ first (pilot) phase (1993-1997); Black: since network expansion/ second large (dissemination) phase (1998-).

In summary, the Slovenian network from early on emphasized *both* networking 'within' and with selected 'others'. Over time the latter was expanded to include the regional level. The former changed differently: in the young, yet small Slovenian network on Health Promoting Schools networking 'within' was concerning *all* members; after the network's expansion it was more or less split into two areas: contacts between national and regional, and regional and local level members (with first signs of reemergence of networking among *all*).

The Slovenian network and 'hard' networking, means of 'soft' networking, and the relative emphasis on 'hard' and 'soft' networking

As said before, in written documents on the Slovenian network **'hard' networking** within the network or with others was not an issue. 'Hard' networking (linking computers/e-mail) did serve the National Support

Center's *international* networking with 'external others' or within the *European* Network. Whether this was sooner or later also the case 'within' the national network itself is not documented. From verbal information received it is known that during the 1990s Slovenian schools (as schools in many other European countries) became increasingly computerized - a first basis for 'hard' networking with its potential to significantly increase the frequency of contacts across a network. However, this potential seems to not have been unfolded, at least this was not documented. **Networking *within* the Slovenian network was oriented towards and apparently depended on the systematic use of 'soft' technologies.** Interestingly, these were mainly applied separately for networking 'within' (or among network members) and with 'others' - with the National Support Center in a *central* role as to the network's *outside* contacts beyond school/community links (as the only member participating in National Advisory Board, selection committee, 'evaluation and dissemination group', and being and maintaining linked to regional Institutes of Public Health, national and international European Network actors.

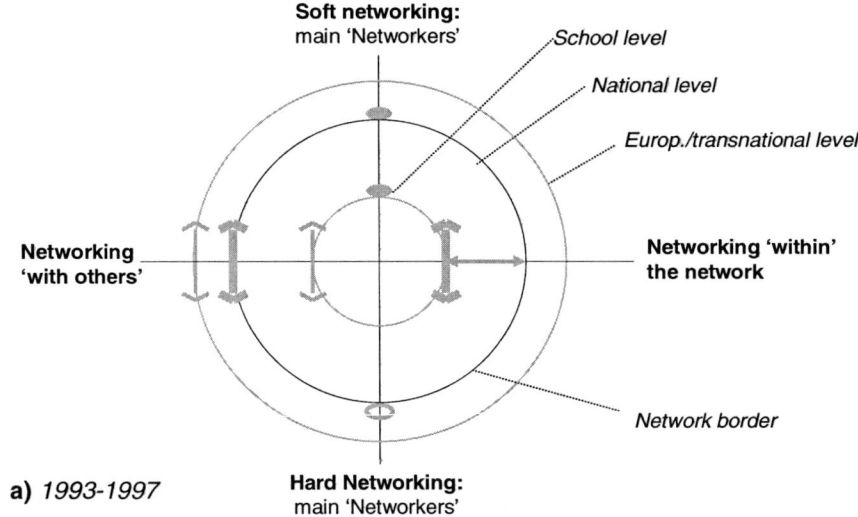

Figure 5.6.5a: "Organizational networking" of the ENHPS in Slovenia (i.e. the Slovenian network for the development of Health Promoting Schools) - Illustration of its emphasis on networking 'within' the net, 'with others', and 'hard' and 'soft' networking by main developmental phases: a) first phase (1993-1997); b) from then on (1998-), i.e. after the network's expansion.

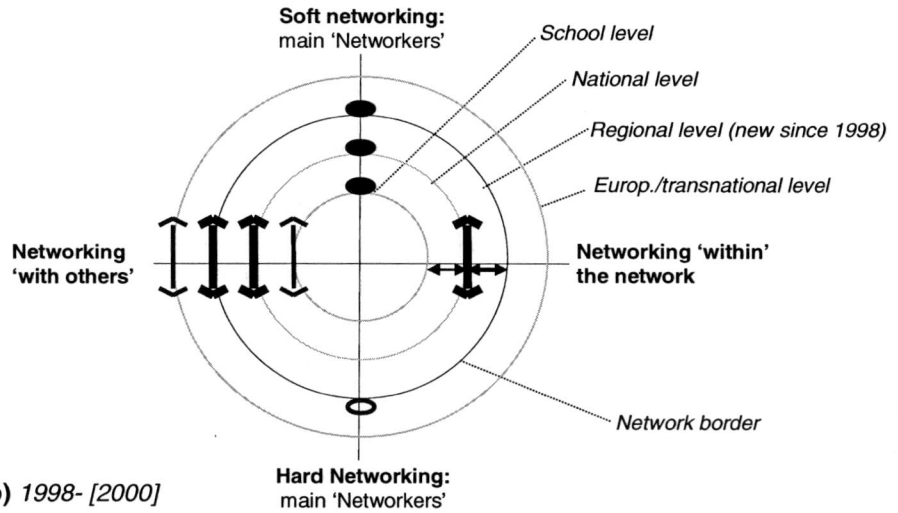

x-axis / left:	The Network's networking with external organizations at local, regional, national and European level
x-axis / right:	The networking within and among groups of members of the Slovenian network (school, regional, national, European)
y-axis / upper half:	The Network's emphasis on soft networking by member groups (i.e. by user groups of 'soft' technologies)
y-axis / lower half:	The Network's emphasis on hard networking by member groups (i.e. by user groups of 'hard' technologies)
Thinner arrows / ellipse unfilled:	less emphasis; thicker arrows/ ellipse filled: more emphasis; no arrow/ ellipse: hardly emphasis

Figure 5.6.5b: "Organizational networking" of the ENHPS in Slovenia (i.e. the Slovenian network for the development of Health Promoting Schools) - Illustration of its emphasis on networking 'within' the net, 'with others', and 'hard' and 'soft' networking by main developmental phases: a) first phase (1993-1997); b) from then on (1998-), i.e. after the network's expansion.

The Slovenian network's "organizational networking" - intermediate synthesis and discussion

Following Hastings' model of the 'new' organization capable of networking, now the overall picture of the "organizational networking" of the Slovenian network as a whole can be summarized - as a picture that emerged out of the analysis of this network as to *each* of the *four* networking processes that together constitute an organization's "organizational networking". Figure 5.6.5 visualizes not only the network's "organizational networking" in general but illustrates the **relative emphasis on each of the four networking processes** as well as **developments over time.**

In sum, from the start (figure 5.6.5 a) the Slovenian network for the development of Health Promoting Schools as a *whole* (which refers to the *ensemble* of its members): a) much emphasized 'soft' networking 'within' the network, but not 'hard' networking; b) emphasized such networking among members first with view to *all* members, since network expansion as to *sub*-groups. With regard to networking with 'external others' the network's main emphasis was first on national level actors, since network expansion also on regional ones. With regard to *changes over time*, a look from the first through the second phase of network development (figure 5.6.5 b) shows that overall there was **neither a reduction in emphasis as to one of the four organizational networking processes nor a shift in the *relative* emphasis** on the x- or y- axis of organizational networking. The emphasis on both networking 'within' and 'with others' was increased by *further differentiation* at the time of the network's first expansion: Networking 'with others' gained a regional dimension as did the networking 'within' the network. The latter gave rise to clear differentiation of networking between national/regional and regional/local level members which (via the double role of pilot schools as regional centers) represents at the same time a selective approach regarding the direct networking of national and local network members. - The regional clustering of network members reduced geographic distance within *sub*-groups of network members.

The reminder of this chapter will round up this 'synthesizing analysis I' of the Slovenian network by addressing: the yet outstanding features of interorganisational networks as identified by Hastings (1993) and/or Alter and Hage (1993), i.e.: geographical distance; the culture of self-reflection/ evaluation/ feed back; and network outcomes in terms of perceived effectiveness and levels of conflict. The schools' "organizational networking", an intrinsic part of creating Health Promoting Schools within a network context, will be looked at, too.

5.6.4 Distance, assessment culture, and satisfaction within the Slovenian Network

Geographical distance among network members

As Hastings pointed out, even with full use of new information technologies (i.e. 'hard' networks) psychological barriers for collaboration increase with geographical distance. Obviously, interorganisational networks with geographically dispersed members that lack access to 'hard' networks have in addition to overcome the *physical* barrier of geographical distance to meet and engage in 'soft' networking. The beginning clustering of the Slovenian network by region after its ten-fold expansion to over 130 members indicates that geographic closeness between network members may be 'better' for their collaboration.

The culture of (self-) reflection, observation, evaluation processes and feed back loops within the network

Both Alter and Hage, and Hastings refer to this issue, the former as part of the network feature 'operational processes' (discussed above), the latter as a central element of his *'radar beam'* model of the "new" organization (see figure 2.4.1). The radar beam symbolizes well the needed culture of *continuous or regularly repeated* self-reflection, self-observation and (self-)evaluation and feed back loops within organizational systems capable of and involved in networking. The reports on the Slovenian network contain several indications that such a culture has emerged: For example, since the second network year network schools systematically document their work in a 3-months-rhythm - (at least during the pilot years) as a basis for joint reviews, evaluation and planning during the regular network meetings and for overall pilot phase evaluation purposes later on. Over the first six years the National Coordinator sent several progress reports per year to the WHO country office; public statements on strengths, weaknesses or 'lessons learned' have been repeatedly found. And since the second network year training course evaluation is a standard activity (Stergar 1997). - This and the general emphasis on participation and learning show that the Slovenian network implemented several of Hastings' 'radar beams' into its network related daily work.

The 'organizational networking' of the Slovenian network *schools*

For two reasons this is an important issue not only as to the ENHPS in Slovenia but in all countries: First, as explained in chapter 4.2 the widespread implementation of the Health Promoting Schools (HPS) concept - the main goal of the Slovenian network as a whole - explicitly expects network schools to develop school-community-links which is a matter of a school's networking 'with others' such as organizations locally. At the same time the school development dimension of the HPS concept and - particularly in Slovenia - the 'education for health'- curriculum development therein, requires much 'networking within' schools. Second, the network approach itself to develop Health Promoting Schools on a larger scale across the country requires capabilities of all members to network 'with other' organizations, and in the ENHPS the majority of network members are schools. Thus, within the ENHPS context **particularly network *schools* face a three-fold innovation challenge** of realizing on the one hand, *'networking within' their organization* to achieve innovations beyond class room walls and subject borders and, on the other hand, *'networking with external others'* and this both *amongst themselves across their country or region* (network approach) and with other *organizations within their local community* (HPS concept).

The Slovenian network's pilot phase evaluation and the ENHPS survey during that phase (see above) have shown: When entering the network the school community groups of the **pilot schools** were much oriented towards school *internal* processes: with motives and widely shared goals directed at health and educational improvements within; activities directed at the *school* community; establishing the school as a 'healthy community' ranking first among 13 activity groups; and the only goal related to links with *external others locally* being that of the 'HPS project team'-members rather than one widely shared. Matching with this is the **emphasis on networking 'within'** pilot schools at the time as indicated by the extent of active contributions to HPS activities by 'HPS project team'-members on the one hand, and other teachers on the other: with of the former 70% constantly contributing and 30% sometimes, and of the latter 25% constantly and 50% sometimes. (Stergar, bevc Stankovic 1998) In comparison to this, pilot schools **emphasized *less* networking with *local* others and *more* networking amongst *each other*** - as shown by the analyses under the headings 'networking with external others' (e) and 'connectivity/networking within the net' (b) above. - In comparison to the pilot schools, the **'new' network schools** of the expanded Slovenian network may show an increased emphasis on networking 'with others' locally: The modified selection criteria applied included more explicitly the school's commitment to interorganisational relations with local services and the local health care service's agreement to cooperate. The emphasis on networking 'within' pilot and 'new' network schools was likely similar as both were and are guided by the same HPS concept. However, the commitment required of 'new' network schools for at least one HPS related training per year for *all* teachers potentially strengthened the networking 'within' these network schools.

Satisfaction of network members - perceived effectiveness and levels of conflict

Following Alter and Hage (1993; chap. 3) it was suggested to take a 'reasonable' network outcome approach and to focus on effectiveness and levels of conflict as *perceived* by key actors within the network. In the case of the Slovenian network for the development of Health Promoting Schools (HPS) the perceptions of National Support Center and network schools are at stake: the network's 'pilot phase evaluation' included the examination of perceptions of pilot school communities of how far their original expectations of 'their' Health Promoting School had been realized (Stergar, bevc Stankovic 1998). As to the perceptions of the National Support Center little information has been found. The *majority of information stems from or refers to the first four network years* (or ENHPS pilot phase). Particularly the levels of satisfaction or perceived effectiveness of the *network schools* during the transition phase and after the network's expansion in early 1998 remains an open question. *Levels of conflict* have been if at all, then only indirectly addressed.

With regard to the twelve **pilot schools** of the Slovenian network for the development of Health Promoting Schools (HPS) the information stems from two sources: the ENHPS Schools Data Base (WHO/EURO 1998) and summaries of evaluation results 'of **the first phase** of the HPS project in the Republic of Slovenia' (Stergar, Bevc Stankovic 1998; Stergar 1996). *During* the pilot phase, all 8 of the 12 pilot schools that responded to a European survey, i.e. *at least two thirds of the pilot schools* reported on usually *a range of 'successful' activities;* the vast majority concerned issues *internal* to the schools but at least a quarter of schools also mentioned successes related to *interorganisational* relations (to the community, other school's, or school medical services). In addition, six (or at least 50%) of the pilot schools reported on activities 'carried out with *difficulties'. At least two thirds of all pilot schools felt 'supported' by other organizations* (the National Center and local others).

At the end of the pilot phase, the Slovenian network conducted a **survey on 'expectations and opinions' of different *groups* involved in the HPS related activities *locally*.** 80% of the members of *'HPS project teams'*, 90% of the *pupils*, 50% of the *teachers* and 60% of the *parents* expressed themselves with view to: goals and expectations at the beginning of the project; perceptions of their school as Health Promoting School after 3 pilot years; the fulfillment of their expectations; contribution to HPS activities; perceived changes at school; successful as well as missing activities; and barriers and incentives. - **T**he members of *school doctor's teams* were also addressed, from a network perspective i.e. 'external others locally'. However, most results shed light on the *pilot schools'* satisfaction or perceived effectiveness regarding the transformation of 'their' school into a Health Promoting School:

After three pilot years, about two thirds of the **pupils** expressed that their (pilot) school matches with their idea of a "Health Promoting School". Similarly, for more than 70% of **parents** their child's school reflected the idea of a Health Promoting School (HPS). The factors referred to were nearly the same in both groups (environmental factors such as food services, other health related activities, building/ surroundings, and good working and learning conditions; and life style or relational factors such as no use of drugs and a sense of "at school we care" for health and better life). However, there was also dissatisfaction: 37 % of pupils stated that their school did not match with their idea of a HPS (for environmental reasons such as poor facilities and food services, and/or lifestyle or relational factors such as drug use or poor interpersonal relations). Almost 30% of parents expressed dissatisfaction, too (but the general quality of lessons and curriculum, and the pupil/teacher- and school/parent-communication). - As to **teachers** and **members of the 'school project teams'** 25% of the former and about 30% of the latter reported that their goals or expectations held at the beginning of the HPS project had been realized or fulfilled. Expectations were partly fulfilled for almost 70 % of the teachers and about 65% of the members of the school project teams. Matching with the HPS concept these school team members mainly referred to issues internal to their school (good relationships, healthy life styles, more attention to health, and better environmental circumstances and nutrition); but better relations towards outside the school (i.e. with pupils' home and the local community) were referred to, too. Similarly, the teachers also referred to healthy life styles and good relationships but in addition, to higher levels of quality of their work and better working conditions.

Overall, this reflects **a somewhat mixed picture** as to the pilot schools' satisfaction or perceived successes; but the majority of individuals making up the (pilot) school communities finds their HPS related expectations fulfilled or partly fulfilled. A comparative look at the different school community groups shows: In Slovenia at the end of the pilot phase, that group that is at the heart of the Health Promoting (pilot) Schools in the making, i.e. the group of members of school project teams did always show the highest percentage of those that perceived positive changes - no matter which category of school related change was examined (teachers-pupils-relations, school meals, teaching methods, and parent's interest for health - with the exception of spare time activities where all groups scored about the same). Where negative changes were perceived, the highest percentage always stemmed from the group of pupils. - A comparative look at all pilot schools did show that members of three or a quarter of the twelve Slovenian pilot schools did show generally lower levels of satisfaction or perceived effectiveness as compared to the others (if measured by the extent of negative assessments of changes in the five areas examined). - When looking at those groups professionally involved with a pilot school from either within or outside (i.e. teachers, members of 'school project teams', and 'school doctors' teams') the evaluation did show: all groups professionally involved perceived several of the 'activities within the HPS program' as successful but not necessarily the same ones (with the exception of nutrition related activities). Professionals were also satisfied with the various training courses, i.e. a core network activity (Stergar 1998 a, b).

Supported by the design of the pilot phase evaluation, hardly any of the perceived successes identified related to *inter*organisational activities of pilot schools or effects *beyond* school walls: Interestingly only school doctors' teams (from a network perspective 'external others') came up with *one successful interorganisational activity* of pilot schools: the school/ health center - cooperation. As to the evaluation area of *parents' interest for health,* positive change clearly emerged: More than one third of pupils noticed positive changes in this regard, a perception shared by more than a third of the teachers and school team members surveyed.

In spite of the variety of findings one may summarize that overall, at the end of the first phase of network development (or pilot phase), the Slovenian pilot schools as network members show higher levels of perceived successes and/or satisfaction than of perceived negative changes or dissatisfaction; and pupils, parents and school doctor's teams overall favored the expansion of the Slovenian network initiative to further disseminate the Health Promoting Schools approach in Slovenia. - The evaluation results such as the above played a crucial role in the National Advisory Board's decision to expand and formally establish the Slovenian Network after four/five network years.

When shifting the attention to successes as perceived by the *second* type of member of the Slovenian network for the development of Health Promoting Schools, i.e. the National Support Center, only a rough picture emerges due to the paucity of written statements: When looking across various documents for statements on progress made, some fall into the category of *Health Promoting Schools development* (such as the network schools' broadened perspective beyond health education towards Health Promotion and 'education for health'). Others address the 'hand in hand'-development of the two innovations 'Health Promoting Schools' and 'education for health' curriculum. With view to the area of *cooperation and 'networking' (however defined)* the true 'team' work among pilot schools and National Center has been perceived as satisfactory. Towards the end of the pilot phase 'lessons learned' covered mainly *interorganisational issues,* for example, that 'those involved' learned to introduce innovations and cooperation between the health and education sector. The importance of 'European support' was stressed as was that of financing and 'avoiding obstacles'. (Stergar 1996) This hints at both perceptions of success as well as challenges. As to the network's *closer environment* the intersectoral cooperation between Ministry of Education and of Health was without 'problem'; and from the start the European Network membership was beneficial.

After about six years of network development the National Coordinator publicly expressed **a certain degree of satisfaction** by pointing to several 'strengths' of the Slovenian network initiative related to *interorganisational relations*: 'the network itself' and the cooperation and technical support in place. The international recognition within the European Network and the WHO award received will also have been a source of satisfaction. However, *dissatisfaction* in the form or 'threats' was expressed, too: Mainly with regard to the network's *environment* (e.g. national policies; lack of resource provision) but *also* lacking motivation among those *teachers* of network schools that are *not* 'HPS project team' members.

Various **actors in the Slovenian network's closer environment expressed satisfaction** with this network: the local school health services as mentioned above; national actors referred to it towards WHO/EURO as 'one of the best' Health Promotion 'programs' in Slovenia and accepted by 'top level' politicians (HEA 1998); the European Network's Technical Secretariat show cased it as model of good practice and WHO/EURO gave the network its 50th anniversary-award.

6. Linking theory and practice: the ION assessment framework and the European Network for the development of Health Promoting Schools

6.1 Introduction (or towards the journey's end)

This research project set out to identify structural and process indicators for international networks for the development of Health Promoting Schools (HPS) and develop a practical tool to assess such networks' in terms of structures and processes. To enhance the assessment dimension, the general *assessment framework for interorganizational networks* (IONs) developed in chapter 3 not only spells out these network features (structure/ processes) but puts them into context: by inclusion of external/environmental factors and network goals as well as 'reasonable' network outcomes. A '3-step'-case study approach was chosen to pilot test this ION assessment framework or 'tool' developed. The previous chapter 5 did, on the one hand, unfold the *overall picture* of each of the complex network systems for Health Promotion in question as to both their network and Health Promotion dimension (Case study step 1). Surprisingly much effort was needed to identify the units of analysis, i.e. "the networks" in question (their borders or members). On the other hand, chapter 5 analyzed - network case by network case - each of the structural and process features identified for interorganizational networks (Case study step 2). *At this point, the core goal of the research project was fulfilled*: a set of indicators of network structures and processes was identified and pilot tested. Nevertheless and as explained in chapter 4, the step 3 of the case study was pursued, because during the course of the research (with its combination of a Health Promotion and a network research perspective elaborated in chapters 2.1 to 2.4) the opportunity arose and the added value was acknowledged to advance the 'assessment dimension' of the desired network assessment tool: *beyond* network structures and processes towards a more *comprehensive* network assessment framework. The literature review allowed to develop comprehensiveness in two regards:

1. with view to **'additional network dimensions'** of the networks of interest, regarding: *factors that influence or shape* network structure and processes (such as external control/ network goals) and their interplay; *links between* structural/ process features and selected network outcomes (perceived effectiveness/ levels of conflict) and the attention to 'reasonable' outcomes ('assessment principle 1'); aspects of network *evolution* ('assessment principle 2'); and issues of sustainable capacity development ('assessment principle 3');

2. with view to **the 'Health Promotion dimension'** of the networks of interest, regarding: the integration of the *social-ecological approach* and the use of a *combination* of strategies; principles such as *participation, empowerment, and continuous learning;* and valued outcomes related to goals set and desired changes in factors that influence or co-determine health.

By including such issues into network assessment an even deeper understanding of interorganizational networks in general and the international networks for the development of Health Promoting Schools in focus would be possible. Therefore, the above two domains are the theme of the 'synthesizing analysis II', which represents the third and last step in the overall case study approach taken. It is the focus of chapter 6.2. **The European Network for the development of Health Promoting Schools as a *whole* moves back into focus**. Therefore, the two examples of national networks examined separately before, will be analyzed as *building blocs of the European Network* rather than as separate networks. The analyses will directly build on the results derived from the case study so far (chap. 5). As before, it not only will further improve the understanding of the networks in focus but also - most importantly - serve as **pilot application for the *remaining* elements of the comprehensive network assessment framework** developed and related assumptions. In line with the core goal of this research project, the network assessment framework developed is more detailed in its 'Part A' on the 'network dimension' of networks, than in 'Part B' on a network's 'Health Promotion' dimension. Accordingly, also this chapter 6 or the last part of the case study gives **most emphasis to the *network* dimension (now the networks as 'a whole' and their 'evolution'); but the *Health Promotion* dimension of the networks will be brought back into view, too.**

Once the comprehensive case study and pilot testing of the network assessment framework is finalized, this research project comes to its closure. The final **chapter 7 will shift the attention back to the overriding issue of this research: the by then pilot tested framework to assess international networks for the development of Health Promoting Schools and similar networks.** In light of the findings, **the assessment framework will be critically reflected upon** with regard to its *applicability* to the networks of interest and similar networks in Health Promotion and beyond, *adaptations needed*, and its *usefulness* as a 'practical tool' for future analyses and assessments.

6.2 The networks as a whole, their evolution and Health Promotion dimension (Synthesizing analysis II)

6.2.1 Network structures and processes in context: The networks as a whole and over time

After having 'deconstructed' the European, German and Slovenian networks' structure and processes (synthesizing analyses I) it is time to look at these networks again as a *whole* system. The European Network for the development of Health Promoting Schools (HPS) as an interorganizational system is *much though not solely characterized by the sub-networks or systems of sub-networks in about 40 countries*. The German and Slovenian networks examined are just two examples. The formations of the 'ENHPS in countries' are not the only sub-clusters of organizations in the bigger European whole. German speaking (national) networks formed *a trans-national network* within the European network. The ENHPS twinning-strategy led to a significant number of *trans-national pairs* of mainly health promoting (pilot) schools but also national networks. As the *whole* of the European Network is again at stake, it is useful to **recall the network definition** derived from the literature review earlier: Interorganizational networks "constitute the basic social form that permits interorganizational interactions of *exchange, concerted action, and joint production* based on *trustful* relationships. Networks are *bounded* clusters of organizations that, by definition, are *non- or less central* collectives of *legally separate, laterally* linked units." And interorganizational networking "is the act of *creating and/or maintaining* such a cluster of organizations *for the purpose of* exchanging, acting, or producing among the member organizations." (chap. 3.1.2, p.161)

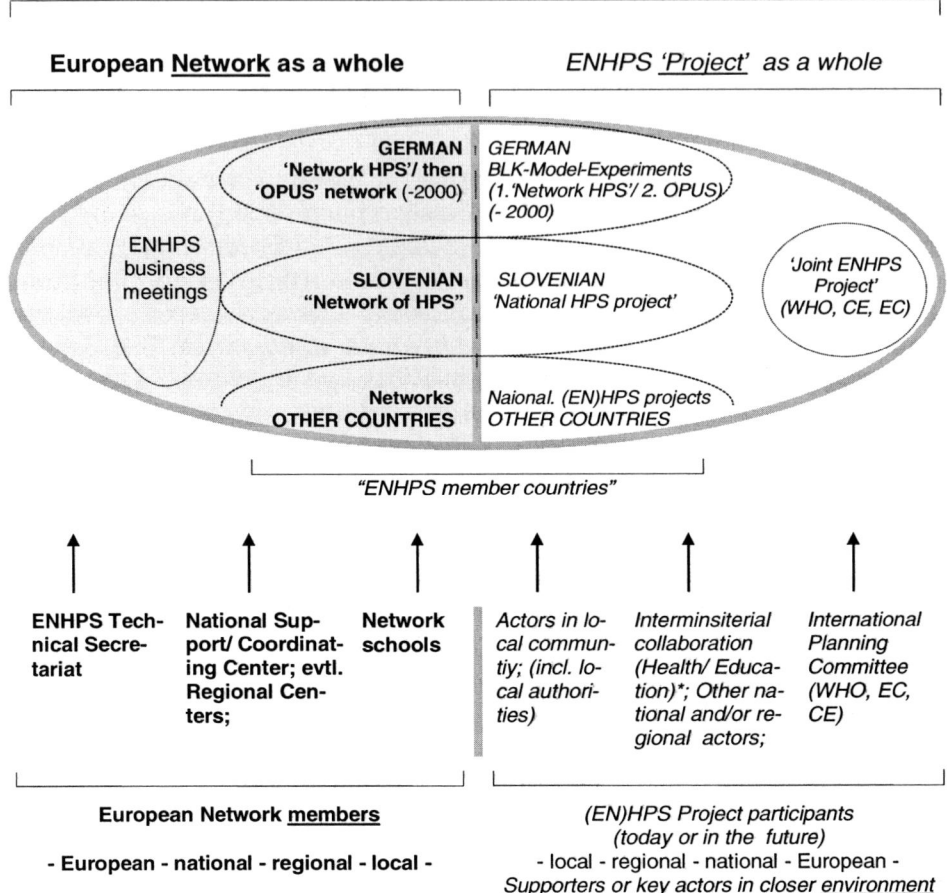

Figure 6.2.1: The "European Network of Health Promoting Schools (ENHPS)"-initiative deconstructed: A two-partite multi-layer entity. - The European interorganizational network and the national networks therein (left side) are to be distinguished from related supportive 'projects' or 'model experiments' (right side). National networks for the development of Health Promoting Schools make up the European network. Each network (gray) is a *distinct* social system on its own that thrives through the related support projects (white) where these exist.
[* not in Germany]

As brought out in chapter 5 through studies of membership and relationships, the European, German and Slovenian network *initiatives* for the development of Health Promoting Schools (HPS) are complex *composite* systems: Each comprises a) **a network** that from the start was meant to be maintained over an *infinite* time span and b) **a complementary support 'project'** or otherwise labeled support system providing essential financial and human resources (see fig. 6.2.1). At *European* level, the latter is the so called 'tripartite ENHPS project of WHO, European Commission and Council of Europe' which from the start was meant to be a longer term endeavor; but nevertheless budget lines and agreements were 'project like' (i.e. to be periodically re-negotiated every some years). At *national* level, 'ENHPS membership' required that at the outset some support project was agreed for a particular time span (of at least 3 years); however, from the European perspective more implicit than explicit these were expected to be somehow prolonged, renewed or sustained (without a clear strategy to achieve this in place). In any case, the support projects form (part of) the networks' closer environment. This 'deconstruction' of the *overall* ENHPS *initiative* illustrated in figure 6.2.1 is the valuable result of the examination of the European Network from an *interorganizational network research perspective* which brought about the need to clearly carve out the units of analysis, the "networks" (i.e. their members or borders). What first seemed to be a network with a kind of double border (European *Network* surrounded by the supportive 'tripartite ENHPS *project*' or alliance of key European agencies (fig. 5.1.3) unfolded as a distinct *double system:*

On the one hand, there is the **European *Network* that links organizations *laterally***, i.e. health promoting schools (HPS), national HPS support or coordinating centers, in some areas over time even regional centers of this kind, and the ENHPS Technical Secretariat. On the other hand, there is **a distinct *second* system** with a strong tradition of hierarchical links but where lateral links play an increasingly important role. This system represents the core part of the **European Networks closer, institutional environment - the public education and health sectors**. It comprises several interlinked building blocs: as of now the formal partnership or tripartite alliance on the ENHPS of WHO, CE and EC (i.e. the European public *health* sector, not that of education); plus - at least during the first three years of a countries ENHPS membership at least but often beyond - formal bilateral cooperative agreements of *Education and Health* Ministries or respective authorities in support of HPS development within a European Network context. (As the German case has shown there are exceptions as to the high level involvement of the public health authorities in ENHPS countries.) Desired and often realized is, that the high level inter-ministerial collaboration *continues* over a *longer* time span beyond the 'three years' that are required when entering the ENHPS. This 'ENHPS project'- system (fig. 6.2.1 right side) has significant development potential and needs yet to be consolidated and expanded to be an effective sustainable support system for large scale

HPS development across Europe. This deconstruction of the overall 'ENHPS initiative' helped to gain a better understanding of factors of *'external control'* concerning the European Network for developing Health Promoting Schools and the national networks therein (see fig. 6.2.2).

Network goal and external control, and their influence on network structure and process

The work by Alter and Hage led to **several assumptions** in this regard which offer some interpretation of particular constellations of individual network features. This raises a twofold question: whether these assumptions contribute to a better understanding also of the network cases in focus here and whether the case studies confirm these assumptions. A first suggestion is that networks that are dependent on *multiple funding sources*, tend to exhibit *highly cooperative, less centralized working modes*.

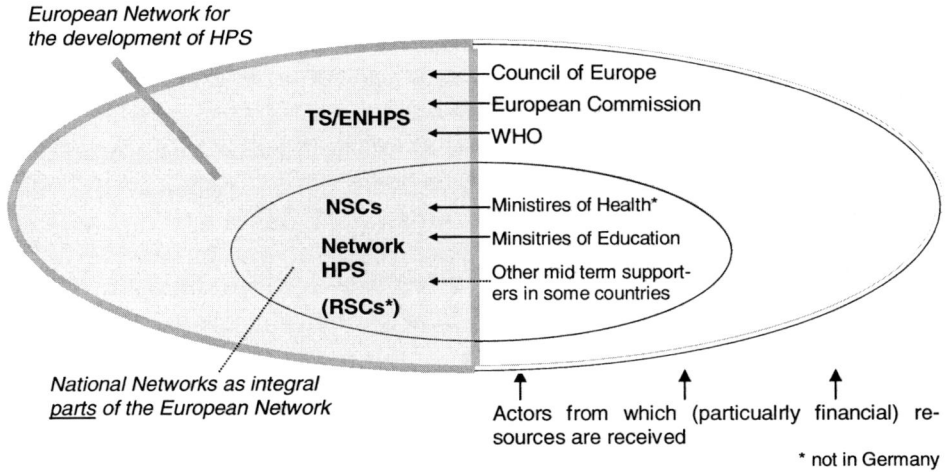

ENHPS:	European Network for the development of HPS
HPS:	Health Promoting Schools/ Network schools
NSCs:	National HPS Support Centers
RSCs:	(Sub-)Regional HPS Support Centers
WHO:	World Health Organizations
TS/ENHPS:	ENHPS Technical Secretariat

Figure 6.2.2: Resource dependency of the European Network for the development of Health Promoting Schools (ENHPS) as a whole. Most external resources (mainly financial) go to specific groups of network members; others to particular network activities.

As illustrated in figure 6.2.2 and particularly elaborated in chapter 5.1, the **European Network as a whole is dependent on multiple sources**

of funding with at European level mainly the intergovernmental *public health* sector involved, at national level usually both the public *education and health* sector (with some variations among countries and over time). At times or for specific purposes *some additional* sources of funding did exist. This does *not* mean that individual (groups of) network *members* are always dependent on multiple funding, too. (E.g. the ENHPS Technical Secretariat is particular dependent on funds from WHO and European Commission, national support centers from their 'host organization' or *one* Ministry only (see Germany and Slovenia), and network schools mainly from their Education Ministries). Dependency on *technical* resources (e.g. as to the Health Promoting Schools approach) is yet another matter. - Triggered through the ENHPS membership criteria for 'countries', *most national networks* will be financially dependent on mainly *two external others,* as nicely mirrored by the **Slovenian Network** for the development of Health Promoting Schools: From the start it was **dependent on both the national Education Ministry and the Health Ministry**. The (financial/human resource) investments of the latter grew slowly over time (in favor of the national network level); that of the former was reduced (to the disadvantage of network schools and regional HPS centers). The **German network**, however, was almost entirely **vertically dependent on *one* actor**, the Federal-State-Commission of the *Education* Ministries (i.e. the public education sector). All human resources at both national and school level came from here (and the leading State Ministry therein). The public health sector as such never got involved. **Although three other** formal 'national cooperating partners' provided important support, the core financial pillar of the countrywide network was with the Commission of Education Ministries. Once this was taken away, the national HPS center had to be closed. (But several State Education Ministries continued the work begun in their States individually.)

Alter and Hage found that **vertical resource dependency** of interorganizational networks could lead to *reduced* **autonomy in decision making** but this must not be; and *low* levels of network *autonomy* were found to be linked with *higher* levels of **conflict** within the net. Thus, network autonomy is an important network feature to be looked at further.

As to the *link between vertical resource dependency and autonomy in decision-making*, the donor's behavior is important. For the ENHPS initiative the European key agencies and donors themselves put forward the motto "partnership as a method and goal". If taken seriously also by other financing agencies, then the autonomy of networks and network members could be rather high - even in case of vertical resource dependency. As far as documentation allows a judgment, the *vertically de-*

pendent **German network** had indeed *nevertheless a relatively high autonomy* in making decisions (with the exception of network school selection particularly at the beginning). The overall 'leading' State Education Ministry was from the start a strong supporter of the German network. It served as bridge and may be mediator towards the Federal/State-Commission of which it was a part and which funded the national 'model-projects' on the network. That Ministry actively participated in the national network meetings and worked closely with the team of the national support center. The impression is that the German network's autonomy at least for the first four network years was almost too high, in the sense of reflecting little interest or involvement of the Education Ministries in the network's undertakings (with the exception of the 'leading' State Ministry). In the following years (as OPUS network) the German network tried to change this situation and the ensemble of State Education Ministries got more involved. (This likely supported the sustainability of the network in several States.) - The **autonomy** to make decisions of the **Slovenian Network** was significantly lower than that in Germany. As recommended for ENHPS 'country members', a National Advisory Board as the main decision making body was in place - with the National HPS Support Center but one of many national actors therein. The Board not only decided on the selection of network members but also, for example, on the composition of groups to develop the network's evaluation and dissemination strategy and these strategies themselves. Also, each of the network's training courses had to be approved by the Education Ministry to achieve cost coverage for network school participants. In contrast to the German Network the Slovenian one is much more anchored within the public (health and education) sector, and it seems that its price for higher sustainability is lower network autonomy. - The **autonomy** to make decisions of the **European Network** as a whole relates much to the annual ENHPS business meetings, the meeting point not only of (national and international level) network *members* but the *core supporters and donors at European level*, too, i.e. the 'International Planning Committee' with WHO, European Commission (EC), and Council of Europe (CE). The business meetings allow joint network related decision-making and formulation of recommendations towards WHO, EC and CE. But, as is the case with the German and Slovenian networks, also the European Network does *not* decide itself on a key network issue: new network members. ('Country' members are selected jointly by the external supporters WHO, CE and EC; members within countries are selected by actors *in* these countries). Remarkably, *not all* groups of network members participate in the business meetings and related decision-making, only the ENHPS Technical Secretariat and all National Support Centers (the latter represent the network schools and potential other sub-national members at European level).

The Alter/Hage study suggests that of the various network features *low* network **autonomy** and *higher* **differentiation** are highly correlated with *higher* levels of **conflict** within the network, but that this influence of high differentiation can be buffered by intense coordination (see also fig. 2.4.8). This point will be taken up again. But first, the analysis of factors that influence a network's structure and processes will be completed, i.e. after that of 'external control' (resource dependency/ autonomy - above) that of the **network's goal or task**.

According to Alter and Hage (1993) the scope of a network's task or the **complexity of a network's goal** influence the **methods of coordination used** by the network, its **complexity and differentiation**. Their findings suggest that more *complex or broader goals* or tasks lead to the use of *group and team methods of coordination*, and to *higher* levels of network *complexity and differentiation*.

In the case of the **European Network** for the development of Health Promoting Schools (HPS) is has been surprisingly difficult to identify the **goals** *of* this *Network*. Not only was it difficult to clarify the network's borders or members, i.e. *whose* goals would be at stake; in addition, there was not the goal to be cited but a range of goal related statements and objectives has been found. But nevertheless it can be said that the European Network (and the ensemble of its members) has among *others* the common goal that network schools transform themselves into 'Health Promoting Schools' (see chap. 5.1.2). Already this is a *complex goal* encompassing a *series* of action programs directed not only at internal changes of schools but also changes of their (interorganizational) relations with others locally. That in addition, this goal was to be pursued in a larger *network* context for the purpose of experience and information exchange and exchange of models of good practice, and this *across* country borders means yet another increase in complexity of the network's goal. There is no need to go into further detail here. For the analysis of the European network as an interorganizational *network* it is sufficient to acknowledge that **its goal *is* very complex** (or the task given by the ENHPS initiators and voluntarily accepted by Network members *is* quite broad in scope). - Similarly, and as elaborated in chapters 5.3.1 and 5.5.1, both the **German and Slovenian networks** for the development of Health Promoting Schools (HPS) pursue **complex goals, too** - in terms of the implementation of the HPS concept in network schools and particularly in the German case, increasingly beyond.

Did the *complex* goals lead to the preferred use of 'group or team' *methods of coordination* as Alter and Hage suggest? And in the case of the combination of complex goal and *low* vertical dependency also to 'personal' methods of coordination?

As to the **European Network** it has been shown in chapter 5.2.3 that from the start there was a focus on both *personal* and *group or team* **methods of coordination**. The former took mainly the form of 'designations of coordinators' required of *each* network member. The latter was realized with the establishment of the ENHPS business meetings. (To use a 'HPS team' approach was even expected from *each* Network member within countries individually.) - The **German and Slovenian network** exemplify, what data within the ENHPS Schools Data Base indicate for many countries: that the European Network not only emphasizes *group* **methods of coordination** at *international* level (business meetings) but at *national or sub-national* level, too. At least during the networks' pilot years (but likely beyond) national network meetings of network schools and National Support Center were held. In Slovenia clearly from early on, and in Germany latest with the second (OPUS) phase, such meetings were places for joint planning and decision making among network members; and the German network from its second (OPUS) phase or decentralization on much stressed the new multi-level "team structure" of the network formally established (table 5.3.1). *As required* by the European Network, in addition both networks used *personal* methods of coordination (designated coordinators per network member), too. In Germany, with the second phase of network development (OPUS) even *impersonal* methods of coordination (e.g. rules and regulations) were consciously used: in the form of a defined set of 'guiding ideas' to which *all* network members had to commit themselves. However, *overall* within the European Network the use of *impersonal* methods of coordination was limited; it was mainly applied to 'regulations of membership' - and this due to decisions by 'external others' (the tripartite ENHPS project).

In sum, the network case studies of this research project support at least parts of Alter's and Hage's goal related assumption that *complex goals* are linked to the *preferred* use of *group or team* methods of coordination. The link found between *low vertical* resource dependency and the use of *personal* methods of coordination for the European and Slovenian networks (equally an assumption by the authors) should not be over-interpreted as supporting this assumption because the European Network *requires* of national networks the use of such personal methods (coordinators). May be therefore, even the German network, *highly vertically* resource dependent, did show such *personal* methods of coordination (a finding contradicting the assumption above).

Now that both the networks' **funding** sources and **methods of coordination** have been synthesized another suggestion by Alter and Hage mentioned earlier can be addressed: that networks dependent on *multiple funding sources* tend to exhibit *highly cooperative* (and less centralized) working modes. Both the European and the Slovenian Networks were and are dependent on multiple funding sources, the German network as to the main financial resources for staffing on one, as to some technical and material resources on three additional ones. All networks used much group or team methods of coordination, which supports the first part of this suggestion by Alter and Hage. The second part related to less centrality is questionable because – as recalled above and explained earlier - interorganizational networks by *definition* are non- or less central systems.

Coming back to *goal* related assumptions, Alter and Hage suggested a second one: that *complex* **goals** lead to *higher* network **complexity and differentiation**. Do the case studies support this?

A look at the networks examined (see chapters 5.2.1, 5.4.2 and 5.6.2) shows that the so called "**European Network** of Health Promoting Schools" or better European Network for the development of Health Promoting Schools (HPS) had a *high* **complexity** - higher than the name and the limited number of three to four *types* of members (ENHPS Technical Secretariat/ National Support Centers/ eventually Regional Centers/ and network schools) suggest. *Many more* different services, sectors, or competencies are present: among National Support Centers i.e. those from education and health, public and non-governmental sectors, from teaching, medical and social science staff, and related to differing experiences and contexts in the different countries, etc. Among network schools i.e. those of (HPS-experienced) 'pilot' and 'new' schools; secondary, primary and other schools; and related to different 'methods needed' to pursue health promoting school development (e.g. project management) and/or 'action areas' (from social climate to nutrition education); etc. - The same applies to the **German Network,** with the *high* **complexity** among National Support Centers across Europe reflected at the level of *Regional* Support Centers, not from the start but after the network's decentralization (as OPUS) and related expansion. - Similarly, the **Slovenian Network** for the development of Health Promoting Schools has also reached fairly *high* **complexity** that as in Germany increased over time (with the network expansion). But apparently network complexity in Slovenia did not rise as much as in Germany as it were the pilot schools that became Regional HPS Centers rather than a range of 'new' organizations joining the net. The latter could happen step by step if Regional Institutes of Public Health unfold their potential or decide to position themselves as *members* of the Slovenian network rather than external supporters in the future.

Besides high complexity another *structural* factor, high **network differentiation** (or the division of labor or function within a network) has been linked to complex network goals. Judging form the analysis of the defined roles and responsibilities of different groups or types of network members (chap. 5.2.2), within the **European Network** the division of labor or function varied as to three areas: networking 'within' the European Network, networking with 'external others', and provision of 'technical support' - of course always directed at supporting the main network *goal*, i.e. creating Health Promoting Schools (HPS), and with little change over time. The networking 'within' the European Network was divided as to the *local* and *national* level (with the former covered by schools and national centers, the latter by national centers and international Secretariat). The networking with 'external others' was divided by systems levels, too (each member was responsible for 'others' at its *own* systems level). Here some change occurred after five to seven network years, when the *international* Technical Secretariat started to plan to shift its focus more towards *national* 'others' (Ministries) in the future. The differentiation within the European Network regarding 'technical support functions' was *first very small* but *rose* over time (first the job of the international Secretariat, it soon became also that of the (now trained) National Centers and increasingly even pilot schools).

The **German Network** had always a clear **differentiation** or division of labor by groups of network members and directed at supporting the main network *goal* (HPS creation); but during the first four years this was less refined, after the network's decentralization and expansion much more: First, schools focused on matters of *their internal* development, the national Support Center on supportive, *network* related tasks. Later (under the OPUS scheme) the division of function or labor was further specified mainly by systems levels: Tasks related to 'networking within' the network were shared as to the supra-regional and regional/sub-regional levels (with the network member *at* a particular level being the *orchestrator* in this regard). Tasks related to networking with 'external others' were shared similarly (with the network members *at* a particular level usually in charge *at* that level, but with Regional Centers filling remaining gaps at the *sub*-regional level and the national center at *supra*-national level). As to (the coordination of) 'technical support functions', the first years only the National Center was in charge, later particular the Regional Centers and each 'actively participating' network school. Overall, the German Network's differentiation *increased significantly* over time. - Similarly to the German development during the first four, five years of the **Slovenian Network,** schools focused on *their internal* development and links with *local* others, and the National Support Center on *network* related and all *supra*-local tasks. With the network's expansion, pilot schools as new Regional HPS Centers started to take over some of the National Center's tasks (but by region). However, this new division of labor was handled flexibly and in general, changes were not as remarkable as in Germany. The Slovenian Network's **differentiation** *increased* over time but to a lesser extent.

Overall, for the **European Network** for the development of Health Promoting Schools (HPS) and two national examples therein it is clear that **network differentiation** has rather increased than decreased over time. The document analyses suggest that the division of labor is mainly *between* (rather than within) *groups* of network members and it increases when new *types* of members occur (e.g. regional level members). A division of labor or function *within* one group of network members *along the lines of different strengths, experiences or interests therein* (e.g. within the heterogeneous group of National Support Centers or pilot schools) appears to be *a yet un-used potential* (see also chap. 7.1).

The case studies of this research project support the suggestion by Alter and Hage that *more complex network goals* or tasks lead to *high network complexity and differentiation.* All networks for HPS development examined show *high and/or increasing* network complexity and differentiation. But the information available does not allow to judge about the suggested causal link (when A, then B and C).

Network autonomy, differentiation and (barriers to resolve) conflicts within a network

Alter and Hage in their network studies found that *low* levels of network autonomy and *high* levels of network differentiation (i.e. of division of function and labor) are *barriers to* conflict *resolution* within a network (see also fig. 2.4.8). While the level of conflict within a network is suggested as 'reasonable' outcome measure (besides perceived effectiveness) and conflict appearance as an unavoidable, natural process in any network over time, the authors draw attention to the importance of *two* network features (low autonomy and high differentiation) as *main barriers* to conflict resolution. Such barriers could lead to levels of conflict that reduce a network's functioning to achieve its goals. However, intense coordination efforts could act as buffer. - The case studies of the **European, German and Slovenian Network** for the development of Health Promoting Schools, unfortunately, do not allow to examine this suggestion further. While the document analyses did allow to examine levels of network autonomy and differentiation in all network cases, and while it found both fairly *high* levels of the latter (i.e. *barriers* to conflict resolution) as well as *high* emphasis on group or team methods and personal methods of coordination (i.e. *buffers*), the information available does not allow a judgment about the levels of conflict themselves in these networks. Thus, this kind of network dynamics remain **an issue for further examination** in the future.

Assessment of the 'organizational networking' of the European Network and two national ones therein

Hastings four 'organizational networking' -processes (chap. 2.4.2), i.e. networking within/with others and soft/hard networking, have been examined network by network case (see chapters 5.2.3/.4, 5.4.3/.4 and 5.4.3/.4). As to their valuation, Hastings makes two suggestions: The first one concerns a network's **relative emphasis on networking 'within' the net and 'with external others'**: If a (multi-)organizational system has *all* resources needed to achieve its goal available *within* its system, then it may solely focus on '*networking within*' the system. If this is *not* the case, or if joint working would lead to a better use of resources or partnerships are desired for other reasons, then (*inter*organizational) *networking 'with external others'* needs to be the focus. Hastings' second suggestion concerns the **relative emphasis** of a network on **'soft' networking (among people) and 'hard' networking**: If the following are desired: innovation and change within a given (multi-) organizational system, *patterns of communication and learning* within and outside this system, and individual self-confidence, *empowerment and 'positive power'* to make desired things happen (i.e. power derived from a culture of *reciprocity* rather than formal authority), then (face-to-face) 'soft' networking among people should be accentuated. If the (multi-)organizational system works *nationally or internationally* and/or with *several* other organizations or systems, 'hard' networking (i.e. links via e-mail and Internet) that *supports* 'soft' networking is particularly important and influential.

In the light of this knowledge, **was the European Network's *relative emphasis* on the four organizational networking processes over time reasonable?** A judgment is of course dependent on the Network's goals for given periods of time. In spite of some lack of clarity in goal definitions (chap. 5.1.2) it can be said: both the European agencies in the 'ENHPS project' (network environment) and the European Network members themselves (including National Centers and pilot schools), during the *first four (pilot) years or so*, clearly aimed at successful *implementation of the Health Promoting Schools-concept* within the 'group of' pilot schools to *demonstrate the 'impact* of health promotion in the school setting'. Afterwards, the experiences and examples of good practice were to be 'disseminated' to other schools.

This needs to be kept in mind when assessing the **relative emphasis on soft and hard networking**. The **European Network** for the development of Health Promoting Schools (HPS) as well as the **German and Slovenian** networks therein all much *emphasized* (and *may* be also realized) *soft networking* - in comparison to 'hard' networking either solely (Slovenia), or more strongly (European Network), or more or less equally strong (Germany*). Some changes occurred over time*: In Germany and Slovenia the regional network level was created and the attention to soft networking within these countries' networks was drawn towards (Germany) or expanded to include this level (Slovenia). At the same time, *hard* networking in Germany was even more emphasized while it remained a non-documented issue in Slovenia. As to the European Network as a whole the situation is somewhat different: the emphasis on hard networking remained stable over time but limited to national and international members. But, while during the Network's first (pilot) phase the *emphasis* on soft networking was equally referring to *all* groups of network members (from network schools to National Support Centers to ENHPS Technical Secretariat), *after that first phase* this changed; during the transition years that followed this broad *emphasis on 'soft networking'* or the overall network dimension of the European Network *faded* (at least in European level documents) and as to a networking 'within' the net it did show mainly in the continued annual business meetings of national and European level members (and European supporters).

Against the background of the main goals over periods of time (above) the following can be synthesized: Hastings stresses that soft networking should be accentuated if innovation within an organizational system, and *patterns of communication and learning* within and outside this system are desired as well as self-confidence, *empowerment* and 'positive power' to make desired things happen. This applies to the European Network and its goal to - during the first (pilot) years or phase - help the self-transformation of pilot schools into Health Promoting Schools and this in a process of experience exchange and mutual learning within a European Network. Thus, the **European Network's and sub-network's strong emphasis on soft networking during the first years or network phase was right**. Also with Hastings' findings **matching is that hard networking was generally less or maximal equally emphasized than soft networking** as the former is a means to *support* the latter, not the other way around. **But, a reduced emphasis on soft networking during the transition years *after* phase 1** by the European Network (or its European level members ?) - as documents indicate - would be **problematic** and a clear contrast to the German Network: On the one hand, it seems reasonable that the European Network did strive to head on to its goal defined for a "second phase", the *dissemination* of the good practice in creating Health Promoting Schools or achieving health promoting school development, i.e. of practice developed by the pilot schools over the first (pilot) years. Many schools in many countries wanted to step into such processes, too. However on the other hand, the goal of the *first* phase of *demonstrating the impact* of this practice in HPS development was not yet achieved; and even if it would have been, the '*dissemination* process', too, represents a continued high innovation and desirably empowerment component of the overall undertaking which needs continued and strengthened patterns of communication and learning within the European Network and its sub-networks in countries. Thus, **'soft' networking in a broad sense** within the European Network was and is **continuously and at *least equally* needed *beyond* the 'pilot' years** or network 'phase 1' - among not only national and international network members but *all* members, including network schools. This is also indicated by the fact that the two national networks examined (Germany/ Slovenia) *did* keep up or even strengthened their soft networking 'within' - however, with a tendency towards increased networking by *regions* and eventually (as in Germany) on the cost of nationwide networking.

As the German and Slovenian network cases illustrate, networking among ENHPS *schools* was in general 'soft' networking (in some cases via cross-border encounters but mainly via *national* meetings, in Germany from the second (OPUS) phase more via regional meetings). However, it can be assumed that the **strong emphasis on *soft* rather than hard networking among network *schools* was not a *strategic* decision by the European Network** as to the network's organizational networking. Even if 'hard' networking (via e-mail etc.) *would* have been wanted, the *opportunities and capacities for this did not exist* for most network schools. Only in recent years, more and more national and European initiatives exist to improve schools' access to the Internet and so called 'e-learning' (see also chap. 5.1.1). Thus, only today the ground may be prepared for the European Network and national sub-networks therein to reflect on and **eventually reconsider** the relative emphasis or extent of realization of soft and hard networking at the level of the network *schools*. Hard networking, or the 'new' information technologies would allow to realize more than before to unfold the overall vision of the European Network's so called "European dimension", i.e. cross-border or trans-national relations and networking, and this not only among *National* Support Canters but network *schools* as well – and also among the number of *Regional* network centers that were created during various efforts of ENHPS expansion in particular countries. This is an issue not only for the European Network as a whole but each national sub-network, the **German and Slovenian Networks** included. But, putting new emphasis on 'hard' networking within the whole of the European Network for HPS development and national networks therein should not reduce the emphasis on soft networking opportunities.

When turning from the organizational networking dimensions of 'hard' and 'soft' networking towards assessing the **relative emphasis on networking 'within' a network and 'with others',** the following can be summarized: The **European Network** for the development of Health Promoting Schools (HPS) during the *first four (pilot) years* was strongly oriented towards *'networking within'* the net (among international and national level members, and among pilot schools). From an international perspective, the European *Network*'s systematic networking *'with others'* was *limited* to its key supporters at European level (WHO, EC, CE). In general, links to national Ministries were limited to the period of a country's ENHPS membership application. Only in *the years that followed* these first four Network years, i.e. a *transition phase*, the ENHPS Technical Secretariat, i.e. *one 'group' of network member* rather than the European Network as a *whole* started to emphasize and plan a shift in focus from 'networking within' the European Network *towards increased linking up with 'external others'*, particularly the national Education and Health Ministries. Here the renewal of their initial cooperative agreements was at stake, but this rather country case by case than as part of an overall strategy directed at the Education and Health Ministries in *Europe* in general. Also the education and health *sectors* as a whole (from national to local level) received more attention (at least in writing).

Following Hastings, the **strong 'networking within'-orientation of the European Network during the first years would have been the strategy of choice if the technical and financial resources needed to achieve the goal would have been available *within* the Network. But this was not fully the case:** Much of the basic **technical resources needed** to *guide or support schools* in this process were available *within* the European Network - first via the ENHPS Technical Secretariat and (to a smaller or larger extent and increasingly) National Support Centers, later increasingly also via the pilot schools. This *justifies a strong focus on 'networking within'* the network. However, the European Network should have engaged more and *complementary* into networking 'with external others' already in these first years: because a *crucial* technical resource, the capability of assessing or evaluating 'the impact' of the Health Promoting Schools (or Settings) approach, was *not* available *within* the network. Even if acknowledging that the whole *field* of Health Promotion of the time faced great evaluation challenges as valuation models and methods were (and still are) insufficient, it can be said: a targeted networking *early* on with a *broader range* of 'external others' to develop an evaluation framework for the Network that would cover the *range* of facets of the guiding HPS concept (organization development included) plus ideally also the intra-network experience exchange and actions in support of this, would likely have helped. This way the *European Network could have made better and more timely progress towards the partial goal of 'demonstrating' valued 'impact' at school level.* - But not only the lack of some *technical* resources within the European Network suggests that an *earlier* emphasis on 'networking with others' (*complementary* to the 'networking within') would have been beneficial. The **financial resources needed** by the European Network (particularly those that secure essential human resources) were almost entirely only available *outside* the network. While those for the *European* level network member and actions were secured by the *highly committed* 'tripartite ENHPS project' (i.e. WHO, CE, EC), those for the network members and activities in *countries* (national and local) were in general *not* secured for a longer term. The cooperative agreements between Health and Education Ministries on time limited 'national HPS projects' (*required* by the ENHPS rather than intrinsically motivated) did secure resources for ENHPS members only for the *first three years* of network membership. This is a fairly short time span if one considers the overall innovations in support of (school) health at stake.

For these reasons, the **European Network already during the first few (pilot) years should have focused not only on networking 'within' the network but increasingly equally on networking with 'others', too,** - both with partners in evaluation development and the network's closer institutional environment (the health and education sectors) - and both in countries and at European level. As to the country level, the European Network did not ignore this dimension but left it to each *individual* National Support Center (or National Advisory Board where in place). A general strategy for 'ENHPS countries' in general in support of this is lacking up to day. In recent years, the Network's response (or may be just the one of the European level?) is to emphasize the need for national *education policies* that support the implementation of the Health Promoting Schools concept in all schools of a country. Other aspects of the European Network's closest environment in countries and beyond are not addressed. For example, ideally the European Network and/or its key European level supporters (i.e. WHO, CE and EC) would strategically work towards that not only the health but the *education* departments of European Commission (EC) and Council of Europe (CE) start to join the ENHPS initiative or 'ENHPS support project' (e.g. by participating in an expanded 'International Planning Committee'). This would then work towards realizing the idea increasingly brought up that the 'ENHPS *Project*' (fig. 6.2.1 right) increasingly includes national and sub-national Ministries and authorities of the education and health sectors in countries or these sectors as a whole. A yet underutilized channel to achieve this are the *European* level Committees of the Ministers concerned. Meanwhile, the *network dimension* of the European 'Network' for the development of Health Promoting Schools (fig. 6.2.1 left) should be *sustained* and even *strengthened* (rather than loosing attention as it seems) - and this in support of effective experience exchange, mutual learning and support, dissemination of examples of good practice across countries and Europe, and joint action (such as advocacy). - **Overall,** the strong emphasis on 'networking within' of the **European Network** for the first network years was a reasonable choice but only for the first *one, two* years. But already *before* the end of the first (pilot) phase (and not only slowly during the years that followed) a *targeted networking with external others* would have been needed to: a) develop early on a joint *evaluation* approach for the European Network and b) act more *timely* on the prolongation of agreements of national education and health sectors to provide essential external resources for the ENHPS in countries beyond the agreed upon three initial years.

In contrast to the apparent shift *from* networking 'within' *to* networking 'with others' of the European Network as a *whole* (judging from European level documents) the **German and Slovenian networks' relative emphasis on networking 'within' and 'with others'** over periods of time was as follows: Both networks *kept up* (Slovenia) or even strengthened (Germany) their emphasis on *networking within* the network *beyond the 'pilot' years* into the (dissemination) years that followed. In Germany, this organizational networking dimension was significantly strengthened over time; in Slovenia a strong emphasis was maintained. But, this emphasis on networking 'within' the networks was *complemented by* an increasing emphasis on *'networking with others'* (in Germany the latter increased significantly from the first to the second network period, in Slovenia less strongly). In Germany and Slovenia the *relative emphasis* on networking 'within' and 'with others' *did not change much; the emphasis on both somewhat increased* over time, most strongly in Germany. This reflects that in comparison to the Slovenian and the European Network, within and around the German Network the reflection and understanding of a "network *approach*" chosen for the development of Health Promoting Schools was most advanced. - The **emphasis of the German and Slovenian networks on *both* networking within and with others match with the fact that, from the start, they had only some but not all resources needed to achieve their goal available within their network**. These orientations of organizational networking of the Network's as a whole also match with the request towards network members, particularly network schools, to equally step into networking 'within' the school *and* 'with others' (in their local community and across their network) - always in support of the main goal of transforming themselves into Health Promoting Schools and letting others learn from their experiences on the way.

The Alter/Hage-network typology and theory of interorganizational network evolution, and the networks examined

As explained in chapter 2.4 the Alter/Hage network theory suggests: There are not only three types of interorganizational networks (exchange/ obligational, promotional, and systemic) but these represent stages of *evolution* of such networks. Do the three network cases examined in this research project support this? How far did they mature or evolve over the observed time span of seven, eight years? Alter and Hage called network's of five years still 'young', and those over 10 years as 'older' networks. - In the primary case studies (chapters 5.1, 5.3 and 5.5) the developments over time of the European, German and Slovenian Networks for the development of Health Promoting Schools (HPS) have been analyzed and the findings show:

The **European Network** during the **first three, four years** (or its 'phase 1') was an **exchange network under development** (or 'obligational' network), with a *slowly increasing frequency and extent* of information and experience exchange *across* the *European* Network: first, only among national and international level network members, later also among network schools (with the latter remaining more limited than the former regarding *cross-border* exchange). The **transition years that followed** (i.e. the less defined second phase) brought about **some joint activities** to accomplish *functional purposes* or solve *supra-ordinate member problems* (such as creating a public data base, joint reviews of progress made and definition of new guiding principles (ENHPS Resolution), etc.). This shows that the **European Network did evolve into a promotional network** of segmented (rather continuous) but concerted action, **while continuing the exchange** relations established. At the end of the time span analyzed (i.e. end of the 1990s) the Network may be best described as a 'promotional network *under development*' because not all (groups of) network members started to engage repeatedly into such joint activities yet. - Similarly, also the transnational 'sub-regional' or better **sub-European network of German-speaking national networks** started up as an **exchange network** but soon did show features of an *emerging* **promotional network** (concerted action for functional purposes such as joint funding applications to donors).

The national networks examined show comparable patterns: The **German Network** during the **first phase** of network development, is best described as an **'exchange network under development'** concerning pilot schools and National Support Center. Later (under the OPUS scheme) the *exchange* dimension of the now reshaped network was overall *strengthened* (with view to school members by region, as to the Regional Centers also across the country). Half way through this **second phase**, *clear indications* were found for both a **wide spread experience exchange among network schools by regions,** and the **sub-national networks' maturing towards a promotional network** for concerted action via its regional sub-networks. The latter is indicated by judgments of network schools: for 25% these networks *did* serve the 'development of *joint plans'*, for another 70% this was true to a low degree. Also, Regional Centers worked towards regional entities for both exchange and *planning* of *joint activities*. - The case of the **Slovenian Network** is a bit different: **Already during the first phase** of network development it was **both an exchange network, and a 'promotional network under development'**. In three monthly national meetings network members from the beginning not only exchanged experience but acted jointly on issues beyond the interest of individual pilot schools (e.g. the establishment of Regional HPS Center, new selection criteria and information material for the time of the network's expansion). After the network's expansion (i.e. the **second phase** of network development) the limited information available suggests that the Slovenian Network's character as an **exchange and promotional network was not equally applying to all network members**: for the *first* generation (or 'old') network members this remained; but regarding the many *'new'* network schools (the second generation) it seems that, if regional network building took place right away then for the purpose of *exchange* of experience and information.

These **findings confirm the Alter/Hage network theory as to its core element of network evolution**. Without an established exchange of some kind, no promotional or joint action network develops; but both network features may occur time wise parallel (as in Slovenia). And, *five network years are not a 'long' life span for interorganizational networks*, and the fact that the networks examined over seven years or so "only" matured as exchange and may be 'promotional networks under development' is, thus, not to be judged negative in any way. This holds even more if one considers the truly double innovation taken up by these networks: the organizational transformation of the *majority* of its members into health promoting organizations (here schools), and this on a large international scale and by means of a 'network approach' that at the time was (and still is up today) not yet well understood, in the field of application, i.e. Health Promotion, and also beyond. **Overall, the European**

Network as a whole remains up today a combined exchange and promotional network - with further development potential in both domains.

The networks' cultures of self-observation, -reflection and/or -evaluation (Hastings 'radar beam' metaphor)

As explained in chapters 2.4 and 3, the assessment of interorganizational networks needs to consider the *establishment of continuous self-reflection, -observation, and -evaluation processes and feed back loops* at both the level of a network as a *whole* and its *member* organizations. This refers to Hastings' "radar beam" in his model of the 'new organization' capable of networking that is integral part of the comprehensive network assessment framework proposed (see chap. 2.4.2 and 3.2). Such a 'radar beam' is essential as the behavior of any organizational system varies and is hardly predictable (be it schools, national organizations or an international network for the development of Health Promoting Schools). A *reflexive culture* is also a criteria of good governance, a key factor in sustainable capacity development. Did the European Network for the development of Health Promoting Schools develop such a culture of continuous self-reflection and (self-)evaluation? The primary case study on this network and its 'synthesizing analysis I' have shown: From early on the Network's **general emphasis on group methods of coordination** has brought about some **opportunity structures for regular self-reflection** among particular groups of network members (annual ENHPS business meetings for national and international level members; regular 'national meetings' for network members within particular countries). How far these were indeed *used* as places for systematic self-reflection and -evaluation is in general not documented. (Unfortunately, minutes of the business meetings could not be analyzed; and analyses of documentation or evaluations of the various ENHPS sub-networks in countries is as of now not available.) But the German and Slovenian network cases demonstrate that this *has* been the case at least in some national networks.

Towards the end of the first phase or 'pilot' years of the European Network and during the transition years that followed, a **few and quite different evaluation or review activities** emerged (see fig. 6.2.3). These reflect the *search and recognized need* for evaluation activities by the *internationally* active network members; but the differing content, coverage of actors and of countries, and also inconsistency of approaches indicate that within the European Network a *culture* of regular (self-) evaluation has not yet emerged: as regards content no clear and agreed upon direction emerged; the network members and geographic regions involved differ from activity to activity; and it seems that main external evaluations were initiated and conceptualized by one or the other key external supporter and donor rather than the European Network itself (European Commission or WHO/EURO).

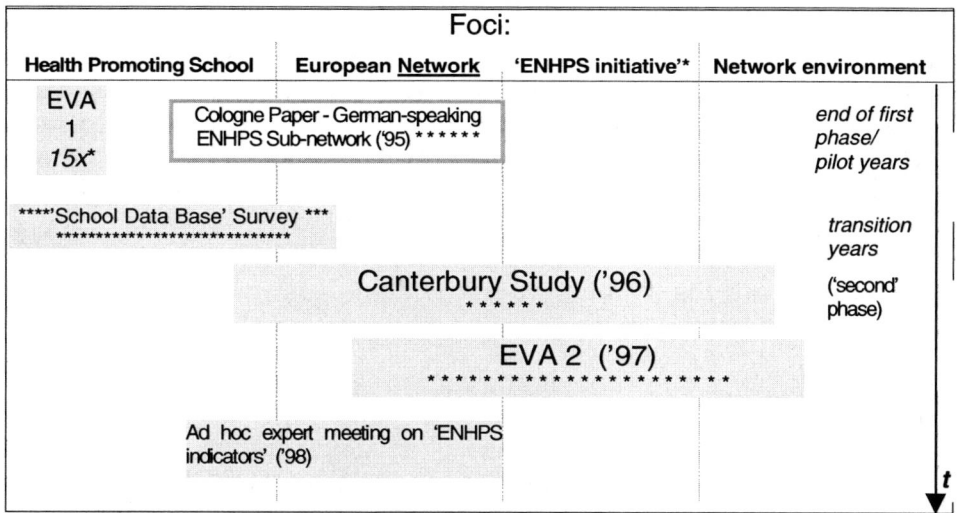

* 'ENHPS initiative': the overall initiative, without that a European *Network* and a supportive 'ENHPS *project*' are being distinguished

☐ Self organized   ▨ Activity of ENHPS initiative   *** No. of countries involved

'EVA': name of evaluations sponsored by the European Commission;

Figure 6.2.3: Illustrative overview of major evaluations, surveys or evaluation development activities of the European Network for the development of Health Promoting Schools (ENHPS) by or on behalf of this European Network and/or the tripartite ENHPS project (gray fields).

The proposed network assessment framework emphasizes a **'reasonable' outcome approach (assessment principle 1).** Alter and Hage suggest to focus on effectiveness and levels of conflict as *perceived* by network *members*. That perceived network effectiveness or levels of satisfaction of network members are a meaningful 'network outcome category' also regarding international networks for the development of Health Promoting Schools is supported by findings of this case study. Both ENHPS evaluation studies (such as the Canterbury and EVA 2 studies) as well as some evaluations by the German and Slovenian network initiatives include in smaller or greater parts issues of *perceived* effectiveness of at least *one* group of network members each. For example, the

Slovenian pilot phase evaluation covered that of the pilot schools' communities; the German OPUS evaluation that of the Regional Coordinators; and some European evaluation studies e.g. that of National Coordinators and 'other key actors' within countries (be they within *or* outside the network in question). That both the European and the German network initiatives included perceived network effectiveness earliest in their second evaluation efforts indicates: The importance of this measure had first to be discovered as a 'valuable' outcome or area of change which is in line with the lacking or less elaborated network concepts of these Networks in their early years and the focus on changes at *pilot school* level at the time. The Slovenian network did measure perceived effectiveness already in its pilot phase evaluation, but with regard to the implementation of the *HPS* concept locally, not to the network approach.

The key factors for developing sustainable (performance) capacity and the European Network

According to the assessment framework for interorganizational networks (IONs) developed (chap. 3) 'assessment principle 3' is to consider the 'key features of sustainable capacity development'. As explained in chapter 2.4.4, sustainable capacity development means the sustainable improvement of the *ability of* an organization or an organizational system (such as a network) to fulfill a task or *to achieve a goal*. It may involve formal projects or activities and/or take place through informal processes such as learning by doing, participation, and experience exchange. And it may be initiated by and involve solely actors *within* the organizational system (or network) concerned and/or external others. Applied to the European Network for the development of Health Promoting Schools (HPS) this leads to the question: **Did or does the European Network as an organizational system exhibit the 'key features' of sustainable capacity development**, i.e. of the sustainable improvement of its ability to achieve its goals? In the following this question is broken down into a set of sub-questions each briefly addressing a key feature in this regard. This way the assessment framework's 'assessment principle 3' is being *tested*. It should be recalled that in the case of the European Network **abilities were needed to achieve two complex goals** set at the *very beginning* by the network *initiators* (WHO/EURO, EC, CE) and into which all future 'network members' had to and did 'buy in':

first, to *help one type of member*, i.e. the first generation of network (or pilot) schools a) to *transform itself* into Health Promoting Schools (HPS) while *actively sharing* their experiences on the way across national borders, and b) to *demonstrate the impact of Health Promotion* in the school setting;

second, to *ensure that a desired next step would follow,* i.e. that this first generation of 'health promoting' network *schools* (so the original intent) *disseminates* their experience, information and 'good practice' to a) *other schools* (i.e. likely but not necessarily to a second generation of 'network' schools) and b) also 'their communities' and health and education sectors or services at all levels (within the country and beyond).

When looking at the key features of sustainable improvement of a system's ability to achieve its goals, a first general question is: **How far did the European Network generally consider** four basic interrelated dimensions: the individual; organizations/groups; interrelationships between the latter; and the enabling environment or broader context? - **Individuals** in the system were much considered from the start as indicated by a) the generally high attention to and provision of training for the National *Coordinators* (rather than National HPS *Centers*), particularly during the first network years; and b) the general emphasis on *school coordinators* and their HPS teams. Also, the Network's core concept of the Health Promoting School (HPS) brings about the general issue of participation and empowerment of all individuals within school communities, and in addition a focus on the following **groups**: *pupils, teachers, and other* members of the 'school communities' (first those of the first generation of network or pilot schools, later these groups in general). The **organizations** in focus were first of all the *network or pilot schools,* less the other organizational members of the European Network identified in this research project, namely the national HPS support centers and the ENHPS Technical Secretariat. The *European* Network did not much consider the group of *'other'* (non-pilot) schools that over time wished to join the ENHPS, too. During the first network years labeled as 'associated' schools they were first *not* considered as ENHPS members, but later counted as such. Inherent in the Network's core goal of implementing the Health Promoting School (HPS) concept, the **interrelations of the groups in focus** were considered, but mainly *individual* school by school. Otherwise, national or international associations of these groupings would likely have moved already more into view as potential collaborating partners. **Interrelations of the organizations in focus**, i.e. the first generation of *network/ pilot schools* were highly emphasized from the start (particularly by emphasizing the so called 'European dimension' and related school twinning). As inter-personal rather than inter-organizational relations emphasized were the annual business meetings of National Coordinators (and, thus, national support centers) and European level actors. Finally, as to **the 'enabling environment' of the European Network,** most attention was given to the supportive environment at *European level*, and here only to the *health* sector (rather than the education sector, too). For most network years (beyond pilot years) European level documents almost solely focus on the 'tripartite ENHPS project' of the Network initiators WHO/EURO, EC, and CE. Only in later years, the potentially but not *necessarily* 'supportive environment' *within countries* has been moved into the foreground, too: after the initially required cooperative agreements of Health and Education Ministries in 'ENHPS countries' ran out in many cases. Particularly emphasized are now the *national education* sector and also the schools' local communities; (the latter is an inherent but yet less realized component of the HPS concept). - In sum, *the European Network did consider* from the start *all four basic interrelated dimensions* of sustainable capacity development, but in parts rather selective and/or with delay.

A second key feature of *sustainable* capacity development would be the **European Network's consensus on a clear vision and goals.** The case studies have shown that **all network members (plus key European level supporters) clearly share *one* vision:** that over time *all* schools in Europe become *'Health Promoting Schools'* (HPS). This is an important strength of the European Network initiative. While attempts to more precisely define 'criteria' for a Health Promoting School for the whole of the European Network failed (the criteria suggested by the network initiators were not accepted equally and/or in all their facets by all members - see chap. 2.2.6), the *overall* idea and concept of a Health Promoting School (HPS) is up today widely shared. This confirms lessons from organization sciences that 'open' concepts are better. **A consensus on *'clear goals'* within the European Network is another matter:** During the *first (pilot) years* or first phase of European Network development, the *overall goal* was *clear and widely shared*: the creation of a network of 'pilot schools' that demonstrate the impact of Health Promotion in the school setting by implementing the concept of the Health Promoting School, and that do so while actively sharing experiences across national borders. However, the *goal for a 'second' phase* of *Europe wide* developments was less clearly defined: the *'pilot schools'* were now expected to somehow "disseminate" their experiences and the HPS concept to others (particularly other schools but the health and education 'sectors', too). Originally, the ENHPS initiators had put forward the expectation that this would somehow 'influence policies and practices' up to the national and international level. The notion of 'dissemination' was not sufficiently clarified and neither were the target groups (except 'other schools') and the role of important network actors (beyond pilot schools). This matches with the lack of a clear 'network' concept or approach (including network membership, borders etc.) found in this research project, and the related lack of distinction between the actors, goals or tasks and planning issues of the supportive 'tripartite ENHPS project' and of the still expanding European Network itself. (During the first years that had not been a problem as both European level support project, European Network and the national networks therein had the same goal and more or less timelines.) - In the light of this it is no surprise that, in the years *after* the 'pilot years' or 'first phase' of the ENHPS initiative, the *European* Network as a whole and its key European supporters (but not necessarily individual national sub-networks) drifted into a kind of *transition* phase (from 1996). This reminds of Alter's and Hage's notion of 'phases of muddling through' that can be expected between network development stages (when networks evolve from exchange to promotional and/or to systemic networks). In the case of the ENHPS initiative, it was mainly the international network level that initiated or engaged in various reviews or assessments of goals or progress made, but without that a clear *strategy* was developed on how to achieve the still desired goal of 'dissemination' of the HPS concept and the pilot schools' experiences to *all* schools in Europe. This may be in parts due to the fact, that at that time a crucial objective of the *first* phase of the European Network was *not yet sufficiently achieved: the 'demonstration of impact* of Health Promotion in the school setting'. At the same time, the importance of also assessing the overall *context* of such developments (including some network dimensions) was slowly recognized. While in some countries such as Germany and Slovenia the *network approach* was over time even *more* emphasized to achieve the European Networks overall goal (i.e. more and more schools stepping into processes of health promoting school development), at European Network level (or at the level of European actors) the 'network' dimension of the ENHPS initiative remained hardly reflected; here the focus of the early years (health promoting development of *schools*) was now complemented by a focus on how to create *national education policies* supportive of HPS development in a country.

A third important factor of sustainable capacity development is **the European Network's goal specific strategic partnerships**. The European Network as an *interorganizational network* can be seen *itself* as a strategic partnership (of selected schools, national support centers and ENHPS Technical Secretariat, and across national borders and various systems levels). This is much of what the 'network approach' is about. But, the European Network as a *whole* had only *limited* strategic partnerships with external *others*. The only one, the partnership with its European level initiators and donors (WHO, EC and CE/ or their so called 'tripartite ENHPS project'), was *installed* and wanted by those donors. As explained earlier, it was structurally well anchored (via the International Planning Committee and annual business meetings of Network and Committee); and it proved to be sustainable for a decade by now. Unfortunately, there were *no comparable developments* with view to the

Health or Education Ministries of European countries – neither from the Network itself nor from the Network initiating, intergovernmental agencies. When looking at the European Network as a whole (not at particular country specific developments!) it has to be stated that from the very beginning, links to the Ministries of Health and of Education within 'ENHPS countries' were limited. European and national actors that were committed to the vision of the ENHPS initiative, motivated these Ministries to *'contract in'* for a defined time span (three years) in support of a nationwide ENHPS or HPS network project (nomination/ resources for national support center and pilot schools). But contracting or buying into an idea for a limited time span (in addition somewhat obligatory as a countries ENHPS membership depended on this) is not to be compared with a *strategic partnership* of European Network and/or international 'ENHPS project' *with* such Ministries. Only in recent years European level documents (written by European level actors) reflect the search for ways to *further or re-involve* particularly the *education* sectors and Ministries in countries. But a clear *Europe wide* strategy has not yet been formulated (or at least not yet communicated in accessible documents). However, there were already partial hints into this direction from ENHPS evaluation studies (see Piette et al 1999; Parsons et al 1997), for example, the proposal to use the system of *European Committees* of national Ministers to gain further support for HPS development across Europe.

Fourth, **the European Network's focus on *existing* capacities** with strategies for their development, maintenance and proper use is another important feature of sustainable capacity development. This point does not need many words to be addressed: Chapter 5.1 analyzed the membership criteria for 'ENHPS countries' and the first generation of ENHPS network schools; related ENHPS recommendations such as on multi-organizational 'National Advisory Boards' for ENHPS initiatives in countries; the series of international ENHPS training seminars for National Coordinators (and may be staff of the ENHPS Technical Secretariat) at least during the *first* years of ENHPS development; and the mechanisms of ENHPS business meetings and *national* meetings of network members in countries (amongst others as places for regular experience exchange and mutual learning within the network). This demonstrates that the overall strategy implemented by the European Network for the development of Health Promoting Schools (called ENHPS) was directed at *building on existing* capacities particularly of (pilot) schools and the nominated national HPS support centers, and more generally of the health and education sectors in countries. The issue for the ENHPS initiators and then the European Network as a whole was rather to *direct, strengthen and in parts complement* those existing resources in ways that would encourage and support health promoting school development of the selected number of pilot schools and afterwards also those 'other' schools that would wish to follow their example. This is well documented at least for the 'first phase' of ENHPS development; for the years that followed the impression remains that overall, the European Network and its European supporters (the tripartite ENHPS project) had no clear response to the much stressed 'diversity' that emerged as to various dimension of the European Network as a whole.

A fifth feature of sustainable capacity development is **the European Network's dealing with the core characteristics of 'good governance'**, i.e. of *the 'how'* of (its) efforts of the sustainable improvement of (the Network's) abilities to achieve its goals (see chap. 2.4.4):

One issue here is **responsiveness.** The European Network for the development of Health Promoting Schools (or ENHPS) as an interorganizational 'network' can, on the one hand, be assumed to be a *flexible* system able to respond to **environmental changes**. Its **closer institutional environment** at *European* level remained quite stable over time (the same three agencies (and individuals except one) in the International Planning Committee); and there were no changes as to the lack of involvement of the education sector at this level. The mechanisms of the '*tripartite* ENHPS project' of WHO, CE and EC seems to have buffered the radical (and not supportive) changes that occurred within some of these agencies over time. As to the *closer institutional* environment at *national* level the situation was different: Over time, several of the national ENHPS sub-networks had to deal with significant changes in this part of their environment, i.e. their education and health sectors or public sector at large. A general challenge was the lack of a European or ENHPS *strategy* on how to deal with the critical and predictable phase of the ending of the initial three-year-cooperative-agreements between Education and Health Ministries 'ENHPS countries'. It seems (and the German and Slovenian case studies illustrate) that this was done more or less individually by national support centers or sub-networks when concerned. But were they, for example, well prepared for this? It is easy to imagine some systematic support from the European Network as a whole. When considering the various backgrounds of National Coordinators and the challenge of the task at stake, i.e. advocacy for *long term*, *intersectoral* support and investment in Health Promoting Schools development within a network contact, it is unlikely that the assumed discussions of such issues during the *annual* business meetings will have been sufficient. – Another important but less discussed element of the European Network's closer environment is that of (Public Health) research knowledge internationally. The Network's **knowledge environment** in the area of social factors that influence or co-determine health and/or health relevant behaviors did change significantly. But, as far the document analysis allows a judgment, the European Network as a whole did *not* respond to this (from a Health Promotion perspective) *positive change*. There is a general lack of reference to this important body of knowledge (chap. 2.1) - with the exception of the repeated reference to the general link between education and health development, and an emerging link to the European HBSC survey system (WHO 2002). This issue will be taken up further when assessing the *Health Promotion* dimension of the European Network and, thus, pilot testing 'Part B' of the proposed network assessment framework (chap. 6.2.2). – Another point to be mentioned is the European Network's responsiveness to **donor's expectations:**

As shown before it was, on the one hand, resource dependent on *European* agencies, i.e. the 'tripartite ENHPS project' of WHO, CE and EC. These were highly committed external *long term supporters* of the Network and, at the same time, providing leadership and *'guidance'* as to the Network's overall development direction. Their regular participation in the Network's 'business meetings' and the Technical Secretariat's participation in the IPC meetings of these donors were the mechanisms to facilitate the Network's responsiveness to donor expectations and related environmental changes. But, most importantly, this worked also vice versa. As the German and Slovenian network cases suggest, at least *some* of the national sub-networks of the European Network exhibit, too, mechanisms that could facilitate those network's responsiveness to their core national donors (particularly the Ministries involved). But again, in comparison to the *European* donor level, the European Network as a *whole* had only a limited strategy to assure its responsiveness to the expectations of those public donors' at *national* level that the Network itself got involved in the first place. A systematic examination of the expectations of (Education and Health) Ministries as key donors of the ENHPS sub-networks in almost *all* countries was not undertaken. The Canterbury and EVA 2 studies brought about only late and minimal and segmented results in this regard; see Parson et al 1997; Piette et al 1999, w.y.). The Slovenian Network case illustrates that the recommended National Advisory Board or similar bodies, when implemented in all participating countries and covering both Education and Health Ministries and other important national actors, are a promising mechanisms in two ways: to facilitate a) the *European Network's* responsiveness to *national* level donors or supporters in countries, and b) the responsiveness of the latter to the former or its national sub-networks. But the strategic use of other, *European* level mechanisms seems to be needed, too (e.g. of European level Committees of national Ministers).

Of course, **responsiveness** does not only refer to the European Network's environment (above) but the **needs of network members**, too. While a more inward oriented system such as the European Network may be reasonably expected to be quite responsive to its members' needs, and while interorganizational networks by their very nature build on *reciprocity* among members, the information available does not allow a judgment. The high level of group or team methods of coordination used within this Network (see above) indicates that the Network as a whole had at least a *high potential* to be responsive to its members' needs. The bits and pieces of information on levels of satisfaction of groups of network members with others signals that responsiveness towards each other was realized at least in parts (see chapters 5.2.4, 5.4.4 and 5.6.4). The overall impression is that satisfaction remained dominant over dissatisfaction as indicated also by remarkably low drop out quotes of members even after five years or more. For example, German and Slovenian network members perceived the transnational information exchange as meaningful and successful and the being part of the European Network as valuable and beneficial.

As to the 'good governance' feature of involvement and **participation and its institutionalization, the European Network** exhibited from the start mechanisms in this regard: the annual *international* business meetings and the usually more frequent *national* network meetings in countries. But, the group of National Support Centers was in a central role as the Centers participated in both. The regular participation of the group of ENHPS (pilot) *schools* was *in general* limited to processes within their *national* (or even regional) ENHPS sub-networks; and that of the *European* Network Secretariat to those of a supra- or *inter*-national scale. The case studies did show that overall and in various ways, the ENHPS motto *'participation as a method and goal'* was taken seriously from the start. In parts, this applies also to the Network's interactions with its closer environment. How far also a **consensus orientation** was implemented within the European Network remains a somewhat *open question*; the document analysis did not find explicit statements on this. But the general emphasis on a 'partnership' approach implies mutual respect and at least fair negotiation of issues if not consensus orientation. Also the principles of **transparency and accountability** have not been spelled out in particular but for many will be seen as implicit elements if working in partnership. Working in an interorganizational network as elaborated in this research project needs a certain level of *trust* among members for which issues such as transparency, participation, and accountability will be crucial.

Good governance as feature of sustainable capacity development of a organizational system also means assuring **equity in access to resources.** How far did the European Network for the development of Health Promoting Schools take care of this? As it from the start was resource dependent on external others, the *European Network was not fully in control* of this dimension. On the one hand, the European Network, via its membership criteria, established for each new sub-national network system in a country, that Ministries of Education and of Health would provide a minimal level of resources to the nominated pilot schools and national support center. However, these would vary according to country specific situations. And also external resources from the ENHPS project partner 'European Commission' (e.g. support for transnational twinning arrangements or participation in the first evaluation study EVA 1) were for the first years only accessible to those ENHPS sub-networks in EU member countries (i.e. to 15 out of close to 40); but during the transition phase of the European Network (after 1996) the circle of countries to benefit from EU programs was fortunately expanded - to the benefit of a significant number of national ENHPS sub-networks though not all.

Inequity in access to resources has been an issue at the *level of member schools*, too. Not only that the resources available to the various pilot schools and national HPS support centers varied country by country; also *within* countries some inequity was perceived. This concerns particularly the generally more generous support given to the first generation of Health promoting (pilot) Schools by the national Ministries while the second generations of schools that would enter the network did receive less or no such external support. This was found to be an issue in the development of both the German and Slovenian network. - However, as far assessable from the document analysis, the European Network *itself* did assure equal access of members to those resources available *within* the Network. But one group of network members (the national support centers) had generally better access to information than the others due to their central position between network schools and the ENHPS Technical Secretariat.

A last feature of good governance and sustainable capacity development is **the European Network's strategic orientation with a long term perspective**. As the case studies have shown, all Network *members,* from schools to ENHPS Technical Secretariat, have definitely entered the network with a long term perspective. Drop out quotes have been found to be very low up today, and most members are already more than five years within the European Network or its sub-networks. Even the donors at *European* level were from the start long term committed to their 'ENHPS project'; however, those *within* countries not necessarily. But membership criteria reflected at least a *mid* term perspective as Ministerial commitments were required for the initial 3 pilot years. - In addition, this case study did identify a 'strategy gap' concerning the European Network and its second phase after the clearly defined first phase of ENHPS development. This is further explained in the final chapter 7 where strengths and weaknesses of the European Network are synthesized. But before doing so the last element of the network assessment framework proposed needs pilot testing: Part B on a network's 'Health Promotion dimension'.

6.2.2 The Networks' Health Promotion dimension

Complementary to Part A of the network assessment framework on a network's 'network dimension', Part B addresses a network's 'Health Promotion dimension'. Elaborated in *less detail* than Part A, Part B of the assessment framework covers *basic characteristics* of *any* Health Promotion program, intervention or initiative (the rational for which has been elaborated in chapters 2.1, 2.2 and 3). The goal is to provide a **general picture** as to the European Network's Health Promotion dimension, and this as before primarily *for the purpose of pilot testing* of the network assessment framework developed.

As explained earlier, the Health Promotion approach is a *social-ecological* approach (responding to a social-ecological model of health). Therefore, **the extent of the integration of the social-ecological approach** into a particular program or initiative to promote health has been chosen as one general indicator of a network's Health Promotion dimension. In light of the range of activities usually captured under the heading 'health promotion' researchers have suggested: The *more* environmental and individual targets are integrated, across a *variety* of settings, the more a program is 'ecological'; and an ecological program should include *at least two* different interventions strategies: one with the 'target individuals' or groups as *direct* target, and *at least one other* that targets a component of their *environment*. Also, more weight is given to a larger number of *targets* than settings. (see Richard, Potvin et al 1996) In the case of the European Network for the development of Health Promoting Schools and the two sub-networks therein, the integration of the ecological approach can be examined only to a limited extent as varying goals (and with this 'targets') have been formulated at different occasions and over time. However, already a look only at the *one* goal that is clearly shared among *all* network members, the creation of 'Health Promoting Schools' (HPS), does show: The European Network and the two national networks therein *integrate an ecological approach to a larger extent*. Although also the HPS concept has been described with some variations (see chapters 5.1.2, 5.3.1 and 5.5.1) it is clear that it typically comprises at *least one* intervention strategy directly targeting individuals or groups (e.g. health education for pupils, or activities on interpersonal relationships) and *several* interventions targeting various aspects of the school as health supportive environment (e.g. social climate, physical aspects of the school as environment, food services, improved school-community-links, etc.). The results of the pilot phase evaluations of the Slovenian and German network support this statement.

Another *general* aspect of assessing the European Network's Health Promotion dimension addresses the **extent to which a *combination* of several strategies is used,** as suggested already in the Ottawa Charter and repeatedly confirmed as most effective by subsequent international Declarations and Resolutions (see chap. 2.2). Of the five Health Promotion strategies widely accepted and usually referred to (i.e. building Healthy Public Policy, creating health supportive environments, strengthening community action for health, developing personal skills, and reorienting health services), the European Network uses several: The *implementation of the 'Health Promoting Schools' concept comprises generally at least the second, third, and forth strategy* - of course with focus on school communities and schools as environments. More seldom references to school policies can be found, as well as - as in the Slovenian network case - special attention to mobilization and even training opportunities for local school health service staff. Also, over recent years the emphasis of the European Network on a particular form of Healthy Public Policies, i.e. *HPS supportive education policies*, has grown - policies already identified in some ENHPS countries. Also in Slovenia there was a high level initiative towards this end. Interestingly, the initiators of the *German Network* at the outset systematically *analyzed the meaning of each of the five Health Promotion strategies above for individual schools* which did shape their 'health promoting school development' -approach from 'within' a school more than the ENHPS criteria of a 'Health Promoting School' of the time (see chap. 5.3.1).

Complementary to the assessment of networks as to the above five Health Promotion strategies, the use of one or more of the *methods or strategic approaches identified in planning* by a network (e.g. health education, organization development, etc.) has been proposed as assessment factor. The European Network for the development of Health Promoting Schools (ENHPS) specified two approaches at the outset: the *Settings approach* (in the form of the 'Health Promoting Schools' (HPS) - concept) and some kind of *network approach.* And as the case study has shown both have been used indeed. However, as discussed below with view to the European Network the emphasis on a network approach weakened somewhat over time, while at the same time the opposite happened in the two national networks examined. Particularly in Germany, after three, four years the network approach moved *significantly* into the foreground in support of large scale HPS development. And less pronounced this happened in Slovenia, too. - Another important strategy identified already in the planning phase of the European Network was *intersectoral collaboration* between national Ministries of Health and of Education; this was achieved through the mechanism of ENHPS membership criteria, which meant its obligatory formal establishment for at least the first three years of the ENHPS in a country.

Network assessment from a Health promotion perspective draws attention to the **principles and processes of participation and empowerment**. It can be clearly said that the European Network established clear mechanisms for participation and joint planning or decision making, most importantly the ENHPS business meetings and regular national level meetings within ENHPS countries (with an advantage for one group of network members, the national HPS support centers). As the two national network cases indicate, the participation principle is also being implemented and even expanded towards actors in the network's *environment* if out of national networks regional sub-networks evolve. From an international perspective, however, more difficult to assess is how far the Networks for the development of Health Promoting Schools examined indeed support or lead to empowerment processes. What can be said is that the ENHPS motto 'partnership as a method and goal' and the organizational form of interorganizational networks is conducive to such processes as are opportunities for participation and their use (see also chap. 2.4 and 3). ENHPS membership criteria for schools such as the agreement of the *whole* school community on their school's participation in the ENHPS initiative (rather than a decision of just some school professionals) indicates the European Network's intention to empower schools as whole organizational systems. Both the German and Slovenian network implemented this 'rule'. The way and extent of consideration given to 'empowerment' is a core issue for further work on the European Network's evaluation strategy and efforts (see below), because empowerment is the core principle of Health Promotion and in an interorganizational network context must apply to both individuals and organizations.

Related to the principle of empowerment and supported by both the Health Promotion perspective and modern organization theory is the assessment issue of how far a network allows and encourages **processes of continuous learning** 'within' the network (at the level of individuals and/or organizations) and with view to 'external others'. From a network perspective this has already been addressed in the previous chapter 6.1 (under the heading self-reflection/ -evaluation etc.). From a Health promotion perspective it should be noted that the principle of supporting continuous learning is an integral part of the European Network's core goal: creating *'Health Promoting Schools'*. These are defined as *schools 'constantly strengthening' their 'capacity as a healthy setting for living, learning and working'* (chap. 2.2.6 and 5.1.2). Also the European Network's character as an information and experience *exchange network* (which was emphasized particularly as to the initial 'pilot schools' and realized among other network members, too) reflects this principle. And so does the preference for methods of *team or group coordination* identified within the European, German and Slovenian networks alike. This was particularly elaborated in the German network's second developmental phase as 'OPUS' network in which mutual and continuous learning was highly emphasized. The Slovenian network accentuates continuous learning through its elaborated system of HPS related *training* provision; this covers even both training for *individual* teachers and at the level of the organization/ *school* as a whole (via the whole staff community). - With view to the European Network as a whole and its *national* level, National *Coordinators* rather than National HPS Support *Centers* have been considered most; and opportunities for continuous learning are directed at these core *individuals* rather than the core national organizations.

A last indicator proposed for assessing a network's consideration of basic Health Promotion *principles and processes* relates to the extent to which the network represents, supports, or encourages **intersectoral collaboration** in support of health development. As said above, this was one of the European Network's strategies identified already in its planning phase. With view to the European Network as a *whole*, this was realized with a bias towards public and national organizations, and *mainly* regarding the Network's *closer supportive environment* (or *'external others'*) - through the initially obligatory but time limited collaborative agreements between national Ministries of Health and Education. Less pronounced it is realized *within* the Network, too, as National Coordinators usually represent either an organization from the health or the education sector. The German and Slovenian Networks demonstrate that *within countries* the situation may be different: Particularly the German Network over time built on both public and *non*-governmental organizations (NGOs) both within the network and as to its supportive environment; and as the Slovenian Network the *sub-national* level is increasingly concerned, too.

Finally, a *very challenging assessment area* covered by Part B of the proposed network assessment framework concerns **valued network**

outcomes from a Health Promotion perspective. Here, three issues are at stake: outcomes in terms of a) the *goals* or objectives *set by* a network; b) the way and extent of *consideration and action upon the range and interplay of those factors that influence or co-determine the health of the target population* (here 'school communities', particularly pupils and teachers); and this most importantly, c) in light of the *level of resources available within or to* the network. As the literature reviews in chapter 2 and the case studies in chapter 5 have shown here lies still an enormous challenge.

The **self set goals of the European *Network*** and its sub-networks could not be clearly identified; documents contain a mix of goal statements related to the 'ENHPS' but do not distinguish between Network members in general, or particular groups of members, and external supporters. When looking again just at the guaranteed minimal consensus that all actors involved have as common goal the implementation of the 'Health Promoting Schools' concept within an increasingly large number of schools that joined the ENHPS initiative or one of its sub-systems, the following can be said: Indeed, the work towards creating 'Health Promoting Schools' has begun in a large number of European schools in about 40 countries (on a scale of thousands rather than hundreds). Over five years or more, these exhibit low drop out rates and are supported by some kind of national HPS support center (and/or increasingly regional ones) in most countries. However, how far these 'health promoting' network schools have made progress in the implementation of the 'Health Promoting Schools' concept and with what results is for the *whole* of the *European* Network not known (as further discussed below). Only once a survey was undertaken, towards the end of the pilot years of the 'first generation' of national ENHPS initiatives (which means the vast majority) did capture a range of activities of the then Health Promoting (pilot) Schools that indicate a rethinking from health education towards Health Promotion in schools (e.g. activities on 'their' school's social or physical environmental features in support of health). However, there are some networks known to be 'well evaluated' such as the German and Slovenian networks that exemplify the progress indeed made by pilot schools, i.e. the first generation of ENHPS schools in Europe, in transforming themselves into 'Health Promoting Schools'. But what these two network case studies exemplify, too, is the explorative and incomparable way such evaluations have been (and may be had to be) done as of now (see chapters 5.3 to 5.6 and further discussions below).

Up to day, the European Network exhibits a clear vision (an important strength!) but from an assessment perspective not a sufficiently clear set of goals 'of the Network' for defined periods of time. And related to this but also other issues (below) it still lacks a sufficient evaluation strategy and framework. The case studies in this research project suggest that the European Network and ENHPS initiative over the years did succeed in implementing important cornerstones for sustainable and large scale development of Health Promoting Schools and in generating new knowledge in various ways but, - it did not yet succeed in finding the right way or approach to 'harvest its many fruits' and present them in a way that assures widespread acknowledgment particularly among core actors in the Network's closest environment, decision makers in the public education and health sectors in countries. In light of the great importance of this issue it is further discussed below - also in order to prevent ad hoc or pre-mature negative judgments of the achievements of the ENHPS initiative so far.

Besides the 'self set goals', Part B of the proposed network assessment framework suggests to look at a *second* area when assessing a network's 'Health Promotion dimension': a network's way and extent of **consideration and action upon the range and interplay of those factors that influence or co-determine the health of the target population** (here school communities, particularly pupils and teachers). **Two groups of factors** should be distinguished: 1. factors that are related to an *individual school* (or local community) and which at least to a certain degree can be influenced *directly* by an individual school community (such as food services, social/school climate, safety on school grounds, school health policies or codes of conduct, conflict resolution, etc.); 2. factors that *concern the main groups of school communities in general*, i.e. the population groups of school-aged children and adolescents, and of teachers (or school staff in general) - and which are more or less *beyond the control* of individual school communities or groups therein (e.g. socio-economic inequity, advertising for health harming life styles, education policies, or other societal factors).

As shown in chapter 2.1, since the European Network's inception the body of scientific knowledge on factors that influence or co-determine health has significantly increased, particularly as to the health of *populations*. Importantly, it confirms the general direction taken by the European Network for the development of 'Health Promoting Schools' and its European initiators, that much more attention than before has to be given to social and other environmental factors than to individual 'health behavior' change - if the goal is improving or sustaining the health of whole populations or large groups therein (e.g. of children). Obviously, a coordinated response is needed by many sectors of society. The ENHPS initiative has outlined, initiated and commenced a coordinated response of public health and school education sectors at *country* level: the large scale implementation of the 'Health Promoting School' concept with systematic knowledge exchange and mutual learning on the way via the European Network for the development of Health Promoting Schools (ENHPS). However, chapter 2.1 and the case studies in this research project have also shown what needs **yet to be done**: **an analysis and synthesis for advocacy and other purposes** of today's knowledge on the *full range* of factors that influence or co-determine health **from an 'education and health' and 'health promoting schools' perspective**, - and with particular attention to both the 'co-determinants' of *'population health'* and of health relevant *behaviors* or lifestyles. The latter concerns a range of social, socio-economic and societal factors. Overall, the analysis should to focus on school aged children or young people as well as teachers or similar (public sector) 'employees' in general. Latest models on evaluating Health Promotion such as by Goodstadt et al (2001) or Nutbeam (1999, 2000) (chap. 3) should be considered as a help to meaningfully *categorize* the range of factors of relevance.

Unfortunately, the *ENHPS initiative* as a whole as one of the few major large scale Health Promotion initiatives in Europe, *did not pay much attention to this area yet,* although it is *one of the two main pillars of scientific knowledge that underpin the European Network's goal and purpose.* The other one is the *intervention knowledge* still to be 'harvested' and improved (regarding both ENHPS innovations, the transformation of European schools into health promoting schools and the network development in support of this).

Here, the *German Network* has shown particular *strengths*: In its *first* years, it worked on both dimensions: On the on hand, it discussed and identified a list of *school related factors that are health relevant* for members of schools communities. Here it could build on recent work done under the leadership of the German Federal Ministry of Education and Science and a published synthesis of such factors (Broesskamp 1994). On the other hand, the German Network evaluated *HPS related interventions of network schools* along a self-developed system of 'steps' towards a Health Promoting School and could prove progress made. - *Later,* after the pilot years, the German Network (now as 'open participation network' OPUS), expanded and shifted its evaluation focus: Now it concentrated on the *second innovation and intervention area* of the ENHPS initiative, that of *network building in support of* large scale sustainable HPS creation. In light of the limited resources available understandable but nevertheless unfortunately, in this phase it left behind its attention to health relevant *factors*. However, the explicit focus on building *interorganizational networks* (of schools, regional support centers, and other organizations) in support of health promoting school development lends itself to be combined with some attention to factors that influence the health of school community members; a strong network could be a good advocate for changes in such factors - particular in those that are either related to schools of a country or region in general, or that are *beyond* the control of any individual school or even local community but could either facilitate or override any school's particular efforts to promote health.

Now, that with the help of the network assessment framework developed in this research project, the European Network for the development of Health Promoting Schools (HPS) and the German and Slovenian sub-networks therein have been assessed as to various dimensions, it is time to conclude. Overall, the pilot testing of the proposed assessment framework has worked out well. It brought about some interesting insights and observations regarding the European Network as a whole. The rather *general* assessment from a Health Promotion perspective above, the more in depths primary case studies of each network on both Health Promotion and network dimensions (chapters 5.1, 5.3 and 5.5), as well as the particular analyses of network structures and processes (chapters 5.2, 5.4. and 5.6) taken together brought about several lessons: on the one hand, lessons learned from and some main suggestions towards the European Network and its German and Slovenian sub-networks; on the other hand, lessons learned with regard to the assessment framework for such (inter)national networks that was developed and pilot tested in this research project. These are the focus of the next and last chapter 7.

PART III

**LESSONS LEARNED,
RECOMMENDATIONS,
AND
OUTLOOK**

- Lessons learned from, and suggestions towards the members of the ENHPS

- Critical appraisal of the proposed network assessment framework

- Outlook

7. Lessons learned, recommendations, and outlook

Now that the comprehensive *network assessment framework developed has been pilot tested* by means of a comprehensive case study approach, it is *time to conclude*: Where did this research project lead to, in terms of both the network cases examined and, most importantly, the network assessment instrument developed. Also the three theses formulated at the outset should be revisited. This final chapter 7 presents the **main conclusions**, with particular attention to the critical reflection of the assessment framework for interorganizational networks (IONs) developed.

7.1 Lessons learned from, and suggestions towards members and supporters of the "European Network of Health Promoting Schools" (ENHPS)

The network analysis undertaken in this research project has clearly shown: The European Network for the development of Health Promoting Schools and its sub-networks have taken up **the challenge of a double innovation**: first, the creation of '**Health Promoting Schools**' across Europe, i.e. the initiation and support of *sustainable health promoting school development* (with health promoting *organizational change* in schools) – and this on a *large scale;* second, the initiation and support of this process within an international or transnational network context, i.e. by means of creating **interorganizational networks** of not only *schools* but, as shown in this study, of *other* organizations, too - *across* not only country borders but, as shown in this study, across *systems* levels, too. While the **Settings approach** chosen (here the Health Promoting Schools concept) is supported by up to date research knowledge from Public Health and Health Promotion (chap. 2.1/2.2), the interorganizational **Network approach** or flexible organizational form chosen is supported by current research knowledge from the organization sciences – particularly when complex goals (as typical in Health Promotion) are at stake (chap. 2.4 and 3). But latest research shows, too, that the sustainable change of the factors co-determining health, the creation of health promoting Settings, and the building and sustaining of interorganizational networks still pose great challenges when assessment, evaluation or 'evidence of effectiveness' of such interventions is at stake.

The European Network for the development of Health Promoting Schools (HPS) and its national (and trans-national) sub-networks were created in the early 1990s on the base of the then scientific and practice knowledge on Public Health challenges and health creation and promising organized social responses to this knowledge woven into the Health Promotion concept. But, the initiators of the European Network to a significant degree had to experiment with both the Settings and network approach, as only little experience existed. The European Network for Health Promoting Schools (HPS) was the first of its kind globally; and its learning opportunities offered by the European Healthy Cities network (the first and only one at the time, too), with a focus on contextual rather organizational Settings and without involvement of the national level, were limited. All of this needs not only to be kept in mind but **should be well acknowledged** and actively communicated, **particularly when it comes to efforts to assess or evaluate** these Networks.

Main strengths, weaknesses and challenges of the European Network

This research project has identified several strengths of the European Network for the development of Health Promoting Schools. An organization research perspective points particularly to the following **strengths**:

- The European Network's *strong vision*, i.e. that all schools in Europe will be 'Health Promoting Schools', and that this will be realized through processes of mutual exchange and learning, - initially among a group of pilot schools (as 'early adopters' of the HPS concept) and later on through their active role in disseminating knowledge and experiences generated on the way; of advantage for broad stakeholder involvement is that the guiding idea of the 'Health Promoting School' is a reasonably *clear but open* concept (but this challenges evaluation efforts; see below);

- The set of membership criteria defined at European level, with:

  o Systematic involvement of a combination of national *and* local level members (through the combination of 'country' and school membership with the former having to provide national HPS or network support centers);

  o Only *voluntary* membership (thus, members can be assumed to see an added value in their joining the European Network; in addition, school membership only if the *whole* school community agreed to participate in the ENHPS;

  o Membership on the base of a *mid* term commitment *only* (at least 3 years);

  o No financial incentives for *national* level members from the European level; incentives are rather the being part of an innovative international network for an important cause that is recognized and

supported by three reputable and major international agencies (WHO, EC, CE), and that provides technical guidance and a framework for mutual support and learning; for this and other reasons, the national organizations serving as ENHPS or HPS support centers in their countries can be assumed to be highly committed (or at least their designated national coordinator).

- The *direct* involvement by the *international* initiative of *schools*, i.e. of the *local* organizations or Settings that are the main 'target' of the European network initiative; this demonstrates:
  o that the implementation of the Health Promotion principles of *participation and empowerment* is possible from the international level;
  o the translation of the HPS *concept* right away into *'real life'* practice which, if succeeding in many cases, is a strong argument for its further dissemination (which has been realized already in many areas);
- Related to the above, the use of a network approach for *international and transnational exchange* of information and experience, and within this framework,
  o Knowledge generation at international level not only on or about schools but also *with* schools (even though this is mostly mediated by the national support centers);
  o Integration of the need for a) support of *locally specific* priorities and ways towards reaching the common goal of sustainable HPS creation and b) *knowledge generation at national and international levels* on best ways to reach this common goal on a *large* scale; work towards mutuality between local and international levels;
  o the use of the potential of peer approaches and mutual learning also at the level of organizations, here a) among 'schools' (among teachers, pupils, school communities, etc.) to *'spread'* the HPS concept and practice among peers and establish peer support, and b) among national HPS support centers;
- Linking up with and/or *involvement of those national level actors* that represent, guide or control an important part of the *closer institutional environment* of the 'target' organizations/ target Settings and the network as a whole, i.e. here the public education and health sectors (Ministries; and also services with a support potential); however, this was ensured only for the first few network years (see below);

- The ENHPS Recommendations (1997), a joint position paper of the members and international supporters of the European Network that positioned the network clearly within the political debates and concerns of the time in the network's political and institutional environment at large (particularly the recognized needs to make progress in the *interrelated* areas of economic, social and health development in Central and Eastern Europe; in its resolution the ENHPS emphasized the links between education, health, and democracy on both technical grounds and the value base shared with European societies.

The case studies on the *ENHPS in Germany and Slovenia*, undertaken as an integral part of the overall case study to pilot test the proposed network assessment framework also as to *national sub*-systems of the European Network in focus, did lead to comparable results (chapters 5.3 to 5.6). This is due to the systematic application of the network assessment framework. Although based on document analysis, the body of knowledge derived and developed is a good basis for a future comparative study of the two national network systems and their evolution over time. Because such a comparison goes beyond the goals of this research project it is planned to be taken up in a separate project, ideally jointly with representatives of the two networks concerned. That project would address the commonalities and differences, strengths, weaknesses and challenges of the Slovenian and German network for the development of Health Promoting Schools in detail which cannot be done here. However, one lesson learned already now from the German and Slovenian case studies is that **the network assessment framework proposed seems applicable to networks that evolved in quite *different* contexts:** *international and national* (and apparently also subnational) ones; *different country contexts* (Western and Central or Eastern European cultures, big and small countries, federalist and more centralized ones); and overall, to networks evolving within *dynamically changing societies or broader environments*. And, from a different perspective these case studies confirm what is often stressed in the literature: that an interorganizational network (ION) is an *organizational form that is flexible enough* to be used in such different and changing contexts or environments.

Besides the above strengths of the European Network for the development of Health Promoting Schools (ENHPS) the European case study and the two national ones therein have also identified **four main weaknesses or challenges** of this Network and in parts its supporters: a) **a 'strategy gap'** of the European Network as to the time *after the well defined 'first phase'* (1992/93 to 1995); related to this, b) **a 'conceptual gap'** as to the *'network'* -approach chosen to achieve desired health promoting innovations in schools on a large scale; c) the **lack of an agreed upon overall evaluation or assessment framework and strategy** for the European Network as a whole and as to both its Health Promotion and network dimension; and d) a **lack of advocacy material** concerning policy and decision makers and potential partners at different levels of society, particularly those in the education and health sectors, of material in support of effective advocacy for long term investments into the sustainable development of 'Health Promoting Schools' by means of interorganizational networks.

A strategy and a conceptual gap

With view to a **'strategy gap' concerning the years after the pilot phase** the case study has shown: After the first three, four years the European Network rightly shifted its attention towards a linking up with 'external others', particularly at the *national or Ministerial* level but also the level of *local communities.* The latter addressed one dimension of the Health Promoting Schools (HPS) concept that network schools had yet to realize (the school-community-link). The former happened somewhat late and, unfortunately, was approached as a rather one-sided emphasis on *national education policy* development in support of HPS creation. At the same time the attention to the interorganizational *network* approach for HPS development faded (at least in the ENHPS documents of the years after the pilot phase). This research suggests that this *fading of the 'network' approach* that at the beginning was consciously chosen to encourage and benefit from mutual exchange and learning among network members in support of the network goal, is *due to a combination of factors*:

- the name given to the European Network at the beginning: '...network *of* Health Promoting *Schools*'; positively, this signals the important role given to the network schools (as 'target Settings' of the ENHPS initiators); negatively, this misleads *network* related reflections to focus on the network's *school members only* (rather than on national HPS centers and Technical Secretariat, too, as done in this research project); this is related to:

- the lack of a clear understanding or conceptualization of the European Network as an '*interorganizational network*' and accordingly a lack of systematic analysis of the European Network from a *network* perspective;

- the fact that after the 'first phase' of the ENHPS, some of the general aims were not yet reached, i.e.:

- there were not yet comparable evaluations across countries to prove the pilot schools' progress in health promoting school development or the implementation of the HPS concept;
- that the pilot schools did not form a *European* network of Health Promoting Schools yet (and that this was done within individual countries was not recognized because of the lack of network related evaluations strategies); this might have caused the fading of the belief or focus on the network approach at European level;

• at the same time, there was the general desire, and in parts even pressure from other (non-pilot) schools in 'ENHPS countries', that the European Network and its national sub-networks should move on and expand or enter the intended 'second' phase of further 'dissemination' of the HPS concept and of 'examples of good practice' developed, beyond the pilot schools;

• in many countries the co-operative agreements of the education and health ministries had run out and further support was yet to be secured;

In light of both the positive potential of the organizational form of 'interorganizational networks' to achieve complex goals (such as a sustainable large scale HPS development), and the positive perceptions by network members *themselves* of the network approach (both of national and school members as shown for the German and Slovenian networks and the transnational 'Sub-regional network' of German speaking networks) it is recommended that: **the network approach chosen by the ENHPS initiative should be re-emphasized particularly by European level actors and in European level documents**. The name "European *Network* of..." is more than a 'name'. A well framed and managed *network*, in strategic cooperation with clearly situated 'external supporters' of the network, will be well placed to prepare the ground and achieve the goal of effective advocacy for national education policies that support HPS development. To realize this potential the actors within and around the ENHPS need to *clearly conceptualize* the 'European Network' and its closer environment.

As of now there is clearly **a 'conceptual gap' as to the network dimension** of the European Network for the development of Health Promoting Schools. Of the two innovations introduced by the ENHPS initiative one was well conceptualized: the Settings approach in the form of the Health Promoting Schools (HPS) concept. But the network approach, the second innovation introduced in support of a sustainable and large-scale implementation of the first, was *not* conceptualized by and for the European Network as a whole. In this regard, and on the base of results of the organization sciences and case studies undertaken, this research project led to a proposal: **the conceptualization of the overall European Network 'initiative' as *two* distinct systems, the European 'Network' and its supportive closer environment, the 'ENHPS project'** (see figures 6.2.1 and 6.2.2). This has several **advantages**:

First, it guides a better *systematization, clarification and potentially reformulation of the division of function and labor* (structural differentiation) among the *range* of actors involved with the ENHPS initiative (from WHO, EC and CE to national advisory boards/ Ministries/ organizations to regional and local education and health authorities/ organizations/ services; from the ENHPS Technical Secretariat to National HPS Centers to the different generations of 'Health Promoting Schools' in the making). The more actors are getting involved the more important is it to clearly communicate: who is *member* of the European *Network* and thus, expected to relate and behave in particular ways, and who is participating in a closely related *support system* such as the 'ENHPS *project*', - and who is external to both. Similarly, the relations between network and support project and their dealing with their joint wider environment need to be clarified. All of this should not be 'carved in stone' but nevertheless agreed upon for periods of time and be subject to regular review and adaptation when desired or needed. As the case studies have shown, the ENHPS is *not* as the name suggests a "European Network *of* Health Promoting Schools (HPS)" but an interorganizational network for the *development* of HPS - with not only schools but also *other* member organizations (national HPS support centers and ENHPS Technical Secretariat) – but nevertheless with the network schools clearly as *core* member group because of their being at the center of the Network's overall goal and an important 'target' for change though not the only one.

This conceptualization of the ENHPS initiative and the European Network therein also *draws attention to the network's true complexity* as defined by Alter and Hage. This way the often stressed *'diversity'* within the European Network *becomes amenable to constructive use to pursue the common goal*; and feelings of 'unmanageable' diversity or complexity that hinder strategy development for the whole of the European Network and leave a 'case-by-case-approach' as the only option can be prevented. From the Healthy Cities Networks stems a useful tool to actively build on the *different* strengths and interests among network members without loosing sight but in support of the common goal and network identity: the so called 'Multi City Action Plans' or 'MCAPs' (chap. 2.2.6). As to the European Network for HPS development, for example, a 'Multi Member Action Plan' could join network members with different capacities to work on particular challenges or issues such as the European

Network's advocacy strategy for HPS supportive national education policies (e.g. the ENHPS Technical Secretariat; some national HPS centers interested, experienced or particularly concerned; and even some schools). Similarly, 'Multi *School* Action Plans' could be a useful tool to build on particular experiences and current interests of some schools and at the same time generate new knowledge for the international field of Health Promotion.

The more it is clear (for a particular period of time) who is 'within' the European Network and who is 'outside', and who of the latter are already in direct supportive roles and who *should* be in the future, a good strategy can be developed as to a *shaping and handling of the Network's closer and wider environment,* and this by making ful use of the range of competencies of the various (groups of) members. For example, if it is agreed within the Network that national Education Ministries should be *long term* partners in the Network's closer environment, i.e. the so called 'ENHPS project', strategies and advocacy material can be developed to convince these agencies to get or stay involved – and this not only country by country but as a European Network effort. Importantly, the Network and existing supporters can offer those agencies a *clear network related identity and positive role without asking them to become a Network member.* For example, they could be invited as donors of the European Network in their *country* and supporters of its overall goal, as actors that actively join WHO, European Commission and Council of Europe in their overall *guiding* role regarding this *European* endeavor.

The illustration (in fig. 6.2.3) of the 'deconstructed' ENHPS initiative by *systems levels,* with the *European Network on the left* and the *supportive ENHPS project on the right* side has additional advantages: First of all it facilitates the Network's strategic decisions and priority setting regarding 'networking within' the network and 'with others' and keeps in mind that *both* is possible and eventually needed for a given period of time. It also facilitates to distinguish between priorities in this regard of the European *Network as a whole*, of particular *member groups*, and (particular groups of) *external supporters* (such as the partners in the 'ENHPS project'). For example, when looking at the Network system in place (fig. 6.2.1, left side) and the desired move beyond the 'first (pilot) phase' towards 'dissemination' of the HPS concept it becomes obvious: On the one hand, a *'network' focus is continuously needed* so that the various groups of European Network members as originally planned actively build on the information and experiences gained and systematically 'reach out' to new schools to join the ENHPS. On the other hand and complementary to this, an *outward orientation is needed* to build up or strengthen the Network's closer supportive *environment particularly at local and national level*. Here, the focus of the European level actors during the last few years on HPS supportive, national education policies is a necessary step in support of the intended dissemination of the HPS concept to more and more (and at the end all) schools in European countries. But, this policy focus should not have the cost of neglecting the network approach itself, a situation indicated by European level documents. A school's sustainable transformation into a health promoting school comes from participation, from voluntary involvement into the 'HPS movement', and it can only be encouraged and facilitated but not commanded. The interorganizational network approach is a concrete organizational form that allows the balancing out of two needs: that *for action to evolve within schools and be shaped 'bottom up'* (from school communities), and that of *initiating and guiding change from outside and even 'top down'* (e.g. from health and education authorities). Thus, today the European level actors of the ENHPS should **give the same level of attention to the network approach itself as to environmental factors such as national education policies** in support of HPS development. The sustainability of health promoting schools development is dependant on both; but the knowledge development needed and knowledge and experiences exchange in support of a more efficient use of limited resources, synergy creation, and mutual learning across Europe is particularly supported by the network approach.

A last advantage of the 'deconstruction' or conceptualization of the European Network for the development of Health Promoting Schools and its environment worth mentioning is, that it draws **attention to the need of a clear European Network strategy concerning the *sub*-national network systems at regional or sub-regional levels** that emerge(d). In federalist countries their emergence is predefined (e.g. in Germany); but also other countries show such development (e.g. Slovenia). This is likely due to the geographic distance as barrier for soft networking (particularly as long as no 'hard' networking via e-mail etc. is a routine part of communication). Without a clear European strategy as to the regional level developments the European Network risks that the latest and future generations of 'Health Promoting Schools' in the making, i.e. the school members of national and particularly sub-national networks, will show a weak ENHPS related identity if any; and this could mean a falling apart of the overall European Network into smaller unrelated networks or clusters of 'Health Promoting Schools' (HPS) or – in the extreme – into a smaller or larger number of individual, not interconnected Health Promoting Schools. Without the network dimension, however, i.e. without a flexible but unifying, motivating and guiding organizational context, effective exchange, mutual support, mutual learning, and synergy creation – systematically and on a large scale, across geographic areas and national borders, and reaching out to *all* schools over time - gets lost; or it relies on chance favoring some and disfavoring others. This risk should and can be minimized or even avoided. Towards this end and with view to its internal cohesion, **the *European Network* as a whole should increase its efforts to clearly and widely communicate the *interrelations* of the various sub-systems, groups of members and external partners as to the overall European Network initiative.** It also should carve out, further **elaborate and clearly communicate the *positive potential* or benefits of network membership for individual member organizations as well as the Network's *potential to create synergy and avoid 'reinventing the wheel'* in the overall 'school and health' domain.** A conceptual frame and **mechanisms are needed to offer and communicate also regional and sub-regional actors, HPS support centers or similar ones, as well as each new generation of Health Promoting (network) Schools, a clear *ENHPS related* position and identity** (preferably as network members or as core network supporters). Also, increased attention to regional sub-networks is needed because here lies the key to a speedier 'reaching out' to many more schools and a faster inclusion of those schools already interested to join the European Network and 'HPS movement'. Regional arrangements are crucial to ensure voluntary participation, high quality (mutual) support and work, and to avoid an equity gap as to HPS development. HPS supportive public policies at national or regional level should ideally support this development and its sustainability.

While this has been realized in some "ENHPS countries" and/or regions therein, a widespread long term ministerial commitment to the European Network initiative and the work of its members remains to be achieved. **A vision of the "ENHPS initiative of the future"** is illustrated in figure 7.1.1. On the one hand, the **European Network** for the development of Health Promoting Schools (left side) would be *further differentiated at the regional level* and this in most countries but within a *clear European* Network context. On the other hand, the **"ENHPS project"** (right side) – as of now encompassing 'only' the health sections of WHO, European Commission (EC), and Council of Europe (CE) – would be *expanded* in several regards: a) at *national* level (with most Ministries of Education *jointly* involved, similarly most Ministries of Health; and eventually European NGOs such as IUHPE and teachers unions); b) at *sub-national* levels (with local and regional governments and education authorities supportively involved as well as other local and regional level organizations with a support potential); and c) and at European level, as to the *education* sections of WHO, EC and CE.

Future "ENHPS initiative" as a whole

Envisioned European Network (ENHPS): a continuously growing, inter-organizational/ inter-school exchange and action network across Europe with differentiation by region

Envisioned 'Network environment': An <u>expanded</u> "ENHPS support project" involving all levels of society, with stronger public sector involvement

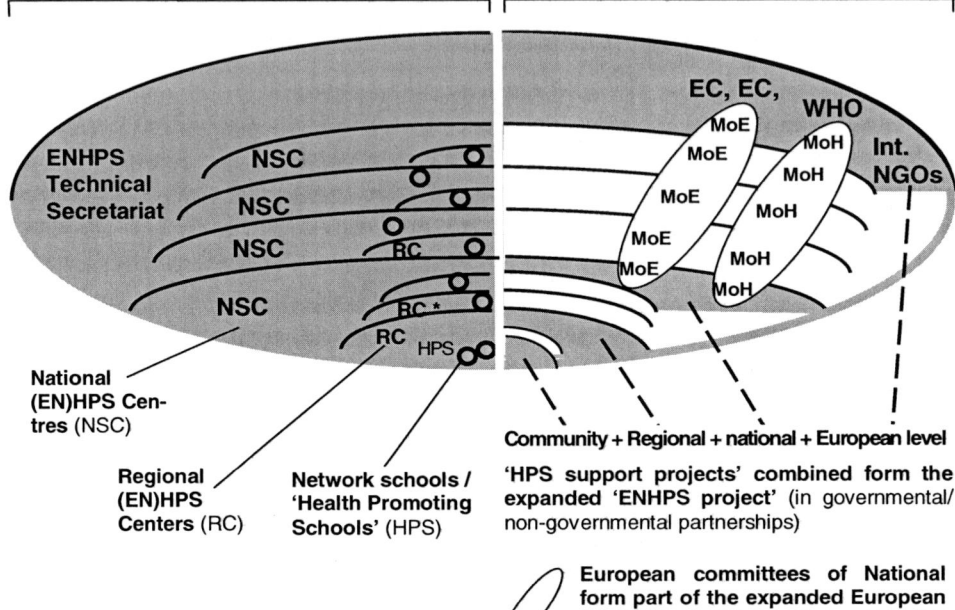

National (EN)HPS Centres (NSC)

Regional (EN)HPS Centers (RC)

Network schools / 'Health Promoting Schools' (HPS)

Community + Regional + national + European level

'HPS support projects' combined form the expanded 'ENHPS project' (in governmental/ non-governmental partnerships)

European committees of National form part of the expanded European ENHPS project (education and health)

CE:	Council of Europe	MoH:	Minister of Health
EC:	European Commission	NGO:	Non-governmental Organization
MoE:	Minister of Health	WHO:	World Health Organization

Figure 7.1.1: Envisioned development directions of the ENHPS initiative.

The lack of an overall assessment and evaluation strategy and framework – a core challenge to be tackled

As the case study has shown, the European Network for the development of Health Promoting Schools (ENHPS) and the still tripartite 'ENHPS project', in spite of some evaluation efforts, did up today not develop or agree upon an overall assessment or evaluation strategy and framework – neither regarding the measurement of progress of network schools in implementing the *Health Promoting Schools* concept (the overall network goal) nor regarding a measurement of progress and effects in terms of implementing the *'network approach'* chosen for achieving large scale HPS development in Europe.

The research findings suggest that this is **for several reasons**: On the one hand, it reflects the *evaluation challenges inherent in social-ecological approaches* to action in general and in the field of Health Promotion and parts of Public Health in particular; there are neither generally agreed upon evaluation models for Health Promotion nor a consensus on how best to evaluate interventions into social systems or Settings in support of health. In the light of this it is understandable, that the European Network received only insufficient guidance in evaluation matters by its initiators and supporters in the International Planning Committee; and that these had even different positions in this regard, as different ENHPS related evaluation projects initiated by them suggest. But the European Network's persistent lack of an evaluation strategy and framework also reflects that it did not engage enough into broader 'networking with external others' on these matters, although latest during the transition years it became clear that the technical resources to adequately respond to the assessment and evaluation challenges of the Network were *only in parts* available within the Network (and some by then experienced national networks) and via its close supporters. That the search direction for additional technical support was not clear is also due to the above-mentioned conceptual gap with regard to the *network* dimension of the ENHPS. Written documents suggest that the European Network as a whole and/or its European level actors, generally quite responsive to network members, did not much respond to work results and suggestions of some of its sub-networks or national members regarding the network dimension and evaluation development needs. While different views as to difficult evaluation and assessment matters are understandable, it is problematic that *no Network strategy* has been developed on how to *overcome* those difficulties and effectively *deal* with the *evaluation challenges* faced. This will also have weakened the Network's potential to respond to the over time increasing need for (scientifically) sound advocacy material on the ENHPS initiative's good cause (see below).

On the base of this research project the following is suggested: **The future ENHPS assessment and evaluation strategy and framework should encompass *two* broad areas**: 1. The level of **individual network schools**: their *transformation into 'Health Promoting Schools'*; 2. The level of the **European Network as a whole**: particularly issues of *network building and functioning* on the basis of a clarified and agreed upon concept of the European Network as an *'interorganizational network'*.

The former was not the main focus of this research project but, nevertheless, the research led to some suggestions: The European Network and

ENHPS initiative as a whole should urgently **undertake a *special* effort to systematically analyze, consolidate, and advance existing efforts to develop an evaluation approach appropriate to the multi-dimensional 'Health Promoting Schools' -concept** and inherent organization or school development processes. Examples or promising elements to build on exist as the German and Slovenian network studies have shown. However, the European Network should also **take into account latest *general* models on evaluating Health Promotion interventions.** These offer valuable categories for (self-)reflection and (self-)evaluation of goals and objectives chosen and potential (intended or unintended) outcomes. These also draw attention to the range of factors that influence health. With view to not only network schools but the European Network and its sub-networks as a whole, a ENHPS assessment or evaluation strategy and framework should **consider** levels of attention, occurrence and results of **activities to achieve positive change in school related factors that jointly influence or co-determine health and health relevant behavior of school community members.**

The second area of a future ENHPS assessment or evaluation strategy and framework *was* the main focus of this research project: i.e. the European Network's *network* dimension. Accordingly, suggestions are more specific. On the one hand, this research project offers a *conceptualization of the ENHPS as a complex interorganizational network* that considers all important actors at all levels of society that emerged as relevant as of now, from school to European level (see above). The actors within and around the European Network are invited to critically reflect on this conceptual frame and how far this, also from their perspective, fills the current conceptual gap as to the European Networks 'network' dimension. The European Network's **future assessment or evaluation strategy and framework should cover the 'network dimension' in two regards: the ENHPS as a *Europe* wide (trans-national and international) system and as a system of multiple sub-networks *within countries* (with both *country* wide and *regional* dimensions).** The pilot application of the assessment framework for interorganizational networks developed in this research project has been overall encouraging. It seems that this assessment framework could serve as the basis of an overall ENHPS assessment framework and assessment strategy yet to be developed. It identifies important *cornerstones* for an ENHPS assessment strategy and framework: particularly with view to the Network's *network* dimension. But it also draws attention to the range of factors that influence health. With view to the European Network and its sub-networks as a whole, a ENHPS assessment or evaluation framework and strategy should **consider** the levels of attention, occurrence and results of **activities to advocate for positive change of those factors** that a) **influence health and health relevant behavior of school communities but b) are** *beyond* **the influence or control of any** *individual* **school** or even local community. - As the network assessment framework is the core outcome of this research project, its elements and related open questions will be critically discussed in more detail below (chap. 7.2).

Related to the above, but nevertheless *independent* from the yet outstanding work on an appropriate assessment and evaluation strategy on HPS development and the network approach, it is recommended to the European Network to **synthesize the current knowledge on health influencing factors or co-determinants of health and health relevant behavior.** The focus should be on the **factors of relevance a) in school Settings** in general (e.g. school climate) and **b) to school aged children and adolescents and school staff in general as far as these are** *beyond* **the influence of any individual school or even local community.** The range of *social and societal* factors should receive special attention. (see chap. 2.1)

Overall, it is recommended that the European Network - in developing its assessment and evaluation strategy and framework - concentrates not only on generating *intervention* knowledge (as to the HPS and network approach) but *also* on synthesizing *health development* knowledge in the 'school/ education and health' domain. This would scientifically underpin advocacy efforts related to the European Network while the evaluation challenges are being tackled and evaluation or intervention research results awaited.

Improving advocacy for sustainable, large scale Health Promoting Schools development within a network context

Several findings of the case study show the **urgent need (**and good potential) today for that the 'European Network for the development of Health Promoting Schools' (ENHPS) develops sound **advocacy material** in support of its goals. The main **reason** is the *Network's general dependency of external resources*, and related to this the over the years observed persisting minimal or decreasing (financial) support of network members in countries (which generally concerns the 'second generation' of Health Promoting (network) Schools and many national support centers, too). Often, in the about 40 countries where the ENHPS is being implemented, the initial three year cooperative agreements between Education and Health Ministries have not been renewed, and complementary and supportive public policies are yet lacking (e.g. HPS supportive education policies although here a positive trend was observed). In *general*, pilot schools and others did not yet succeed to create the desired school-community-links and mobilize external resources needed and locally available in support of their transformation into Health Promoting Schools. And the European Network cannot rely on that the majority of network members in countries have already acquired the knowledge and skills needed (and a good position) for effective advocacy towards the Network's core actors in its closer environment, particularly in the education and health sectors.

Overall, **advocacy material is needed for two purposes:** First, the desired *expansion* and strengthening of the European Network's (and sub-networks') *supportive environment.* This is most pressing at the national or in federalist countries sub-national levels (particularly as to Ministries of Education and of Health) and related to this at European level (here as to the 'education' sections of European Commission and Council of Europe and related Committees of Ministers); here, the overall work context of the Health Promoting (network) Schools is being shaped. In addition, local governments and communities need to be reached out to, to mobilize their potentials as supportive environments for individual Health Promoting Schools. - The second purpose is the desired further *expansion* of the overall 'European *Network* for the development of Health Promoting Schools' (ENHPS), first of the national and sub-national networks already therein. The issue at stake is one of equity: to be more and more inclusive as to *school members*, whether via 'open participation' mechanisms as developed in Germany or a consistent 'step by step' approach as in Slovenia, but without giving up the principle of *voluntary* participation and network membership. However, a strategy to mobilize the remaining 25% of European countries currently not participating in the ENHPS initiative needs to be developed, too.

This research suggests that the following advocacy material is much needed and can be prepared today much better than in the early years of the European Network as the **knowledge basis** for this has been strengthened: a) Today, eight to ten *years of practice development and knowledge generation* of many competent organizations and actors within the European Network can be harnessed; the two national network cases examined have demonstrated this clearly. b) The vast body of scientific *knowledge of factors that influence or co-determine health* and health relevant behavior is better understood; there is growing agreement on main categories of factors which can be used meaningfully to systematize and generally assess the *diversity* of activities and (self set) goals of both Health Promoting (network) Schools (HPS) and the networks for the development of HPS as a whole. (The use of the adapted 'Nutbeam model' of outcome areas in Health Promotion in this research project was just a little test in this direction.)

The **advocacy material should cover:**

- An updated synthesis of the **benefits and positive potential of implementing the 'Health Promoting Schools' concept** on a large scale in European countries – for both *individual schools* as well as the *education sectors* and *societies* at large;

For example, the overlap of the features of good learning environments or effective schools and health promoting schools can be shown as can the be a general health and education link.

- A synthesis of the **benefits and positive potential of the 'network approach' for the large scale development of Health Promoting Schools** in European countries - for the current and 'next generations' of Health Promoting Schools *and* the national or regional HPS/network centers in countries;

Some ENHPS sub-networks such as the Slovenian, German, and transnational one did already some work in this direction and results of the EVA 2 study may include valuable information, too.

- a synthesis of *two groups* of **factors that influence or co-determine health** and health relevant behavior **of school aged children and adolescents, and school staff**: a) the factors *within* the direct influence or control of an individual school and b) major factors that are *beyond* the direct influence or control of any *individual* school (or even local community).

Examples of the former are school climate or a school's health policy. Examples of the latter are general working conditions of school staff, advertising for harmful lifestyles, or socio-economic inequity – areas in which the individual organizations concerned through a network approach can gain a stronger public 'voice'.

- an overview and synthesis of the **inherent challenges of evaluating the comprehensive interventions into schools (and other social systems)** *needed* **to sustain and promote health and progress made in the field of Health Promotion to tackle these challenges;**

To be harnessed are on the one hand, practical evaluation *tools* and related results achieved *within* the European *Network* (e.g. measurable steps towards a Health Promoting School) and latest *general evaluation frameworks* for Health Promotion interventions developed *outside* the network. - A combination of these technical issues will help to appropriately respond to the calls for the 'evidence base' of the Network's actions. A lot has been done within and by the European Network but the fruits have not yet been all harvested to strengthen advocacy efforts for sustainable and expanded support. Of course, generally decision-making takes place on many other grounds than technical reasons only. Therefore, the European Network's advocacy strategy and material needs also to cover:

- the **current political 'entry points' or societal challenges** that the European Network for the large scale development of Health Promoting Schools can *help* to solve, with special attention to persisting differences between Central and Eastern Europe and Western Europe.

Linking up with 'Investment for Health' initiatives seems promising in this regard. The mechanism of Multi-Member-Action-Plans (similar to the 'MCAPs' of the Healthy Cities Networks) may facilitate the European Network's ability to respond to particular external demands or needs without giving up its basic features and principles such as voluntary participation, self set goals locally, flexibility, etc.

The advocacy material is to be prepared for at least **two target groups:** First, **Education and Health Ministries or authorities** particularly at *national or regional* level, i.e. key actors in the *European Network's closer institutional environment* that need to be kept or brought into the European Network's *supportive* environment or the overall 'ENHPS project'; second, the **members of the European Network** themselves, to strengthen their advocacy capabilities for the common goal in their direct environments (e.g. that of schools towards local organizations, that of regional and national HPS support centers or network co-ordination centers towards not only public authorities but a range of other potential partners). To act on the latter will also help to strengthen the European Network's *cohesion* and identity as one European, though multi-faceted network system and its capability to speak with 'one strong voice'. As the case studies have shown the European Network and the two national sub-networks therein have evolved already beyond the level of pure exchange networks towards promotional or joint action networks. This indicates that the European Network today would be able to *jointly act* on the creation of such advocacy material, in collaboration with external others where needed.

7.2 Critical appraisal of the new assessment framework for inter-organisational networks for the development of Health Promoting schools and similar networks

The goal of this research project was to develop an instrument for the assessment of international networks for the development of Health Promoting Schools and similar networks in terms of both network structures and processes. To achieve the goal a broad body of knowledge was built upon which accounts for the **major strengths** of the instrument developed: its compatibility with and *reflection of core knowledge from both the field of Health Promotion and interorganizational relations (IOR)*. Bringing these two knowledge strands together to initiate and strengthen network assessment in the field of Health Promotion and beyond is *a major innovative step* of this research project. This had to be done in an explorative and somewhat pragmatic way because theory development in both fields (particularly action or intervention theory) is still under way, empirical research on interventions into social systems such as organizations and interorganizational networks to enhance health is still rare, and existing intervention knowledge or models are not well integrated yet. But in general the common ground between the two fields did lie at hand: with Health Promotion as a social-ecological (or systems) intervention approach (due to the underlying social-ecological understanding of health) and the systems theoretic perspective of modern approaches to organization development and interorganizational relations and networks.

To achieve the research goal, and based on the above knowledge strands, a conceptual framework for network assessment was developed that centered around structural and process indicators (objective 1) but also covered factors that *influence* network structure and processes. The *guide* created for enhanced efforts of systematic comparable documentation, analyses or monitoring of *structures and processes* of the networks of interest was in light of the limited understanding in the field **an intended and already valuable result**. But in addition, the ground was prepared for assessing network structures and processes in light of a network's relevant *environments* and the type of *goals set*, and this while taking into account some *general network outcomes*. Importantly, *changes over time* were considered (particularly network evolution). Here lies **a particular strength** of the assessment framework (as of now covered in its 'Part A'). **Another strong point** is the complementary 'Part B' that *accounts for the particular field of application* of the network assessment instrument being developed, i.e. Health Promotion. However, the *lack of integration of the two parts* of the instrument (on a network's network and Health Promotion dimension) **has also its weaknesses** as the pilot testing of the at the end comprehensive draft network assessment instrument (research objective 2) has shown. The pilot tested version or 'original' network assessment instrument will now be critically reviewed in more detail and adapted where needed. *The yet unresolved objective 3 will be accounted for now* - by including a reflection on both 'key' characteristics of the networks of interest and the notion of 'practicality' of the assessment tool.

7.2.1 Critical appraisal of the main assessment categories, adaptations, and recommendations

The guiding question for this appraisal is: Does the framework to assess interorganizational networks (IONs) provide appropriate indicators or categories of indicators for a systematic, comparable documentation, analysis and assessment of the networks of interest – in terms of network structure and processes, and beyond? The appraisal of the main assessment categories and related issues of the multi-facetted network assessment instrument will provide an answer by addressing:

- the two foci of this research project defined at the outset, i.e. *the structural*, and *the process features* of networks; and related to this,
- *relationships within the network*, as well as 'network *evolution*';
- the issues of *interrelatedness* of network features and *'key' characteristics* of interorganizational networks;
- the assessment framework's coverage of a network's '*Health Promotion dimension*', and aspects of *integrating network and Health Promotion perspectives*; and finally,
- the notion of a '*reasonable outcome approach*'.

The ION assessment framework's consideration of network structure

The set of *structural* indicators of interorganizational networks (IONs) covered by the ION assessment framework's element 'network structure' was taken from Alter and Hage (1993). The literature review had shown that it is compatible with, supported by, and in parts leading beyond related findings of others. The application of this indicator set during the 'synthesising analyses I' of the European, German and Slovenian network for the development of Health Promoting Schools (HPS) did show: **The indicators of 'network structure' in the ION assessment framework are of great value for a meaningful systematic documentation and analysis of such international and national networks** to promote health. All structural aspects of the 'real life' network cases examined, that were repeatedly documented or studied in particular evaluations or review efforts by or on these networks are covered; some are positively refined (e.g. connectivity in the context of 'networking within' a network); important ones are added (e.g. centrality, only discussed in the German Network). In addition, relations to other network features are proposed: on the one hand, to network processes (here Hastings' 'organisational networking' and Alter's and Hage's 'operational processes'), on the other hand, to network goals and some environmental factors.

A look at the whole *set* of structural network indicators raises the question whether there are some indicators more important than others. For example, network *size* was much emphasised by ENHPS actors during the first network years; and in the *phase of newly creating* such an innovative network system for Health Promotion this is certainly an important indicator of success. However, when it comes to the point that an *existing network* wishes to achieve health promoting changes (e.g. in schools) at a larger scale, with the inherent challenges of long term outcomes and sustainability, the case studies show that *other structural features* are more important at the beginning: the division of labour or function within a network (*differentiation*); the composition or types of members to achieve a often complex goal (captured with network *complexity*); and also *'geographic distance'* between members, a quite important factor as the case studies have shown. The original assessment framework (the one that was pilot tested) addresses the latter separately from the framework element 'network structure': as an integral element of Hastings' 'radar screen' model of organisations (see also fig. 7.2.1, bottom left). 'Geographic distance' between members was found to be a limiting factor particularly regarding the important 'soft' networking and face-to-face encounters among persons within a net. As the German and Slovenian network cases indicate, in both highly federalist and more centralist countries, bigger or smaller ones, *geographic distance combined with network growth* leads quite likely sooner rather than later to a sub-differentiation of networks (here at regional/sub-national level) and this way to higher network complexity and/or differentiation. In light of its importance, **the adapted version of the assessment framework will better highlight the indicator 'geographic distance'** by integrating it into the assessment category 'network structure'.

In chapter 3, inconsistencies in the literature regarding the network issues of centrality and hierarchy were discussed and it was decided to define networks as "based on trustful relationships" and as "bounded clusters of organisations that, by definition, are *non or less central* collectives of legally separate, *laterally linked* units". The case studies in this research project support this decision. As far as document analysis can tell (and as explained around figures 5.2.1, 5.4.3 and 5.6.3) the networks for the development of Health Promoting Schools examined were, if not from the start then latest after the 'pilot years' *explicit* (Germany) or *clearly observable* (Slovenia) *multi-centred networks*. The *European* Network as a *whole* was fairly stable in this regard. This supports the **definition of interorganizational networks** (IONs) as "non or less central collectives" which **predefines the value of network centrality as**

'low' or close to zero. Even the Health Promotion networks examined - with their strong participation and empowerment orientation due to their conceptual basis 'Health Promotion' – did exhibit in their early years more or less *some* centrality but this *did decline* over time if it was not low from the start. However, within the European Network one *group* of about 40 members (the national HPS support or coordinating centres) was found to have a *central role.* Thus, when assessing or monitoring network centrality attention should be paid not only to the dominance or not of 'one or a few' *individual* network members but of particular *groups* of members, too. This is directly related to the structural network features complexity and differentiation.

The network indicator 'connectivity' turned out to be a challenging one. It is a rather compound indicator that commonly captures network structure in simple quantitative terms: as the *extent to which each channel between members is used* ('who has contact with whom'), plus the *percentage of these contacts that is reciprocal.* Ideally, also the *frequency* of such contacts would be measured. To measure the connectivity of an "interorganizational network" at least the *first two* indicators must be used. And, **by definition the relative level of *reciprocal* contacts within an interorganizational network should be high. The *absolute* level of (reciprocal) connectivity should only be judged in connection with an examination of the network's overall organisational networking**. The results of the network case studies, particular the German one, suggest: An examination of a) the relative emphasis given to (and as far as possible the realisation of) each of the four organisational networking processes, *combined with* b) an examination of connectivity in the above discussed terms, can help to prevent to step too far into quantitative data collection on connectivity or intra-network relations and interactions which is not only impractical for practitioners but in any case has its built in limits as discussed and demonstrated by German network actors themselves (see case study chapter 5.4.2).

In sum, with regard to assessing network structure the pilot testing of the assessment framework has shown: The original assessment framework covers the important indicators of network structure; a modification of the framework as regards content is not needed. There is no rational for ranking the indicators as regards importance; but it is advisable to **start assessments with examinations of network complexity, differentiation, and centrality** (and the latter should be low). **Two slight adaptations of the original assessment framework enhance its conciseness and practicality**: a) the 'move' of 'geographic distance' (inherent in the element on organisational networking) into the element on 'network structure' so that all indicators of network structure are *grouped* in *one* framework element; b) making explicit that network 'centrality' *by definition* of an interorganizational network should be *low* if not zero. (see fig. 7.2.1)

The assessment framework's consideration of 'network processes'

The original version of the network assessment framework covers *process* features of a network within *several* framework elements - due to the fact that the framework Part A on assessing a network's 'network dimension' (fig. 3.1.1) was made up of the Alter/Hage study frame for interorganizational networks, the 'radar screen' model of the 'new' organization capable of networking by Hastings, and three 'assessment principles' number 3 of which ('considering key factors for sustainable capacity development') covers mainly process related factors. Obviously, also 'assessment principle 2' on network evolution addresses a process but this one will be addressed separately below as it concerns the *maturing* of a network system *as a whole*, an overriding issue.

The case studies and 'synthesizing analyses I' of the European, German and Slovenian networks for the development of Health Promoting Schools have shown that **the following process indicators (originating from different models or research areas) do complement each other well**: the assessment of a) a *network's "organizational networking"* in terms of Hastings' four networking processes (within the net/with others; 'soft'/'hard' networking); b) the extent to which there is a *culture of (self-) reflection and observation* within a network (Hastings' "radar beam" metaphor); and c) a network's *'operational processes'* (suggested by Alter and Hage). As the case studies have shown the lack of integration of these various process features of a network leads to redundancies if the assessment framework is applied as a whole. Therefore, another adaptation of the framework is suggested, again more in terms of a regrouping of indicators than as regards content: **The former assessment category 'operational processes' is now broadened and relabeled; as assessment category 'processes' it includes now *three* elements: first of all, a network's "organizational networking"** (including that of member organizations); then as before **"operational processes"** (with a focus on methods of coordination used). The former should be looked at first, as it is the more comprehensive process. The third element is **"regular (self-) reflection, observation, assessment, evaluation and feed back"** which are to be assessed as to their integration or not into the network's culture and its concrete activities; (this captures the 'radar beam' of Hastings' model, most items from 'assessment principle 3' on 'key factors for sustainable capacity development', as well as the fact that the behavior of organizational systems generally is not predictable. Also this adaptation enhances the framework's conciseness and practicability (fig. 7.2.1).

The regrouping of some (sets of) indicators has strengthened the original network assessment framework in the two focal areas of this research project: network structure and processes. However, a related issue needs further reflection: that of quality relationships. 'Connectivity' as indicator of network structure addresses this only in parts.

The assessment framework's consideration of relationships and climate within a network

The network case studies have highlighted the importance of paying attention to *quality relations* in a network and that these more than formal status define network membership. The great importance of qualities of interactions and relations in interorganizational network assessment is due to two interrelated facts: a) Intra-network relations are *defining criteria* of interorganizational networks and the basis to assess whether a multi-organizational system is a "network" or not. b) *Sustainability* in terms of sustainable capacity development depends largely on the realization of principles that refer to interorganizational relations and interactions (particularly those of good governance). In the original network assessment framework the former are addressed, but somewhat dispersed and hidden in parts: 'Assessment principle 3' on considering 'key features of sustainable capacity development' covers a range of factors most of which are *principles* such as participation, transparency, equity, etc. The original framework's network processes captured relational qualities: 'operational processes' refer to methods of coordination used and coordination refers to the extent of 'joint decision making' and 'reliance on mutuality and feed back'. And Part B of the original assessment framework on a network's 'Health Promotion dimension' includes the encouraging or facilitating of 'participation', 'empowerment', and 'continuous learning'. - During the case studies, this proved to be inconvenient and in parts redundant. To make the network assessment instrument more practical and concise also in this assessment area, it is further adapted as follows:

'Assessment principle 3' is dissolved and a new framework element added instead which covers only network *'principles' related to the qualities of relations within a network* discussed. Thereby, *normative statements* receive a clear place within the overall framework - *without* affecting the *other* assessment framework elements for which a particular extent or value can not be defined as generally 'better' than others (as e.g. for network size and complexity). Also, this complements the one normative statement already integrated into the adapted framework (i.e. centrality by definition to be low). **Figure 7.2.1 shows the *adapted* version of the network assessment framework** (to be compared with the original version presented in chapter 3.2). It still holds that, overall, the adaptations refer less to the content as such, and more to enhanced conciseness of categories and related practicability of the original assessment framework, and now also to **transparency as to normative statements and principles related to 'network' features: The indicator categories network 'structure' and 'processes' are now complemented by network 'principles'** (with the former 'assessment principle 3' being dissolved). The 'new' assessment category on *'network principles/ sustainability principles'* contains: nurturing *trustful* relations; remaining *lateral* intra-network links; *avoiding* network centrality; and implementing the 'law' of *reciprocity*; (Networks should apply these principles by their very definition.) The new assessment category also contains: *participation/* wide spread ownership; *transparency*; *sharing* of information, resources, risks/ equity in access to resources; *accountability*; *consensus orientation*; strategic, *long term* orientation with reflection of the full range of opportunities; and enabling *continuous learning* for individuals and organizational systems alike.

Introducing **the assessment category 'principles' allows to partially integrate the two parts of the assessment framework on a network's 'network dimension' and its 'Health Promotion dimension'.** The indicator 'extent to which processes allow or encourage *continuous learning...*' will be moved into the new element on 'principles' as will be the one on *'participation'*. It could be argued that this should be done with the Health Promotion principle of 'empowerment', too; but in light of both its *central* role in the Health Promotion concept and that only some organization analysts refer to this concept, it will be kept in the Health Promotion specific part of the assessment framework. *'Empowerment' issues remain to be assessed in the context and from the perspective of Health Promotion*. This makes even more sense if considering that necessary further clarifications of this concept and its application are more likely to arise from Health Promotion research than organization or network research.

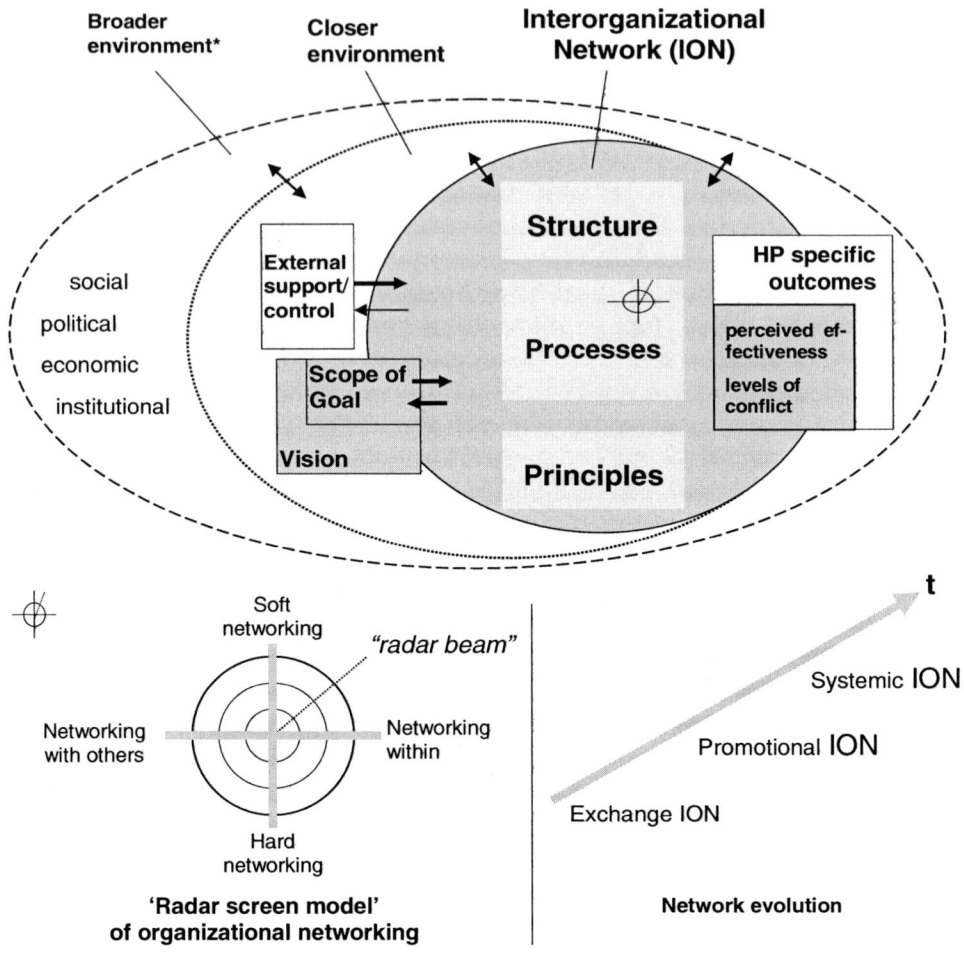

Figure 7.2.1: The comprehensive assessment framework for interorganisational networks - key elements. Adapted version with special attention to Health Promotion as the field of application. (bottom left: 'Radar screen' model by Hastings 1993 / bottom right: Network evolution based on ION-evolution-theory by Alter and Hage 1993).

Not only from a practical standpoint the various principles should be taken as categories of (self-) reflection and observation of the overall network 'climate' rather than a list of distinct network indicators - also because several of these concepts need yet further clarification or agreement on a common definition. What Marmot (1999) stressed with view to the social environment at large and health influencing factors therein applies to the social climate within (and around) a network, too: It is a challenge to 'unpick' the social environment in a way that is susceptible to scientific assessment efforts *and* relevant to policy and practice; and *the more one attempts to unpick social environments and separates them into discrete analytical categories, the further one retreats from reality*.

Therefore, when undertaking a first network assessment it is recommended to use the sets of indicators in the three core network assessment categories 'structure', 'processes', and 'principles' not one after the next and in full each time but rather take a step wise approach focusing on some indicators each while examining the network in a 'radar beam' mode. The structural indicators identified above as to be first, a network's organizational networking, and network climate in terms of the four principles that define interorganizational networks (trustful, lateral, non-central, reciprocal relations…) should be reflected upon first; together and complemented by network goal and objectives they provide a very meaningful overall picture of a network in focus. This is best complemented by a short look at its evolutionary stage.

'Network evolution' as element of the network assessment framework

The main innovation introduced to interorganizational network research by Alter and Hage is their theory of *network evolution* and the closely linked *network typology* (obligational/ promotional/ systemic networks, i.e. exchange/ concerted action/ joint production networks). Such network evolution was integrated into the original network assessment framework as a promising assessment category; but **it was originally subsumed under the heading 'assessment principle 2: attention to development stages/ levels'. The latter turned out to be too all encompassing** at least for assessment efforts from an international level. It could not be pilot tested in its entirety, i.e. regarding stages of the *initial* setting-up of *new* networks, and stages of organizational change *within* member *organizations* of a network (such as network schools). This was due to the paucity of documentation of such developments at international level regarding the three network cases examined combined with the lack of theoretical or consistent empirical knowledge. The latter indicates that even a better level of documentation would not have fully solved the problem. Also - in light of the limited understanding of the phase of newly creating a network - the inclusion of some aspects related to the time before a network has come into being, into an instrument to assess *existing* networks makes not yet much sense. However, 'assessment principle 2' *was* pilot tested, but with concentration on the assessment of 'network development as a continuous process of evolving and maturing over time with three identifiable but overlapping network development stages', i.e. the Alter/Hage-theory of 'network evolution' that applies once a network is in place. In light of the yet limited empirical basis of the network evolution theory one questions needs to be answered before adapting the assessment framework accordingly:

Do the case study results of this research project support the 'network evolution' theory and the related network typology? This can be confirmed, at least as to the *first two* levels of network evolution: exchange/ obligational network, and promotional/ concerted action network. As expected, the former was found to be always realized first, the latter always some time after a certain level of exchange relations had been established. Also the three network cases studied, the European, German and Slovenian network for the development of Health Promoting Schools, exhibit the predicted continuity of such network evolution. While exchange relations were still being enhanced and expanded, network sections (or sub-groups of network members) started to develop concerted action in several cases. When considering Alter's and Hage's categorization of networks from 10 years of age on as 'older' networks, and those up to 5 years as 'young', it is no surprise that the networks examined (7 to 8 years of age) did not show signs of maturing into systemic, joint production networks yet. Also, from the perspective on large scale networks 'for the development of Health Promoting Schools' with schools concerned being integral *part* of such networks rather than an object to be transformed or 'produced' by a network of outside actors, this evolutionary step may not be of relevance anyway. In addition, goals such joint action of all network members in support of the creation of (policy) environments supportive of the network's goals (such as today at stake for the European Network ENHPS) would be achieved via '*concerted action'* in the area of advocacy (ENHPS as promotional network) rather than jointly 'produced by' that network.

Overall, the case studies have shown that **the inclusion of 'network evolution' into the network assessment framework is meaningful and practical.** Importantly, it draws attention to the fact that any established network has still development potentials at any time; that well established exchange relations should not be considered as signal for 'still stand' but as a good platform for selected, concerted action in support of particular network goals or objectives. Assessing a network's evolutionary level helps to identify, free and build on the full potential of particular member organizations, as it recognizes the importance of establishing and nurturing good exchange relations among all network members while at the same time encouraging (particularly interested and/or qualified) members to involve into concerted action on particular issues of importance to achieve the network goals. The strategic use of mechanisms such as Multi Member Action Plans is a promising one as Healthy Cities Networks have shown.

In sum, also 'assessment principle 2' ('attention to development stages') can be transformed into a specific network assessment category. In contrast to the modification of 'principle 3' and the few other small adaptations of the ION assessment framework presented above, here not just a regrouping or better illustration of indicators and assessment framework is at stake but *a change of content*. For the above reasons the focus of 'assessment principle 2' is now limited to the issue of network evolution and the inherent sequence of unfolding general *purposes* of networking within a net (exchange, concerted action, joint production). **The former 'assessment principle 2' is now one *concise* network assessment category labeled 'network evolution (and purposes)'.** This strengthens the framework's character as practical instrument and better highlights the important assessment dimension of *changes over time* (see fig. 7.2.1, bottom right).

By now, the critical appraisal of Part A of the proposed network assessment framework (on a network's 'network dimension') led to some adaptations of the framework. With one exception, the specific adaptations did not concern the content areas covered but the *grouping of indicators, dissolving a few overlaps of assessment categories, and the overall illustration* of the assessment framework. Figure 7.2.1 (as compared to fig. 3.1.1) shows that **this re-grouping or re-shaping of selected elements or indicators led to an adapted Part A of the network assessment framework that is more clear and practical and still covers almost all assessment areas as before.** And a few overlaps with framework Part B on a network's 'Health Promotion dimension' have been dissolved, too.

From a 'logic model' for studying networks towards an interactive model for network assessment

The case studies have shown that attempts like those by Alter and Hage to identify particular causal links between different network features in the direction of creating a 'logic model' of network functioning do not lead too far. Nevertheless, the Alter/Hage studies and the results of the European, German and Slovenian case studies support an interesting assumption: that *complex* network goals – typical in Health Promotion - are linked to a) the occurrence of *high network complexity and high differentiation* (a causal relationship seems plausible) and b) the *preferred use of group or team methods of coordination.* And that *high differentiation may best be combined with intense coordination* to avoid dysfunctional levels of conflict within a net. This matches with the systems theoretic view of (multi-) organizational systems as self-regulatory systems. **Feed back loops such as coordinating mechanisms are important - not only *within* a system but also towards its *environment*.** Also the three network cases studied demonstrate that *network assessment must consider network-environment-interactions* which leads to **another simple but important adaptation** of that part of the original network assessment framework that builds on the 'network study frame' by Alter and Hage: There must be **two-way arrows between network and environment** (see the adapted framework in fig. 7.2.1). Similarly, not only the scope of network goals influences network structure and processes but, vice versa, complex or long term goals are being influenced by the latter - ideally while the network's *vision* is kept as a *stabilizing force* (such as the idea of creating "Health Promoting Schools" all over Europe). Explicitly illustrating the *interaction* between networks and their environments (rather than focusing one sided on network dependency as did Alter and Hage) helps to emphasize not only the importance of decisions by any network regarding its relative emphasis on 'organizational networking' within the net and with external others; it also draws attention to the notion of empowerment: by highlighting that any network *can* actively influence at least to a certain degree its environment, 'external control'-factors included – either directly or via additional cooperative links and advocacy efforts with external others. Even if this might take time.

Overall, when taking into account: a systems theoretic or social ecological perspective on social systems; Alter's and Hage's own findings; the network case studies undertaken; and also the yet limited understanding of interorganizational networks in general, **it can be concluded: a general assessment framework for interorganizational networks as strived for in this research project should - if interrelations between elements are addressed - follow an *interactive* rather than 'logic model' approach.**

In the light of this, it is no surprise that **the intended identification of "key characteristics"** of international networks for the development of Health Promoting Schools and similar networks **has its limits**: The third objective of this research project concerns the identification of "key characteristics" of such networks in terms of both network structures and processes. How far this objective could be achieved can be asked from two perspectives: looking at key characteristics of interorganizational networks *in general* (at least as to structures and processes), and at key characteristics *specific* to those interorganizational networks for the development of Health Promoting Schools or similar Settings. - With view to the former, i.e. **in general**, network characteristics may be judged as "key" on two grounds: a) if they are *defining* characteristics of an 'interorganizational network' per se; b) if there is good reason to judge that they are particularly important in achieving a network's goal or some kind of *valued* (even intermediate) network outcomes. As to point a), the research identified **some <u>defining</u> characteristics of interorganizational networks** as clusters or organizations:

- particular *qualities of interactions* and relations among network members: interactions for the *purpose* of at least exchange, eventually also concerted action, or even joint production; interactions based on *trustful* relations; and *lateral* links;
- two *structural features*: (one or more) defined boundaries for periods of time, i.e. clarity regarding network *(one or more) categories of members*; in addition, *low centrality* if any.

With view to the wide spread use of the term 'network' as a buzz word with little or no definition (also within and around the field of Health Promotion and networks for the development of health promoting Settings) the identification of these defining features of interorganizational networks is already a quite valuable step. It *allows to assess whether or not any so called "network" is indeed an interorganizational network (ION)* to which the proposed network assessment framework can be meaningfully applied.

A look at the whole set of indicators identified in the assessment framework and related discussions above show **several sub-sets of (often compound) indicators**: six indicators of *network structure* (including 'low centrality' as a defining network characteristic); three indicators of *network processes* of which the compound indicator 'organizational networking' encompasses six indicators alone: the extent of four networking processes (soft/ hard/ 'within' a net/ 'with others') and their relative emphasis twice (soft vs. hard/ 'within' vs. 'with others'); in addition, there is overall *'network evolution'*, a compound indicator, too. None of these indicators has been identified as being generally more important or more 'key' for network functioning and goal achievement than others. Rather it is clear that **various factors do interact, but the 'how' remains an open question**. Interestingly and as mentioned above, a few constellations of factors were found to be correlated to complex network goals. –

But in sum, there is no rational to select some of the indicators of network structure and processes generally as 'key' indicators of network functioning or success, not even if the focus is on 'reasonable' outcomes such as perceived effectiveness or levels of conflict within the network. This is no surprise as interorganizational networks and their member organizations are complex *social systems* the behaviors of which are, strictly spoken, unpredictable. **The whole sets of (structural and process) indicators are important research based categories for systematic (self-) reflection, observation and assessment of interorganizational networks**, be they networks for the development of Health Promoting Schools or other ones. **Attempts to identify 'key' indicators of interorganizational networks in *general*, beyond their defining characteristics, seem to be as elusive as the attempts to identify 'the key determinants of health'.** Nevertheless, it may be that for a *particular* network, context and period of time some network features need more attention than others – something to be identified by means of 'radar beam' type of self-observation and (self-) assessment. In the case of networks for the large scale development of Health Promoting Schools it will be of particular importance to look at the network's complexity, differentiation and networking with external others, as part of the resources for goal achievement will be influenced by or even in the hands of a range of actors across society.

Asking for the 'key' indicators concerning the range of **'principles'** that, in the *adapted* version of the assessment framework (fig. 7.2.1) have been made explicit in *one* assessment category is a different issue. Eight of the eleven network principles or principles to assure sustainability (not to be confused with the three 'assessment principles' of the original version of the framework) are known to be *"key factors for sustainable capacity development"*; the other three are *defining* features of interorganizational networks. Thus, **all of these principles are quite important in network assessment, at least if maintaining or improving a network's ability to achieve its goal is at stake or that of member organizations**. The latter is always the case if network organizations implement the 'health promoting Settings' approach and strive to enhance their capacity to promote health. This leads to the second perspective on a search for 'key characteristics' of networks: those that may be *specific* to interorganizational networks *for the development of Health Promoting Schools or similar Settings*.

Critical appraisal of the assessment frameworks consideration of a network's 'Health Promotion dimension'

The indicators proposed to assess a network's 'Health Promotion dimension' in Part B of the original assessment framework mirror two facts:

first, the general challenge posed to research and practice in the Health Promotion field that originates from the limited understanding and lack of consensus in the area of evaluating or assessing *complex interventions into social systems*; second, the main focus of this research project on identifying network indicators in terms of *structure and processes*.

The case studies confirmed that **from a Health Promotion perspective, the indicators of network structure do not need expansion or adaptation, and those on network processes only to a small extent**. Indicators of the application of the above-discussed 'principles' are of particular relevance also from a Health Promotion perspective. Basic principles and sustainability factors inherent in the Health Promotion concept such as 'participation' as well as factors often highlighted such as 'continuous learning' *are* covered when network assessment takes into account the set of 'principles' identified above from a *network* research perspective. If for some reason an assessment of a network needs to take a selective approach then, from a Health Promotion perspective, **the implementation of the principle of 'participation' must *always* be assessed. But - assessing a network's 'Health Promotion dimension' means that indicators of 'empowerment' must be added** and their potential overlaps with the *general* network indicators above have to be made explicit. Unfortunately, up today understandings or concepts of 'empowerment' vary in the field and *there is not the preeminent definition or concept of empowerment to build on when striving to enhance the proposed network assessment framework in this regard*. Should a network express it's understanding of empowerment, that one would be a reference point for assessment. But this is not yet common practice. Also the networks examined, i.e. the European network for the development of Health Promoting Schools and two national networks therein, did not yet document their particular understanding of 'empowerment'. (Documents on the 'later' German network, however, highlight links between empowerment and network functioning). To encourage these and other Health Promotion networks to clarify and make transparent how *they* understand and consider the core Health Promotion principle of 'empowerment', the indicator 'extent to which processes of empowerment are supported or facilitated' is not only kept as a main *Health Promotion specific 'process indicator';* **in the adapted network assessment framework empowerment is even more highlighted:** as a *Health Promotion specific* expansion of the newly shaped assessment category *'principles'*. The latter could be assessed at a minimal level with the help of indicators such as whether or not 'empowerment' is referred to in core network documents, and the extent to which members have reflected upon the meaning of this concept in relation to the network's goal and functioning. (see fig. 7.2.1)

After the pilot testing of the network assessment framework, of the originally four process indicators suggested as 'Health Promotion specific' remains not only the one on empowerment. Also the indicator 'extent to which a network represents, supports or encourages **intersectoral collaboration**' stays. This compound indicator is *measured in various facets by means of assessing the following structural and process indicators of an interorganizational network in general*: network *complexity* (which might show organizational members to represent more than one sector); and network *differentiation* (which might show a division of labor among network members that supports or encourages intersectoral collaboration, whether within the network or with 'other sectors' outside). Should the collaboration of different sectors within the network be an issue, further qualities could be assessed - by means of examining: *'networking within'* the net/ *connectivity* and/or networking *'with others'* (relative emphasis, extent); and *'operational processes'* (with methods of coordination used between sectors as quality indicator of intersectoral collaboration). But also other network features such as membership criteria, goal definition, and underlying concepts (e.g. the 'Health Promoting School' or other Settings concepts) could indicate the extent to which a network 'supports or encourages' intersectoral collaboration. Therefore, the **extent of intersectoral collaboration is kept as a separate, Health Promotion specific *process* indicator** also in the adapted version of the network assessment framework. Another important reason is: As explained earlier any network implementing the Health Promotion concept should early on reflect on the importance and type of intersectoral collaboration needed or aimed at - *after* it analyzed the *range* of factors that influence or co-determine the health of the population groups in focus (e.g. pupils and school staff) and the actors that influence these factors, too (from particular groups to local organizations to societal sectors).

Beyond indicators of network structure and processes, the network assessment framework covers two **other groups of 'Health Promotion specific' indicators**. A critical look at the first group of **'general indicators'** shows: Measuring the 'extent of the **integration of the ecological approach**' seems less important if a network is implementing (not only advocating for) the 'health promoting Settings'-approach, a genuinely social ecological approach to promote health. However, its measurement might unravel tendencies to target environmental factors *only* and not also directly the selected groups of people within these environments. This could indicate tendencies to regulate 'key determinants of health' *for* people rather than with them, which - in light of the long term over emphasis on individual health behaviors and the increased knowledge of social and socio-economic factors that influence health - would be an understandable, but potentially misleading direction. – To assess 'whether and how a network works in one or more of **the five Health Promotion action areas'** (from personal skills to healthy public policies, chap. 2.2) was a rather pragmatic suggestion of some Health Promotion researchers. It accounts for far reaching experiential knowledge and reflects international consensus documents such as the Jakarta Declaration (1997) and World Health Assembly Resolution on Health Promotion (WHA 1998) - and this with regard to the need to combine a range of (social) change strategies to sustainably modify the range of interrelated factors that co-determine the health of population groups (e.g. of school communities). *As long as there is a lack of guidance in the field* due to the lack of a consistent set of 'Health Promotion action theories' or models of social change for sustaining and promoting health, and/or due to the lack of appropriate evaluations of complex, multi-strategic Health Promotion interventions that could guide a network's Health Promotion practice, the *indicator concerning the five Health Promotion action areas should be simplified but kept:* as a point for (self-) reflection on a network's 'Health Promotion dimension'. **The adapted framework contains the adapted indicator '*whether or not* each of the five so called Health Promotion action strategies have been *considered* in a network's action planning'**, and similarly one on **whether or not these are being *acted upon* in one way or the other.** Results should be interpreted with caution.

The last set of Health Promotion specific network indicators refers to network outcomes and is best discussed jointly with indicators of general network outcomes.

Critical appraisal of the assessment framework's consideration of 'network outcomes'

The search for indicators to assess international networks for the development of Health Promoting Schools in terms of both structure and processes led to a comprehensive assessment framework that puts network structure and processes in context, i.e. in relation to network goals and factors in the network's closer environment as well as network outcomes. Neither from a network research nor a Health Promotion research perspective there is the approach to measuring network outcomes. A 'reasonable' outcome approach has been argued for in both fields which – in the original version of the network assessment framework developed - was taken on board in the form of an 'assessment principle 1'.

From a *practical* point of view, the **general network outcome indicators** taken from Alter and Hage (1993), i.e. levels of *'perceived effectiveness'* and of *'conflict'* within a network, seem to be a good starting point.

- Even though the case studies have shown that levels of conflict cannot be expected to be documented, **in networks with sufficient levels of trust or mutual acceptance assessing and reflecting on perceived levels of conflict should be possible**. - Obviously, measuring 'perceived effectiveness' becomes a tricky task if network goals and objectives are not clear and/or a wide range of desired outcomes is defined. Therefore, **network assessment efforts should only include perceived effectiveness if network goals and objectives are assessed, too** (with regard to their quantity and quality and in relation to resources available). However, the case studies have shown that in any case it is meaningful to **at least assess the overall level of satisfaction** of (groups of) network members with regard to their participation in the network at stake. Wide spread low levels or contradictive results would signal the need for further examinations.

Already a quick look at the assessment framework in terms of **indicators of network outcomes from a Health Promotion perspective** (framework Part B) points to a major challenge of the field of Health Promotion at large. As the case studies have demonstrated, the indicator, or better the implicit *sets* of indicators, related to assessing *the 'extent of achievement of goals and objectives set by a network'* leads to **a cascade of difficult issues and open questions** – at least in the case of networks for the development of health promoting schools or other Settings. While there is good scientific reason to *pursue* such goals there is little knowledge about appropriate approaches to evaluate intervention effectiveness. And problems start even earlier. Goals and objectives *set by* a network and those of others or of individual members only, need to be distinguished – but this is not necessarily easy. One indicator per goal and objective is unlikely enough. The inherent long term perspective of complex interventions such as those to create 'health promoting schools' call for *intermediate or short term* outcome measurement, but a widely agreeable evaluation model is yet lacking. At least, a model by Nutbeam (1999, 2000) provides some practical *categories* of potential or desired outcomes in Health Promotion or of intervention points; in the network case studies these proved useful for systematizing the range of goals, objectives or desired outcomes put forward related to the networks. While there will be much agreement that the general network assessment framework developed, rightly suggests to assess as far as possible the extent of achievement of *self set* network goals and objectives, the case studies have also shown: Even a focus on 'only' those desired outcomes that together reflect the creation of 'Health Promoting Schools' (HPS) makes the task of assessing self set goal achievement not much easier. – Although assessing the extent of achievement of goals and objectives of networks for HPS development and similar 'Settings networks' (beyond 'overall perceived effectiveness') remains a difficult task, the network assessment framework from a Health Promotion perspective must continue to ask for it.

Similarly, the assessment of a network's Health Promotion dimension has to include the *extent of consideration of up to date knowledge about the range of factors that influence or co-determine the health of the groups or communities in focus.* A range of indicators could be useful, from whether or not documents refer to such factors in one way or the other, to the extent of a network's knowledge development in this area (literature reviews, data collection), to whether action is undertaken to positively change or maintain the level of one or more of such factors and to what extent and with which results.

In conclusion, indicators to assess an interorganizational network's 'Health Promotion dimension' need clearly further elaboration - a challenging but worthwhile focus for a follow-up research project on assessing networks for the development of health promoting Settings such as schools. It would be no surprise if an examination of social or societal factors that co-determine health in this context would show a significant overlap between features of 'social capital' or similar factors and interorganizational networks for the development of health promoting Settings. As said before, the same is assumed for the feature 'empowerment'. If research would indeed unravel such overlaps, this would indicate an inherent health promotion potential of such interorganizational networks per se.

Now, that the various *elements* of the network assessment framework developed have been critically reviewed and some adaptations have been undertaken, the attention will be shifted to the assessment framework as a *whole*.

7.2.2 Critical appraisal of the network assessment framework as a whole

Besides a reflection on the value of the assessment framework as a concrete 'practical' instrument for network assessment in the field of Health Promotion and beyond, another point is of interest: that of the **general advantages of systematically applying an interorganizational network perspective** when examining *networks for the development of health promoting Settings such as schools*. The former will be addressed first.

The analysis of the "European Network of Health Promoting Schools" (ENHPS) and the Slovenian and German sub-networks therein from a network perspective was based on the assumption that these 'real life' networks are interorganizational networks, a thesis supported by all three network case studies. The case studies have shown that an important general advantage of the network research perspective is that, first of all, attention is drawn to a differentiated view on network 'members' and potential 'others' and, thus, on the *various* actors and their roles, responsibilities and relations. This way, as well demonstrated by the case studies, the **range of relevant actors within or around a network in focus becomes amenable to systematic analysis** and thereby, the **network-environment-interaction, too**. *Meaningful categories for systematic (self-) reflection, analysis and assessment* as offered by the network assessment framework developed help **reducing complexity** of network systems. In the case of the 'European Network for the development of Health Promoting Schools' and the overall ENHPS initiative it led to a differentiated view and understanding of the 'network' component and related support 'projects' as supportive network environments to be distinguished from the broader network environment (see figures 5.2.1, 5.4.1 and 5.6.1).

Assigning to a complex initiative such as the 'ENHPS initiative' an *ordering, consistent set of sub-categories* that is easy to understand and communicate provides a good basis for a crucial step in network assessment: to identify or further clarify and **distinguish between 'network goals' and goals of particular stakeholders related to the network.** The former refers to goals *of* the network, shared and agreed upon by all network members. The latter refers to *additional* goals related to the network, i.e. goals of particular stakeholders. Here, goals of both particular (groups of) network *members* and of 'external *others*' (e.g. network 'partners', or donors) are at stake. The three network cases examined have shown that currently **clarity of 'network goals' can *not* be presumed to exist in all network cases**. While multiple goals and objectives (and even modifications over time) are likely to occur not only in large scale Health Promotion interventions but any intervention into social systems with a long term perspective, it must be made transparent *whose* goals these are and in case of changes, *when* these occurred and ideally, why. Only then the increasingly recognized need and challenge of evaluating the effects of networks for the development of Health Promoting Schools and similar networks can be successfully tackled (see also below).

In the field of Public Health today as in other fields the term 'network' has become a buzz word. And there are at least three broad network categories, inter*organizational* networks, inter*personal* networks (e.g. expert networks, social networks), and a *mix* of both. As the network assessment framework developed in this research project is one for inter*organizational* networks (IONs), the question arises: **How far does the**

network assessment framework help to judge about whether a system labeled as a "network" is indeed an interorganizational network? How far does it help to clarify whether the whole network assessment tool could be meaningfully applied? To do so it should clearly identify those *defining 'core' characteristics* of interorganizational networks. This research project builds on the definition of interorganizational networks (IONs) as constituting 'the basic social form that permits interorganizational interactions of exchange, concerted action, and joint production based on *trustful* relations. Networks are bounded (…) clusters of organizations that, by definition, are *non- or less central collectives* of *legally separate, laterally linked* units. Therefore it is suggested: **Any network assessment using the assessment framework developed in this research project should start with a) an analysis of the *types* of network *members*** (considering both formally declared members and others that may be an *integral part* of a network but not *labeled* as network 'members' for whatever reason). **If network members are organizations or legally separate units** (or persons with a formal mandate to represent their organizations in the network), **then b) their relations and interactions should be examined**: first of all the level of **centrality** - which by definition of interorganizational networks should be low - and related to this, whether the interorganizational links are **lateral links** (as opposed to hierarchical ones) - which also by definition should be so and inherently means that member organizations do network in 'partnership' and voluntarily. - As the case of the German network nicely demonstrates, it may well be that in the *early* phase of network establishment centrality may be higher. However, particularly if goals of Health Promotion are pursued and its core principles of participation and empowerment, it can be reasonably assumed that centrality will soon be decreased and a true interorganizational *network* as defined above realized.

With view to 'very young' networks that are just being set up it should be noted, that **the network assessment framework developed is not laid out to assess the *initial* phases of *newly creating* interorganizational networks** whatever there purpose may be. As elaborated in chapter 2.4, such phases are up today not well understood. In light of the wide spread and increasing interest and conviction of the great *potential* of such organizational forms to successfully tackle *complex* (long term) goals such as those in Health Promotion, this is an important research area. Systematically deriving the 'lessons to be learned' on the initial setting up of networks from both a range of existing interorganizational networks in Public Health and networks just being created with context sensitivity would be a valuable step forward. This should include the main *reasons or motives* of organizations (e.g. schools or national centers) to *enter* a network or apply for network membership, as well as *processes of decision making* towards this end (within applicant organizations and the network at stake). That such knowledge is useful also for *existing* networks is demonstrated by the Slovenian network for the development of Health Promoting Schools: In preparation of the first wave of formal '*network expansion*' existing members synthesized the 'pro's and con's' of network membership to enable new schools to apply better informed for network membership.

After this look at some general advantages and attention points concerning the proposed network assessment framework as a whole, the attention will be shifted towards the notion of 'practicality'. This research project did strive for developing a '*practical*' instrument to assess international networks for the development of Health Promoting Schools and similar networks in terms of both structure and processes. How far this was achieved is reflected upon now.

The notion of 'practicality' and the adapted network assessment framework

There are **several possible indicators** to measure whether the network assessment framework is a 'practical' tool: First of all, the framework as a 'practical assessment instrument' *should serve practical purposes* such as enhanced network *documentation*; network *comparison*; systematic *self-reflection, -analysis and -assessment* efforts by network members; or even network *monitoring*. And as outlined below, it does. - As a 'practical' assessment instrument is meant to be meaningful for and used by actors or practitioners within networks, the assessment framework should be able to *accommodate network features that network actors perceive as important*. And when judging from that what has been documented over the years on the European, German and Slovenian networks for Health Promoting Schools development, the framework developed fulfills this criteria of 'practicality'. - Categories of indicators should be not only concise but also easy to understand. And after some introductory training network *actors themselves should be able to measure or well estimate* most if not all of the network features at stake (in quantitative or qualitative terms). This is taken up below. - An appropriate *visualization* would be helpful, too, and has therefore been done (fig. 7.2.1). - Also, a 'practical' network assessment framework should not only reduce complexity of the 'real world' of networks (by offering meaningful categories of reflection on them); it also should help to systematically reflect on and assess *general network functioning and development directions* over time. And as discussed below the network assessment framework meets also these criteria of 'practicality' to a good extent. - Finally, from a

Health Promotion perspective the 'practicality' of a network assessment framework is higher if there is a higher level of *integration of categories of general network indicators and Health Promotion specific indicators* – a step that has been done as part of the above critical appraisal of the various elements of the original assessment framework. However, *general and Health Promotion specific indicators should nevertheless be (and indeed remain) distinguishable*: on the one hand, in order to allow more informed decisions of network assessment initiatives that wish or need to focus on selected indicators only; on the other hand, to prepare for targeted adaptations of the framework in the future (which quite likely will occur as the areas of 'network assessment' and 'evaluating Health Promotion' are still under development).

Obviously, network *members* of the networks examined (i.e. the European, German and Slovenian networks for the development of Health Promoting Schools) **as well as members of similar networks will have to judge about the 'practicality' of the network assessment framework** developed within this research project; it is them to say how far it meets *their* practical needs when it comes to network documentation, analysis and appraisal. **The above and following conclusions as to the assessment framework's 'practicality' are those of a well informed 'external expert'** that since years is part of the supportive environments of the networks examined. A further look from this perspective at the *original*, pilot tested network assessment framework (chap. 3.2) and the *adapted* version elaborated above and illustrated in figure 7.2.1 leads to the following conclusions on 'practicality':

The network assessment framework developed is **well suited to guide network documentation efforts** in ways that make them more systematic, directed to core network dimensions, and also comparable. The **same applies to the identification of commonalities and differences** in basic terms: network vision, goals/objectives, structure, processes, basic principles of work, external resources available and related dependencies, and internal resources. (Internal resources, however, are indirectly assessed, by means of assessing network 'complexity' and 'differentiation', and eventually also membership criteria.) Should a network's Health Promotion related goals and objectives need systematization, the *complementary use of models that categorize desired or potential Health Promotion outcomes* is recommended; the adapted model originating from Nutbeam (fig. 3.1.3) has in the case studies proven to be useful. **With view to network monitoring**, the adapted assessment framework with its six categories of indicators provides **a good basis and general direction**; but which indicators of the large set of indicators would be useful for particular monitoring purposes needs to be negotiated and decided jointly by the various stakeholders.

In comparison to the original (pilot tested) version, and as a result of the above critical appraisal **the <u>adapted</u> version of the comprehensive network assessment framework has a reduced number of more concise elements or assessment categories, which – at least at a general level - should be easy to understand for network members.** As visualized in figure 7.2.1, *the complex world of interorganizational networks* such as large scale networks for the development of Health Promoting Schools *is well captured by six categories*: vision and goals; external support or control; network structure, processes, and principles; as well as network outcomes (at least two general ones: perceived effectiveness and levels of conflict within the net).

While Health Promotion specific *processes and principles* (such as participation and empowerment) are already sufficiently accommodated by this framework, Health Promotion specific *outcomes* are not yet. This is not because the framework is not able to do so (figure 7.2.1 offers already a place for them). But there is a) no agreement in the field as to *general* categories of potential or desired outcomes of Health Promotion interventions to which this general network assessment framework should refer to; (even the understanding of the term 'outcome' is in flux). b) For the particular networks in focus of this research project, the about 40 national networks that make up the European network for the development of Health Promoting Schools, *neither a common approach* to the categorization and evaluation of network outcomes has been found, *nor a common set of (categories of) indicators* to measure a school's progress in transforming itself into a 'Health Promoting School'. Therefore, **also the adapted version of the network assessment framework developed has to remain fairly general when it comes to indicators of 'Health Promotion specific outcomes'.** There are three suggestions in this regard:

a) to focus on the extent of achievement of 'network goals' as discussed above, *at least* in terms of members' *perceptions* of effectiveness; complementary to this

b) to assess how far preconditions of *empowerment* processes on the side of member organizations and people therein have been realized (e.g. mechanisms for participation); and

c) to *at least* assess the extent of *awareness* of up-to-date knowledge about the range of factors that jointly influence or co-determine health, and ideally also the extent of their consideration (n discussions, documents, etc.) – with focus on those factors particularly related to a network's goal (see also chap. 7.1).

Overall, with view to the notion of 'practicality' of the assessment framework it can be said that **the adapted network assessment framework reduces complexity without neglecting the interplay of various network features**. Particularly the integration of Hastings 'radar screen model' of organizational networking **facilitates first interpretations of a network's functioning as a whole in a comprehensive and yet practical way** - by guiding into a (radar beam like) systematic reflection on extent and relative weight of core networking processes and the assessment of the findings in relation to the resources available to a network to achieve its goals. The 'radar screen model' (in fig. 7.2.1 bottom left) links, and to a certain degree even integrates the assessment of 'network structure' and 'network processes'.

As the case studies have shown, the proposed **network assessment framework is applicable to different types of networks in different contexts**. It is applicable to *networks for the development of Health Promoting Schools* in Europe; and there is no reason to believe that this does not apply to networks for the same purpose in other world regions and countries. (Those networks that unlike the European Network do *not* encompass the target Settings/ schools as members will just show differences in network 'complexity' and 'differentiation'.) The assessment framework did also prove to be applicable to both *international* and *national* networks; and there is no reason to assume, that it would not be applicable to sub-national or *regional* networks, too. Also, it proved to be applicable to networks that occurred in *different political systems and cultural contexts:* for example, in a large, federalist country (Germany) as well as in a small, more centralized country (Slovenia), in a 'Western' as well as 'Eastern' European country; and from what is known of their European 'parent' network ENHPS there is no reason to assume that the framework would not apply to networks that occurred in other European countries, too. It seems also applicable not only to networks for the development of health promoting *schools* but *other Settings, too,* at least to other formal elemental Settings/ organizations; but there is no reason to assume that this would not apply to contextual/ multi-organizational Settings such as Healthy Cities or Municipalities, too. Thus, the network assessment framework developed is **from an international perspective promising and practical for network assessment initiatives**. - It seems a *major strengths* of the framework to clearly distinguish between the core 'interorganizational *networks*' for the development of Health Promoting Schools, and closely related support systems or 'projects'. The latter seem to differ more strongly depending on variations in the political contexts than the former; or the other way around, networks are flexible enough organizational forms to adapt to different environmental circumstances without loosing their genuine shape.

A last issue of 'practicality' is of course, **how far network members themselves would be able to measure or at least well estimate the scale of the various network features suggested by the network assessment framework.** With regard to the assessment categories **network 'structure' and 'processes'**, the foci of this research project, it can be said: Almost all network *characteristics can be measured to a meaningful degree without complicate measurement procedures* or tools. But as to several network features, particularly 'organizational networking' and 'connectivity', 'differentiation', and 'continuous self-reflection, observation and assessment', it is advisable to approach measurements or estimations *by main groups* of network member organizations, not by individual organizations (as has been demonstrated in the three case studies). – However, it needs to be noted that the assessment framework does include some concepts that are not necessarily clearly defined in the field or the understanding of which will vary. These need to be made explicit in *each* individual assessment effort and indicators need to be identified accordingly. This refers mainly to the assessment category **'network principles/ sustainability principles'**, particularly to the concept of 'empowerment' but also concepts such as 'transparency', 'accountability' or 'enabling continues learning'.

But with or without such conceptual issues, Health Promotion evaluation in general as well as interorganizational network assessment in the field of Health Promotion in particular remain quite challenging action areas. Those who wish to use the proposed network assessment framework should gain sufficient understanding of networks as multi-organizational systems and the various network features identified. This will be easier for those that not only have experience as network members or close partners but a high level of *awareness* of 'their' network's character as an *interorganizational network* for exchange and may be joint action, as a flexible mechanism to pursue complex goals. In addition, they should have some experience in the area of evaluating complex projects or interventions. Obviously, **the comprehensive network assessment framework as a whole is not meant to be a 'tool for the hand of practitioners' in general.** But its elements **can be used to guide step by step into a deeper understanding of a network.** The 'gray' assessment categories in figure 7.2.1 (top) are good areas for self-reflection and observation; also the 'radar screen model' (bottom left) can be used quite easily and meaningfully to reflect on networking practices of either an individual network member organization or a network as a whole.

Conclusion

After this critical appraisal of the network assessment framework developed it can be concluded that: a) the objectives of this research project have been achieved; b) the pilot testing of the original network assessment framework did hardly give reason to adaptations as regards content; but it did lead to important adaptations in terms of regrouping of indicators and improving the conciseness of assessment categories; c) the adaptations enhanced the framework's practicability; the adapted network assessment framework illustrated in figure 7.2.1 is practical enough to be offered to the networks in focus and their partners (in support of systematic reflection and assessment efforts on the networks as particular organizational systems to achieve goals, and for a *further testing* of the proposed assessment framework); d) the case studies have helped to further integrate various elements of the original network assessment framework that stemmed from different research areas; this includes the originally separate framework parts 'A' and 'B' on a network's 'interorganizational network dimension' and its 'Health Promotion dimension'; however, the integration was done more on pragmatic than theoretical grounds for reasons elaborated above (state of theory development in interorganizational relations and Health Promotion/ paucity of appropriate and comparable empirical studies/ etc.).

7.3   Theses and outlook

This comprehensive *pilot* project on assessing interorganizational networks for the large-scale development of Health Promoting Schools and similar networks has been brought to a closure. It remains to check on the three theses put forward at the very beginning and to look ahead towards future research and action areas.

Thesis 1 had been a quite complex one with multiple facets: **"The sustainable creation of 'health promoting Settings' (such as Health Promoting Schools) on a *large scale* across countries is enabled and facilitated by a *network approach* for mutual benefit and learning."** Its *underlying assumption has been supported* by the analyses of the scientific and value basis of the Health Promotion concept and developments of the field (chap. 2.1/ 2.2): that 'since Ottawa' the field of Health Promotion did evolve beyond the Settings approach; while latest health research has confirmed the relevance and potential of that approach, the field brought about new *complementary* approaches, particularly the 'network approach'. - But *thesis 1 itself* needs yet a closer look – an easier task once the less complex theses 2 and 3 are confirmed or disproved.

Thesis 2 was the following: **"International networks for the development of 'health promoting Settings' (such as the "European Network of Health Promoting Schools") are *inter-organisational* networks. Therefore, their assessment requires the use of *general interorganizational network indicators* besides those related to Health Promotion goals."** The *first part of the thesis has been clearly confirmed*: Informed by network research (chap. 2.4 and 3), the case studies of the European Network and its German and Slovenian sub-networks (chap. 5) did confirm these networks' character as interorganizational networks (IONs). - As to the *second part of the thesis* it should be recalled that Health Promotion through a network approach is a practice hardly analysed yet. In order to understand how and why networks as interventions to promote health do or do not achieve particular results, their resources, processes, and environmental factors have to be assessed in more detail - besides Health Promotion specific processes or outcomes (such as empowerment or changes in resources and co-determinants of health). This is required even more if networks explicitly aim at 'disseminating' experiences and results. Considering general network features in the assessment of Health Promotion networks also *makes sense* in light of the interesting similarities between features of 'interorganizational networks' as defined in this research project and 'social capital' (see below).

Thesis 3 formulated at the outset was: **"The organisational form of 'interorganizational networks' matches well with Health Promotion goals, strategies and principles in general and the 'health promoting settings' -approach in particular."** The *first part has been confirmed* already by the analysis in chapter 3.1, and the *second part has been supported*, too, at least on theoretical or conceptual grounds. The above critical appraisal of the now pilot tested assessment framework (chap. 7.2) *supports this thesis* even more: it identified particular overlaps as to process features and principles of interorganizational networks and Health Promotion programs in general (e.g. participation, and long term commitment to a shared vision and goal and continuous learning). As was shown, the organisational form of an interorganizational network (ION) is particularly well matching with two typical features of Health Promotion interventions: certainly with complex goals pursued in changing environments; and apparently with empowerment processes, too. Empowerment processes will be supported or facilitated by interactions based on trustful relations, mutuality and voluntary participation, i.e. interactions typical for interorganizational 'networks' but further research is definitely needed in this regard. - That the ION approach is particularly matching with the 'Settings approach', i.e. the *second part of the thesis, has been confirmed in parts*: the organisational form of interorganizational networks serves well if a linking of 'formal Settings' (i.e. mono- or multi-organisational systems) for the purpose of information and experience exchange, mutual learning, and avoidance of "reinventing the wheel" is desired; as to 'informal Settings' (such as quarters of towns), however, this remains to be examined.

When looking now **back to thesis 1** and its various *facets,* the following can be concluded: The existence of a *'network approach'* has been confirmed (in the form of an *interorganizational* network approach). That this supports among others *'mutual benefit and learning'* has been demonstrated, too: On the one hand, mutuality is a defining characteristic of the networks in question; on the other hand, several case study findings support this statement (i.e. voluntary network membership, low drop out quotes in spite of financial incentives, widespread general satisfaction, mutual relations among pilot schools and 'their' national support centers, and sub-networks jointly expressing the relevance and importance of mutuality and learning in the network). The case studies also confirm that the networks examined facilitate *'across countries'* the *'large scale' development* of - let's say - "Health Promoting Schools in the making" (with remarkable 70% of European countries voluntarily involved as well as, first hundreds, today thousands of schools). Unfortunately, the evaluations undertaken as of now are not appropriate enough to allow a judgment about the extent to which network schools do or did indeed transform themselves into *'Health Promoting Schools'* (HPS); but some data on pilot schools, particularly from the first network evaluation in Germany but also from the ENHPS Schools Data Base and Slovenian network evaluation, indicate that schools do develop into this direction. That the school's HPS related efforts might be *'sustainable'* is indicated by low drop out quotes at the level of network schools and national support centers alike, and the emergence of sub-national/ regional level support or coordinating centers in some countries. Thus, **overall thesis 1 holds but to be confirmed in its entirety further research is needed**, particularly on: appropriate evaluation approaches to measure progress towards the desired network outcome of 'schools becoming Health Promoting Schools'; the sustainability of such results; and the assumed transferability of the findings to other Settings networks.

Looking ahead

This research project amalgamated two research perspectives: interorganizational relations and network research (with capacity development) on the one hand, and Health Promotion research and research on health factors on the other. The development and pilot testing of the new assessment framework for interorganizational networks (IONs) has shown that inter-*organizational* relations research (on private/ public sectors), *macro*-perspective capacity development research (on public/ NGO sectors/ society at large), and research on collaborative Health Promotion practice (on communities/ organizations *locally*) confirm or at least well complement each other. And combined with some fundamental Health Promotion research this provides the scientific basis for the comprehensive assessment framework for interorganizational networks for the development of Health Promoting Settings and similar networks.

Similarities of these domains were identified not only as to network features but also remaining challenges: **Theory development** needs to be advanced and the carving out of implicit theories. Social-ecological and social change theories are of particular interest to interorganizational network and Health Promotion research alike. Network research and assessment is not sufficiently guided by theory yet. – In addition, **more empirical research on interorganizational networks** is needed, in general and with view to the field of Health Promotion and 'Settings-networks' in particular. However, the abovementioned research domains identified already matching or complementary sets of network features and assessment categories. - Interorganizational network research and Health Promotion intervention research share the **evaluation challenges related to interventions into complex social systems or social-ecological approaches** to action. Appropriate evaluation approaches are yet to be developed, for both the health-promoting Settings approach and interorganizational network approach. While Health Promotion research since the 1990s paid increased attention to the former (particularly to organization development in support of health), the latter is hardly examined.

The pilot research on network assessment undertaken in this research project points to several **research areas whose results remain to be harvested** to advance interorganizational network research and assessment: From a network perspective, this refers to *policy network research*; it likely bares some valuable lessons to be learned: as to understanding interorganizational networks in general, and the potential of networks (for the development of Health Promotion Schools) to successfully influence policies in support of health. - From a Health Promotion but also organization development perspective, results of *empowerment research* should be systematically examined as to their contributions to advancing the understanding and assessment of interorganizational networks (IONs). As this research project has shown, *process* features of IONs, and trustful and mutual *relations and interactions* between members and with external others, are key features of such networks. These need particular attention. It remains to be examined how far key features and conditions for empowerment processes overlap with features of interorganizational networks, particularly process features and network and sustainability principles. Interorganizational networks (IONs) by their very nature seem to offer opportunities for empowerment processes on the side of organizations and people; and the Health Promotion principle of empowerment seems to facilitate that Health Promotion actors engage in demanding processes of interorganizational networking. – A third exciting research area whose potential contribution to the advancement of ION assessment should be explored is *social capital research.* It is separately addressed below.

With view to **particular 'network issues'** some need special research attention in the future - for the benefit of networks for the development of Health Promoting Schools (HPS) and interorganizational networks (IONs) in general: Not much is known about the *initial creation* of such networks, a phase not covered by the assessment framework developed. But even more important is research on *mid and long term network functioning,* 'good practice', network *evolution,* and valued network *outcomes.* While as to the former experiential knowledge of a range of networks still waits to be analyzed, as to the latter the focus should first of all be on analyses by 'families' of networks, such as the several year "old" networks for HPS development. - The potential of the ION approach or *network initiation as a goal specific, large-scale intervention* (to, for example, promote health), as opposed to the 'spontaneous' emergence of such networks or traditional 'top down' initiatives, needs further examination. Research on reasons to enter and, most importantly, to *remain* over years in networks for the development of Health Promoting Schools and similar networks is still scarce and particularly needed as to 'intervention *target* organizations' (e.g. schools) as network *members.* Related to this, network *evolution* is an important research area to be advanced; it highlights that interorganizational "networks" that deserve their name are not just short term or 'one off' projects but long term interorganizational arrangements and investments; they allow to not only pursue one complex goal agreed upon at a particular point in time but the taking up of any joint succeeding or future goal on the way; this is possible a) without that the organizational set up needs change and, most importantly b) while allowing to effectively build on the quality relations and trust among member organizations that all those involved did invest in and develop in the pursuit of their first joint goal.

Overall, future research must look at the **comparative advantage** of the organizational form of **interorganizational networks (IONs) and other multi-organizational forms** such as 'intersectoral action' or '- collaboration' (much called for in Public Health today). Decisions on implementing the network approach and related investments (or the lack thereof) should be better informed (decisions by members, external supporters, and particularly those that are yet to get involved). A general 'public health argument' for the flexible form of interorganizational networks is the need of *sustainable* improvements in spite of the dynamic interplay of a range of factors that influence or co-determine health. This cannot be achieved by any one organization, sector or societal level alone; and inter-organizational collaboration needs a long term but flexible framework. It would be of great value to systematically derive from current network practice the *specific* answers of organizations, and individuals in organizations, to questions such as: 'why such networks?' and 'why we in such networks?' This applies not only to the field of Health Promotion but beyond. Answers lie not only in the area of field specific goal achievement but also in the linking of the latter to important other societal needs or goals, and to overall societal and global changes that influence field specific goal achievement. Examples in Europe are needs to improve *education* systems and the *quality of life* of populations.

From a Health Promotion perspective, the li**nk between 'interorganizational networks' (IONs)** and factors that are known to be **social resources or co-determinants of health** is quite exciting. Do such networks as defined in this research project not only match with Health Promotion approaches and principles but also have the potential to make a direct contribution to the health of populations? In particular interesting are similarities in features of interorganizational networks for the development of health promoting Settings and 'social capital'. Are such networks structures, in which social capital manifests itself? Are they even mechanisms to build social capital? If social capital is indeed a health resource or co-determinant of the health of populations (as recent studies in 'developed' countries after controlling for income have shown), any interorganizational network for the development of local Settings and similar networks could have a genuine health promotion potential – no matter whether it pursues health related goals or not. Already other researchers pointed into this direction (e.g. Roussos, Fawcett 2000). Social capital may be both facilitating the relationships needed *for* collaboration and a byproduct *of* collaborative partnerships that influences valued outcomes related to community health and development. Possible 'side effects' of collaborative partnerships include enhanced trust. - Although overall still loosely defined, current conceptualizations of social capital show a common conceptual core such as distinctions between a structural and a cognitive dimension (the extent and intensity of social ties and functioning within or across societal levels, and *perceptions* of these social ties and functioning). A quick comparative look at the defining characteristics, process indicators and principles of interorganizational networks (IONs) identified in this research project, and existing measures of social capital (e.g. Dimakakos 2002) show interesting overlaps: measures on both sides relate to *trust*ful relations, social and institutional *links, reciprocity, voluntary membership* in groups or organizational systems, *participation, sharing, collective or concerted* action, and the notion of *equity or perceived fairness*. This supports the above-assumed links between IONs and social capital. - In addition, it is interesting that some of the indicators remind of conditions for empowerment processes to take place, for example, people-to-people interactions based on mutual respect, tolerance and social support, or participatory processes. Network assessment in the field of *Health Promotion* would much benefit from further research into the exciting **triangle of interorganizational network building and networking, social capital (or other social co-determinants of health), and empowerment.** However, both potential synergies and contradictions should receive attention.

The network approach in Health Promotion seems to well advance the field as to the core goal of *enabling* people to gain control over the factors that influence their health, by serving not only as a platform for mutual learning and exchange about *local* solutions, but as a mechanism for local organizations and people to join forces, jointly advocate for and act towards improvements in those resources or co-determinants of health that are *beyond* local control. It is one of the great strengths of the organizational form of **interorganizational networks** (IONs) to be **able to formally but flexibly link organizations not only from public and non-public sectors but *different levels* of society (local to global) - in *lateral* ways** and in the pursuit of a *common* goal. As such the network (ION) approach offers opportunities to get *locally defined priorities* and perceived needs better accepted by macro-level societal actors, and to *buffer contradictory priority setting* for health related action at *higher* hierarchical or systems levels. But again, much further research is needed into the particular strengths of the network approach in Health Promotion and beyond.

In light of the complexity of network research and practice and the lack of appropriate evaluation approaches it is important to *link future empirical research and network theory development* more closely. **Interdisciplinary efforts** are crucial to make significant progress. This would further strengthen the scientific underpinning of the assessment instrument for networks for the development of Health Promoting Settings and similar networks developed in this research project. It would guide further refinements of indicator categories and indicators, and also strengthen the overall rational for the interorganizational network approach in Health Promotion.

Meanwhile, it is important to **support and advance ongoing practice of interorganizational networks** in the field of Health Promotion or Public Health. One important point is to support their response to *external pressures to prove the value of their existence*. In the case of networks for Health Promotion such as Health Promoting Schools this is closely related but not at all limited to proving outcomes in terms of HPS development. Measured and communicated as to their value must be also achievements such as in joint working and mutual learning, in improved interorganizational and interpersonal links, policies, social activation levels of core people or groups in support of the network's goal, in social cohesion and trust – whether at the level of schools, regional and/or national level network members, or other organizations. Nutbeam (1999) has made this point very clearly: there are many outcomes in Health Promotion (and Public Health) that are to be achieved first or in conjunction with action directed at a) *sustainable* and b) *positive changes* in health resources or co-determinants of health and their interplay at various life stages. An appropriate and widely agreed upon *typology of Health Promotion outcomes* is much needed and ideally includes outcomes in terms of improved inter-organizational (network) practice in support of health, too. Anyway, networks for the development of Health Promoting Settings and other interorganizational networks are not *only* to be assessed as to their *current* network goal but *also* as to the capacity being built to achieve *future* goals. The network assessment framework developed in this research project is a helping tool towards this end that now needs further testing in 'real life' assessment efforts.

References

- Abelin T/ Brzezinski Z J/ Carstaits Vera D L (Eds.) (1987) Measurement in health promotion and protection. (WHO Regional Publications, European Series No.22). WHO/EURO: Copenhagen
- Adelaide Recommendations on Healthy Public Policy (1988) Recommendations from the 2nd International Conference on Health Promotion, Adelaide, Australia. WHO/HPR/HEP/95.2. WHO: Geneva (www.who.int/hpr/conference)
- Alter Catherine/ Hage Jerald (1993) Organizations working together. Thousand Oaks, California
- Anderson Rob/ Kickbusch Ilona (1990) Health Promotion. A resource book. WHO/EURO, Copenhagen.
- Ansell Christopher K/ Parsons Craig A/ Darden Keith A (1997) Dual networks in European Regional Development Policy. In: Journal of Common Market Studies 35(3): 347-375
- Antonovsky Aaron (1979) Health, stress and coping: new perspectives on mental and physical wellbeing. San Francisco
- Antonovsky Aaron (1987) Unraveling the mystery of health. How people manage stress and stay well. San Francisco.
- Antonovsky Aaron (1996) The salutogenic model as a theory to guide health promotion. In: Health Promotion International 11(1): 11-18
- Arnhold Wolfgang (1997) Let's learn together. Collaboration. - Case study Germany. In: ENHPS (1997b) First Conference of the European Network of Health Promoting Schools "The Health Promoting School – an investment... (Case study book). ENHPS, WHO/EURO: Copenhagen, p.7
- Arnold Wolfgang/ Barkholz Ulrich/ Gabriel Regine/ Heindl Ines/ Paulus Peter (1994) Netzwerk Gesundheitsfoerdernde Schulen. Erster Zwischenbericht der Projektleitung und der wissenschaftlichen Beratung (Berichtszeitraum 1.8.1993-31.7.1994). Flensburg, Kiel, Magdeburg: NGS/ Projektunterstuetzungszentrum Deutschland: Rostockerstr. 6, D-24944 Flensburg, Germany.
- Arnold Wolfgang/ Barkholz Ulrich/ Gabriel Regine/ Heindl Ines/ Paulus Peter (1995) Netzwerk Gesundheitsfoerdernde Schulen. Zweiter Zwischenbericht der Projektleitung und der wissenschaftlichen Begleitung (Berichtszeitraum 1.8.1994-31.7.1995). Flensburg, Kiel, Magdeburg: NGS/ Projektunterstuetzungszentrum Deutschland: Rostockerstr. 6, D-24944 Flensburg, Germany.
- Badura Bernard/ Kickbusch Ilona (Eds.) (1991) Health promotion research: Toward a new social epidemiology. (WHO Regional Publications, European Series, No.37) WHO/EURO: Copenhagen
- Baird PA (1994) The role of genetics in population health. In: Evans, RG/ Barer ML/ Marmor Th.R (Eds.) (1994) Why are some people healthy and others not? New York, pp133-159
- Barham Kevin (1991) Networking – the corporate way round international discord. In: Multinational Business, No.4
- Baric Leo (1994) Health promotion and health education practice. Module 2. The organizational model. Altrincham
- Baric Leo (1996) Health promotion and health eduction. Handbook for students and practitioners. Altrinsham/Cheshire
- Baric Leo (1997) Accountability and the Settings Approach. In: EuroNEWS - Quarterly newsbulletin for IUHPE-members in Europe, Dec.1997. Vol.V(4): 5-8
- Barkholz Ulrich/ Gabriel Regine (Eds.) (1994) Spuren zeigen – Spuren suchen. Gesundheitsfoerderung im schulischen Alltag. (Dokumentation einer internationalen Fachtagung in Senkelmark/ Flensburg, 22-27August 1993). Flensburg: Netzwerk Gesundheitsfoerdernde Schulen, Projektunterstuetzungszentrum Deutschland.

- Barkholz Ulrich/ Gabriel Regine/ Jahn Holger/ Paulus Peter (1998) OPUS - Offenes Partizipationsnetz und Schulgesundheit. Gesundheitsfoerderung durch vernetztes lernen. Erster Zwischenbericht der Projektleitung und der wissenschaftlichen Begleitung (Berichtszeitraum 1.6..1997-30.6.1998) Flensburg, Lueneburg: OPUS Nationales Koordinierungszentrum Deutschland, Rostockerstr.6, D-224944 Flensburg
- Barkholz Ulrich/ Gabriel Regine/ Jahn Holger/ Paulus Peter (2001) Offenes Partizipationsnetz und Schulgesundheit. Gesundheitsfoerderung durch vernetztes lernen. Bundesministerium fuer Bildung und Forschung: Bonn-Bad Godesberg
- Barkholz Ulrich/ Paulus Peter (1998) Gesundheitsfoerdernde Schulen. Konzept, Projektergebnisse, Moeglichkeiten der Beteiligung. Gamburg
- Barmer Ersatzkasse (Ed.) (w.y.) Netzwerk Gesundheitsfoerdernde Schulen. Ein europaeisches Projekt. (gedruckt zwischen 1995 und Sommer 1996)
- Barnekow Rasmussen Vivian (1996) How the Network is financed. In: ENHPS Technical Secretariat (1996) Network News (Newsletter of the ENHPS). ENHPS, WHO/EURO: Copenhagen, p19
- Barnekow Rasmussen Vivian (1997) Editorial. In: ENHPS Technical Secretariat (1997) Network News (Newsletter of the ENHPS). ENHPS, WHO/EURO: Copenhagen, p2
- Barnekow Rasmussen Vivian/ Rivett David/ Ziglio Erio (1996) The European Network of Health Promoting Schools A joint WHO-CEC-CE project. In: World Health Magazine (March 1996). WHO: Geneva
- Barnekow Rasmussen Vivian/ Rivett David/ Ziglio Erio (1996b) Innovation in a fast changing Europe. In: World Health (July-August 1996). 49(4), pp8-9. WHO: Geneva
- Belz-Merkel Martina, Bengel Juergen, Strittmatter Regine (1992) Subjektive Gesundheitskonzepte und gesundheitliche Protektivfaktoren. In: Ztschr. f. Medizinische Psychologie 1992,(4): 153-171
- Bengel Juergen/ Strittmeier Regine/ Willmann Hildegard (1999) What keeps people healhty? The current state of discussion and the relevance of Antonovsky's salutogenic model of health. Expert report commissioned by the Federal Center for Health Education, Germany (FCHE). Cologne
- Ben-Sira Zeev (1994) Professor Aaron Antonovsky (1923-1994). In: European Journal of Public Health 1994, (4): 304
- Benzeval M/ Judge K/ Whitehead M (Eds.) (1995) Tackling inequalities in health: an agenda for action. Kings Fund Institute: London
- Berkman Lisa F/ Glass Thomas (2000) Social integration, social networks, social support and health. In: Berkman LF/ Kawachi I (Eds.) (2000) Social epidemiology. New York, pp137-173
- Berkman Lisa F/ Kawachi Ichiro (Eds.) (2000) Social epidemiology. New York
- Birdthistle Isolde (Ed.) (1999) Improving health through schools: national and international strategies. WHO/NMH/HPS/00.1. WHO: Geneva, pp20-23
- Birley Martin H (1995) The health impact assessment of development projects. (Glossary). London
- Blaettner Beate (1994) Gesundheitsfoerderung und Gesundheitsbildung - Aktueller Stand der Diskussion - Literaturrecherche, Deutsches Institut fuer Erwachsenenbildung: Hamburg
- Blane David/ Brunner Eric/ Wilkinson Richard (Eds.) (1996) Health and Social Organization. Toward a health policy for the 21st Century. London, New York
- BLK Modellversuch Netzwerk Gesundheitsfoerdernde Schulen (1993) Der BLK Modellversuch Netzwerk Gesundheitsfoerdernde Schulen. (Ein gemeinsamer Schulversuch der Kultus- und Senatsverwaltungen von 12 Laendern der Bundesrepublik Deutschland) Information Nr.1 (Stand August 1993). Ohne Ort
- BMBF (Bundesministerium für Bildung, Wissenschaft, Forschung und Technologie, Germany) (Ed.) (1997) Gesundheit und Allgemeine Weiterbildung. Beitrag zu einer neuen Perspektive der Gesundheitsförderung. BMBF, Bonn

- Boppel Werner (2001) Bundesministerium fuer Bildung und Forschung, Kapitel 5.9 in: Barkholz et al (2001) Offenes Partizipationsnetz und Schulsgesundheit. Bundesministerium fuer Bildung und Forschung: Bonn-Bad Godesberg, pp402-406
- Bowes John E (1997) Communication and community development for health information: constructs and models for evaluation. Review prepared for the National Network of Libraries of Medicine, Pacific Northwest Region, Seattle, December 1997; Graph 'The innovation process in an organization'. Jbowes@u.washington.edu www.commminit.com/power_point/change_theories/index.html
- Brackhahn Bernhard (2001) Statement in 'Zusammenarbeit der wissenschaftlichen Begleitung mit der nationalen Koordinierungsstelle'. Kapitel 5.8 in: Barkholz et al (2001) Offenes Partizipationsnetz und Schulgesundheit. Bundesministerium fuer Bildung und Forschung: Bonn-Bad Godesberg. pp400-402
- Blane David (1999) The life course, the social gradient, and health. In: Marmot M/ Wilkinson RG (Eds.) (1999) Social determinants of health. New York, pp64-80
- Broesskamp Ursel (1992) Gesundheitsförderung in und mit Schulen. (Gesundheitswissenschaftliche Diplomarbeit Jan.1992). University of Bielefeld, School of Public Health: Bielefeld, Germany (Unpublished document)
- Broesskamp Ursel (1994) Gesundheit und Schule (Health and School) - Beitrag zu einer neuen Perspektive der Gesundheitsfoerderung. Reihe „Bildung - Wissenschaft - Aktuell" 6/94, Herausgegeben vom BMBW (German Federal Ministry of Education and Science). BMBW, Bonn, Germany.
- Broesskamp-Stone Ursel (2000) Zusammendenken, was zusammen gehoert. Die Bundesempfehlungen "Gesundheit und Schule". In: Paulus P/ Brueckner G (2000) Wege zu einer gesuenderen Schule. Handlungsebenen - Handlungsfelder - Bewertungen. Tuebingen, pp.45-53
- Broesskamp-Stone Ursel/ Kickbusch Ilona/ Walter Ulla (1998) Gesundheitsfoerderung und Praevention. In: Schwartz et al (Eds.) (1998) Das Public Health Buch. Muenchen, Wien, Baltimore, pp141-150
- Broesskamp-Stone Ursel/ Kickbusch Ilona/ Walter Ulla (1998) Gesundheitsfoerderung. In: Schwartz FW et al (Eds.) (1998) Das Public Health Buch. Muenchen, Wien, Baltimore, pp141-150
- Brundtland Gro Harlem (2000) Health. The key to human development. Frankfurt/M., New York
- Brunner Eric/ Marmot Michael (1999) Social organization, stress, and health. In: Marmot M/ Wilkinson R (1999) Social determinants of health. Oxford, pp17-43
- Buechel Bettina (1996) Partnerships for Health Promotion. Background paper prepared for the 4th International Conference on Health Promotion (Jakarta, 21-25 July 1997). Unpublished draft (Sept. 1996). WHO: Geneva
- Bundeszentrale fuer gesundheitliche Aufklaerung (Hg) (1996) Leitbegriffe der Gesundheitsfoerderung. Schwabenheim a. d. Selz
- Bunton Richard/ Macdonalds Gordon (Eds.) (1992) Health promotion: disciplines and diversity. London
- Burgher Mary Stewart, Barnekow Rasmussen Vivian, Rivett David (1999) The European Network of Health Promoting Schools – the alliance of education and health. EUR/ICP/IVST060305. ENHPS: WHO/EURO, Copenhagen (www.who.dk/document/e62361.pdf)
- BzgA (Bundeszentrale für gesundheitliche Aufklärung) (Ed.) (1996) Leitbegriffe der Gesundheitsförderung. Schwabenheim
- Castells Manuel (1996) The rise of the network society. (The Information age: economy, society and culture – Volume I). Oxford

- Castells Manuel (1998) Information Technology, globalisation and social development. (Paper prepared for the UNRISD Conference on Information Technologies and Social Development, Palais des Nations, Geneva, 22-24.June1998.) UNRISD: Geneva (www.unrisd.org/infotech/conferen/castelp1.html) (downloaded 20Nov.1998)
- Catford John (1999) Editorial: WHO is making a difference through health promotion. In: Health Promotion International 14(1): 1-4
- CE, EC, WHO/EURO (Eds.) (1995) Towards an evaluation of the European Network of Health Promoting Schools. The EVA project. (A manual for national coordinators of the ENHPS and their collaborators.) IPC c/o WHO/EURO: Copenhagen
- Conrad Günter/ Schmidt Werner (Eds.) (1990) Health Promotion/ Gesundheitsförderung. Glossary/ Glossar (Prepared on behalf of WHO/EURO for the International Conference ‚Investment in health', 17-19 December 1990, Bonn, Germany). Gamburg/ Berlin
- Cook K S/ Whitmeyer J M (1992) Two approaches to social structure: exchange theory and network analysis. In: Annual Review Sociology 1992. 18: 109-127
- Corin E (1994) The social and cultural matrix of health and disease. In: Evans RG/ Barer ML/ Marmor Th.R (Eds) (1994) Why are some people healthy and others not? New York, pp93-132
- Council of Europe (2001) Website of the Council of Europe: Overview. Council of Europe: Strasbourg (www.coe.international - downloaded on 8.June 2001)
- Daft Richard L (1992) Organization theory and design. Saint Paul, NY, LA, San Francisco
- Dahlgreen Goeran/ Whitehead Margret (1991) Tackling inequalities: a review of policy initiatives. In: Benzeval M et al (Eds.) (1995) Tackling inequalities in health: an agenda for action. Kings Fund Institute: London
- Davies John Kenneth/ Macdonald Gordon (1998) Beyond uncertainty. Leading health promotion into the 21st century. In: Davies JK/ Macdonald G (Eds.) (1998b) Quality, evidence and effectiveness in health promotion. Striving for certainties. London, New York, pp 207-216
- Davies John Kenneth/ Macdonald Gordon (Eds.) (1998b) Quality, evidence and effectiveness in health promotion. Striving for certainties. London, New York, pp189-206
- Decache Alain/ Laperche Jean (1998) Paradigms, values and quality criteria in health promotion: an application to primary health care. In: Davies JK/ Macdonald G (Eds.) (1998b) Quality, evidence and effectiveness in health promotion. Striving for certainties. London, New York, pp 149-164
- Dimakakos, Panagiotis Th. (2002) Measuring social capital. EUHPID Working Paper (for the 3rd meeting of the "EU Health Promotion Indicator Development" (EUHPID) -Project financed by the European Union, 8-9Nov.2002, Lisbon, Portugal). EUHPID secretariat: Dr J.K.Davies, University of Brighton, UK. (Unpublished document)
- Dlugosch Gabriele E. (1994) Modelle der Gesundheitspsychologie. In: Schwenkmezger P/ Schmidt L R (Eds.) (1994) Lehrbuch der Gesundheitspsychologie. Stuttgart, pp.101-117
- Downie R. S./ Fyfe Carol/ Tannahill Andrew (1990) Health promotion: models and values. Oxford
- Doyle Yvonne/ Tsouros Agis/ Cryer P. Colin/ Hedley S/ Russell-Hodgson C (1999) Practical lessons in using indicators of determinants of health across 47 European cities. In: Health Promotion International 14(4): 289-299
- Drofenik Marinka (1999) Extending the idea of the European Network to the regional level in the region Celje, Slovenia. In: ENHPS Technical Secretariat (1999) Network News (Newsletter of the ENHPS). ENHPS, WHO/EURO: Copenhagen, pp23
- EC/ CE/ WHO/EURO (1993) Resource manual – The European Network of Health Promoting Schools. ENHPS Technical Secretariat, WHO/EURO: Copenhagen
- EC/ CE/ WHO/EURO / Health Education Board for Scotland (Eds.) (1994) Promoting the health of young people in Europe; a training manual for teachers and others working with young people. nal

- ECHP (European Center for Health Policy) (2000) Country profiles. (last updated on Dec. 2000) ECHP (www.who.dk/hs/echp/cprofiles/ - downloaded on 7 May 2001)
- Eis Dieter (1998) Gesundheit und Krankheit: Welchen Einfluss hat die Umwelt? Schwartz FW et al (1998) Das Public Health Buch. Gesundheit und Gesundheitswesen. Muenchen, Wien, Baltimore, pp51-80
- ENHPS (1996) Development plan 1996-2000 for the ENHPS - A joint project of the WHO/EURO, EC, CE. (A working document settings out the strategy, aims, and priorities for the ENHPS 1996-2000. Where do we come from? Where are we now? Where do we want to be?) WHO/EURO: Copenhagen, Jan.1996. Unpublished
- ENHPS (1997) Development plan 1996-2000 for the ENHPS - A joint project of the WHO/EURO, EC, CE. (Revised version of ENHPS 1996 from January 1997) WHO/EURO: Copenhagen. Unpublished
- ENHPS (1997a) The ENHPS Conference Resolution. Resolution passed at the First European Conference "The Health Promoting School - An Investment in Education, Health and Democracy" (1-5 May 1997, Greece). WHO/EURO: Copenhagen
- ENHPS (1997b) First Conference of the European Network of Health Promoting Schools "The Health Promoting School – an investment into education, health and democracy", Thessaloniki-Halkidiki, Greece, 1-5 May 1997 (Case study book). ENHPS: WHO/EURO, Copenhagen
- ENHPS (1999) ENHPS website: "Organization". WHO/EURO: Copenhagen (www.who.dk/enhps/page/ org.html - last updated 17 June 1999)
- ENHPS (1999a) Report of the meeting of an Expert Working Group on the integration of ENHPS evaluation tools and processes. (Copenhagen, Denmark, 5th October 1999). WHO/EURO: Copenhagen
- ENHPS (1999b) About the European Network of Health Promoting Schools. (Introduction on the ENHPS website, updated 17 June 1999). WHO/EURO: Copenhagen (www.who.dk/enhps - downloaded 16 November 2000)
- ENHPS (w.y.) The ENHPS indicators for a health promoting school. (document received in 1999) ENHPS: Copenhagen. Unpublished document.
- ENHPS Technical Secretariat (Ed.) (1995) Network News. The European Network of Health Promoting Schools. (Newsletter of the ENHPS) WHO/EURO: Copenhagen *(www.who.dk/ enhps/ Publication)*
- ENHPS Technical Secretariat (Ed.) (1996) Network News. The European Network of Health Promoting Schools. (Newsletter of the ENHPS) WHO/EURO: Copenhagen *(www.who.dk/enhps/Publication)*
- ENHPS Technical Secretariat (Ed.) (1997) Network News. The European Network of Health Promoting Schools. (Newsletter of the ENHPS) WHO/EURO: Copenhagen *(www.who.dk/enhps/Publication)*
- ENHPS Technical Secretariat (Ed.) (1998) Network News. The European Network of Health Promoting Schools. (Newsletter of the ENHPS) WHO/EURO: Copenhagen *(www.who.dk/enhps/Publication)*
- ENHPS Technical Secretariat (Ed.) (1999) Network News. The European Network of Health Promoting Schools. (Newsletter of the ENHPS) WHO/EURO: Copenhagen *(www.who.dk/enhps/Publication)*
- ENHPS Technical Secretariat (Ed.) (2000) Network News. The European Network of Health Promoting Schools. (Newsletter of the ENHPS) WHO/EURO: Copenhagen *(www.who.dk/enhps/Publication)*

- ENHPS Workshop Task Force (Ed.) (1998) First workshop on practice of evaluation of the Health Promoting School - models, experiences and perspectives (held in Bern/Thun, Switzerland, 19-22 November 1998). Executive Summary. ENHPS Technical Secretariat c/o WHO/EURO: Copenhagen

- ENHPS/TS (ENHPS Technical Secretariat) (1997) The European Network of Health Promoting Schools. (Project brochure, 11 pages) WHO/EURO: Copenhagen

- ENHPS/TS (ENHPS Technical Secretariat) (1998a) "The Health Promoting School - an investment in education, health and democracy". Conference Report of the First Conference of the European Network of Health Promoting Schools (1-5 May 1997, Thessaloniki-Halkidiki, Greece). EUR/ICP/IVST 06 01 02 (A). WHO/EURO: Copenhagen

- ENHPS/TS (ENHPS Technical Secretariat) (1998b) "The Health Promoting School - an investment in education, health and democracy". Case study book. First Conference of the European Network of Health Promoting Schools (1-5 May 1997, Thessaloniki-Halkidiki, Greece). EUR/ICP/IVST 06 01 02 (B). WHO/EURO: Copenhagen

- ENHPS/TS (ENHPS Technical Secretariat) (Ed.) (1993a) Resource manual: The European Network of Health Promoting Schools. WHO/EURO: Copenhagen

- ENHPS/TS (ENHPS Technical Secretariat) (Ed.) (1993b) Extracts from Resource manual: The European Network of Health Promoting Schools. WHO/EURO: Copenhagen

- ENHPS/TS (ENHPS Technical Secretariat) (w.y.) (-before 1997) The European Network of Health Promoting Schools. (Project brochure 11p.) WHO/EURO: Copenhagen

- Eoyang Glenda H/ Berkas Thomas H (1998) Evaluation in a complex adaptive system. (dated April 30, 1998). Circle Pines, Minneapolis; USA (Unpublished document)

- European Union (2001) Website of the European Union: Europe - activities - education - overview. European Union: Brussels (http://europea.eu.international/scadplus/leg/en/cha/ c00003.htm – downloaded: 8 June 2001)

- Evans Robert G (1994) Preface. In: Evans RG/ Barer ML/ Marmor Th.R (Eds.) (1994) Why are some people healthy and others not? New York, pp ix-xix

- Evans Robert G (1994a) Introduction. Preface. In: Evans RG/ Barer ML/ Marmor Th.R (Eds.) (1994) Why are some people healthy and others not? New York, pp 3-26

- Evans Robert G /Hodge M/ Pless I B (1994) If not genetics, then what? Biological pathways and population health. In: Evans RG/ Barer ML/ Marmor Th.R (Eds) (1994) Why are some people healthy and others not? New York:, pp161-188

- Evans Robert G/ Barer, Morris L/ Marmor, Theodore R (Eds) (1994) Why are some people healthy and others not? New York

- Evans Robert G/ Stoddart G L (1990) Producing health, consuming health care. In: Social Science and Medicine 31(12): 1347-1363

- Evans Robert G/ Stoddart G L (1994) Producing health, consuming health care. (slight authorial and editorial revision of 1990 version). In: Evans RG/ Barer ML/ Marmor Th.R (Eds.) (1994) Why are some people healthy and others not? New York, pp27-64

- Faltermaier Toni (1994) Gesundheitsbewusstsein und Gesundheitshandeln. Ueber den Umgang mit Gesundheit im Alter. Weinheim.

- Federal, Provincial and Territorial Advisory Committee on Population Health (1999) Toward a healhty future: Second report on the health of Canadians. (Prepared for the Meeting of Ministers of Health, Charlottetown, September 1999). Health Canada: Ottawa , Info@www.hc-sc.gc.ca

- Freitag Marcus (1998) Was ist eine gesunde Schule? Einfluesse des Schulklimas auf Schueler- und Lehrergesundheit. (What is a healthy school? Influences of the school climate on pupils and teachers health). /Weinheim, Muenchen: Juventa Verlag.

- Funnel Rachel/ Oldfield Katherine (1998) An evaluation tool for the self-assessment of healthy alliances. In: Scriven A (Ed.) (1998) Alliances in health promotion. Theory and practice. London, pp70-76
- Gabriel Regine (1999) OPUS – open participation network and school health. In: ENHPS Technical Secretariat (Ed.) (1999) Network News. (Newsletter of the ENHPS). WHO/EURO: Copenhagen, p8-9
- Galea Gauden/ Powis Brent/ Tamplin Stephen (2000) Healthy Islands in the Western Pacific – international Settings development. In: Health Promotion International 15(2): 169-178
- Garbarino J (1995) Raising Children in a socially toxic environment. San Francisco
- Geiger Andreas/ Kreuter H (1997) Handlungsfeld Gesundheitsfoerderung. 10 Jahre nach Ottawa. Gamburg
- Gesundheitsförderung Schweiz (2000) Quint essenz. Bern, Lausanne (www.quint-essenz.ch:8080/de/topics/projektzielformulierung - downloaded last on 15Dec.2002)
- Gillies Pamela (1998) Effectiveness of alliances and partnerships for health promotion. In: Health Promotion International 13(2): 99-120
- Glanz Karen/ Lewis Frances Marcus/ Rimer Barbara K (1997) Health behavior and health education. Theory, research, and practice. San Francisco
- GNHPS (German Network of Health-Promoting Schools) (1994) FSC Model Project - The German Network of Health-Promoting Schools. A multi-state project by the Ministries for Education of the Laender. (Yellow brochure dated March 1994)
- Goldstein Greg (1997) WHO Travelreport summary from 26 Sept. 1997 on: "Workshop for environmental health advisors on Healthy Islands, Healthy Municipalities and Negotiation, Washington DC, 8-12 Dec1997" and on "1997 International health congress: Investment Strategies for healthy uraban communities: innovative partnerships for a healthy future, Baltimore Maryland, 15-17Sept.1997". WHO: Geneva (Unpublished paper)
- Goldstein Greg (1998) International networks and settings development. Healthy Cities. (A global review by WHO/HPR Geneva) WHO/HPR, Geneva (Unpublished document)
- Goodman Robert M/ Steckler Allan/ Kegler Michelle (1997) Mobilizing organizations for health enhancement. Theories or organizational change. In: Glanz K et al (1997) Health behavior and health education. Theory, research, and practice. San Francisco, pp287-312
- Goodstadt Michael S/ Hyndman Brian/ McQueen David V/ Potvin Louise/ Rootman Irving/ Springett Jane (2001) Evaluation in health promotion; synthesis and recommendations. In: Rootman I et al (2001b) Evaluation in health promotion. WHO/EURO: Copenhagen, pp517-533
- Goumans Marleen (1993) What about healthy networks ? An analysis of structure and organization of national Healthy Cities networks in Europe. RHC Monograph Series 3. RHC Clearing House, School of Health Sciences, University of Limburg: Maastricht, NL
- Government of Canada, Ministry of National Health and Welfare (Ed.) (1994) A new perspective on the health of Canadians. A working document. Ministry of National Health and Welfare, Ottawa
- Green L W/ George A/ Daniel M/ Frankish C J/ Herbert C P/ Bowie W/ O'Neill M (1995) Participatory research in health promotion. Ottawa, Ontario
- Green Lawrence W./ Richard Lucie/ Potvin Louise (1996) Ecological foundations of health promotion. In: American Journal of Health Promotion 10(4): 270-281
- Green Lawrence W/ Kreuter Marshall W (1991) Health promotion planning. An educational and environmental approach. Mountain View, Toronto, London (pp150-177)
- Green Lawrence W/ Kreuter Marshall W (1999) Health promotion planning. An educational and environmental approach. Mountain View, Toronto, London

- Green Lawrence W/ Poland Blake D/ Rootman Irving (2000) The settings approach to health promotion. In: Poland BD/Green LW/ Rootman I (Eds) (2000) Settings for health promotion. Linking theory and practice. Thousand Oaks, London, New Delhi, pp1-43
- Green Lawrence W/ Raeburn John (1988) Health Promotion. What is it? What will it become? In: J. Health Promotion 3(2): 151-159
- Gregory D/ Urry J (1985) Social relations and spacial structures. London
- Grossman Ralf/ Scala Klaus (1993) Health promotion and organizational development: developing settings for health. WHO/EURO, IFF Health Organisation Development: Copenhagen, Vienna
- Grossmann Ralf/ Scala Klaus (1994) Gesundheit durch Projekte foerdern. Ein Konzept zur Gesundheitsfoerderung durch Organisationsentwicklung und Projektmanagement. Weinheim
- Grossmann Ralf/ Scala Klaus (1996) Settingsansatz in der Gesundheitsfoerderung. In: BzgA (1996) Leitbegriffe der Gesundheitsförderung. Schwabenheim, pp100-101
- Grossmann Ralph (Ed) (1997) Besser Billiger Mehr - Zur Reform der Expertenorgansisationen Krankenhaus, Schule, Univeristaet. iff texte. Wien, NY
- Grossmann Ralph/ Pellert Ada/ Gotwald Victor (1997) Krankenhaus, Schule, Universitaet: Charakteristika und Optimierungspotentiale. In: Grossmann R (Ed) (1997) Besser Billiger Mehr - Zur Reform der Expertenorgansisationen Krankenhaus, Schule, Univeristaet. pp24-35
- Grundboeck Alice/ Nowak Peter/ Pelikan Juergen (1997) Das Oesterreichische Netzwerk Gesundheitsfoerdernder Krankenhaeuser: ein WHO-Netzwerk. In: Grundboeck A/ Nowak P/ Pelikan J (Eds) (1997) Gesundheitsfoerderung - eine Strategie fuer Krankenhaeuser im Umburch. Wien, pp54-62
- Grundboeck Alice/ Nowak Peter/ Pelikan Juergen (Eds) (1997) Gesundheitsfoerderung - eine Strategie fuer Krankenhaeuser im Umburch. Wien
- Gumucio Dagron, Alfonso (2001) Making waves. Stories of participatory communication for social change. (A report to the Rockefeller Foundation.) Rockefeller Foundation: New York; pp5-13
- Haggerty Robert (1990) Changing lifestyles to improve health. In: WHO/EURO (1990) Health Promotion. A resource book. WHO, Copenhagen. pp69-90.
- Hancock, Trevor (1990) The mandala of health: a model of the human ecosystem. In: Anderson R/ Kickbusch I (1990) Health Promotion. A resource book. EUR/ICP/HSR 612. WHO/EURO: Copenhagen, pp129-138.
- Harris Elisabeth/ Wise Marylin/ Hawe Penelope/ Finlay Penelope/ Nutbeam Don (1995) Working together: intersectoral action for health. Commonwealth of Australia: Canberra
- Hastings Collin (1993) The New Organization. Growing the culture of organizational networking. London
- Hayes Roger (1996) Systematic Networking. A guide for personal and corporate success. London, New York
- HEA (Health Education Authority)/ WHO/EURO (Ed.) (1996) WHO Europe health promotion profiles. A survey for internal use only by members of the European Committee for Health Promotion Development (ECHPD). (Update 1.Sept.1996). WHO/EURO, HEA: Copenhagen, London. (Published, but limited distribution)
- HEA (Health Education Authority)/ WHO/EURO (Ed.) (1998) WHO Europe health promotion profiles. A survey for internal use only by members of the European Committee for Health Promotion Development (ECHPD). (Update 1998). HEA, London. (Unpublished document)
- Health Canada/ Sante Canada (2000) Intersectoral action ... towards population health. Health Canada: Ottawa. (www/hc-sc.gc.ca/hppb/phdd/resources/index.html – downloaded: 21 December 2000)

- Health Promotion Unit (1992) Draft strategic proposal European Network of Health Promoting Schools. (prepared by the Health Promotion Unit of WHO/EURO for the IPC meeting on 11 December 1992.) ICP/HSC 639 3 Dec.1992. WHO/EURO: Copenhagen (Unpublished document)
- Heclo H (1987) Issue networks and the executive establishment. In: King A (Ed.) (1987) The new american political system. Washington
- Hertzman C/ Frank J/ Evans RG (1994) Heterogeneities in health status and the determinants of population health. In: Evans RG/ Barer ML/ Marmor Th.R (Eds.) (1994) Why are some people healthy and others not? New York, pp67-92
- Hilderbrand Mary E/ Grindle Merilee S. (1994) Building sustainable capacity: Challenges for the public sector. (Pilot study of capacity building INT/92/676 - prepared for the United Nations Development Programme by Harvard Institute for International Development, Harvard University). UNDP: New York (http://magnet.undp.org/cdrb/parti.html - downloaded 8Oct.1998)
- Homfeldt Hans Guenther/ Barkholz Ulrich (1993) Eckpunkte schulpraktischer Gersundheitsfoerderung. In: Priebe B et al (Eds.) (1993) Gesunde Schule. Weinheim, Basel, pp76-97
- Homfeldt Hans Guenther/ Barkholz Ulrich (1994) Schule zwischen Bewegung und Erstarrung. Erfahrungen und Ergebnisse des BLK-Modellversucs 'Gesundheitsfoerderung im schulischen Alltag'. In: PaedExtra Juli/August 1994, pp15-18
- Homfeldt Hans Guenther/ Huenersdorf Bettina (1997) Soziale Arbeit und Gesundheit. Neuwied
- Hurrelmann Klaus (1990) Familienstress, Schulstress, Freizeitstress – Gesundheitsfoerderung fuer Kinder und Jugendliche. Weinheim
- Hurrelmann Klaus (1991) Sozialisation und Gesundheit. Somatische, psychische und soziale Risikofaktoren im Lebenslauf. Weinheim, Muenchen
- Hurrelmann Klaus (1993) Lebensphase Jugend. Eine Einfuehrung in die sozialwissenschaftliche Jugendforschung. Weinheim, Muenchen
- Hurrelmann Klaus (2000) Gesundheitssoziologie. Weinheim, München
- Hurrelmann Klaus/ Laaser Ulrich (Hg) (1993) Gesundheitswissenschaften. Handbuch fuer Lehre, Forschung und Praxis. Weinheim, Basel
- Hyndman Brian (1997) Health promotion in action: What works? What needs to be changed? - A review of the effectiveness of health promotion strategies (1986-present). (Draft for discussion, 30April 1997) Centre for Health Promotion, University of Toronto
- IPC (International Planning Committee of the ENHPS) (1993) The European Network of Health Promoting Schools. A joint WHO-CE-CEC project. (Project brochure 11p.) WHO/EURO: Copenhagen
- IPC (International Planning Committee of the ENHPS) (w.y.) European Network of Health Promoting Schools. Entry Form. WHO/EURO: Copenhagen. (Unpublished)
- IUHPE (International Union for Health Promotion and Education) (1999a) The evidence of health promotion effectiveness. Shaping public health in a new Europe. Part one - core document. A report for the European Commission. ECSC-EC-EAEC: Brussels, Luxembourg
- IUHPE (International Union for Health Promotion and Education) (1999b) The evidence of health promotion effectiveness. Shaping public health in a new Europe. Part two - evidence book. A report for the European Commission. ECSC-EC-EAEC: Brussels, Luxembourg
- Jakarta Declaration on Leading Health Promotion into the 21st Century (1997) Declaration adopted at the 4th International Conference for Health Promotion, Jakarta, Indonesia. WHO/HPR/HEP/4ICHP/BR/97.4. WHO: Geneva (www.who.int/hpr/conference)
- Jordan Grant/ Schubert Klaus (1992) A preliminary ordering of policy network labels. In: European Journal of Political Research 21(1-2): 7-27

- Kaba-Schoenstein Lotte (1996) Gesundheitsfoerderung I, II, III. In: Bundeszentrale fuer gesundheitliche Aufklaerung (Hg.) (1996) Leitbegriffe der Gesundheitsfoerderung. Schwabenheim a. d. Selz. pp39-47
- Kahan Barbara/ Goodstadt Michael (1997) Best practices in health promotion. (Draft paper from 27.Oct.1997, with the support of the Centre of Health Promotion). Toronto, Canada (Unpublished document)
- Kahan Barbara/ Goodstadt Michael (1999) Continuous quality improvement and health promotion: can CQI lead to better outcomes? In: Health Promotion International 14(1): 83-91
- Kassim Hussein (1994) Policy networks, networks and European Union policy making: a skeptical view. In: West European Politics 17(4): 15-27
- Kawachi Ichiro/ Colditz G A/ Ascherio A (1996) A prospective study of social networks in relation to total mortality and cardiovascular disease in men in the USA. In: Journal of Epidemiology and Community Health 1996, 50: 245-251
- Kenis Patrick/ Schneider Volker (1989) Policy networks as an analytical tool for polica analysis. (Paper for a conference at the Max-Planck-Institute, Cologne, 4-5 Dec.1989). Cologne
- Kickbusch Ilona (1989) Approaches to an ecological base for public health. In: J. Health Promotion 4(4): 265-268
- Kickbusch Ilona (1991) Implementing a social model of helath. Presentation at "The window of opportunity" congress, Adelaide, Australia, 2-6 December 1991. Unpublished document.
- Kickbusch Ilona (1992) Health, lifestyle and the environment - human and ethical dimensions. Presentation at the tenths Commonwealth Health Ministers Meeting, Nicosia, Cyprus, 19-23 October 1992) London: Commonwealth Secretariat, paragraphs 26-29.
- Kickbusch Ilona (1993) Vorwort. In: Pelikan JM/ Demmer H/ Hurrelmann K (Hrsg.) (1993) Gesundheitsfoerderung durch Organisationsentwicklung. Weinheim, Muenchen
- Kickbusch Ilona (1994) Introduction: Tell me a story. In: Pederson A/O'Neill M/ Rootman I (Eds.) (1994) Health Promotion in Canada: Provincial, national and international perspectives. Toronto
- Kickbusch Ilona (1994b) Social networks and health policies. (Presentation at the Symposium on Social Networks and Health, Schaeffergarden, Copenhagen, 24-25 November 1994). Unpublished document (IK/hs/5.9.1995)
- Kickbusch Ilona (1994c) Foreword In: Baric L (1994) Health promotion and health education in practice. Module 2. The organizational model. Altrincham
- Kickbusch Ilona (1995) An overview to the settings based approach to health promotion. In: Theaker T/ Thompson J (Eds.) (1995) The settings-based approach to heath promotion: report of an international working conference. Hertfordshire, UK: Hertfordshire Health Promotion
- Kickbusch Ilona (1996) Editorial. New players for a new era: how up to date is health promotion? In: Health Promotion International 11(4): 259-262
- Kickbusch Ilona (1997) Think health: What makes the difference? Keynote address given at the 4th International Conference on Health Promotion, Jakarta, Indonesia, 21-25 July 1997. In: Health Promotion International 12(4): 265-272
- Kickbusch Ilona (1997b) New players for a new era: responding to the global public health challenges. In: Journal of Public Health Medicine 19(2): 171-178
- KMK (Kultusminister Konferenz) (1992) Zur Situation der Gesundheitserziehung in Schulen. (Veröffentlichungen der Kultusminister-Konferenz). Bericht der KMK vom 5./6.11.1992. Bonn
- Krech Ruediger (1999) Health Promotion – European experiences with regard to intersectoral policies to improve the health of the public. Inaugural dissertation. University of Bielefeld, Faculty of Health Sciences/School of Public Health: Bielefeld, Germany.

- Kreiner Kristian/ Schultz Maijken (1990) 'Crossing the institutional divide... Networking in biotechnology. EUREKA Managemetn Research Initiative, Copenhagen, Business School. Summarized in: Hastings (1993) The New Organization. Growing the culture of organizational networking. London, p60-78
- Kuh Diana/ Ben-Shlomo Yoav (Eds.) (1997) A life course perspective to chronic disease epidemiology. Oxford
- Labonte Ronald (1994) Health Promotion and empowerment: reflections on professional practice. In: J. Health Education Quarterly 21(2): 253-268
- Lalonde Marc (1994) A new perspective on the health of Canadians. (A report of the Minister of Health and Welfare, Canada). Ottawa: Ministry of Supply and Services
- Laverack Glenn (1999) Addressing the contradiction between discourse and practice in health promotion. (Doctoral theses, July 1999). Deakin University, Australia
- Laverack Glenn/ Labonte Ronald (2000) A planning framework for community empowerment goals within health promotion. In: Health Policy and Planning 15(3): 255-262
- Lavis John N/ Sullivan Terrence J (2000) The State as a Settings. In: Poland B et al (2000) Settings for Health Promotion. Thousand Oaks, London, New Delhi, pp308-332
- Leeuw de Evelyne (2000) Commentary: Beyond communtiy action: communication arrangements and policy networks. In Poland et al (2000) Settings for health promotion. Thousand Oaks, London, New Delhi, pp287-300
- Lehmann Harald (1997) Entwicklungen der Gesundheitsfoerderung und Gesundheitsaufklaerung in Deutschland. In: Geiger A/ Kreuter H (1997) Handlungsfeld Gesundheitsfoerderung. Gamburg, pp37-44
- Levin Lowell S/ Ziglio Erio (1996) Health promotion as an investment strategy: considerations of theory and practice. In: Health Promotion International 11(1): 33-40
- Levin Lowell S/ Ziglio Erio (1997) Health promotion as an investment strategy: a perspective for the 21st century. In: Sidell M et al (Eds.) (1997) Debates and dilemmas in promoting health. London, pp363-368
- Lobnig Hubert/ Novak Peter/ Pelikan Juergen (1997) Das Gesundheitsfoerdernde Krankenhaus als Lernende Organization. In: Grundboeck et al (Eds) Gesundheitsfoerderung - eine Strategie fuer Krankenhaeuser im Umburch. Wien, pp195-210
- Lohaus Arnold (1993) Gesundheitsfoerderung und Krankheitspraevention im Kindes- und Jugendalter. (Hogrefe Reihe Gesundheitspsychologie, Band 2) Goettingen, Bern, Toronto, Seattle
- Lopez-Acuna Daniel/ Pittman Patricia/ Gomez Paulina/ de Souza Heloiza Machado/ Lopez Fernandez, Luis Andres (2000) Reorienting health systems and services with health promotion cirteria:a critical component of health sector reforms. Technical paper prepared for the 5th Global Conference on Health Promotion, 5-9 June 2000, Mexico City, Mexico. WHO: Geneva. www.who.org/hpr/conference
- Macdonald Heather/ Williams Trefor/ Ziglio Erio (1992) Reprot of the first consultative meeting of the national coordinators or the European Network of Healht Promoting Schools, Strasbourg, 21-22 May 1992. (July 1992) WHO/EURO: Copenhagen. (Unpublished document)
- MacDonald Gordon (1996) Indicateur de qualite et efficacite de la promotion de la sante: la necessite de les epouser. (Paper presented at the 3rd European Effectiveness Conference, 12-14Sept.1996, Turin, Italy). (Unpublished paper)
- MacDonald Gordon/ Bunton Richard (1992) Health Promotion: Discipline or disciplines. In: Bunton R/ Macdonald G (Eds) (1992) Health promotion: disciplines and diversity. London, pp6-19
- Makara Peter (1997) Partnerships for health promotion. Conference working paper for the 4th International Conference on Health Promotion "New Players for a New Era: Leading Health Promotion into the 21st Century", Jakarta, Indonesia, 21-25 July 1997. HPR/HEP/4ICHP/PT/97.4 Distribution: limited. WHO: Geneva

- Marmot et al (1991) Health inequities among British Civil Servants: the Whitehall II study. Lancet 337: pp1387-1393
- Marmot Michael (1996) The social pattern of health and disease. In: Blane D/ Brunner E/ Wilkinson R (Eds.) (1996) Health and Social Organization. Toward a health policy for the 21st Century. London, New York, pp42-67
- Marmot Michael (1999) Introduction. In: Marmot M/ Wilkinson RG (Eds.) (1999) Social determinants of health. New York, pp1-16
- Marmot Michael (2000) Understanding social determinants. In: Berkmann L/ Kawachi I (2000) Social Epidemiology. Oxford, pp349-367
- Marmot M C/ Kogevinas M/ Elston M A (1991) Socioeconomic status and disease. In: Badura B/ Kickbusch I (Eds.) (1991) Health promotion research: Toward a new social epidemiology. WHO EURO: Copenhagen. pp113-146
- Marmot Michael/ Wilkinson Richard G (Eds.) (1999) Social determinants of health. New York
- Mayntz Renate (1993) Policy-Netzwerke und die Logik von Verhandlungssystemen. In: Mayntz R (1997) Soziale Dynamik und politische Steuerung. Frankfurt/Main, New York, pp239-262
- Mayntz Renate (1997) Soziale Dynamik und politische Steuerung. Theoretische und methodologische Überlegungen. Frankfurt/Main, New York
- McKay Lindsey (2000) Making the Lalonde Report. Towards a new perspective on health policy project, Health Network, CPRN, Background paper Oct.2000. CPRN: Canada. (www.cprn.com/cprn.html - downloaded last Nov. 2002)
- McMichael Antony J (2000) The world's widening social, economic and health inequalities: The "globalisation" factor. Paper prepared for the WHO/CDC/HEA workshop on 'Theory and Action for Health', London, 27-29 March 2000. Geneva, London. (Unpublished paper)
- McQueen David (2000) Perspectives on health promotion: theory, evidence, practice and the emergence of complexity. In: Health Promotion International 15(2): 95-97
- McQueen David (2000a) Strengthening the evidence base for health promotion. Technical background report and presentation at the 5th Global Conference for Health Promotion: Bridging the equity gap", 5-9 June 2000, Mexico City, Mexico. (www.who.int/hpr/conference)
- McQueen David (2001) Strengthening the evidence base for health promotion. In: Health Promotion International 16(3): 261-268
- Meierjuergen Juergen (2001) Probleme des Managemetns von Netzwerken der Gesundheitsfoerderung. In: Barkholz U et al (2001) Offenes Partizipationsnetz und Schulsgesundheit. Bonn-Bad Godesberg, pp120-137
- Meierjuergen Juergen (2001b) Der BLK-Modellversuch "Offenes Partizipationsnetz und Schulgesundheit (OPUS)" aus Sicht des Kooeprationspartners BARMER Ersatzkasse. In: Barkholz U et al (2001) Offenes Partizipationsnetz und Schulsgesundheit: Bonn-Bad Godesberg. pp428-435
- Michaelis Heinz (2001) Arbeitszufriedenhiet der Netzwerkkoordinatoren. In: Barkholz U et al (2001) Offenes Partizipationsnetz und Schulsgesundheit: Bonn-Bad Godesberg. pp93-96
- Mielck Andreas (2001) Soziale Ungleichheit und Gesundheit: ein zentales Theam der Public-Health-Diskussion. In: Ztschr. Public Health Forum 9, Heft 33, pp2-4 (www.urbanfischer.de/journals/phf)
- Mielck Andreas/ Bloomfield Kim (Eds.) (2001) Sozial-Epidemiologie. Eine Einführung in die Grundlagen, Ergebnisse und Umsetzungsmoeglichkeiten. Weinheim, Muenchen
- Millio Nancy (1990) A framework for prevention: changing health -damaging to health-generating life patters. In: WHO/EURO (1990) Health Promotion. A resource book. WHO: Copenhagen, pp169-177

- Millstein Susan G/ Petersen Anne C/ Nightingale Elena O (1993) Promoting the health of adolescents. New directions for the 21st Century. New York, Oxford
- Moss Kanter, Rosabeth (1983) The change masters. London
- Moy Gerald (1998) Healthy Marketplaces. (A global review of international networks and settings development by WHO/HPR Geneva.) WHO/HPR, Geneva (Unpublished document)
- Mullen PD/ Evans D/ Forster J/ Gottlieb NH/ Kreuter M/ Moon R/ O'Rourke T/ Strecher VJ (1995) Settings as an important dimension in health education/promotion policy, programs, and research. In: Health Education Quarterly 22(3): 329-345
- Murray Chris/ Lopez Alan (Eds.) (1996) The global burden of disease. A comprehensive assessment of mortality and disability from disease, injuries and risk factors in 1990 and projected. Boston
- NGS (Netzwerk Gesundheitsfoerdernde Schulen) (1994) Netzwerk Gesundheitsfoerdernde Schulen. Ein gemeinsamer Schulversuch der Kultus- und Senatsverwaltungen von 13 Laendern der Bundesrepublik Deutschland (Stand: Maerz 1994). ohne Ort
- NGS (Netzwerk Gesundheitsfoerdernde Schulen) (w.y.) Sich wohlfuehlen in der Schule. Netzwerk Gesundheitsfoerdernde Schulen. (Faltblatt/ leaflet)
- Noack Horst (2002) A rational for the development of Health Promotion indicators. Draft - EUHPID Project Working Paper (for the 2nd meeting of the "EU Health Promotion Indicator Development" (EUHPID) -Project financed by the European Union, 8.-9. June 2002, London, UK). EUHPID secretariat: Dr J.K.Davies, University of Brighton, UK. (Unpublished document)
- Noack Horst (1987) Concepts of health and health promotion. In: Abelin T et al (Eds.) (1987) Measurement in health promotion and protection. WHO/EURO: Copenhagen, pp5-28
- Noack Horst (1997) Research for Health Promotion: A challenge for the 21st Century. In: WHO (Ed.) (1997b) Review and evaluation of health promotion. WHO/HPR/HEP/4ICHP/RET/97.3. WHO: Geneva, pp57-92
- NSC (National HPS Support Center in Slovenia) (1998a) The dissemination of the HPS project in Slovenia. (Presentation for the 1998 business meeting of National Coordinators of the ENHPS.) National HPS Support Center: Ljubljana (Unpublished document)
- NSC (National HPS Support Center in Slovenia) (2000a) Slide presentation prepared in March 2000 for the presentation of the network to representatives of Wales. National HPS Support Center: Ljubljana (Unpublished document) (HPS30.ppt)
- Nutbeam Don (1986) Health Promotion Glossary. In: J. Health Promotion 1(1), pp113-127
- Nutbeam Don (1996) Healthy Islands - a truly ecological model of health promotion. In: Health Promotion International 11(4): 263-264
- Nutbeam Don (1997) Evaluating Health Promoting - Progress, Problems and solutions. In: WHO (Ed.) (1997b) Review and evaluation of health promotion. Series: New Players for a New Era - conference background documents. WHO/HPR/HEP/4ICHP/RET/ 97.3. WHO: Geneva, pp11-51
- Nutbeam Don (1998) Evaluating Health Promotion - Progress, problems, and solution. In: Health Promotion International 13(1): pp27-44
- Nutbeam Don (1998a) Health Promotion Glossary. (see also WHO 1998a) In: Health Promotion International 13(4): 349-364
- Nutbeam Don (1999) Health Promotion effectiveness - The questions to be answered. In: IUHPE (for the European Commission) (Ed.) (1999b) The evidence of health promotion effectiveness. - Part II: Evidence Book. (A report by the IUHPE for the European commission.) ECSC-EC-EAEC: Brussels, Luxembourg, pp1-11
- Nutbeam Don (2000) Health literacy as a public health goal: a challenge of contemporary health education and communication strategies into the 21st Century. In: Health Promotion International 15(3): 259-267

- Nutbeam Don/ Harris Elizabeth (1998) Theory in a nutshell. A practitioner's guide to commonly used theories and models in health promotion. (Chapter 5) University of Sydney, National Center for Health Promotion: Sydney, pp56-65

- Nutbeam, Don (1997b) Comprehensive approaches to the prevention of tobacco use among young people: Research challenges into the 21st Century. Paper presented at the 14th Int. Symposium: Health Risk Behaviour in Adolescence: Theoretical concepts and the evaluation of prevention programmes. Bielefeld, 26-27 September 1997. University of Bielefeld, Bielefeld. (Unpublished paper)

- O'Neill Michel/ Lemieux Vincent/ Groleau Gisele/ Fortin Jean-Paul/ Lamarche Paul A (1997) Coalition theory as a framework for understanding and implementing intersectoral health-related interventions. In: Health Promotion International 12(1): 79-87

- Oldenburg B F/ Sallis J F/ French M L/ Owen N (1999) Health promotion research and the diffusion and institutionalization of interventions. In: Health Education Research 14(1): pp121-130

- Oldenburg Brian/ Hardcastle Deborah M/ Kok Gerjo (1997) Diffusion of innovations. In: Glanz K/ Lewis F M/ Rimer B K (1997) Health behavior and health education. Theory, research, and practice. San Francisco, pp270-286

- Ottawa Charter for Health Promotion (1986) Charter released at the 1st International Conference for Health Promotion, 17-21 November 1986, Ottawa, Canada (jointly held by WHO, Health and Welfare Canada, and the Canadian Public Health Association). WHO/HPR/HEP/1995.1. WHO: Geneva (www.who.int/hpr/conference)

- Parsons Carl/ Stears David/ Thomas Caroline/ Thomas Lynette/ Holland Jennifer (1997) The implementation of ENHPS in different national contexts. Canterbury. WHO/EURO, ENHPS Technical Secretariat: Copenhagen

- Pattenden Jill (1998) Indicators for the health promoting school. In: ENHPS Workshop Task Force (Ed.) (1998) First workshop on practice of evaluation of the Health Promoting School - models, experiences and perspectives. Executive Summary. ENHPS Technical Secretariat c/o WHO/EURO: Copenhagen, pp39-41

- Paulus Peter (1997) Soziale Netzwerke, soziale Unterstuetzung und Gesundheit. In: Homfeldt HG/ Huenersdorf B (1997) Soziale Arbeit und Gesundheit. Neuwied

- Paulus Peter (2000) Von der Ottawa-Charter zur Resolution von Thessaloniki und darueber hinaus. Gesundheitserziehung in der Schule im Wandel zur schulischen Gesundheitsfoerderung. In: Paulus P/ Brueckner G (Eds) (2000) Wege zu einer gesunederen Schule. Tuebingen

- Paulus Peter (2001) verbal information in November 2001

- Paulus Peter/ Brueckner Gerhard (2000) Wege zu einer gesuenderen Schule. Handlungsebenen - Handlungsfelder - Bewertungen. Tuebingen, pp.45-53

- Pederson Ann/ O'Neill Michel/ Rootman Irving (Eds) (1994) Health Promotion in Canada: Provincial, national and international perspectives. Toronto

- Pelikan Juergen M (1997) Das Gesundheitsfoerdernde Krankenhaus - Vision, Anwendungen, Projekterfahrungen. In: Grundboeck A/ Nowak P/ Pelikan J (Eds.) (1997) Gesundheitsfoerderung - eine Strategie fuer Krankenhaeuser im Umburch. Wien, pp27-35

- Pelikan Juergen M/ Demmer Hildegard/ Hurrelmann Klaus (Hrsg.) (1993) Gesundheitsfoerderung durch Organisationsentwicklung. Konzepte, Strategien und Projekte fuer Betriebe, Krankenhaeuser und Schulen. Weinheim, Muenchen

- Pelikan Juergen M/Krajic Karl/ Dietscher Christina (1999) The evaluation of health promotion interventions in social systems and settings. WHO, Geneva. (Unpublished technical paper - version 21.11.1999)

- Petermann Franz (1994) In: Broesskamp U: Gesundheit und Schule. Beitrag zu einer neuen Perspektive der Gesundheitsfoerderung. Bonn, Germany, p29

- Piette Danielle/ Roberts Chris/ Prevost Marianne/ Tudor–Smith Chris/ Tort I Badolet, Jaume (1998) Tracking down ENHPS successes. The EVA 2 project. (Report, Dec. 1998) ENHPS, WHO/EURO: Copenhagen (Unpublished document)

- Piette Danielle/ Roberts Chris/ Prevost Marianne/ Tudor–Smith Chris/ Tort I Badolet, Jaume (w.y.) (after 1999) Tracking down ENHPS successes in sustainable development and dissemination. The EVA 2 project. (Final report) ENHPS, WHO/EURO: Copenhagen (Unpublished document) (www.who.dk - see 'health topics', 'health promotion', 'European Network of Health Promoting Schools')

- Piette Danielle/ Roberts Chris/ Tudor–Smith Chris/ Prevost Marianne/ Tort I Badolet, Jaume (1999) Auto diagnosis towards sustainable development of school health promotion. Guidelines for national and regional coordinators of the European Network of Health Promoting Schools. ENHPS, WHO/EURO: Copenhagen (Unpublished document)

- Pirnat Proza (1999) Disseminating the health-promoting school at the local level in Slovenia. In: ENHPS Technical Secretariat (1999) Network News (Newlsetter of the ENHPS). ENHPS, WHO/EURO: Copenhagen, p23

- Poland, Blake D/Green, Lawrence W/ Rootman, Irving (2000a) Reflections on settings for health promotion. In: Poland B D/Green L W/ Rootman I (Eds.) (2000) Settings for health promotion. Linking theory and practice. Thousand Oaks, London, New Delhi, pp341-3).

- Poland, Blake D/Green, Lawrence W/ Rootman, Irving (Eds) (2000) Settings for health promotion. Linking theory and practice. Thousand Oaks, London, New Delhi

- Potvin Louise/ Haddad Slim/ Frohlich Katharine L (2001) Beyond process and outcome evaluation: a comprehensive approach for evaluating health promotion programs. In: Rootman I et al (Eds.) (2001) Evaluation in Health Promotion. Principles and perspectives. CDC, Health Canada, WHO/EURO. WHO/EURO: Copenhagen, pp45-62

- Priebe Botho, Israel Georg, Hurrelmann Klaus (Eds.) (1993) Gesunde Schule. Gesundheitserziehung, Gesundheitsfoerderung, Schulentwicklung. Weinheim, Basel

- PUZ (Projekt Unterstuetzungs-Zentrum NGS) (1994) Empfehlungen zur Regionalisierung des BLK-Modellversuches Netzwerk Gesundhietsfoerdernde Schulen. (Ueberarbeiteter Entwurf aufgrund der Ergebnisse der Tagung der regionalen BeraterInnen am 30./31.Mai 1994 in Rissen/Hamburg und der Sitzung der ReferentInnen fuer Gesundheitserziehung in den Senats- und Kultusverwaltungen der Laender (Stand: 15.9.1994) In: Arnold W et al (1994) Netzwerk Gesundhietsfoerdernde Schulen. Erster Zwischenbericht... (Berichtszeitraum 1.8.1993-31.7.1994). Flensburg, Kiel, Magdeburg: NGS/ Projektunterstuetzungszentrum Deutschland: Rostockerstr. 6, D-24944 Flensburg, Germany; Anlage 3

- Raeburn John/ Rootman Irving (1998) People-centered health promotion. Chicaster, New York, Weinheim

- Rasmussen Vivian, Rivett David, Ziglio Erio (1996) Foreword to EVA manual. In: CE, EC, WHO/EURO (Eds.) (1996) Towards an evaluation of the European Network of Health Promoting Schools. The EVA project. IPC c/o WHO/EURO: Copenhagen

- Resolution (1997) Resolution of the First Conference of the European Network of Health Promoting Schools: "The Health Promoting School - an investment in education, health and democracy" (1-5 May 1997, Thessaloniki-Halkidiki, Greece). In: Burgher MS (1999) The European Network of Health Promoting Schools – the alliance of education and health. ENHPS, WHO/EURO: Copenhagen, pp16-18

- Restrepo Helena (2000) Increasing community capacity and empowering communities for promoting health. Technical background report and presentation at the 5th Global Conference for Health Promotion: Bridging the equity gap", 5-9 June 2000, Mexico City, Mexico. (www.who.int/hpr/conference)

- Richard Lucie/ Potvin Louise/ Kishchuk Natalie/ Prlic Helen/ Green Lawrence W (1996) Assessment of the integration of the ecological approach in health promotion programs. In: American Journal of Health Promotion 10(4): 318-328

- Rivett David (2000) European Network of Health Promoting Schools (ENHPS) in Slovenia. Technical report from the ENHPS Technical Secretariat. (Report written after WHO/ ENHPS site visit to Slovenia in March 2000) WHO/EURO: Copenhagen (Unpublished document)
- Rootman Irving (2001) Introduction to the book. In: Rootman I et al (Eds.) (2001b) Evaluation in health promotion. WHO/EURO: Copenhagen
- Rootman Irving/ Goodstadt Michael/ Hyndman Brian/ McQueen David V/ Potvin Louise/ Springett Jane/ Ziglio Erio (Eds.) (2001b) Evaluation in health promotion. (WHO Regional Publications, European Series No.92). WHO/EURO: Copenhagen
- Rootman Irving/ Goodstadt Michael/ Hyndman Bryan/ McQueen David/ Potvin Louise/ Springett Jane/ Ziglio Erio (Eds.) (2001b) Evaluation in Health Promotion. Principles and perspectives. WHO Regional Publications, European Series, No.92. CDC, Health Canada, WHO/EURO. WHO/EURO: Copenhagen
- Rootman Irving/ Goodstadt Michael/ Potvin Louise/ Springett Jane (1997) Toward a framework for health promotion evaluation. (WHO Regional Office for Europe, Copenhagen). In: WHO (1997b) Review and evaluation of health promotion. WHO: Geneva
- Rootman Irving/ Goodstadt Michael/ Potvin Louise/ Springett Jane (2001) A framework for health promotion evaluation. (Pre-print of chapter) In: Rootman I et al (2001b) Evaluation in health promotion. WHO/EURO: Copenhagen
- Rootman Irving/ Ziglio Erio (1998) Quality and effectiveness. International perspectives. In: Davies J K/ Macdonald G (Eds.) (1998b) Quality, evidence and effectiveness in health promotion. London, New York, pp189-206
- Rose G (1981) Strategy of prevention: lessons from cardiovascular disease. In: British Medical Journal (Clin Res Ed) 1981 June 6. 282(6279): 1847-1851
- Roussos Stergios Tsai/ Fawcett Stephen B (2000) A review of collaborative partnerships as a strategy for improving community health. In: Ann. Rev. Public Health 2000, 21: 369-402
- Samdal Oddrum/ Wold Bente (1997) The importance of school experiences for student's health and subjective well-being. In: ENHPS Technical Secretariat (1997) Network News (Newsletter of the ENHPS). ENHPS, WHO/EURO: Copenhagen, pp5-6
- Schwartz Friedrich W/ Badura Bernhard/ Leidl Reiner/ Raspe Heiner/ Siegrist Johannes (Eds.) (1998) Das Public Health Buch. Gesundheit und Gesundheitswesen, Muenchen, Wien, Baltimore
- Schwarzer Ralf (1990) Gesundheitspsychologie. Goettingen
- Schwarzer Ralf (1992) Psychologie des Gesundheitsverhaltens. Goettingen
- Schwarzer Ralf (1997^2) Gesundheitspsychologie. Goettingen
- Schwenkmezger Peter/ Schmidt Lothar (1994) Lehrbuch der Gesundheitspsychologie. Stuttgart
- Scicluna Henry (1997) Democracy and freedom: the role of health education. In: ENHPS Technical Secretariat (1997) Network News (Newsletter of the ENHPS). ENHPS, WHO/EURO: Copenhagen, p3
- Scicluna Henry (1999) Council of Europe involvement in the European Network of Health Promoting Schools - expansion to the social and educational sectors. In: ENHPS Technical Secretariat (1999) ENHPS Technical Secretariat (1999) Network News. ENHPS, WHO/EURO: Copenhagen, p4
- Scriven Angela (Ed.) (1998) Alliances in health promotion. Theory and practice. London
- Senge Peter (1990) The fifhts discipline. New York
- Senge Peter (1996) The leader's new work: building learning organizations. In: Starkey K (Ed.) How organizations learn. London, Bonn, pp288-315.
- Sidell Moyra/ Johns Linda/ Katz Jeanne/ Peberdy Alyson (Eds.) (1997) Debates and dilemmas in promoting health. London

- Siegrist Johannes (1998) Gesundheit und Krankheit: Machen wir uns selbst krank? In: Schwartz et al (1998) Das Public Health Buch. Gesundheit und Gesundheitswesen. Muenchen, Wien, Baltimore, pp110-123
- SLNHPS (Slovenian network of Health Prompting Schools) (Ed.) (1995) Bulletin of the Slovenian Network of Health Prompting Schools - 1/1995. National IPH: Ljubljana
- Soester Thesen und Leitlinien zur Gesundheitserziehung und Gesundheitsfoerderung in Schulen (1991) In: Priebe B/ Israel G/ Hurrelmann K (Eds.) (1993) Gesunde Schule. Weinheim, Basel, pp145-151
- Speller Viv (1998) Future developments of healthy alliances. In: Scriven A (Ed.) (1998) Alliances in health promotion. Theory and practice. London, pp85-93
- Speller Viv/ Learmonth Alyson/ Harrison Dominic (1998) Evaluating health promotion is complex. (Letters) In: British Medical Journal 9May1998, 316: p1463
- Speller Viv/ Rogers Liz/ Rushmere Annette (1998b) Quality assessment in health promotion settings. In: Davies J K/ Macdonald G (Eds.) (1998b) Quality, evidence and effectiveness in health promotion. Striving for certainties. London, New York, pp 130-146
- St Leger (1997) Health promoting settings: from Ottawa to Jarkarta. In: Health Promotion International 12(2): 99-101
- Stergar Eva (1993a) The ENHPS: Activities in 1993. Report to the WHO Representative. National HPS Support Center, Slovenia: Ljubljana. (Unpublished report)
- Stergar Eva (1994a-d) The ENHPS: Activities in 1994 (a) beginning; b) April -June; July -c) September; d) October -December;). Reports to the WHO Representative. National HPS Support Center, Slovenia: Ljubljana. (Unpublished reports)
- Stergar Eva (1995) Letter to the reader "Dear friends, ..." In: Turnsek N/ Stergar E (Eds.) (1995a) Bulletin of the Slovene Network of Health-Promoting Schools, 1/95. (English translation of the 1st Bulletin, Sept. 1994) Institute of Public Health of the Republic of Slovenia (IPH): Ljubljana, p4
- Stergar Eva (1995a/b) The ENHPS: "Six monthly reports" (a) January-June 1995; b) July- December 1995;). Reports to the WHO Representative. National HPS Support Center, Slovenia: Ljubljana. (Unpublished reports)
- Stergar Eva (1995c/d) The ENHPS: Activities in 1995 (a) January-June 1995; b) July- December 1995;). Reports to the WHO Representative. National HPS Support Center, Slovenia: Ljubljana. (Unpublished reports)
- Stergar Eva (1996) "The Slovenian Network of Health Promoting Schools" - Presentation at the Council of Europe (June 196). National HPS Support Center, Slovenia: Ljubljana. (Unpublished document)
- Stergar Eva (1996a) Slovene Network of Health Promoting Schools. January-March 1996. Report to the WHO Representative in Slovenia. National HPS Support Center, Slovenia: Ljubljana. (Unpublished reports)
- Stergar Eva (1996b) The ENHPS: Activities in 1996. Report to the WHO Representative in Slovenia. National HPS Support Center, Slovenia: Ljubljana. (Unpublished reports)
- Stergar Eva (1997) Drug use prevention within the Slovenian Network of Health Promoting Schools. (Presentation written in Sept. 1997 for the 'methadone conference' held in Slovenia.) National HPS Support Center, Slovenia: Ljubljana. (Unpublished document)
- Stergar Eva (1997a-d) Slovenian Network of Health Promoting Schools. Reports on activities. (a = January-March 1997; b = April -June 1997; c = July-September 1997; d = October - December 1997). Reports to the WHO Representative in Slovenia. National HPS Support Center, Slovenia: Ljubljana. (Unpublished reports)
- Stergar Eva (1997e) 'Case Study: Slovenia'. In: ENHPS (1997b) First Conference of the European Network of Health Promoting Schools "The Health Promoting School..." (Case study book). ENHPS, WHO/EURO: Copenhagen, p27

- Stergar Eva (1998a-d) Slovenian Network of Health Promoting Schools. Reports on activities. (a = January-March 1998; b = April -June 1998; c = July-September 1998; d = October -December 1998). Reports to the WHO Representative in Slovenia. National HPS Support Center, Slovenia: Ljubljana. (Unpublished reports)

- Stergar Eva (1999) National dissemination of the Slovenian project. (Article written for 'Network News, the ENHPS newsletter.) In: ENHPS Technical Secretariat (1999) Network News (Newletter of the ENHPS). ENHPS, WHO/EURO: Copenhagen, p14

- Stergar Eva (2000) The health promoting school concept used by the Slovenian Network of Health Promoting Schools. (text prepared for the Danish Royal School of Education, spring 2000). National HPS Support Center, Slovenia: Ljubljana. (Unpublished document)

- Stergar Eva (2001) verbal information in May 2001

- Stergar Eva/ bevc Stankovic, Mojca (1998) The outcomes of the first phase of the HPS project in the Republic of Slovenia. (Presentation held at the XVI IUHPE World Conference, 21-26 June 1998, San Juan, Puerto Rico) National HPS Support Center, Ljubljana. (Unpublished document)

- Stokols Daniel (1996) Translating socialecological theory into guidelines for community health promotion. In: American Journal of Health Promotion 10 (4): 282-298

- Stokols Daniel/ Allen Judd/ Bellingham Richard L. (1996) The social ecology of health promotion: implications for research and practice. In: American Journal of Health Promotion 10(4): 247-250

- Subregional network of German-speaking Networks of Health Promoting Schools (NHPS) in Germany, Austria, Luxembourg, Belgium and Switzerland (1995) The Cologne Recommendations. A joint position paper. In: "Subregional" network... (1997) A network within the network. Netzwerk Gesundheitsfoerdernde Schulen: Flensburg, Germany.

- Subregional network of German-speaking Networks of Health Promoting Schools (1997) A network within the network. The "subregional" network of Austria, Belgium, Germany, Luxembourg and Switzerland. (Leaflet) Netzwerk Gesundheitsfoerdernde Schulen: Flensburg, Germany.

- Sundsvall Statement on Supportive Environments for Health (1991) Statement adopted at the 3rd International Conference for Health Promotion, Sundsvall, Sweden. WHO/HPR/HEP/95.3. WHO: Geneva (www.who.int/hpr/backgroundhp/sundsvall)

- Syme S Leonard (1994) The social environment and health. In: Daedalus 1994, Fall: 79-86

- Syme S Leonard (1996) Rethinking disease: where do we go from here? In: American Epidemiological Review 6(5): 463-468

- Tavlov Alvin (1996) Social determinants of health. the sociobiological translation. In: Blane D/ Brunner E/ Wilkinson R (1996) Health and Social Organization. London, New York, pp71-93

- Tennyson Ros (w.y.) Managing partnerships: Tools for mobilising the public sector, business and civil society as partners in development. Prince of Wales Business Leaders Forum, London, UK. London (info@pwblf.org.uk)

- Theesen Gottfried (1997) ENHPS - A priority for the European Commission. In: ENHPS Technical Secretariat (Ed.) (1997) Network News (Newsletter of the ENHPS). WHO/EURO: Copenhagen, p4

- Tones Keith/ Tilford Sylvia (1994) Health educaiton: effectiveness, efficiency, and equity. Referred to in: ENHPS (w.y.) The ENHPS indicators for a health promoting school. (Document received in 1999) ENHPS, WHO/EURO: Copenhagen (Unpublished document)

- Trojan Alf (1996) Soziale Netzwerke und Gesundheitsförderung. In: BzgA (Ed.) (1996) Leitbegriffe der Gesundheitsförderung. Schwabenheim, pp104-105

- Troschke von Juergen (1993) Gesundheits - und Krankheitsverhalten. In: Hurrelmann K/ Laaser U (Eds.) (1993) Gesundheitswissenschaften. Handbuch fuer Lehre, Forschung und Praxis. Weinheim, Basel, pp155-175

- Tsouros Agis (1997) Foreword. In: WHO/EURO (1997) The solid facts. Social determinants of health. (Edited by R. Wilkinson and M. Marmot) EUR/ICP/CHVD 030901. WHO/EURO: Copenhagen, pp1-2
- Tsouros Agis D/ Farrington Jill L (1999) Epilogue. In: Marmot M/ Wilkinson RG (Eds.) (1999) Social determinants of health. New York, pp275-279
- Turnsek Nada (1995a) Letter to the reader "Dear colleagues, ..." In: Turnsek N/ Stergar E (Eds.) (1995a) Bulletin of the Slovene Network of Health-Promoting Schools, 1/95. Institute of Public Health of the Republic of Slovenia (IPH): Ljubljana, p4
- Turnsek Nada/ Stergar Eva (Eds.) (1994) Bulletin of the Slovene Network of Health-Promoting Schools (in Slovenian). Sept. 1994. Institute of Public Health of the Republic of Slovenia (IPH): Ljubljana
- Turnsek Nada/ Stergar Eva (Eds.) (1995a) Bulletin of the Slovene Network of Health-Promoting Schools, 1/95. (English translation of the first Bulletin from Sept. 1994) Institute of Public Health of the Republic of Slovenia (IPH): Ljubljana
- UNDP (1995) Capacity development for sustainable human development: conceptual and operational signposts. Working paper (9Sept.1995). UNDP: New York (http://magnet.undp.org/CAPDEV.htm)
- UNDP (1997) Capacity development. Technical advisory paper 2. UNDP, Management development and Governance Division, Bureau for Policy Development. UNDP: New York
- UNDP (w.y. –1997 or later) Capacity assessment and development – in a systems and strategic management context. Technical advisory paper 3. UNDP, Management development and Governance Division, Bureau for Policy Development. UNDP: New York (http://magnet.undp.org/Docs/cap/Main.htm - downloaded 4Dec.2000)
- UNEP/ WHO/ Nordic Council of Ministers (Eds.) (1996) Playing for time... Creating supportive environments for health. Report from the third International Conference on Health Promotion. Sundsvall, Sweden, 9th-15th June 1991. WHO: Geneva
- Van den Broucke, Stephan (2002) Health promotion indicators and health inequalities. (Presentation at 2nd meeting of the European Health Promotion Indicators Development (EUHPID) Consortium, 8-9 June 2002, London). Contact: St. Van den Broucke, Flemish Institute for Health Promotion, Brussels (Unpublished document)
- Waller Heiko (1995) Gesundheitswissenschaft - Eine Einfuehrung in Grundlagen und Praxis. Stuttgart, Berlin, Koeln
- Wenzel Eberhard (1997) A comment on settings in health promotion. In: Internet Journal of Health Promotion 1997/1 (www.ldb.org/setting.htm - downloaded last on 31 Nov.02)
- WHA (1977) Resolution WHA 30.43. WHO Genf (www.who.int)
- WHA (1998) Fifty first World Health Assembly: WHA51.12 Resolution on Health Promotion (16 May 1998). WHO: Geneva (also published in: J. Health Promotion International 1998, 13(3): 266)
- WHA (1998b) World Health Declaration. Adopted by the world health community at the Fifty-first World Health Assembly May 1998. WHO, Geneva. In: WHO/EURO (w.y.) Health 21 - health for all in the 21st Century. An introduction. (European Health for All Series No.5 - published in 1998). WHO/EURO: Copenhagen, pp1-2
- WHO (1948) Constitution of the World Health Organization. WHO: Geneva
- WHO (1986) Ottawa Charter for Health Promotion. (Released at the 1st International Conference for Health Promotion, 17-21Nov.1986, Ottawa, Canada - held by WHO, Health and Welfare Canada, and the Canadian Public Health Association) WHO/HPR/HEP/1995.1, WHO, Geneva
- WHO (1986) Ottawa Charter for Health Promotion. (Released at the 1st International Conference for Health Promotion, 17-21Nov.1986, Ottawa, Canada - held by WHO, Health and Welfare Canada, and the Canadian Public Health Association.) In: J. Health Promotion 1(4): i-v

- WHO (1988b) Adelaide Recommendations on Healthy Public Policy. WHO/HPR/HEP/95.2. Geneva
- WHO (1990) Promoting health in developing countries. A call for Action. Summary report of the 'Working Group on Health Promotion in Developing Countries', Geneva, 9-13 October 1989. WHO/HEP/90.1 Distr.: limited. WHO: Geneva
- WHO (1991) Sundsvall Statement on Supportive Environments for Health. WHO/HPR/HEP/95.3. WHO: Geneva (www.who.int/hpr/backgroundhp/sundsvall)
- WHO (1991b) Sundsvall Briefing book. WHO/HED/91.1 WHO: Geneva
- WHO (1993) Life skills education in schools. (unpublished document 1991) WHO/MNH/PSF/93.7A. WHO: Geneva. (also quoted in WHO 1998a p15)
- WHO (1995) The World Health Report 1995. Bridging the gaps. WHO: Geneva
- WHO (1996a) The status of school health. (Background Document for the WHO Expert Committee on Comprehensive School Health Education and Health Promotion.) WHO/HPR/HEP 96.1 - Distribution: limited. WHO: Geneva
- WHO (1996b) Improving school health programmes: barriers and strategies. (Background Document for the WHO Expert Committee on Comprehensive School Health Education and Health Promotion.) WHO/HPR/HEP/96.2 - Distribution: limited. WHO: Geneva
- WHO (1996d) Promoting Health through Schools. The WHO's Global School Health Initiative. WHO/HPR/HEP 96.4. WHO: Geneva
- WHO (1997) The Jakarta Declaration on Leading Health Promotion into the 21st Century. Adopted at the 4th International Conference on Health Promotion, July 21-25 1997, Jakarta, Republic of Indonesia. WHO/HPR/HEP/4ICHP/BR/97.4 Distribution: General. WHO: Geneva
- WHO (1997a) Promoting health through schools. Report of a WHO Expert Committee on Comprehensive School Health Education and Promotion (WHO Technical Report Series 870). WHO: Geneva
- WHO (1997b) Review and evaluation of health promotion. (Reader for the 4th International Conference on Health Promotion, Jakarta 1997. Collected by Ilona Kickbusch and Ursel Broesskamp-Stone) HPR/HEP/4ICHP/RET/97.3. WHO: Geneva
- WHO (1997c) Intersectoral action for health: addressing heaslth and environmet concerns in sustainable development. WHO/PPE/PAC/97.1 (Distr.: limited). WHO: Geneva
- WHO (1998a) Health Promotion Glossary. WHO/HPR/HEP/98.1. WHO: Geneva
- WHO (2000) The Fifth Global Conference on Health Promotion - Health Promotion: Bridging the Equity Gap (5-9 June 2000, Mexico City, Mexico). Conference Report of the Technical Program (Report writing team: Don Nutbeam, Ursel Broesskamp-Stone, Maria Teresa Cerqueira, Jane Springett). WHO: Geneva. www.who.international/hpr/conference
- WHO (2002) Website of the WHO Global School Health Initiative (www.who.org/hpr/archive/gshi - on 20 May 2002)
- WHO Healthy Cities Project (1998) Healthy Cities baseline indicators. (Revised in March 1998). Downloaded from the WHO/EURO website on 16 November 2000 www.who.dk/healthy%2Dcities
- WHO Kobe Center (1997/1998) Preliminary core set of determinants and indicators of (urban) health. (Unpublished document) WHO Center Kobe, Japan
- WHO/EURO (1984a) Health promotion - A discussion document on the concept and principles. Document ICP/HSR 602 (m01), September 1994. WHO/EURO: Copenhagen. (Unpublished document)
- WHO/EURO (1984b) Health promotion concept and principles - a policy framework. Health for all 2000 booklet. WHO/EURO: Copenhagen
- WHO/EURO (1985) Targets for Health for All. WHO: Copenhagen

- WHO/EURO (1991) Targets for health for all. The health policy for Europe. (Summary of the updated edition September 1991) WHO/EURO: Copenhagen
- WHO/EURO (1993) Ziele zur "Gesundheit fuer alle" Die Gesundheitspolitik fuer Europa. Aktualisierte Fassung September 1991. WHO: Copenhagen
- WHO/EURO (1994) The Health Promoting Hospitals Movement - Working for health. WHO: Copenhagen
- WHO/EURO (1995) Terminology for the European Health Policy Conference. A glossary with equivalents in French, German, and Russian. WHO/EURO: Copenhagen
- WHO/EURO (1996) Networking the networks. (Regions fo rHealth Network.) POLC 050102. WHO/EURO, Copenhagen pp5-6
- WHO/EURO (1997) "Networking for health" - Report of the 4th Annual Conference of the Regiosn for Health Network, Duesseldorf, Germany, 11/12 October 1996. EUR/ICP/POLC 05 01 02. WHO/EURO: Copenhagen, p38-42
- WHO/EURO (1997a) Auditing health promotion capacity: an action framework. In: WHO (1997b) Review and evaluation of health promotion. (Reader for the 4th International Conference...). WHO: Geneva
- WHO/EURO (1998) The Schools Data Base. WHO/EURO: Copenhagen. (see www.who.dk >> health topics >> education for health >> Health Promoting Schools >> Infobase. Or: www.who.dk >> 'The ENHPS' >> 'Network' - downloaded May 2001)
- WHO/EURO (1998a) Gesundheit21. Eine Einfuehrung zum Rahmenkonzept 'Gesundheit fuer alle' fuer die Europaeische Region der WHO. WHO/EURO: Copenhagen (www.who.dk/cpa/H21/H21long.htm)
- WHO/EURO (1999) Gesundheit 21. Das Rahmenkonzept 'Gesundheit für alle' für die Europäische Region der WHO. (Europäische Schriftenreihe ‚Gesundheit für alle', Nr.6). WHO/EURO: Copenhagen. (www.who.dk/cpa/H21/H21long.htm)
- WHO/EURO (1999) Health 21. The Health for All policy framework for the WHO European Region. WHO/EURO: Copenhagen (www.who.dk/cpa/H21/H21long.htm)
- WHO/EURO (2000) About us. Key word 'networks'. (Website: www.who.dk/WHO-Euro/about/networks.htm - updated 23 August 2000). WHO/EURO: Copenhagen. (downloaded Dec.2000)
- WHO/EURO (2002) Health Behavior in School Aged Children (HBSC). A World Health Oranisation Cross-National Study. WHO/EURO: Copenhagen (www.ruhbc.ed.ac.uk/hbsc/)
- WHO/EURO (Ed.) (1990) Health Promotion - A ressource book. Collected by Anderson Ronald/ Kickbusch Ilona. EUR/ICP/HSR 612. WHO/EURO: Copenhagen
- WHO/EURO (Ed.) (1997) The solid facts. Social determinants of health. EUR/ICP/CHVD 030901, WHO/EURO: Copenhagen.
- WHO/EURO (w.y.) Health 21 - health for all in the 21st Century. An introduction. European Health for All Series No.5 (published in 1998). WHO/EURO: Copenhagen
- WHO/SEARO (2000) Resolution of the WHO Regional Committee for South-Est Asia on 'Healthy Settings' (SEA/RC53/R4 - 7Sept.2000). WHO/SEARO: New Delhi
- WHO/UNICEF International Conference on Primary Health Care (1978) Declaration of Alma Ata (adopted at the conference). Alma Ata (www.who.int/hpr/archive/docs/almaata.html)
- WHO/WPRO (1995) New horizons in health. (Policy document for the Western Pacific Region. Revised version, June 1995). WHO/WPRO: Manila
- WHO/WPRO (Ed.) (1996) Regional guidelines. Development of health-promoting schools - A framework for action. WHO/WPRO: Manila

- Wilkinson Richard G (1994) The epidemiological transition: from material scarcity to social disadvantage? In: Daedalus (Journal of the American Academy of Arts and Sciences) 123(4): 61-77
- Wilkinson Richard G (1996) Unhealthy societies: the afflictions of inequality. London, New York
- Wilkinson Richard G (1999) Putting the picture together: prosperity, redistribution, health, and welfare. In: Marmot M/ Wilkinson RG (Eds.) (1999) Social determinants of health. New York, pp256-274
- Wilkinson Richard/ Marmot Michael (Eds) (1998) Social determinants of health. The solid facts. EUR/ICP/CHVD 03 09 01. WHO/EURO, Copenhagen.
- Wimbush Erica/ Watson Jonathan (2000) Developing Nutbeam's outcome model for evaluating health promotion initiatives. (Presentation at the 3rd Nordic Health Promotion Research Conference 'Outcomes in Health Promotion – key questions for research and polic', 6.-9.September 2000, Tampere, Finland. Presentation No. A1:5) Contact: E. Winbush, Health Education Board for Scotland, Edinburgh, Scotland (Unpublished document)
- Wold Bente (1996) Health Behavior in School-aged Children – a WHO cross-national survey. In: ENHPS Technical Secretariat (Ed.) (1996) Network News (Newsletter of the ENHPS). ENHPS, WHO/EURO: Copenhagen, p4
- Working Group on Partnerships at WHO/HQ in the Context of the Health for All Renewal (1997) Partnerships for health in the 21st Century: 2 + 2 = 5. Conference working paper for the 4th International Conference on Health Promotion "New Players for a New Era: Leading Health Promotion into the 21st Century", Jakarta, Indonesia, 21-25 July 1997. HPR/HEP/4ICHP/PT/97.1 Distribution: limited. WHO: Geneva
- World Bank (1993) World Development Report 'Investing in Health'. World Bank: New York
- World Commission on Environment and Development (1987) Our Common Future (Final report of the UN Commission on Environment and Development). Oxford
- Ziglio Erio (1996) How to move towards evidence-based health promotion interventions. (Presentation on the 3rd European Conference on Effectiveness 'Quality Assessment in Health Promotion and Health Education', Sept. 12-14 1996, Turin, Italy.) WHO/EURO, Intersectoral Health Development Unit, Health Promotion and Investment Programme: Copenhagen
- Ziglio Erio, Rivett David, Barnekow Rasmussen Vivian (1995) Managing innovation and change. WHO/EURO: Copenhagen. Unpublished
- Ziglio Erio/ Hagard, Spencer/ Griffiths John (2000b) Health Promotion development in Europe: achievements and challenges. In: Health Promotion International 15(2): 143-154
- Ziglio Erio/ Hagard, Spencer/ McMahon Laurie/ Harvey Sarah/ Levin Lowell (2000) Investment for health. (Technical background report for the 5th Global Conference for Health Promotion: Bridging the equity gap, 5-9 June 2000, Mexico City, Mexico.) WHO, Geneva (www.who.int/hpr/conference/products)
- Ziglio Erio/ Hagard Spencer (1998) Appraising investment for health opportunities. World Health Organization, Health Promotion and Investment Programme, unit document. According to: Krech Ruediger (1999)